Sodium-glucose Cotransporter-2 (SGLT2) Inhibitors in Heart Failure

Mukesh Nandave
Editor

Sodium-glucose Cotransporter-2 (SGLT2) Inhibitors in Heart Failure

Mechanisms and Clinical Applications: A Machine-Generated Literature Overview

Springer

Editor
Mukesh Nandave
Delhi Pharmaceutical Sciences & Research University (DPSRU)
Department of Pharmacology and Pharmaceutical Biotechnology
New Delhi, Delhi, India

ISBN 978-981-97-7567-5 ISBN 978-981-97-7568-2 (eBook)
https://doi.org/10.1007/978-981-97-7568-2

This Springer imprint is published by the registered company Springer Nature Singapore Pte Ltd.
The registered company address is: 152 Beach Road, #21-01/04 Gateway East, Singapore 189721, Singapore

Foreword

It is with great pleasure that I introduce this comprehensive and meticulously crafted book, *Sodium-Glucose Cotransporter-2 (SGLT2) Inhibitors in Heart Failure: Mechanisms and Clinical Applications: A Machine-Generated Literature Overview*, edited by Dr. Mukesh Nandave and published by Springer Nature. The advent of SGLT2 inhibitors has marked a paradigm shift in the management of type 2 diabetes mellitus (T2DM), particularly concerning cardiovascular and renal outcomes. This volume offers a comprehensive exploration of the multifaceted benefits of SGLT2 inhibitors beyond glycemic control.

The nine chapters within this book present a deep dive into the historical, mechanistic, and clinical dimensions of SGLT2 inhibitors. Chapter 1, "The History of the Development of SGLT2 Inhibitors for the Treatment of Diabetes: From Biology to Chemistry," sets the stage by tracing the journey from the biological discovery to the chemical synthesis of these groundbreaking drugs. Following this, Chap. 2, "SGLT2 Inhibitors and Mechanism of Cardiovascular Benefits in Type 2 Diabetes," elucidates the underlying mechanisms that confer cardiovascular protection in patients with T2DM.

In Chap. 3, "SGLT2 Inhibitors for Primary and Secondary Protection from Cardiovascular and Renal Diseases in Type 2 Diabetes," the focus shifts to the dual role these inhibitors play in both primary and secondary prevention of cardiovascular and renal diseases. Chapter 4, "SGLT2 Inhibitors: Emerging Opportunities for the Treatment of Myocardial Infarction," explores novel therapeutic avenues, highlighting the potential of these inhibitors in the context of acute myocardial infarction.

Chapter 5, "Potential Role of SGLT2 Inhibitors in the Treatment and Prevention of Diabetic Cardiomyopathy," addresses the critical issue of diabetic cardiomyopathy, offering insights into how SGLT2 inhibitors can alter its course. Chapter 6, "Role of Therapeutic Potential, Contemporary Management, Unmet Needs of SGLT2 Inhibitors in Congestive Heart Failure," delves into the evolving role of these drugs in managing congestive heart failure, highlighting ongoing challenges and future directions.

"A Comprehensive Review of Preclinical and Clinical Information on the Cardiovascular Advantages of SGLT2 Inhibitors," presented in Chap. 7, synthesizes preclinical and clinical data, underscoring the broad cardiovascular benefits. Chapter 8, "Exploring the Current Selective Drugs of SGLT2 Inhibitors for the Treatment of Cardiovascular Disease in Type 2 Diabetes," provides an in-depth analysis of currently available SGLT2 inhibitors, emphasizing their specific cardiovascular effects.

Finally, Chap. 9 offers "A Comprehensive Review of SGLT2 Inhibitors' Effects on Cardiovascular Events, Mortality, and Significant Safety Outcomes in Individuals with Type 2 Diabetes," compiling critical evidence on efficacy and safety.

This book stands as an indispensable resource for clinicians, researchers, and students, providing an extensive understanding of the role of SGLT2 inhibitors in heart failure and their broader implications in cardiovascular and renal health. Dr. Mukesh Nandave and the contributing authors have succeeded in crafting a text that is both informative and transformative, offering a detailed roadmap for future research and clinical practice.

Department of Endocrinology, Metabolism and Diabetes
All India Institute of Medical Sciences (AIIMS),
New Delhi, India
Nikhil Tandon

Preface

The landscape of cardiovascular and renal disease management in patients with type 2 diabetes has undergone a transformative evolution over the past decade, significantly driven by advancements in pharmacotherapy. Among these advancements, sodium-glucose cotransporter-2 (SGLT2) inhibitors have emerged as a groundbreaking class of medications, demonstrating remarkable benefits that extend beyond glycemic control. This book, *Sodium-Glucose Cotransporter-2 (SGLT2) Inhibitors in Heart Failure: Mechanisms and Clinical Applications: A Machine-Generated Literature Overview*, offers an in-depth exploration of the multifaceted roles of SGLT2 inhibitors in managing heart failure and related cardiovascular conditions.

Edited by Dr. Mukesh Nandave and published by Springer Nature, this comprehensive volume brings together leading experts to provide a thorough analysis of the current understanding and future potential of SGLT2 inhibitors. This book is structured into ten meticulously curated chapters, each contributing a unique perspective to the overarching theme of cardiovascular and renal protection in patients with type 2 diabetes.

Chapter 1, "The History of the Development of SGLT2 Inhibitors for the Treatment of Diabetes: From Biology to Chemistry," sets the stage by tracing the journey of SGLT2 inhibitors from their biological roots to their chemical innovation. This historical context provides a foundation for appreciating the subsequent clinical developments.

In Chap. 2, "SGLT2 Inhibitors and Mechanism of Cardiovascular Benefits in Type 2 Diabetes," the authors delve into the underlying mechanisms including improved glycemic control, weight loss, reduction in blood pressure and arterial stiffness, enhanced diuresis and natriuresis, thereby alleviating cardiac workload and improving cardiac function. This chapter offering insights into how these drugs exert cardioprotective effects beyond glucose lowering.

Chapter 3, "SGLT2 Inhibitors for Primary and Secondary Protection from Cardiovascular and Renal Diseases in Type 2 Diabetes," expands on the dual role of these inhibitors in providing both primary and secondary prevention of cardiovascular and renal complications through increased glucose excretion in urine, thereby preserving kidney function, retarding the progression of diabetic nephropathy, and decreasing the risk of end-stage renal disease.

Emerging opportunities are explored in Chap. 4, "SGLT2 Inhibitors: Emerging Opportunities for the Treatment of Myocardial Infarction," where the potential of these drugs in acute cardiac events is examined, highlighting a novel frontier in cardiovascular therapeutics.

Chapter 5, "Potential Role of SGLT2 Inhibitors in the Treatment and Prevention of Diabetic Cardiomyopathy," focuses on the specific context of diabetic cardiomyopathy, providing a detailed review of how SGLT2 inhibitors may modify disease progression by reducing blood glucose levels and improving insulin sensitivity, they alleviate cardiac stress and improve heart function. This chapter also includes studies that demonstrated that these inhibitors can also reduce myocardial fibrosis and inflammation, key factors in diabetic cardiomyopathy.

In Chap. 6, "Role of Therapeutic Potential, Contemporary Management, Unmet Needs of SGLT2 Inhibitors in Congestive Heart Failure," the discussion turns to heart failure, addressing the current management strategies and the unmet needs that SGLT2 inhibitors are poised to fulfill.

The cardiovascular advantages of SGLT2 inhibitors are comprehensively reviewed in Chap. 7, "A Comprehensive Review of Preclinical and Clinical Information on the Cardiovascular Advantages of SGLT2 Inhibitors," integrating both preclinical and clinical data to present a holistic view of their benefits.

Chapter 8, "Exploring the Current Selective Drugs of SGLT2 Inhibitors for the Treatment of Cardiovascular Disease in Type 2 Diabetes," evaluates the specific agents within the SGLT2 inhibitor class, comparing their efficacy and safety profiles in the context of cardiovascular disease management.

The effects of SGLT2 inhibitors on cardiovascular events, mortality, and significant safety outcomes are meticulously detailed in Chap. 9, ensuring that readers gain a comprehensive understanding of the evidence base supporting these medications.

Finally, this book discusses "Future Trends in the Use of SGLT2 Inhibitors," offering a forward-looking perspective on the evolving role of these agents in clinical practice.

By providing a detailed and authoritative exploration of SGLT2 inhibitors, this book aims to serve as an invaluable resource for clinicians, researchers, and students interested in the intersection of diabetes, cardiovascular disease, and renal health. It is our hope that this compilation of expert insights will inspire continued research and innovation in this promising field, ultimately improving patient outcomes and quality of life.

New Delhi, Delhi, India Mukesh Nandave

The original version of this book has been revised: The titles of chapters 3 to 9 have been updated. The erratum to the book is available at https://doi.org/10.1007/978-981-97-7568-2_10

Disclaimer

Auto-summaries can be generated by either an abstractive or extractive auto-summarization:

- An extraction-based summarizer identifies the most important sentences of a text and uses the original sentences to create the summary.
- An abstraction-based summarizer creates new text based on deep learning. New phrases are created to summarize the content.

The auto-summaries you will find in this book have been generated via an extractive summarization approach.

Each chapter was carefully edited by Dr. Mukesh Nandave. The editors selected the papers which were then auto-summarized. The editors have not edited the auto-summaries due to the extraction-based approach and have not changed the original sentences. You will find the editors' reviews and guidance on the auto-summaries in their chapter introductions.

In machine-generated books, editors are defined as those who curate the content for the book by selecting the papers to be auto-summarized and by organizing the output into a meaningful order. Next to the thoughtful curation of the papers, editors should guide the readers through the auto-summaries and make transparent why they selected the papers.

The ultimate goal is to provide a current literature review of Springer Nature publications on a given topic in order to support readers in overcoming information overload and to help them dive into a topic faster; to identify interdisciplinary overlaps; and to present papers which might not have been on the readers' radar.

Please note that the selected papers are not used to train a LLM while the auto-summaries are created.

Contents

About the Editor

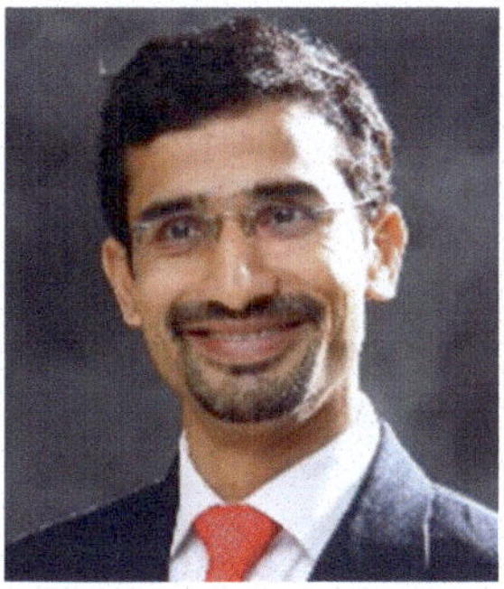

Mukesh Nandave is Associate Dean (Research), Officiating Director of School of Pharmaceutical Sciences and Head of the Department of Pharmacology and Pharmaceutical Biotechnology at the Delhi Pharmaceutical Sciences and Research University, Govt of NCT of Delhi, New Delhi. He has earlier served as Associate Professor and Head in the Department of Pharmacology at NMIMS University, Mumbai (2010–2017). Dr. Nandave earned his Ph.D. in pharmacology from AIIMS, Delhi, and received his postdoctoral training from the Ohio State University Medical Center, Columbus, USA.For over 20 years, Dr. Nandave has been actively engaged in investigating the role of nutraceuticals, herbomineral formulations, and phytoconstituents in mitigating myocardial ischemia and reperfusion injury, diabetes, obesity, and pain management. He has published more than 100 papers in peer-reviewed national and international journals. His lab received more than 3.5 crore in total funding from government (DBT, DST, ICMR, and AYUSH) as well as industry (Pharmazz, Dabur, Charak, Madhavbaug, and Sandu).Dr. Nandave has received numerous awards, including the Distinguished Leadership Award from the International Academy of Cardiovascular Sciences; Prof. S. C. Lahiri Oration and G. Achari Gold Medal from the Indian Pharmacological Society; Young Pharmacy Teacher of the Year Award from the Association of Pharmaceutical Teachers of India (APTI); Early Investigator Award from the International Society for Heart Research; Prof. Duggirala Visweswaram and Prof. Sreemantula Satyanarayana

Prize; Best Research Output of the Year for 2014–2015, 2013–2014, and 2012–2013 Award from SVKM's NMIMS University.Dr. Nandave is the Secretary General of the India Section of the International Academy of Cardiovascular Sciences (IACS) and Treasurer of the Society for Promotion and Research of Cardiovascular Sciences (SPARCS). He is a life member of various professional bodies, including the International Society for Heart Research (ISHR), International Academy of Cardiovascular Sciences (IACS), Indian Pharmacological Society (IPS), Indian Pharmaceutical Association (IPA), Association of Physiologists and Pharmacologists of India (APPI), Association of Pharmaceutical Teachers of India (APTI), and Society for Ethnopharmacology.He is also a BOS member at various institutes and expert member in project review panels of ICMR, AYUSH, SERB, and DBT.

Chapter 1
The History of the Development of SGLT2 Inhibitors for the Treatment of Diabetes: From Biology to Chemistry

Mukesh Nandave

Introduction by the Editor

The World Health Organization (WHO) introduced diabetes mellitus (DM) as one of the leading causes of death in 2019. It also plays a significant role in the development of other diseases like coronary artery disease, stroke, renal disease, eyesight loss, and lower limb amputation. Around 90% of the glucose in plasma is reabsorbable by a sodium-glucose co-transporter 2 (SGLT2) protein, which can be used for the treatment of diabetes.

The human body contains six SGLT proteins, each of which prefers to bind sugar differently. SGLT is transport proteins that move glucose into cells via a sodium concentration gradient created by a Na+/K+ ATPase pump. Within the SGLT family, SGLT1 and SGLT2 are the two important transport proteins. The high affinity/low capacity protein SGLT1 is expressed in the S3 segment of the renal proximal tubule and 10–20% glucose reabsorb that wasn't absorbed in the S1 and S2 segments. Moreover, SGLT1 is present in the brain, heart, and small intestine with the brush boundary membrane of the small intestine, cardiac cardiomyocytes, Purkinje and pyramidal cells, the blood-brain barrier, and the endothelium of intracerebral capillaries among the places it may be found.

Whereas, SGLT2 expression occurs in the proximal convoluted tubules in which 80–90% of glucose reabsorption via kidneys with low affinity/high capacity protein is found in the apical membrane of the renal proximal tubules at S1 & S2 segment shown in Fig. 1.1. SGLT2 is easily absorbed by the digestive system and their plasma protein binding (PPB) is high and distributed across large tissues. As urine is expelled after SGLT2i are biotransformed by UDP-glucuronosyltransferases (UGTs)-mediated glucuronidation, with negligible cytochrome P450 metabolism.

M. Nandave (✉)
Department of Pharmacology and Pharmaceutical Biotechnology, Delhi Pharmaceutical Sciences and Research University (DPSRU), New Delhi, Delhi, India

M. Nandave (ed.), *Sodium-glucose Cotransporter-2 (SGLT2) Inhibitors in Heart Failure*, https://doi.org/10.1007/978-981-97-7568-2_1

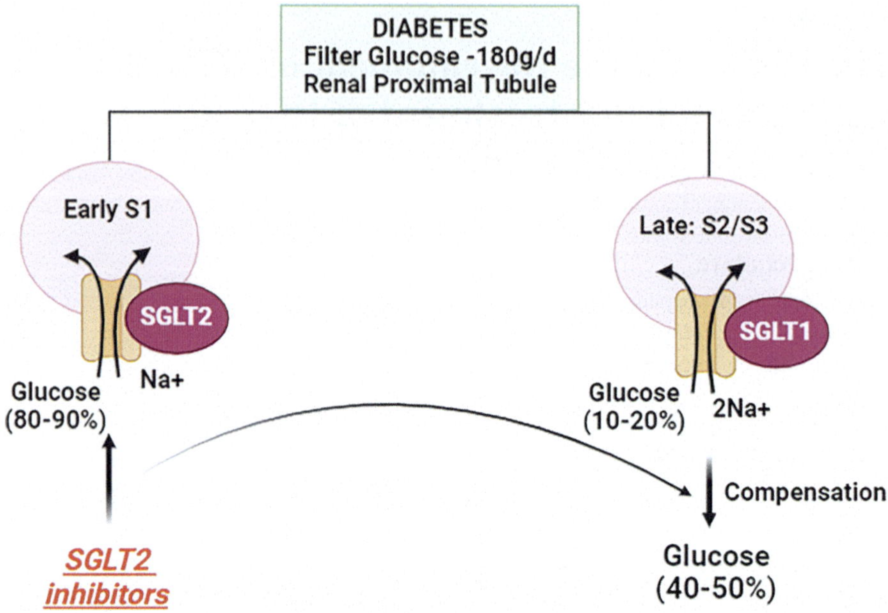

Fig. 1.1 SGLT2 inhibitors mechanism of action in diabetes. Approximately 180 g of filtered glucose is absorbed daily by the renal proximal tubule, whereas 80–90% of filtered glucose reabsorption is accounted for by SGLT2, which is situated in the early portion of the proximal tubule (S1). In light of this, SGLT2Is raise urine glucose excretion and inhibit the early proximal tubule's significant reabsorption of filtered glucose (80–90%)

In the diabetic condition, increased glucose reabsorption results in hyperglycemia as SGLT2 expression and capillary glucose load increase. SGLT2i causes an increase in the excretion of glucose through the urine while inhibiting the subsequent absorption of glucose into the renal tubule.

According to a historical account, its discovery started in 1835 when French scientist C. Petersen extracted phlorizin—the first drug used to cure malaria—from the apple tree's root bark. German medical professor von Mering found that phlorizin has glucosuric properties, which reduce plasma glucose levels. This was first identified in 1886 [1]. It was reported that the proximal renal tubules virtually entirely reabsorb glucose, which is typically filtered in the glomerulus, came about during the first part of the 1900s. Evidence of co-transport reabsorption of sodium and glucose and the need for active transport were shown in the 1960s. It was concluded that sodium and glucose are both eliminated in the urine when the cotransporter and molecule responsible for reabsorption, is blocked. The rival inhibitor of this enzyme-mediated transport was demonstrated by Alvarado and Crane in 1962. Phlorizin was by then recognized to be a sugar molecule connected to two aromatic rings [2].

It was then observed that phlorizin decreased plasma glucose levels when administered to diabetic mice. The hunt for orally effective co-transporter inhibitors was started since phlorizin fails to be absorbed from the gastrointestinal system. The first chemically manufactured SGLT2i were created in 1996 by researchers at Tanuba Seiygyu Co. in Japan and Kyoto University. These analogs were called phlorizin. When administered orally to diabetic rats, T-1095, an SGLT2i, decreased hyperglycemia, indicating that it could be helpful in the treatment of people with T2D which was created in 2000 [3].

Based on the clinical trial database, it was concluded that SGLT2i was thoroughly investigated and shown to be both safe and efficient in improving glucose regulation in persons with T2D. Therefore, the US Food and Drug Administration (FDA) and the European Medicine Agency (EMA) authorized dapagliflozin, canagliflozin, and empagliflozin, three SGLT2is, between 2012 and 2015 to lower plasma glucose in people with type 2 diabetes.

Canagliflozin, also known as Invokana®, was the first SGLT2i to get FDA clearance in March 2013. Dapagliflozin, also known as Farxiga®, received approval in January 2014, and empagliflozin, also known as Jardiance®, received approval in August 2014. For people with T2D, these drugs provide innovative methods for blood glucose management.

Bexagliflozin and Enavogliflozin, two similar drugs, will shortly be approved. Phase 3 clinical studies for DWP16001 (Envogliflozin), a selective SGLTi, are now taking place at the Yongin, Korea-based Daewoong Pharmaceutical Co. Ltd. Bexagliflozin, a highly selective SGLT2i that lowers blood sugar when taken orally, is the subject of phase 3 clinical investigations [3].

Haemoglobin A1c (HbA1c) is a marker of blood glucose levels, and the authorised SGLT2 inhibitors can lower it easily. Other injectable or oral diabetic treatments, such as insulin, can be taken with SGLT2 inhibitors. This is critical because, as insulin production declines, diabetes is a progressive illness that frequently necessitates the use of additional medications. Furthermore, in the absence of other medications that have this adverse effect, SGLT2 inhibitors do not result in hypoglycemia or low blood sugar. Since SGLTs reabsorbed salt as well as glucose, SGLT inhibition also causes an increase in sodium loss in the urine.

In addition to its primary function in the management of diabetes, SGLT-2i has shown promise in several other areas of health, offering benefits beyond reduced blood sugar. Improved cardiovascular (CV) results, a distinct kidney protective activity, and further physical advantages have been seen with this medication family.

It generates its action via proper diet and exercise that can not only improve the glycemic index but also treat diabetes. It can be used single or in grouping with other diabetes prescriptions as it is not prescribed to patients with type 1 diabetes due to the elevation of risk of diabetic ketoacidosis (DKA).

In this chapter, we focused on several novel SGLT2-specific inhibitors that are undergoing clinical trial studies and a few of them have already received approval in other nations for the treatment of T2D. Information on the safety and efficacy of SGLT2i in individuals with type 1 diabetes will come from ongoing research [4].

Therefore, the discovery and development of selective SGLT2i offer hope for controlling and treating DM. This allows researchers to develop more inventive SGLT2i–based medications to treat diabetes. The FDA and manufacturers are still collaborating closely to keep an eye on new evidence on the safety of the three SGLT2i medications that have recently received approval and to notify patients and carers of any updates.

Machine-generated keywords: docking, molecular, trial, carbasugar, insulin, cause, tdm, synthetic, icg, carbasugar sglt, sglti, hsglt, prevent, mutation, coupling.

Development of SGLT1 and SGLT2 Inhibitors

https://doi.org/10.1007/s00125-018-4654-7

A machine generated summary based on the work of Rieg, Timo; Vallon, Volker 2018 in Diabetologia

Abstract-Summary Sodium–glucose cotransporters SGLT1 (encoded by SGLT1, also known as SLC5A1) and SGLT2 (encoded by SGLT2, also known as SLC5A2) are important mediators of epithelial glucose transport.

Phlorizin, a naturally occurring competitive inhibitor of SGLT1 and SGLT2, provided the first insights into potential efficacy, but its use was hampered by intestinal side effects and a short half-life.

It was a starting point for the development of specific inhibitors of SGLT1 and SGLT2, as well as dual SGLT1/2 inhibitors.

Since the approval of the first SGLT2 inhibitor in 2013 by the US Food and Drug Administration, SGLT2 inhibitors have become a new mainstay in the treatment of type 2 diabetes mellitus.

This review focuses on the rationale for the development of individual SGLT2 and SGLT1 inhibitors, as well as dual SGLT1/2 inhibition, including, but not limited to, aspects of genetics, genetically modified mouse models, mathematical modelling and general considerations of drug discovery in the field of metabolism.

Introduction

Multiple drug classes are available for the treatment of diabetes mellitus (e.g. insulin, metformin, sulfonylureas, glitazones); however, significant drawbacks include limited effectiveness with regard to improving cardiovascular outcome, and some may even increase the risk of cardiovascular mortality.

Sodium–glucose cotransporter 2 (SGLT2) inhibitors, including canagliflozin (Invokana, Janssen pharmaceuticals), dapagliflozin (Forxiga [known as Farxiga in the USA]), empagliflozin (Jardiance), and ertugliflozin (Steglatro), have recently been approved by the US Food and Drug Administration as a new class of glucose-lowering compounds (known as the gliflozins) for the treatment of type 2 diabetes mellitus.

The basic concept of the therapeutic strategy is to lower the glucose burden by inhibiting the uptake of dietary glucose in the intestine or excreting the glucose filtered by the kidneys into the urine.

Easy access to exogenous energy resources is a much more recent development, it is not surprising that the body's responses to excess exogenous energy resources can be maladaptive.

Why Target Glucose Handling in the Kidney?

Potential protective mechanisms include the diuretic and natriuretic effects of SGLT2 inhibition, which reduce volume overload and blood pressure, and body weight reduction [5].

The blood pressure-lowering effect of SGLT2 inhibitors and protective effect against heart failure are preserved in individuals with CKD and reduced eGFR [6, 7].

Published modelling studies of CKD and nephron loss predicted that SGLT2 inhibition in remaining nephrons with increased single nephron GFR markedly decreases net proximal tubule Na^+ reabsorption and induces a natriuretic and diuretic effect [8].

Modelling predicted that, in a diabetic normal and diabetic CKD kidney, SGLT2 inhibition shifts glucose and Na^+ transport to segments further downstream in the outer medulla, and that SGLT2 inhibition may further reduce the already physiologically low O_2 availability in the renal outer medulla [9, 10].

The influence on medullary transport and oxygenation would be attenuated by the blood glucose- and GFR-lowering effect of SGLT2 inhibition.

Why Target Glucose Handling in the Intestine?

Rodent studies have indicated that diabetes increases intestinal SGLT1 expression [11, 12] and glucose uptake [13, 14].

Consistent with the importance of SGLT1 in intestinal glucose uptake and, consequently, postprandial hyperglycaemia, $Sglt1^{-/-}$ mice show a strongly reduced blood glucose increase during an OGTT [15, 16].

Consistent with this, pre-meal, in contrast to post-meal, dosing of the selective SGLT1 inhibitor GSK-1614235 in healthy volunteers delayed intestinal glucose absorption [17].

Somewhat unexpectedly, the selective SGLT1 inhibitor GSK-1614235 and the dual SGLT1/2 inhibitor sotagliflozin (LX4211) can be taken orally at doses that measurably inhibit glucose transport in the intestine without severe gastrointestinal side effects [17, 18].

Based on studies in rodents, SGLT1 inhibition in the diabetic heart could be a two-edged sword (for review see [19]): SGLT1 might be involved in the progression of diabetic cardiomyopathy by triggering reactive oxygen species and/or facilitating the accumulation of glycogen in cardiomyocytes, but could also protect against ischaemia reperfusion injury by replenishing ATP stores in ischaemic cardiac tissues by enhancing glucose availability.

Development of SGLT Inhibitors

Sotagliflozin (LX4211) shows only a 20 times higher potency for SGLT2 over SGLT1 and is considered a dual SGLT1/2 inhibitor [20]; it is currently undergoing Phase 3 clinical trials.

Hyperleptinaemia (db/db mice), but not hypoleptinaemia (ob/ob mice), reduces intestinal SGLT1 abundance and blood glucose elevations in response to oral glucose loading [21].

This effect, however, is increased up to the transport maximum of SGLT1 when more glucose is delivered to the late proximal tubule, which may occur in hyperglycaemia or in response to SGLT2 inhibition.

Simultaneously blocking SGLT1 and SGLT2 in the kidney could be advantageous compared with SGLT2 inhibition alone with regard to blood glucose lowering [22].

The impact of intestinal SGLT1 inhibition on blood glucose control discussed above is expected to be additive to the renal effects.

Perspectives

Large clinical outcome trials will be needed for selective SGLT1 and dual SGLT1/2 inhibitors.

Selective SGLT2 and dual SGLT1/2 inhibitors are also currently being tested in individuals with type 1 diabetes as an add on to insulin.

Since the effects of SGLT2 inhibitors on GFR, natriuresis and diuresis can occur in the absence of hyperglycaemia [23], they are also being tested in non-diabetic people with heart failure or CKD [24].

Pharmacodynamic Model of Sodium–Glucose Transporter 2 (SGLT2) Inhibition: Implications for Quantitative Translational Pharmacology

https://doi.org/10.1208/s12248-011-9297-2

A machine generated summary based on the work of Maurer, Tristan S.; Ghosh, Avijit; Haddish-Berhane, Nahor; Sawant-Basak, Aarti; Boustany-Kari, Carine M.; She, Li; Leininger, Michael T.; Zhu, Tong; Tugnait, Meera; Yang, Xin; Kimoto, Emi; Mascitti, Vincent; Robinson, Ralph P.

2011 in The AAPS Journal

Abstract-Summary A biologically based pharmacokinetic/pharmacodynamic (PK/PD) model of SGLT2 inhibitor-mediated UGE was developed.

The derived model was used to characterize the acute PK/PD relationship of the SGLT2 inhibitor, dapagliflozin, in rats.

Direct modeling provided an improved characterization of the data and precise parameter estimates which were reasonably consistent with those predicted from preclinical data.

These results indicate that the acute clinical pharmacology of SGLT2 inhibitors in healthy subjects can be reasonably well predicted from preclinical data through rational accounting of species differences in pharmacokinetics, physiology, and SGLT2 pharmacology.

Because these data can be generated at the earliest stages of drug discovery, the proposed model is useful in the design and development of novel SGLT2 inhibitors.

This model is expected to serve as a useful foundation for future efforts to understand and predict the effects of SGLT2 inhibition under chronic administration and in other patient populations.

Introduction

Considerable efforts have been made to develop and apply biologically based mathematical models in support of quantitative human pharmacokinetic predictions from in vitro and in vivo data generated preclinically [25, 26].

To date, far less attention has been paid to the development and application of biologically based mathematical models to support quantitative pharmacology predictions from in vitro and in vivo data generated preclinically.

It is one of the top eight targets being pursued in the pharmaceutical industry and there are several novel SGLT2 inhibitors currently in clinical development [27, 28].

The objective of this work is to quantitatively examine the translational pharmacology of SGLT2 inhibition between the preclinical and clinical setting using a simple, physiologically based pharmacokinetic/pharmacodynamic (PK/PD) model.

The results of this work indicate that the acute clinical pharmacology of SGLT2-mediated UGE can be reasonably well predicted from preclinical data using the proposed PKPD model.

Materials and Methods

Mean human plasma dapagliflozin concentrations following single doses of 2.5, 10, 50, 100, and 250 mg and associated urinary glucose excretion over 120 h in healthy subjects were obtained from a literature report [29] via digitization using Grab It!

The reported mean concentration-time profiles of dapagliflozin in healthy subjects were described using a two-compartment linear disposition model with first-order absorption: where k_a is the first-order absorption rate constant after oral dosing, k_{pt} and k_{tp} are the first-order rate constants for non-specific distribution of the drug to and from a peripheral compartment, and k_{el} is the first-order elimination rate constant.

GluFR was fixed to a population mean value of 7.5 g/h commensurate with typical mean plasma glucose concentrations (i.e. 100 mg/dl, 5 mM) and GFR (i.e. 125 ml/min) in healthy subjects [30].

Results

Both the data and model indicate less than dose proportional increase in UGE at doses above 1 mg/kg.

Slightly greater increases in UGE were observed at the 3 and 10 mg/kg dose levels than were fitted by the model.

This bias was modest in nature, with the error in UGE prediction at 120 h being 23%, 28%, 7%, 28%, and 23% at dapagliflozin doses of 2.5, 10, 50, 100, and 250 mg, respectively.

Post hoc estimates of glucose filtration rate in the 2.5, 10, 50, 100, and 250 mg dose groups were 6.6, 7.7, 6.8, 8.6, and 8.6 g/h, respectively.

Discussion

This work suggests that the acute clinical pharmacology of SGLT2 inhibitors in healthy subjects can be predicted from preclinical data using the proposed biologically based PK/PD model of UGE with sufficient accuracy to support decision making (compound rank ordering, candidate selection, early clinical trial design).

This work suggests that SGLT2 inhibitor-mediated UGE can be predicted in humans from the following data which can be obtained preclinically: (1) a prediction of human pharmacokinetics, (2) parameters describing the normal physiological process of glucose filtration and reabsorption (GFR, plasma glucose concentration, f_{reabs}), and (3) parameters describing the intrinsic efficacy (I_{max}) and potency (IC_{50}) of the SGLT2 inhibitor for UGE.

The current work suggests that the in vivo potency of SGLT2 inhibitors can be reasonably well predicted from in vitro assays and mechanism-based PK/PD modeling of UGE data obtained in rats.

Conclusion

A simple biologically based PK/PD model has been developed, which was useful in characterizing the PK/PD data of dapagliflozin in rats and humans.

This model provides a structure by which species differences in pharmacokinetics, physiology, and pharmacology can be accounted in order to support clinical pharmacology predictions from preclinical data.

Application of this model to preclinical and clinical dapagliflozin data indicates the general predictive utility of in vitro pharmacology assays and rat pharmacology.

New Oral Antidiabetic Agents

https://doi.org/10.1007/s11739-011-0677-5

A machine generated summary based on the work of Cavallo Perin, Paolo; Fornengo, Paolo

2011 in Internal and Emergency Medicine

Abstract-Summary These include agents that stimulate insulin secretion, reduce hepatic glucose production, delay digestion and absorption of intestinal carbohydrate or improve insulin action.

We focus on the new agents used in the latest years and the overcoming ones in future, in particular incretin-based therapies, drugs inhibiting kidney glucose reabsorption (SGLT2 inhibitors), and glucokinase activators.

The strategy for new drug development advocated here is to establish a broad range of anti-diabetic medicines with different mechanisms of action and potential opportunities for effective combination therapies.

Introduction

The pathophysiology of hyperglycemia in type 2 diabetes involves three main defects: insulin deficiency due to insufficient pancreatic insulin release, excess hepatic glucose output, and insulin resistance (decreased glucose uptake) in peripheral tissues (including muscle and fat) and the liver.

These include agents that stimulate insulin secretion (sulphonylureas and rapid-acting secretagogues), reduce hepatic glucose production (biguanides), delay digestion and absorption of intestinal carbohydrates (alpha-glucosidase inhibitors) or improve insulin action (glitazones) [31].

Pharmacological therapy of type 2 diabetes is changing because of improved knowledge of pathophysiology and of long-term efficacy of traditional oral agents.

Glitazones

Glitazones uniquely target insulin resistance, a core physiologic defect in those with type 2 diabetes, significantly improving blood glucose control.

Glitazones increase nonoxidative glucose disposal, increase triglyceride synthesis, and improve free fatty acid metabolism [32].

They have similar glucose-lowering effects as all the others commonly used oral agents (generally reducing A1C levels by 1–2%), but they can maintain stable blood glucose control over periods of 2 years [33, 34].

Weight gain with glitazone therapy averages 3 kg over the first year of therapy, a rate comparable to that seen with initiation of insulin.

Incretin-Based Therapies

Incretins are gut-derived hormones, principally glucagone-like peptide 1 (GLP-1) and glucose-dependent insulinotropic peptide (GIP), that are secreted at low basal levels in the fasting state.

The DPP-4 inhibitors (DPP-4i) have a greater effect on postprandial hyperglycemia; they also have a lesser effect on fasting hyperglycemia because high, sustained levels of GLP-1 are required to improve fasting blood glucose [35].

Since the levels of endogenous intact GLP-1 achieved following DPP-4 inhibition are at the upper limit of the normal physiological range DPP-4i therapy is not associated with nausea or vomiting, nor with inhibition of gastric emptying or weight loss.

Compared to DPP-4i, long-acting GLP-1 receptor agonists (exenatide, liraglutide) produce a more potent control of hyperglycemia and are associated to weight loss due to more potent and sustained GLP-1 receptor activation, but they are given subcutaneously.

SGLT2 Inhibitors

This process contributes to the sustained elevated serum glucose levels observed in individuals with diabetes, as they have an increased capacity for renal glucose reabsorption [36].

Inhibiting this glucose reabsorption, thereby allowing its excretion in the urine (glucosuria), is therefore emerging as a potential new approach to the treatment of diabetes.

SGLT2 inhibition would lower the maximum glucose reabsorption capacity of the proximal tubule.

The threshold for urinary glucose excretion would be decreased, leading to glucosuria at plasma glucose levels lower than 180 md/dl.

Like other anti-diabetes drugs, the glucose lowering by SGLT2 inhibitors may reduce glucotoxicity, with a theoretical benefit of an increase in insulin sensitivity.

SGLT2 inhibition reduces glucose levels only during hyperglycaemia, because the amount of glucose excreted is related to the plasma glucose level.

The insulin independence of SGLT2-mediated glucose reabsorption means that the action of SGLT2 inhibitors should not be affected by insulin resistance or insulin deficiency.

Glucokinase Activators

The discovery of the allosteric activator site in glucokinase and the development of drugs that interact with this site are important milestones in research related to glucose homeostasis and diabetes mellitus [37, 38].

Although glucokinase activators have a high potential for improving current treatment of type 2 diabetes, full development of glucokinase-based antidiabetic therapy remains challenging.

Considering the limitations of current antidiabetic drug therapy, and on the basis of the knowledge that type 2 diabetes is caused by a large number of pathogenetic defects, a strategy for new drug development is needed.

The challenge for the future is to establish a broad range of antidiabetic drugs with different mechanisms of action and potential opportunities for more effective combination therapies.

Pharmacodynamics, Efficacy and Safety of Sodium–Glucose Co-transporter Type 2 (SGLT2) Inhibitors for the Treatment of Type 2 Diabetes Mellitus

https://doi.org/10.1007/s40265-014-0337-y
A machine generated summary based on the work of Scheen, André J.
2014 in Drugs

Abstract-Summary The available SGLT2 inhibitors share similar pharmacokinetic characteristics, with a rapid oral absorption, a long elimination half-life allowing once-daily administration, an extensive hepatic metabolism mainly via glucuronidation to inactive metabolites, the absence of clinically relevant drug–drug interactions and a low renal elimination as parent drug.

The pharmacological inhibition of SGLT2 co-transporters reduces hyperglycaemia by decreasing renal glucose threshold and thereby increasing urinary glucose excretion.

Results of numerous placebo-controlled randomised clinical trials of 12–104 weeks duration have shown significant reductions in glycated haemoglobin (HbA_{1c}), resulting in a significant increase in the proportion of patients reaching HbA_{1c} targets, and a significant lowering of fasting plasma glucose when SGLT2 inhibitors were administered as monotherapy or in addition to other glucose-lowering therapies including insulin in patients with T2DM.

In head-to-head trials of up to 2 years, SGLT2 inhibitors exerted similar glucose-lowering activity to metformin, sulphonylureas or sitagliptin.

The durability of the glucose-lowering effect of SGLT2 inhibitors appears to be better; however, this remains to be more extensively investigated.

The risk of hypoglycaemia was much lower with SGLT2 inhibitors than with sulphonylureas and was similarly low as that reported with metformin, pioglitazone or sitagliptin.

Both effects were very consistent across the trials and they represent some advantages for SGLT2 inhibitors when compared with other oral glucose-lowering agents.

SGLT2 inhibitors are generally well-tolerated.

Although SGLT2 inhibitors have already been extensively investigated, further studies should even better delineate the best place of these new glucose-lowering agents in the already rich armamentarium for the management of T2DM.

Introduction

Despite a large armamentarium already being available for the management of hyperglycaemia in T2DM, glucose-lowering agents are not adequately effective in maintaining long-term glycaemic control in a majority of patients, even when used in combination [39].

Inhibitors of sodium–glucose co-transporter type 2 (SGLT2) are new glucose-lowering agents with an original insulin-independent mode of action [40, 41].

This mechanism of action holds promise for patients with T2DM not only in terms of improvements in glycaemic control, with a limited risk of hypoglycaemia, but also considering the potential benefits of weight loss resulting from increased glucosuria and arterial blood pressure reduction associated with the osmotic effect [41, 42].

SGLT2 inhibitors may be used as monotherapy in diet-treated patients or in combination with any other glucose-lowering agent [43, 44].

A leading article on SGLT2 inhibitors was published in 2011 discussing the progress and therapeutic potential of this drug class in T2DM, at a time when development was advanced (especially for dapagliflozin) but no agents had yet been approved for use [45].

Dapagliflozin

In another meta-analysis of ten RCTs, dapagliflozin treatment was associated with a reduction in HbA_{1c} [weighted mean difference (WMD): −0.53%; 95% CI −0.58 to −0.47; $p < 0.00001$] and fasting plasma glucose (WMD: −1.06 mmol/L; 95% CI −1.20 to −0.92; $p < 0.00001$).

After 24 weeks, dapagliflozin 10 mg/day was non-inferior to metformin in reducing HbA_{1c} in treatment-naive patients with T2DM and combination therapy was statistically superior to either monotherapy in controlling blood glucose [46].

Despite similar 52-week glycaemic efficacy (HbA_{1c} reduction of 0.52% in both arms), dapagliflozin 5–10 mg/day produced much less hypoglycaemia than glipizide (3.5% of patients vs. 40.8%; $p < 0.0001$) in T2DM patients inadequately controlled with metformin [18].

Canagliflozin

In patients with T2DM, canagliflozin pharmacokinetics were dose dependent, and the $t_{½}$ ranged from 12 to 15 h. After 28 days, the renal threshold for glucose excretion was reduced, UGE was increased, and both HbA_{1c} and fasting plasma glucose decreased in subjects administered canagliflozin [47].

According to a meta-analysis of ten trials including 6701 patients, compared with placebo, canagliflozin produced absolute reductions in HbA_{1c} levels when used as monotherapy (WMD −1.08%, 95% CI −1.25 to −0.90; $p < 0.00001$) or add-on treatment (WMD −0.73%, 95% CI −0.84 to −0.61; $p < 0.00001$) [48].

In a short-term 12-week trial evaluating five doses of canagliflozin (50 mg, 100 mg, 200 mg, 300 mg daily, or 300 mg twice daily), when compared with control subjects (placebo or sitagliptin 100 mg/day), canagliflozin increased UGE but was not associated with increased bacteriuria or adverse event reports of UTIs [49].

Empagliflozin

Increases in empagliflozin exposure were roughly dose-proportional and a dose-dependent increase in UGE was observed for empagliflozin doses up to 100 mg [50].

Empagliflozin exposure increased dose proportionally over the dose range 10–100 mg and showed linear pharmacokinetics with respect to time.

Oral administration of empagliflozin at doses of 10, 25 or 100 mg once daily over 28 days resulted in significant increases in UGE and reductions in blood glucose compared with placebo in patients with T2DM [51].

Because the increase in drug exposure remained rather limited, no dose adjustment of empagliflozin is required in patients with RI.

In a meta-analysis of RCTs with more than 6000 participants, an increased risk of genital tract infections (OR 3.31; 95% CI 1.55–7.09) was observed with empagliflozin compared with placebo or other glucose-lowering agents [52].

Ipragliflozin

A multiple ascending-dose study assessed the pharmacokinetics/pharmacodynamics of ipragliflozin in healthy subjects after single doses and multiple once-daily doses for 10 days (dose levels 5–600 mg).

Ipragliflozin did not affect the pharmacokinetics of sitagliptin, pioglitazone or glimepiride, and vice versa, suggesting that no dose adjustments are likely to be required when ipragliflozin is given in combination with other glucose-lowering drugs in patients with T2DM [53, 54].

These pharmacokinetic findings were confirmed in drug-naïve T2DM patients who were randomised to placebo or ipragliflozin once daily at doses of 50, 100, 200 or 300 mg for 28 days.

In a study designed to investigate the effects of RI on the pharmacokinetics of ipragliflozin in Japanese T2DM patients, C_{max} and AUC were 1.17 and 1.21 times higher, respectively, in subjects with moderate RI than in subjects with normal renal function [55, 56].

A placebo-controlled RCT examined the efficacy and safety of ipragliflozin in combination with metformin in Japanese patients with T2DM.

Other Sodium–Glucose Co-transporter Type 2 Inhibitors in Development

Several other SGLT2 inhibitors, mostly developed by Japanese companies, have received first global approval in Japan [57, 58].

Luseogliflozin [Lusefi® (Japan)] is an orally active second-generation SGLT2 inhibitor developed by Taisho Pharmaceutical for the treatment of patients with T2DM.

Randomised, single-blind, placebo-controlled, single ascending-dose (1–25 mg) and multiple ascending-dose (5 or 10 mg/day, 7 days) trials were conducted in healthy male Japanese subjects to investigate the safety, pharmacokinetics and pharmacodynamics of luseogliflozin [21].

Tofogliflozin [Apleway®, Deberza® (Japan)], an orally active small molecule SGLT2 inhibitor, has been developed by Chugai Pharmaceutical for the treatment of T2DM, and a marketing authorisation application was filed in Japan in 2013 by licensees Sanofi K. K. and Kowa.

In March 2014, tofogliflozin (20 mg once-daily dose) received its first global approval for this indication in Japan as either monotherapy or in combination with other antihyperglycaemic agents [59].

Discussion

SGLT2 inhibitors are the only oral antidiabetic agents that improve glycaemic control while reducing body weight, an interesting combined effect due to the increasing dual burden of obesity and T2DM [39].

Another interesting question concerns the potential effects of SGLT2 inhibitors on renal function itself and whether this novel pharmacological effect may influence the development of diabetic/hypertensive nephropathy in at-risk patients [60].

Even if SGLT2 inhibitors have been shown to be efficacious and safe in diabetic patients with mild to moderate CKD [61, 62], all drugs that may interfere with renal function, by decreasing GFR (for instance, NSAIDs), may reduce the glucose-lowering effects of SGLT2 inhibitors in fragile patients.

A number of large-scale prospective trials are now ongoing to demonstrate the safety and possibly the efficacy of SGLT2 inhibitors on CV outcomes in T2DM patients at CV risk [63].

Conclusion

SGLT2 inhibitors have proven their efficacy in numerous placebo-controlled trials as monotherapy or in combination with various other glucose-lowering agents.

SGLT2 inhibitors may offer the advantage of a better glucose-lowering durability, although this remains to be proven in long-term comparative studies.

A number of large-scale prospective trials are now ongoing to evaluate the clinical effects of SGLT2 inhibitors, especially on CV outcomes in high-risk patients with T2DM.

If positive findings were obtained with SGLT2 inhibitors regarding glucose-lowering durability, CV outcomes or decreased risk of diabetic nephropathy, these results would be considered as major breakthroughs in the management of T2DM.

Results from these clinical studies will help define the role for this new class of oral antidiabetic agents, with its unique mechanism of action, as a treatment option for reducing hyperglycaemia in patients with T2DM.

Initiation of the SGLT2 Inhibitor Canagliflozin to Prevent Kidney and Heart Failure Outcomes Guided by HbA1c, Albuminuria, and Predicted Risk of Kidney Failure

https://doi.org/10.1186/s12933-022-01619-0

A machine generated summary based on the work of Tye, Sok Cin; Jongs, Niels; Coca, Steven G.; Sundström, Johan; Arnott, Clare; Neal, Bruce; Perkovic, Vlado; Mahaffey, Kenneth W.; Vart, Priya; Heerspink, Hiddo. J. L.

2022 in Cardiovascular Diabetology

Abstract-Summary Sodium glucose co-transporter-2 (SGLT2) inhibitors reduce the risk of kidney and heart failure events independent of glycemic effects.

We assessed whether initiation of the SGLT2 inhibitor canagliflozin guided by multivariable predicted risk based on clinical characteristics and novel biomarkers is more efficient to prevent clinical outcomes compared to a strategy guided by HbA1c or urinary-albumin-creatinine ratio (UACR) alone.

We compared the number of composite kidney (defined as a sustained 40% decline in eGFR, chronic dialysis, kidney transplantation, or kidney death) and composite heart failure outcomes (defined as heart failure hospitalization or cardiovascular (CV) death) prevented per 1000 patients treated for 5 years when canagliflozin was initiated in patients according to HbA1c $\geq$ 7.5%, UACR, or multivariable risk models consisting of: (1) clinical characteristics, or (2) clinical characteristics and novel biomarkers.

The combined biomarkers model included all clinical characteristics, tumor necrosis factor receptor-1, kidney injury molecule-1, matrix metallopeptidase-7 and interleukin-6.

Treating all patients with HbA1c ≥ 7.5% (n = 2809) would prevent 33.0 (95% CI 18.8 to 43.3) kidney events at a rate of 9.6 (95% CI 5.5 to 12.6) events prevented per 1000 patients treated for 5 years.

Initiation of canagliflozin based on an estimated risk-based approach prevented more kidney and heart failure outcomes compared to a strategy based on HbA1c or UACR alone.

There was no apparent gain from adding novel biomarkers to the clinical risk model.

These findings support the use of risk-based assessment using clinical markers to guide initiation of SGLT2 inhibitors in patients with type 2 diabetes.

Introduction

Clinical practice guidelines recommend the use of SGLT2 inhibitors in patients with type 2 diabetes and atherosclerotic CV disease, CKD, or heart failure as second-line treatment on top of metformin [64, 65].

Despite the efficacy of SGLT2 inhibitors in patients with and without type 2 diabetes, the initiation of these agents in clinical practice is slow and treatment is centered around isolated risk marker improvement such as glycated hemoglobin (HbA1c) or albuminuria [66–68].

Analyses from CV and kidney outcome trials have demonstrated that the relative benefits of SGLT2 inhibitors are consistent across many patient subgroups including those with or without type 2 diabetes, severity of kidney disease or the presence of heart failure [69, 70].

We first assessed if a treatment strategy to initiate the SGLT2 inhibitor canagliflozin using the multivariable predicted risk of kidney outcome based on clinical risk markers is more efficient for preventing clinical outcomes compared to a strategy based on HbA1c or albuminuria alone.

Methods

This study included data from the Canagliflozin Cardiovascular Assessment Study (CANVAS) program consisting of two multicentre, randomized, double-blind placebo-controlled trials (CANVAS and CANVAS-R) to assess the CV safety and kidney outcomes of canagliflozin in type 2 diabetes patients with an established CV disease or multiple CV risk factors.

For model development, Cox proportional hazards regression models were used for prediction of the 5-year risk and treatment effect of canagliflozin on the composite kidney outcome (defined as a sustained 40% decline in eGFR, end-stage kidney disease with eGFR <15 mL/min/1/.73m^2, or the need of dialysis, kidney transplantation, or kidney death) and the composite heart failure outcome (defined as heart failure hospitalization or CV death).

The 5-year predicted risk for the composite kidney outcome for all patients was calculated by setting the treatment status to zero in the development model (irrespective of patient's actual treatment allocation).

Results

The bootstrap validation of the clinical model to predict the kidney outcome showed calibration with Chi^2-goodness of fit test, P = 0.931 and good discrimination with C-statistics 0.80 (95% CI 0.75 to 0.84).

Adding novel biomarkers to the clinical risk prediction model, TNFR1, KIM-1, MMP-7 and IL-6 were retained after backward selection for prediction of the composite kidney outcome.

The discrimination index to predict the 5-year composite kidney risk was good [C-statistics 0.81 (95% CI 0.76 to 0.86; difference versus clinical model 0.01 (95% CI − 0.01 to 0.04)], and moderately good for the composite heart failure outcome [C-statistics 0.74 (95% CI 0.71 to 0.77; difference versus clinical model 0.01 (95% CI 0.00 to 0.02)].

Discussion

We demonstrated a large variation in the predicted 5-year benefit of the SGLT2 inhibitor canagliflozin for the composite kidney and heart failure or CV death outcomes and that treating patients with type 2 diabetes with the SGLT2 inhibitor canagliflozin according to a multivariable risk prediction model is more effective than a treatment strategy based on HbA1c or UACR alone.

Using the multivariable risk models, we demonstrated a large variation in the predicted 5-year risk for the composite kidney and the composite heart failure outcome alongside a large variation in absolute treatment effects.

Our results demonstrating that a multivariable risk-strategy is more efficient to guide SGLT2 initiation than a strategy based on a single risk marker (i.e., HbA1c or albuminuria) are consistent with previous studies showing the micro- and macrovascular complications in patients with type 2 diabetes are determined by multiple risk markers, and support the measurement of biomarker panels to adequately capture individual risk and guide individualized treatment decisions [71, 72].

Conclusion

This post-hoc analysis of the CANVAS trial suggests that the use of a clinical risk-based assessment is more efficient to guide the initiation of SGLT2 inhibitors for patients with type 2 diabetes instead of using HbA1c or UACR alone.

This would result in the prevention of more kidney and heart failure event for the same number of patients treated compared to the HbA1c or UACR guided initiation of SGLT2 inhibitors across a broad range of potential thresholds to initiate treatment.

Validation in an independent study would support clinical implementation.

Insight into the Interaction Mechanism of Human SGLT2 with Its Inhibitors: 3D-QSAR Studies, Homology Modeling, and Molecular Docking and Molecular Dynamics Simulations

https://doi.org/10.1007/s00894-018-3582-2

A machine generated summary based on the work of Dong, Lili; Feng, Ruirui; Bi, Jiawei; Shen, Shengqiang; Lu, Huizhe; Zhang, Jianjun

2018 in Journal of Molecular Modeling

Abstract-Summary Both comparative molecular field analysis (CoMFA) and comparative molecular similarity indices analysis (CoMSIA) were applied to generate three-dimensional quantitative structure–activity relationship (3D-QSAR) models.

Molecular docking was performed to explore the bonding mode of inhibitors to the active site of hSGLT2.

With regards to binding affinity, we found that hydrogen-bond interactions of Asn51 and Glu75, located in the active site of hSGLT2, with compound 40 were critical.

Hydrophobic and electrostatic interactions were shown to enhance activity, in agreement with the results obtained from docking and 3D-QSAR analysis.

Our study results shed light on the interaction mode between inhibitors and hSGLT2 and may aid in the development of C-aryl glucoside SGLT2 inhibitors.

Introduction

Elucidating the interaction mechanism of SGLT2 with inhibitors could provide crucial information for the development and optimization of improved T2DM therapeutics.

In the absence of an X-ray crystal structure for human SGLT2 (hSGLT2), homology modeling—which is the most precise method of constructing a three-dimensional structure—can be applied to gain insights into the interaction mode of hSGLT2 with its inhibitors [73].

Molecular docking can provide information that helps us to understand the mechanisms of action of inhibitors and may therefore be useful in the development of novel effective inhibitors [74, 75].

3D-QSAR studies, homology modeling, and molecular docking and molecular dynamics simulations were performed to study the interaction mechanism of hSGLT2 with its inhibitors.

Taken in concert, these results provide a significant amount of information on the fundamental interaction mechanism of inhibitors with hSGLT2, which may ultimately contribute to the future development of potent hSGLT2 inhibitors and T2DM treatment options.

Materials and Methods

The Surflex-Dock program in the SYBYL 7.3 [76] software package was used to characterize the binding site of hSGLT2 as well as to complement 3D-QSAR model generation.

During the sampling process, coordinate trajectories were saved every 20 ps, and the conformations generated during the last 2 ns of each simulation were used for binding free energy calculations and analyses.

The stable MD trajectory of compound 40 bound to the hSGLT2 system was used to estimate the binding free energy (ΔG_{bind}) using the MM/PBSA and MM/GBSA methods implemented in Amber14.

In MM/PBSA and MM/GBSA, the binding free energy (ΔG_{bind}) is calculated as follows:where $G_{complex}$, $G_{receptor}$, and G_{ligand} are the free energies of the complex, protein, and ligand, respectively.

ΔG_{bind} was estimated from the change in solvation energy ($\Delta G_{solvation}$), the change of conformational entropy upon ligand binding ($T\Delta S$), and the gas-phase interaction energy (ΔE_{MM}) between compound 40 and the receptor.

Results and Discussion

The compounds were randomly divided into a training set consisting of 33 compounds and a test set consisting of 7 compounds.

The training set was used to generate the CoMFA-based and CoMSIA-based QSAR models, and the test set was used to check the reliability of those models.

The training and test sets, including all of the features of the compounds, were found to be representative.

3D-QSAR Study

By analyzing the steric and electrostatic field contour maps for compound 40 in the model, we found that introducing an electronegative group that is not too small (e.g., CH_3) nor too bulky (e.g., naphthalene or anthracene) at the R position had a favorable effect on the inhibitory activity.

Upon analyzing the hydrophobic and hydrogen-bond field contour maps of compound 40 in the CoMSIA-based QSAR model, we found that increasing the hydrophobicity of the groups at the X and R positions could enhance the receptor-binding affinity.

At the active site of hSGLT2, Tyr266 and His56 were found to be close to the chlorophenyl group of compound 40, resulting in the formation of hydrophobic and electrostatic interactions.

We also found that the hydrophobic interactions of Tyr266, Trp267, and Gln433, located in the active site of hSGLT2, with compound 40 are crucial to receptor binding.

Conclusions

The results obtained indicate that the presence of electronegative and lipophilic substituents at the X position on the inhibitor improves the SGLT2-inhibitory activity by an order of magnitude.

We also showed that electrostatic, steric, and hydrophobic interactions play crucial roles in the inhibitory activity, a finding that was found to be consistent with a subsequent analysis of docking and binding free energy calculations.

The binding modes of the ligand galactose and the most active compound, compound 40 (dapagliflozin), to hSGLT2 were highlighted by molecular docking experiments.

40-ns MD simulations and binding free energy calculations of compounds 40, 14, and 32 bound to hSGLT2 were carried out to further analyze the dynamic binding process and to verify the docking results, respectively.

The interaction between compound 40 and hSGLT2 eventually changed during the simulations, resulting in the formation of stronger H-bonds with the key residues Asn51 and Glu75.

Development of Sodium Glucose Co-transporter 2 (SGLT2) Inhibitors with Novel Structure by Molecular Docking and Dynamics Simulation

https://doi.org/10.1007/s00894-019-4067-7

A machine generated summary based on the work of Feng, Ruirui; Dong, Lili; Wang, Leng; Xu, Yefei; Lu, Huizhe; Zhang, Jianjun

2019 in Journal of Molecular Modeling

Abstract-Summary Molecular docking studies were carried out to explore the binding interactions of sodium glucose co-transporter 2 (SGLT2) with its inhibitors.

In order to understand the structure–activity correlation of compound 1 m (the highest score of docking) and compound 1 t (the lowest score), we carried out a combined molecular dynamics simulation and MM-GBSA method.

This study is expected to shed light on the mechanism of action of compound 1 m, leading to development of active drug candidates targeting SGLT2.

Introduction

SGLT2 can be used as the molecular targets for the treatment of T2DM.

Compared with other diabetic targets, SGLT2 has the following advantages [77–80]: (i) the use of a wide range; (ii) does not easily cause hypoglycemia; (iii) low risk of cardiovascular disease; (iv) glucose excretion from the urine to achieve a negative balance of energy, reduce the weight of diabetic patients; and (v) SGLT2 inhibitors generate fewer adverse reactions.

The SGLT2 inhibitors can effectively treat T2DM by controlling blood glucose levels [81] with almost no side effects.

The SGLT2 inhibitors are classified into C-glucoside [82], O-glucoside [83], N-glucoside [84], and non-glucoside [85].

The clinical research indicated that none of these SGLT2 inhibitors can exert more than 50% renal glucose reabsorption in humans [86], and the research found that dapagliflozin might increase the risk of adverse renal events [87].

It is essential to quickly design a few novel and efficient SGLT2 inhibitors.

The aim of this study was to find novel SGLT2 inhibitors by computational guidance.

Materials and Methods

The newly designed SGLT2 inhibitors were docked, and then the two complexes, SGLT2-1 m and SGLT2-1 t, were chosen for dynamics simulations to calculate the thermodynamic parameters.

The binding free energy calculation was performed to investigate the binding affinity of the inhibitor with protein.

The binding free energy (ΔG_{bind}) between inhibitors (lig) and SGLT2 (rec) was calculated using the following equations: where G_{com}, G_{rec}, and G_{lig} are the free energies of complex, receptor, and ligand, respectively.

The ΔG_{bind} is split into several terms: the gas phase enthalpy (ΔE_{MM}), which is the sum of the internal energy (ΔE_{int}), the electrostatic interaction (ΔE_{ele}), and the van der Waals interaction (ΔE_{vdw}); the solvation free energy (ΔG_{sol}), which includes the polar (ΔG_{GB}) and nonpolar (ΔG_{SA}) parts; and the conformational entropy ($-T\Delta S$) upon ligand binding.

To obtain detailed information about the protein–ligand binding, the interaction energies between inhibitors and SGLT2 were decomposed to each residue using the MM-GBSA method in AMBER14 [87].

Results and Discussion

The inwardly extending pyranose ring of compound 13 showed hydrogen bonds interactions (red dotted lines) with Lys297, Phe74, and Tyr266 in the active site of SGLT2.

Compound 1 m was better able to extend into the active site, which could sufficiently fill the cavity of active site and form more hydrogen bonds, which might be the cause of its high docking score.

The polar residues Lys130, Asp270, and Gln271 could provide strong electrostatic interaction for the stability of SGLT2-1 m. However, the polar solvation energy of residues Lys130 and Asp270 were unfavorable for the stability of SGLT2-1 m. Then the polar residues Asn51, Glu75, Lys130, and Gln433 could offer strong electrostatic interaction for the stability of SGLT2-1 t. The residues that play an important role in the binding of compound 1 m were calculated as Tyr266, Trp267, and Gln271 by decomposing free energy.

Conclusions

We designed a series of novel SGLT2 inhibitors and studied their binding mode by docking and molecular dynamics simulation.

The bioactivity of compound 1 m predicted was higher than dapagliflozin (compound 1), which might help to design more active SGLT2 inhibitors.

Some new SGLT2 protein inhibitors were designed using the 3D-QSAR method, and the molecular dynamics simulations, free energy calculations, and decomposition free energy calculations were performed on the best-predicted bioactivity compound 1 m and the worst compound 1 t. These methods were used to study the differences in the binding mode between compounds 1 m and 1 t in the active site.

The results displayed that the two systems of SGLT2-1 m and SGLT2-1 t were stable after 35 ns, and the RMSF value of the residues constituting the active site were only slightly changed.

Concise and Stereodivergent Synthesis of Carbasugars Reveals Unexpected Structure-Activity Relationship (SAR) of SGLT2 Inhibition

https://doi.org/10.1038/s41598-017-05895-9

A machine generated summary based on the work of Ng, Wai-Lung; Li, Ho-Chuen; Lau, Kit-Man; Chan, Anthony K. N.; Lau, Clara Bik-San; Shing, Tony K. M.

2017 in Scientific Reports

Abstract-Summary The clinical usage of carbasugar SGLT2 inhibitors has been underexplored, due to the lengthy synthetic routes and the lack of structure-activity relationship (SAR) studies of these compounds.

This synthetic strategy, together with computational modeling, revealed the unexpected SAR of these carbasugar SGLT2 inhibitors, and enabled the discovery of a highly selective and potent SGLT2 inhibitor.

Introduction

Departing from this trend, we have pioneered the design and syntheses of carbasugar SGLT2 inhibitors, in which we modify the sugar core rather than the aglycone [88, 89].

We found that some of the carbasugar analogues of sergliflozin (1), such as pseudo-O-glycoside 5 and pseudo-N-glycoside 6, exert a high inhibitory activity/selectivity towards SGLT2 [88, 89], and also exhibit a prolonged blood glucose lowering effect [88].

After the initial success of 5 & 6, we set out to further expand the synthetic toolkit towards carbasugars, and also to enhance the drug-like properties of carbasugar SGLT2 inhibitors.

We report herein a concise and stereodivergent synthetic route towards these challenging synthetic targets, and also the unexpected SAR of carbasugar SGLT2 inhibition.

Results and Discussions

We therefore utilized an underexploited, stereospecific palladium-catalyzed allyl-aryl coupling reaction to address this challenge.

This phosphine-free Pd-catalyzed allyl-aryl coupling reaction is stereospecific and regioselective, with arylated C-1-α-cyclohexene 18 and C-1-β-cyclohexene 20 obtained as single products.

After the transmetalation step, the aryl group on the π-allyl Pd complex is delivered internally to the less-hindered C-1 position of the carbocycle, resulting a net-inversion of configuration and an exclusive regioselection (pathway III).

Another piece of unexpected SAR information came from the activity profiles of aryl pseudo-O-glycosides 28, 29, and 30 (β-O series), in which an exocyclic oxygen atom connects the carbasugar and aglycone moiety.

The exocyclic oxygen atom in 28 effectively disrupts the π-π interactions and also withholds the carbasugar core from forming an extensive hydrogen bond network, resulting in the observed lack of SGLT2 inhibitory activity of 28.

Conclusions

We have developed a concise and stereodivergent synthetic route towards some novel carbasugar analogues of dapagliflozin.

This synthetic study revealed unexpected structure-activity relationship (SAR) of carbasugar SGLT2 inhibitors, and also enabled the discovery of the highly potent and selective inhibitor, cyclohexene 8.

Our study will therefore guide the future design and syntheses of carbasugar SGLT2 inhibitors, thereby unlocking their potential as novel diabetes therapeutics and beyond.

Methods

To a stirred solution of cyclohexene 20 (66.6 mg, 0.105 mmol) in EtOH (1.5 mL) was added 1 M HCl (aq) (1.5 mL) at rt.

The reaction mixture was stirred at 50 °C for 3 h. Concentration of the reaction mixture under reduced pressure followed by flash chromatography ($CHCl_3$:MeOH, 9:1) yield tetraol 8 (36.9 mg, 87%) as a white solid.

Concentration of the reaction mixture under reduced pressured followed by flash chromatography (hexane: EtOAc, 7:2) yielded cyclohexene 20 (82.8 mg, 85%) as a colourless oil.

The cells were cultured in DMEM supplemented with 10% FBS, 1% PS and G418 (1 mg/ml), and kept in 37 °C humidified incubator supplied with 5% CO_2.

The cells were incubated in sodium buffer (140 mM NaCl, 2 mM KCl, 1 mM $MgCl_2$, 1 mM $CaCl_2$, and 10 mM Hepes/Tris, pH 7.5) at 37 °C for 2 h.

Effects of the SGLT2 Inhibitor Dapagliflozin on Cardiac Function Evaluated by Impedance Cardiography in Patients with Type 2 Diabetes. Secondary Analysis of a Randomized Placebo-Controlled Trial

https://doi.org/10.1186/s12933-019-0910-5

A machine generated summary based on the work of Bonora, Benedetta Maria; Vigili de Kreutzenberg, Saula; Avogaro, Angelo; Fadini, Gian Paolo

2019 in Cardiovascular Diabetology

Abstract-Summary Cardiovascular outcome trials have documented a strong benefit of sodium glucose cotransporter-2 inhibitors (SGLT2i) on the risk of hospitalization for heart failure (HF) in patients with type 2 diabetes (T2D) with or without established cardiovascular disease or prior history of HF.

We aimed to evaluate whether treatment with SGLT2i affected cardiac function using impedance cardiography (ICG) in a randomized placebo-controlled trial.

Thirty-three patients with T2D were randomized to receive blind dapagliflozin 10 mg or matching placebo for 12-week on top of their ongoing glucose lowering medication regimen.

Cardiac function was evaluated by resting ICG at baseline and at the end of the 12-week treatment period.

ICG is a non-invasive technology based on the continuous measurement of thoracic electrical conductivity to process a cardiodynamic parameters related to fluid content, blood flow, cardiac function, and circulatory function.

After 12 weeks, patients randomized to dapagliflozin, as compared to those randomized to placebo, showed improvements in HbA1c (− 1.2%; 13 mmol/mol), systolic blood pressure (− 3.7 mmHg), and body weight (− 3.3 kg).

Based on ICG, in both groups, we detected no significant change in parameters of blood flow (stroke volume, cardiac output, cardiac index), systolic function (ejection fraction, acceleration and velocity indexes, systolic time ratio), circulatory function (systemic vascular resistance index), and fluid status (thoracic fluid content) after treatment.

This is the first study exploring cardiac effects of SGLT2i using ICG in T2D. We observed no change in cardiac function parameters estimated by ICG in T2D patients who received dapagliflozin versus placebo for 12 weeks.

Background

Patients with type 2 diabetes (T2D) have a two-to-fivefold increased risk of developing heart failure (HF) compare to non-diabetic patients [90].

Patients with T2D are more likely to be hospitalized for HF [91], to be rehospitalized for HF [39], and to experience a longer hospital stay [92] compared to patients without diabetes.

Patients with T2D and HF have a higher risk of cardiovascular and all-cause mortality than HF patients without T2D [93].

The recent results of the four cardiovascular outcome trials (CVOTs) with SGLT2i have shown remarkable benefits in reducing HF hospitalization by about 30% in patients with T2D with or without established cardiovascular disease and also in patient with or without history of heart failure [94–97].

Large retrospective studies confirmed that treatment with SGLT2i, when compared with other glucose-lowering medications (GLMs), was associated with lower rates of hospitalization for HF among patients with and without history of cardiovascular disease [98–100].

Materials and Methods

The Medis Niccomo ICG device processed these changes with a dedicated algorithm (physiologic adaptive signal analysis) coupling impedance signal and waveform with ECG, noninvasively and continuously provided the following hemodynamic variables: heart rate (HR); systolic blood pressure (SBP), diastolic blood pressure (DBP); SV, stroke index [SI (SV normalized for body surface area)]; CO (SV × HR); cardiac index [CI (CO normalized for body surface area)]; ejection fraction (EF); acceleration index [AI (the maximum acceleration of blood flow in the aorta during systole)]; velocity index [VI (the peak velocity of blood flow in the aorta during systole)]; systolic time ratio (STR); LVET [the time interval between the opening and the closing of the aortic valve (i.e., mechanical systole)]; left cardiac work (LCW) and LCW index (LCWI), which reflected the myocardial oxygen demand; systemic vascular resistance [SVR (estimate of "afterload)] and SVR index [SVRI (SVR normalised to body size); TFC (indicator of chest fluid status); TFC Index [TFCI (TFC, normalized for body surface area)]; total arterial compliance [TAC (indicator of the degree of peripheral arterial stiffness/compliance)], TAC index, [TACI (TAC normalised to body size)]; ICG variables were calculated by using the mean of 2-min beat-to-beat values for 20 min.

Results

In the placebo group, HbA1c increased non-significantly by 0.4% and body weight remained stable (+0.2 kg).

Compared with baseline, SBP declined by 4.7 ± 1.3 mmHg in the dapagliflozin group and by 1.0 ± 2.3 mmHg in the placebo group ($p = 0.035$).

Diastolic dysfunction based on the STR cut-off of 0.31 was present in 63.3% of patients (66.7% in the dapagliflozin group and 60% in the placebo group).

At follow-up, the prevalence of diastolic dysfunction based on STR declined by 6.7% in the dapagliflozin group and remained stable in the placebo group ($p = 0.325$).

No significant correlation was detected between change in HbA1c or body weight from baseline to the end of follow-up and change in ICG parameters (not shown).

Discussion

We found no significant effect of the SGLT2i dapagliflozin on measures of cardiac function evaluated by ICG.

A small observational study showed that in patients with T2D and established cardiovascular disease, a short-term empagliflozin treatment was associated with a significant reduction in LV mass index and improved diastolic function measured by 2D echocardiography.

This is the first study exploring the cardiac effects of SGLT2i using ICG in T2D. This study suggests that, in T2D patients without a history of HF, a 12-week treatment with dapagliflozin exerted no overt effect on haemodynamic and cardiac function parameters compared to placebo.

Previous observational studies documented effects of SGLT2i on diastolic cardiac function in T2D, but a recent re-analysis of the DECLARE-TIMI58 study reported that dapagliflozin prevented HF in patients with a normal or reduced EF and improved survival especially in patients with reduced EF [48].

Conclusions

Despite strong evidence that SGLT2i prevent HF in T2D with or without prior HF episodes, we found no effects of dapagliflozin on parameters of cardiac function measured by ICG.

Short duration of treatment, small sample size, lack or specific diastolic function measures, limited correlation of ICG parameters with gold standard examination of cardiac function, and the masking diuretic effects of SGLT2i are all possible explanations of these negative results.

We also speculate that SGLT2i exert no effects on cardiac function parameters in patients with normal cardiac function but may play a major role at the very early onset of cardiac disfunction, preventing hospitalization and mortality.

Further studies are needed to address this hypothesis.

Bibliography

1. Von Mering J (1886) Über künstlichen diabetes. Centralbl Med Wiss 22:5
2. Rossetti L, Smith D, Shulman GI, Papachristou D, DeFronzo RA (1987) Correction of hyperglycemia with phlorizin normalizes tissue sensitivity to insulin in diabetic rats. J Clin Invest 79(5):1510–1515
3. Braunwald E. SGLT2 inhibitors: the statins of the 21st century
4. https://www.niddk.nih.gov/news/archive/2016/story-discovery-sglt2-inhibitors-harnessing-kidneys-help-treat-diabetes
5. Inzucchi SE, Zinman B, Wanner C et al (2015) SGLT-2 inhibitors and cardiovascular risk: proposed pathways and review of ongoing outcome trials. Diab Vasc Dis Res 12:90–100
6. Wanner C, Lachin JM, Inzucchi SE et al (2018) Empagliflozin and clinical outcomes in patients with type 2 diabetes mellitus, established cardiovascular disease, and chronic kidney disease. Circulation 137:119–129
7. Petrykiv S, Sjostrom CD, Greasley PJ, Xu J, Persson F, Heerspink HJL (2017) Differential effects of dapagliflozin on cardiovascular risk factors at varying degrees of renal function. Clin J Am Soc Nephrol 12:751–759
8. Layton AT, Vallon V (2018) SGLT2 inhibition in a kidney with reduced nephron number: modeling and analysis of solute transport and metabolism. Am J Physiol Ren Physiol 314:F969. https://doi.org/10.1152/ajprenal.00551.2017

9. Layton AT, Vallon V, Edwards A (2016) Predicted consequences of diabetes and SGLT inhibition on transport and oxygen consumption along a rat nephron. Am J Physiol Ren Physiol 310:F1269–F1283
10. Layton AT, Vallon V, Edwards A (2015) Modeling oxygen consumption in the proximal tubule: effects of NHE and SGLT2 inhibition. Am J Physiol Ren Physiol 308:F1343–F1357
11. Miyamoto K, Hase K, Taketani Y et al (1991) Diabetes and glucose transporter gene expression in rat small intestine. Biochem Biophys Res Commun 181:1110–1117
12. Ogata H, Seino Y, Harada N et al (2014) KATP channel as well as SGLT1 participates in GIP secretion in the diabetic state. J Endocrinol 222:191–200
13. Grempler R, Thomas L, Eckhardt M et al (2012) Empagliflozin, a novel selective sodium glucose cotransporter-2 (SGLT-2) inhibitor: characterisation and comparison with other SGLT-2 inhibitors. Diabetes Obes Metab 14:83–90
14. Fujita Y, Kojima H, Hidaka H, Fujimiya M, Kashiwagi A, Kikkawa R (1998) Increased intestinal glucose absorption and postprandial hyperglycaemia at the early step of glucose intolerance in Otsuka Long-Evans Tokushima Fatty Rats. Diabetologia 41:1459–1466
15. Dominguez Rieg JA, Chirasani VR, Koepsell H, Senapati S, Mahata SK, Rieg T (2016) Regulation of intestinal SGLT1 by catestatin in hyperleptinemic type 2 diabetic mice. Lab Investig 96:98–111
16. Roder PV, Geillinger KE, Zietek TS, Thorens B, Koepsell H, Daniel H (2014) The role of SGLT1 and GLUT2 in intestinal glucose transport and sensing. PLoS One 9:e89977
17. Dobbins RL, Greenway FL, Chen L et al (2015) Selective sodium-dependent glucose transporter 1 inhibitors block glucose absorption and impair glucose-dependent insulinotropic peptide release. Am J Physiol Gastrointest Liver Physiol 308:G946–G954
18. Zambrowicz B, Freiman J, Brown PM et al (2012) LX4211, a dual SGLT1/SGLT2 inhibitor, improved glycemic control in patients with type 2 diabetes in a randomized, placebo-controlled trial. Clin Pharmacol Ther 92:158–169
19. Song P, Onishi A, Koepsell H, Vallon V (2016) Sodium glucose cotransporter SGLT1 as a therapeutic target in diabetes mellitus. Expert Opin Ther Targets 20:1109–1125
20. Lapuerta P, Zambrowicz B, Strumph P, Sands A (2015) Development of sotagliflozin, a dual sodium-dependent glucose transporter 1/2 inhibitor. Diab Vasc Dis Res 12:101–110
21. Kurosaki E, Ogasawara H (2013) Ipragliflozin and other sodium-glucose cotransporter-2 (SGLT2) inhibitors in the treatment of type 2 diabetes: preclinical and clinical data. Pharmacol Ther 139(1):51–59
22. Powell DR, DaCosta CM, Gay J et al (2013) Improved glycemic control in mice lacking Sglt1 and Sglt2. Am J Physiol Endocrinol Metab 304:E117–E130
23. Vallon V, Thomson SC (2017) Targeting renal glucose reabsorption to treat hyperglycaemia: the pleiotropic effects of SGLT2 inhibition. Diabetologia 60:215–225
24. Heerspink HJ, Desai M, Jardine M, Balis D, Meininger G, Perkovic V (2017) Canagliflozin slows progression of renal function decline independently of glycemic effects. J Am Soc Nephrol 28:368–375
25. Houston JB (1994) Utility of in vitro drug metabolism data in predicting in vivo metabolic clearance. Biochem Pharmacol 47(9):1469–1479
26. Carpino PA, Goodwin B (2010) Diabetes area participation analysis: a review of companies and targets described in the 2008–2010 patent literature. Expert Opin Ther Pat 20(12):1627–1651
27. Washburn WN (2009) Evolution of sodium glucose co-transporter 2 inhibitors as anti-diabetic agents. Expert Opin Ther Pat 19(11):1485–1499
28. Komoroski B, Vachharajani N, Boulton D et al (2009) Dapagliflozin, a novel SGLT2 inhibitor, induces dose-dependent glucosuria in healthy subjects. Clin Pharmacol Ther 85:520–526
29. Rohlfing CL, Wiedmeyer H-M, Little RR, England JD, Tennill A, Goldstein DE (2002) Defining the relationship between plasma glucose and HbA1c: analysis of glucose profiles and HbA1c in the diabetes control and complications trial. Diabetes Care 25(2):275–278
30. DeWoskin RS, Thompson CM (2008) Renal clearance parameters for PBPK model analysis of early lifestage differences in the disposition of environmental toxicants. Regul Toxicol Pharmacol 51(1):66–86

31. Krentz AJ, Bailey CJ (2005) Oral antidiabetic agents: current role in type 2 diabetes mellitus. Drugs 65:385–411
32. Miyazaki Y, Mahankali A, Matsuda M, Glass L, Mahankali S, Ferrannini E, Cusi K, Mandarino LJ, DeFronzo RA (2001) Improved glycemic control and enhanced insulin sensitivity in type 2 diabetic subjects treated with pioglitazone. Diabetes Care 24:710–719
33. Tan MH, Baksi A, Krahulec B, Kubalski P, Stankiewicz A, Urquhart R, Edwards G, Johns D, The GLAL Study Group (2005) Comparison of pioglitazone and gliclazide in sustaining glycemic control over 2 years in patients with type 2 diabetes. Diabetes Care 28:544–550
34. Durbin RJ (2004) Thiazolidinedione therapy in the prevention/delay of type 2 diabetes in patients with impaired glucose tolerance and insulin resistance. Diabetes Obes Metab 6:280–285
35. Trujillo J (2006) Incretin hormones in the treatment of type 2 diabetes. Formulary 41:130–141
36. Wright EM, Hirayama BA, Loo DF (2007) Active sugar transport in health and disease. J Intern Med 261:32–43
37. Grimsbt J, Sarabu R, Corbett WL et al (2003) Allosteric activators of glucokinase: potential role in diabetes therapy. Science 301:370–373
38. Leighton B, Atkinson A, Coghlan MP (2005) Small molecule glucokinase activators as novel anti-diabetic agents. Biochem Soc Trans 33:371–374
39. Inzucchi SE, Bergenstal RM, Buse JB et al (2012) Management of hyperglycaemia in type 2 diabetes: a patient-centered approach. Position statement of the American Diabetes Association (ADA) and the European Association for the Study of Diabetes (EASD). Diabetologia 55(6):1577–1596
40. Tahrani AA, Barnett AH, Bailey CJ (2013) SGLT inhibitors in management of diabetes. Lancet Diabetes Endocrinol 1(2):140–151
41. Hasan FM, Alsahli M, Gerich JE (2014) SGLT2 inhibitors in the treatment of type 2 diabetes. Diabetes Res Clin Pract 104(3):297–322
42. Bailey CJ (2011) Renal glucose reabsorption inhibitors to treat diabetes. Trends Pharmacol Sci 32(2):63–71
43. Abdul-Ghani MA, Norton L, Defronzo RA (2011) Role of sodium-glucose cotransporter 2 (SGLT 2) inhibitors in the treatment of type 2 diabetes. Endocr Rev 32(4):515–531
44. Vasilakou D, Karagiannis T, Athanasiadou E et al (2013) Sodium-glucose cotransporter 2 inhibitors for type 2 diabetes: a systematic review and meta-analysis. Ann Intern Med 159(4):262–274
45. Berhan A, Barker A (2013) Sodium glucose co-transport 2 inhibitors in the treatment of type 2 diabetes mellitus: a meta-analysis of randomized double-blind controlled trials. BMC Endocr Disord 13(1):58
46. Neumiller JJ, White JR Jr, Campbell RK (2010) Sodium-glucose co-transport inhibitors: progress and therapeutic potential in type 2 diabetes mellitus. Drugs 70(4):377–385
47. Henry RR, Murray AV, Marmolejo MH et al (2012) Dapagliflozin, metformin XR, or both: initial pharmacotherapy for type 2 diabetes, a randomised controlled trial. Int J Clin Pract 66(5):446–456
48. Nauck MA, Del Prato S, Meier JJ et al (2011) Dapagliflozin versus glipizide as add-on therapy in patients with type 2 diabetes who have inadequate glycemic control with metformin: a randomized, 52-week, double-blind, active-controlled noninferiority trial. Diabetes Care 34(9):2015–2022
49. Devineni D, Morrow L, Hompesch M et al (2012) Canagliflozin improves glycaemic control over 28 days in subjects with type 2 diabetes not optimally controlled on insulin. Diabetes Obes Metab 14(6):539–545
50. Yang XP, Lai D, Zhong XY et al (2014) Efficacy and safety of canagliflozin in subjects with type 2 diabetes: systematic review and meta-analysis. Eur J Clin Pharmacol 70(10):1149–1158
51. Nicolle LE, Capuano G, Ways K et al (2012) Effect of canagliflozin, a sodium glucose co-transporter 2 (SGLT2) inhibitor, on bacteriuria and urinary tract infection in subjects with type 2 diabetes enrolled in a 12-week, phase 2 study. Curr Med Res Opin 28(7):1167–1171

52. Seman L, Macha S, Nehmiz G et al (2013) Empagliflozin (BI 10773), a potent and selective SGLT2 inhibitor, induces dose-dependent glucosuria in healthy subjects. Clin Pharmacol Drug Dev 2(2):152–161
53. Heise T, Seewaldt-Becker E, Macha S et al (2013) Safety, tolerability, pharmacokinetics and pharmacodynamics following 4 weeks' treatment with empagliflozin once daily in patients with type 2 diabetes. Diabetes Obes Metab 15(7):613–621
54. Liakos A, Karagiannis T, Athanasiadou E et al (2014) Efficacy and safety of empagliflozin for type 2 diabetes: a systematic review and meta-analysis. Diabetes Obes Metab 16(10):984–993
55. Kadokura T, Zhang W, Krauwinkel W et al (2014) Clinical pharmacokinetics and pharmacodynamics of the novel SGLT2 inhibitor ipragliflozin. Clin Pharmacokinet 53(11):975–988
56. Smulders RA, Zhang W, Veltkamp SA et al (2012) No pharmacokinetic interaction between ipragliflozin and sitagliptin, pioglitazone, or glimepiride in healthy subjects. Diabetes Obes Metab 14(10):937–943
57. Ferrannini E, Veltkamp SA, Smulders RA et al (2013) Renal glucose handling: impact of chronic kidney disease and sodium-glucose cotransporter 2 inhibition in patients with type 2 diabetes. Diabetes Care 36(5):1260–1265
58. Nauck MA (2014) Update on developments with SGLT2 inhibitors in the management of type 2 diabetes. Drug Des Devel Ther 8:1335–1380
59. Sasaki T, Seino Y, Fukatsu A et al (2014) Safety, pharmacokinetics, and pharmacodynamics of single and multiple luseogliflozin dosing in healthy Japanese males: a randomized, single-blind, placebo-controlled trial. Adv Ther 31(3):345–361
60. Stanton RC (2014) Sodium glucose transport 2 (SGLT2) inhibition decreases glomerular hyperfiltration: is there a role for SGLT2 inhibitors in diabetic kidney disease? Circulation 129(5):542–544
61. Yale JF, Bakris G, Cariou B et al (2013) Efficacy and safety of canagliflozin in subjects with type 2 diabetes and chronic kidney disease. Diabetes Obes Metab 15(5):463–473
62. Yale JF, Bakris G, Cariou B et al (2014) Efficacy and safety of canagliflozin over 52 weeks in patients with type 2 diabetes mellitus and chronic kidney disease. Diabetes Obes Metab 16(10):1016–1027
63. Foote C, Perkovic V, Neal B (2012) Effects of SGLT2 inhibitors on cardiovascular outcomes. Diab Vasc Dis Res 9(2):117–123
64. American Diabetes Association (2021) 9. Pharmacologic approaches to glycemic treatment: standards of medical care in diabetes—2021. Diabetes Care 44(Suppl 1):111–124
65. Cosentino F, Grant PJ, Aboyans V, Bailey CJ, Ceriello A, Delgado V, Federici M, Filippatos G, Grobbee DE, Hansen TB et al (2020) 2019 ESC guidelines on diabetes, pre-diabetes, and cardiovascular diseases developed in collaboration with the EASD. Eur Heart J 41(2):255–323
66. Arnold SV, Inzucchi SE, Tang F, McGuire DK, Mehta SN, Maddox TM, Goyal A, Sperling LS, Einhorn D, Wong ND et al (2017) Real-world use and modeled impact of glucose-lowering therapies evaluated in recent cardiovascular outcomes trials: an NCDR(R) research to practice project. Eur J Prev Cardiol 24(15):1637–1645
67. Mahtta D, Ramsey DJ, Lee MT, Chen L, Al Rifai M, Akeroyd JM, Vaughan EM, Matheny ME, Santo K, Navaneethan SD et al (2022) Utilization rates of SGLT2 inhibitors and GLP-1 receptor agonists and their facility-level variation among patients with atherosclerotic cardiovascular disease and type 2 diabetes: insights from the department of veterans affairs. Diabetes Care 45(2):372–380
68. Reaven PD, Emanuele NV, Wiitala WL, Bahn GD, Reda DJ, McCarren M, Duckworth WC, Hayward RA, Investigators VADT (2019) Intensive glucose control in patients with type 2 diabetes—15-year follow-up. N Engl J Med 380(23):2215–2224
69. Young TK, Li JW, Kang A, Heerspink HJL, Hockham C, Arnott C, Neuen BL, Zoungas S, Mahaffey KW, Perkovic V et al (2021) Effects of canagliflozin compared with placebo on major adverse cardiovascular and kidney events in patient groups with different baseline levels of HbA1c, disease duration and treatment intensity: results from the CANVAS program. Diabetologia 64:2402. https://doi.org/10.1007/s00125-021-05524-1

70. Waijer SW, Vart P, Cherney DZI, Chertow GM, Jongs N, Langkilde AM, Mann JFE, Mosenzon O, McMurray JJV, Rossing P et al (2022) Effect of dapagliflozin on kidney and cardiovascular outcomes by baseline KDIGO risk categories: a post hoc analysis of the DAPA-CKD trial. Diabetologia 65:1085. https://doi.org/10.1007/s00125-022-05694-6
71. Oellgaard J, Gaede P, Rossing P, Rorth R, Kober L, Parving HH, Pedersen O (2018) Reduced risk of heart failure with intensified multifactorial intervention in individuals with type 2 diabetes and microalbuminuria: 21 years of follow-up in the randomised Steno-2 study. Diabetologia 61(8):1724–1733
72. Oellgaard J, Gaede P, Rossing P, Persson F, Parving HH, Pedersen O (2017) Intensified multifactorial intervention in type 2 diabetics with microalbuminuria leads to long-term renal benefits. Kidney Int 91(4):982–988
73. Rodriguez R, Chinea G, Lopez N, Pons T, Vriend G (1998) Homology modeling, model and software evaluation: three related resources. Bioinformatics 14(6):523–528. https://doi.org/10.1093/bioinformatics/14.6.523
74. Udatha DB, Sugaya N, Olsson L, Panagiotou G (2012) How well do the substrates KISS the enzyme? Molecular docking program selection for feruloyl esterases. Sci Rep 2:323. https://doi.org/10.1038/srep00323
75. Forli S, Huey R, Pique ME, Sanner MF, Goodsell DS, Olson AJ (2016) Computational protein–ligand docking and virtual drug screening with the AutoDock suite. Nat Protoc 11(5):905–919
76. Tripos, Inc. (2006) Sybyl 7.3. Tripos, Inc., St. Louis
77. Kinne RKH, Castaneda F (2011) SGLT inhibitors as new therapeutic tools in the treatment of diabetes. Handb Exp Pharmacol 203(203):105–126. https://doi.org/10.1007/978-3-642-17214-4_5
78. Pajor A, Randolph KS, Smith C (2008) Inhibitor binding in the human renal low- and high-affinity Na+/glucose cotransporters. J Pharmacol Exp Ther 324(3):985–991. https://doi.org/10.1124/jpet.107.129825
79. Kipnes MS (2011) Sodium–glucose cotransporter 2 inhibitors in the treatment of type 2 diabetes: a review of phase II and III trials. Clin Investig 1(1):145–156. https://doi.org/10.4155/cli.10.12
80. Kanai Y, Lee WS, You G, Brown D, Hediger MA (1994) The human kidney low affinity Na+/glucose cotransporter SGLT2. Delineation of the major renal reabsorptive mechanism for D-glucose. J Clin Invest 93(1):397–404. https://doi.org/10.1172/JCI116972
81. Han S, Hagan DL, Taylor JR, Xin L, Meng W, Biller SA et al (2008) Dapagliflozin, a selective SGLT2 inhibitor, improves glucose homeostasis in normal and diabetic rats. Diabetes 57(6):1723–1729
82. Washburn WN (2009) Development of the renal glucose reabsorption inhibitors: a new mechanism for the pharmacotherapy of diabetes mellitus type 2. J Med Chem 40(29):1785–1794. https://doi.org/10.1021/jm8013019
83. Gao Y, Zhao G, Liu W, Wang Y, Xu W, Wang J (2010) Thiadizole-based thiaglycosides as sodium-glucose co-transporter 2 (SGLT2) inhibitors. Chin J Chem 28(4):605–612. https://doi.org/10.1002/cjoc.201090120
84. Li AR, Zhang J, Greenberg J, Lee T, Liu J (2011) Discovery of non-glucoside SGLT2 inhibitors. Bioorg Med Chem Lett 21(8):2472. https://doi.org/10.1016/j.bmcl.2011.02.056
85. Liu J, Lee TW (2012) Why do SGLT2 inhibitors inhibit only 30–50% of renal glucose reabsorption in humans? Diabetes 61:2199–2204. https://doi.org/10.2337/db12-0052
86. Tang H, Li D, Zhang J, Li Y, Wang T, Zhai S, Song Y (2017) Sodium-glucose co-transporter-2 inhibitors and risk of adverse renal outcomes among patients with type 2 diabetes: a network and cumulative meta-analysis of randomized controlled trials. Diabetes Obes Metab 19:1106. https://doi.org/10.1111/dom.12917
87. Greenidge PA, Kramer C, Mozziconacci JC, Wolf RM (2013) MM/GBSA binding energy prediction on the PDB bind data set: successes, failures, and directions for further improvement. J Chem Inf Model 53(1):201–209. https://doi.org/10.1021/ci300425v

88. Shing TKM, Ng WL, Chan JY, Lau CB (2013) Design, syntheses, and SAR studies of carbocyclic analogues of sergliflozin as potent sodium-dependent glucose cotransporter 2 inhibitors. Angew Chem Int Ed 52:8401–8405
89. Ng WL, Lau KM, Lau CB, Shing TKM (2016) Palladium-catalyzed arylation of carbasugars enables the discovery of potent and selective SGLT2 inhibitors. Angew Chem Int Ed 55:13818–13821
90. Kannel WB, Hjortland M, Castelli WP (1974) Role of diabetes in congestive heart failure: the Framingham study. Am J Cardiol 34:29–34
91. MacDonald MR, Petrie MC, Varyani F, Östergren J, Michelson EL, Young JB et al (2008) Impact of diabetes on outcomes in patients with low and preserved ejection fraction heart failure: an analysis of the Candesartan in Heart failure: Assessment of Reduction in Mortality and Morbidity (CHARM) programme. Eur Heart J 29:1377–1385
92. Targher G, Dauriz M, Laroche C, Temporelli PL, Hassanein M, Seferovic PM et al (2017) In-hospital and 1-year mortality associated with diabetes in patients with acute heart failure: results from the ESC-HFA heart failure long-term registry. Eur J Heart Fail 19:54–65
93. Kapoor JR, Fonarow GC, Zhao X, Kapoor R, Hernandez AF, Heidenreich PA (2011) Diabetes, quality of care, and in-hospital outcomes in patients hospitalized with heart failure. Am Heart J 162(480–486):e3
94. Zinman B, Wanner C, Lachin JM, Fitchett D, Bluhmki E, Hantel S et al (2015) Empagliflozin, cardiovascular outcomes, and mortality in type 2 diabetes. N Engl J Med 373:2117–2128
95. Neal B, Perkovic V, Mahaffey KW, de Zeeuw D, Fulcher G, Erondu N et al (2017) Canagliflozin and cardiovascular and renal events in type 2 diabetes. N Engl J Med 377:644–657
96. Wiviott SD, Raz I, Bonaca MP, Mosenzon O, Kato ET, Cahn A et al (2019) Dapagliflozin and cardiovascular outcomes in type 2 diabetes. N Engl J Med 380:347–357
97. Perkovic V, Jardine MJ, Neal B, Bompoint S, Heerspink HJL, Charytan DM et al (2019) Canagliflozin and renal outcomes in type 2 diabetes and nephropathy. N Engl J Med 380:2295–2306
98. Birkeland KI, Jørgensen ME, Carstensen B, Persson F, Gulseth HL, Thuresson M et al (2017) Cardiovascular mortality and morbidity in patients with type 2 diabetes following initiation of sodium-glucose co-transporter-2 inhibitors versus other glucose-lowering drugs (CVD-REAL Nordic): a multinational observational analysis. Lancet Diabetes Endocrinol 5:709–717
99. Elisabetta P, Ajinkya P, Mehdi N, Anouk D-L et al (2019) Empagliflozin and the risk of heart failure hospitalization in routine clinical care: a first analysis from the empagliflozin comparative Effectiveness and Safety (EMPRISE) study. Circulation 139:2822–2830
100. Hosea NA, Collard WT, Cole S, Maurer TS, Fang RX, Jones H et al (2009) Prediction of human pharmacokinetics from preclinical information: comparative accuracy of quantitative prediction approaches. J Clin Pharmacol 49(5):513–533
101. Poole RM, Prossler JE (2014) Tofogliflozin: first global approval. Drugs 74(8):939–944
102. Kosiborod M, Cavender MA, Fu AZ, Wilding JP, Khunti K, Holl RW et al (2017) Lower risk of heart failure and death in patients initiated on sodium-glucose cotransporter-2 inhibitors versus other glucose-lowering drugs: the CVD-REAL study. Circulation 136:249–259
103. Kato ET, Silverman MG, Mosenzon O, Zelniker TA, Cahn A, Furtado RHM, Kuder J, Murphy SA, Bhatt DL, Leiter LA, McGuire DK, Wilding JPH, Bonaca MP, Ruff CT, Desai AS, Goto S, Johansson PA, Gause-Nilsson I, Johanson P, Langkilde AM, Raz I, Sabatine MS, Wiviott SD (2019) Effect of dapagliflozin on heart failure and mortality in type 2 diabetes mellitus. Circulation 28(139):2528–2536

Chapter 2
SGLT2 Inhibitors and Mechanism of Cardiovascular Benefits in Type 2 Diabetes

Mukesh Nandave

Introduction by the Editor

Since SGLT2i are used to treat diabetes, which has a low risk of hypoglycemia and cardiovascular events, SGLT2 is a very attractive target for treating heart failure (HF) and other cardiovascular disorders. Along with the drop in blood glucose levels, it also regulates the excretion of glucose in urine. Various mechanisms considerably treat cardiovascular disorders, including hemodynamic, anti-inflammatory, anti-fibrotic, antioxidant, and metabolic activities, as shown in Fig. 2.1.

Based on research, it has been found that SGLT2i enhances diastolic function in human and animal models of diabetic heart disease especially when HF ejection fraction remains intact. SGLT2i improved the numerous harmful pathways including free radical damage, apoptosis, inflammation, and fibrosis. Systolic function is crucial in patients with HF and decreased ejection fraction, both with and without diabetes, despite the limited and variable effects on systolic function in investigations of diabetic heart ailments and HF with intact ejection fraction, respectively. The systolic function appears to be significantly improved, followed by a large decrease in left ventricular volume and a corresponding drop in pulmonary stress, resulting in structural remodeling of the heart.

In addition to its ability to reduce blood sugar, SGLT2i has been proven to have a significant role in preventing cardiovascular illnesses in both diabetic and non-diabetic people. In terms of reducing the likelihood of heart failure in diabetic individuals, bexagliflozin, empagliflozin, canagliflozin, and dapagliflozin are the drugs that demonstrated the most striking outcomes in which bexagliflozin is considered the most anticipated medication based on the study, as it demonstrated the rising

M. Nandave (✉)
Department of Pharmacology and Pharmaceutical Biotechnology, Delhi Pharmaceutical Sciences and Research University (DPSRU), New Delhi, Delhi, India

M. Nandave (ed.), *Sodium-glucose Cotransporter-2 (SGLT2) Inhibitors in Heart Failure*, https://doi.org/10.1007/978-981-97-7568-2_2

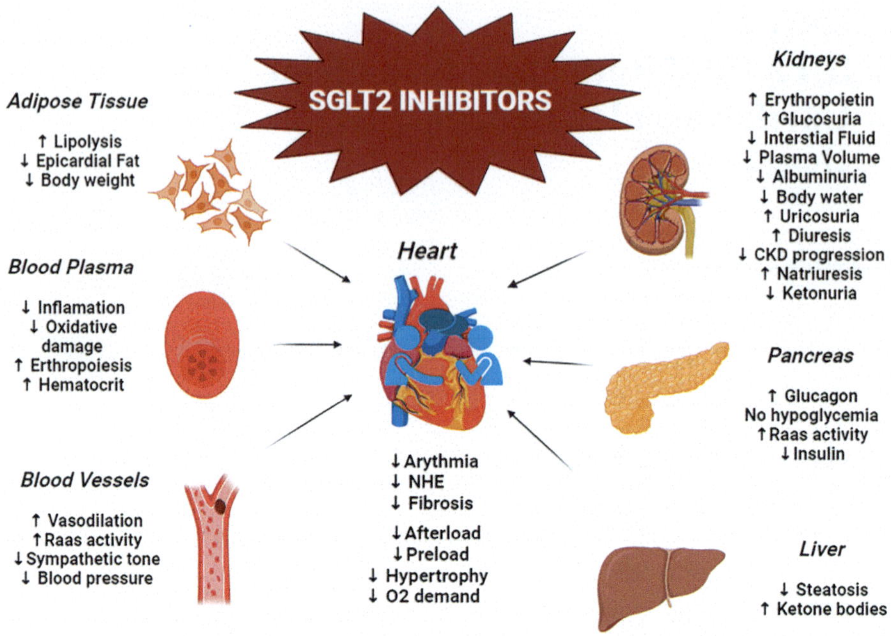

Fig. 2.1 A schematic representation of the different mechanisms implicated in the cardiovascular benefits of SGLT2 inhibitors

incidence of T2D and an increase in the risk of morbidity and death from cardiovascular illnesses [1].

These drugs were first developed to treat T2D by lowering blood sugar levels, but research has revealed that they also have significant cardiovascular benefits.

This chapter focused on the newly approved drugs for the treatment of type 2 diabetes associated with cardiovascular outcomes and their collection of clinical research shown in Table 2.1. All the details of clinical trials were extracted from https://clinicaltrials.gov/. A mixture of "randomised clinical trials," or "RCTs," "SGLT2 inhibitors AND cardiovascular outcomes," or "SGLT2i AND cardiovascular benefits," was employed in the search approach. Out of the 303 investigations that were conducted, only 10 studies were chosen for extraction based on their early phase I status, completed status, and protective action of SGLT2i in cardiovascular diseases. These clinical trials demonstrated significant cardiovascular benefits for individuals with or without T2D.

The main objectives of this chapter are to enumerate, analyze, and contrast all SGLT2i medications that treat cardiovascular illnesses. Diabetes affects several target organs, but the National Health System is most burdened with cardiovascular repercussions in terms of morbidity and death [2].

Therefore, these innovative beneficial approaches goal to advance stronger drugs that improve patient outcomes and mitigate the effects of these diseases. However,

Table 2.1 Summary of all latest status clinical trials of SGLT2i associated cardiovascular outcome

Aim	Identifier	Intervention	Phase	Cardiovascular outcome
Based on heart failure due to reduced ejection fraction				
Compare the efficacy of canagliflozin against a vehicle in improving the total symptom score (TSS) in patients with typical heart failure (HF) on the Kansas City Cardiomyopathy Questionnaire (KCCQ)	NCT04252287	Canagliflzon (100 mg) + Placebo	Completed	Reduced the symptoms of HF despite EF Based on the data, it was found that 4.3 ($P = 0.016$) had higher points over 12 weeks for patients with and without diabetes, HFpEF, and HFrEF
Empagliflozin decreased heart failure and preserved ejection fraction to assess the patient's survival rate	NCT03057951	Empagliflozin + Placebo	III	Reduced CV mortality or hospitalization for HF, maintained EF, despite of presence or absence of diabetes
Analyze the dapagliflozin's impact on mortality, ejection fraction, and deteriorating heart failure in people with chronic heart failure	NCT03036124	Dapagliflozin + Placebo	III	Dapagliflozin medication was linked to a higher risk of developing progressive heart failure or dying from cardiovascular disease in individuals with HF and a decreased EF, regardless of a history of diabetes
Following are the parameters that evaluate the effects of SGLT2i in high-risk type diabetes patients with heart failure such as: (A) Left ventricular diastolic and systolic function (B) Raised plasma ketone levels	NCT06229678	Empagliflozin + Placebo + Acipimox	Early phase I	Not reported yet

(continued)

Table 2.1 (continued)

Aim	Identifier	Intervention	Phase	Cardiovascular outcome
Assessment of the feasibility and efficacy of a polypill-based approach for treating heart failure at a single centre with randomized, mixed demographic individuals	NCT04633005	Polypill + Control Rx	Early Phase I	Not reported yet
Based on high CV risk in T2D patients				
To determine the safety of BI 10773 therapy for those who have high cardiovascular risk and T2D	NCT01131676	Low dose: BI 10773 High dose: Placebo BI 10773 High dose: BI 10773 Low dose: Placebo BI 10773	III	Patients with T2D who were at high risk for cardiovascular events had a lower likelihood of primary composite cardiovascular outcome and death from all causes when empagliflozin was given as standard medication
To determine the significance of dapagliflozin on type 2 diabetes with cardiovascular patients and cardiovascular risk factors.	NCT01730534	Dapagliflozin 10 mg + Placebo	III	Dapagliflozin reduced the rate of hospitalization for individuals with heart failure, and cardiovascular death.
To evaluate the effects, safety, and efficacy of canagliflozin (JNJ-28431754) on cardiovascular (CV) risk for major adverse cardiac events (MACE) in individuals with T2D	NCT01032629	Placebo + Canagliflozin (JNJ-28431754/100 mg) and placebo + Canagliflozin (JNJ-28431754/300 mg)	III	Lower the risk of cardiovascular complications than placebo but they have a chance of amputation, mostly at the toe or metatarsal level

Based on cardioprotective effects via SGLT2i				
This study aims to determine if insulin sensitivity, decreased cell size, decreased inflammation, and metabolic flexibility of epicardial adipose tissue are all improved by sodium-glucose cotransporter 2 inhibitor (SGLT2i) therapy	NCT04167761	Ertugliflozin + Glipizide	Early Phase I	Not reported yet
To investigate the relation of SGLT2i with cardiac, skeletal muscle ketone, bioenergetics, cardiopulmonary exercise capacity, and absorption and also focused on the elevation in plasma ketone concentration	NCT05057806	Empagliflozin + Placebo	Early phase 1	Not reported yet

a thorough analysis and more investigation are still required for the many procedures and important scientific breakthroughs of previous decades [3].

Based on research, SGLT2i has been shown as the most reliable marker for the treatment of T2D who are susceptible to heart failure and cardiovascular disease. The exact selection among these medications should be determined in cooperation with a healthcare professional and may be based on unique patient considerations, such as comorbidities and tolerance. Furthermore, additional studies could yield insightful information on how these medications are used in various patient populations.

Machine generated keywords: sglti, tdm, sgltis, function, cvd, hfpef, cell, database, hfref, diabetic patient, diagnosis, month, treatment sglt, safety, acute.

SGLT2 Inhibitors and Mechanisms of Cardiovascular Benefit: A State-of-the-Art Review

https://doi.org/10.1007/s00125-018-4670-7

A machine generated summary based on the work of Verma, Subodh; McMurray, John J. V.

2018 in Diabetologia

Abstract-Summary Sodium–glucose cotransporter (SGLT)2 inhibitors have been demonstrated to reduce cardiovascular events, particularly heart failure, in cardiovascular outcome trials.

We discuss two emerging themes: how SGLT2 inhibitors may regulate Na^+/H^+ exchange at the level of the heart and kidney and how they may modulate adipokine production.

The mechanistic discussion is placed in the context of completed and ongoing trials of SGLT2 inhibitors in the prevention and treatment of heart failure in individuals with and without diabetes.

SGLT2 Inhibitors and Cardiovascular Protection: Setting the Stage

The thesis that heart failure was the outcome most sensitive to SGLT2 inhibition was confirmed in the Canagliflozin Cardiovascular Assessment Study (CANVAS) Program wherein 10,142 individuals with type 2 diabetes and either established cardiovascular disease or multiple cardiovascular risk factors received canagliflozin or placebo [4].

The concept that SGLT2 inhibitors reduced cardiovascular events primarily through prevention of heart failure (vs atherothrombotic events) has gained broad acceptance, but several questions remained unanswered, the most important being: ‘how’?

Another important and unanswered question arising from previous trials relates to whether the observed cardiovascular benefit of SGLT2 inhibitors occurred primarily in individuals with a history of heart failure and whether a specific phenotype (heart failure with a preserved ejection fraction [HFpEF] or heart failure with a reduced ejection fraction [HFrEF]) was more sensitive to the observed benefits.

Mechanisms of Cardiovascular Protection by SGLT2 Inhibitors

Individuals with diabetes are known to have an increase in whole-body sodium content and, in recently completed translational studies in humans, the SGLT2 inhibitor dapagliflozin has been demonstrated to reduce tissue sodium content in people with type 2 diabetes [5].

Whereas SGLT2 inhibitors are uricosuric, loop diuretics are associated with an increase in uric acid levels, possibly mediating differences in cardiovascular outcomes [6].

Baartscheer et al. showed that the SGLT2 inhibitor empagliflozin inhibited cardiomyocyte NHE and, through this mechanism, reduced cytoplasmic sodium and calcium levels, while increasing mitochondrial calcium levels [7].

An emerging postulate is that SGLT2 inhibition, independent of hyperglycaemia, may have direct and favourable effects on cardiac fibroblast phenotype and function, one of the most important factors of heart failure.

SGLT2 inhibitors were postulated to reduce the levels of the adipokine leptin, which may have a pathophysiological role in sodium regulation as well as cardiac inflammation and fibrosis [8].

Unanswered Mechanistic and Translational Themes

NCT02998970), evaluating the effects of empagliflozin on left ventricular mass by cardiac magnetic resonance imaging, represents an important step in understanding the effects of SGLT2 inhibitors on ventricular remodelling.

There is a paucity of data with respect to the effects of SGLT2 inhibitors on serum and renal biomarkers.

It is also important to determine whether the effects of SGLT2 inhibitors are more pronounced in individuals with evidence of structural remodelling (such as left ventricular hypertrophy) or in those with higher levels of natriuretic peptides.

This area of research would also benefit from translational studies evaluating the effects of SGLT2 inhibitors on mechanisms of arrhythmias.

Physiological studies that evaluate the effects of SGLT2 inhibitors on the sympathetic nervous system and neurohumoral activation are needed.

Mechanistic and functional studies that evaluate the effects of SGLT2 inhibitors on peripheral arterial disease and amputation risk are also urgently required.

Conclusions

SGLT2 inhibitors have emerged as powerful pharmacological tools in the prevention of heart failure, with the suggestion that, unlike with other glucose-lowering agents [9], this benefit may be observed across the spectrum of people with type 2 diabetes with and without established cardiovascular disease.

The largest outcome study on the effects of SGLT2 inhibitors on cardiovascular disease, the Multicenter Trial to Evaluate the Effect of Dapagliflozin on the Incidence of Cardiovascular Events (DECLARE-TIMI 58), which has enrolled about 10,000 participants within a so-called primary prevention cohort, will provide further insights in this regard [10].

We have outlined some of the key mechanisms that may explain the notable cardioprotective benefits of SGLT2 inhibitors, including effects on volume and diuresis, myocardial metabolism and the potentially direct myocardial effects, with some preliminary observations suggesting an effect on myocardial metabolism and adipokine kinetics.

SGLT2 Inhibitors: A Focus on Cardiac Benefits and Potential Mechanisms

A machine generated summary based on the work of Nikolic, Maja; Zivkovic, Vladimir; Jovic, Jovana Joksimovic; Sretenovic, Jasmina; Davidovic, Goran; Simovic, Stefan; Djokovic, Danijela; Muric, Nemanja; Bolevich, Sergey; Jakovljevic, Vladimir

2021 in Heart Failure Reviews

Abstract-Summary As novel hypoglycemics, SGLT2i showed exceptional cardiovascular benefits, reflected through robust reductions of cardiovascular mortality and hospitalization for HF in T2DM patients.

Those effects have been reported even in patients with HF and reduced ejection fraction irrespectively of diabetic status, suggesting that cardioprotective effects of SGLT2i are driven independently of their hypoglycemic actions.

SGLT2i exerted hemodynamic and metabolic effects, partially driven by natriuresis and osmotic diuresis.

Those systemic effects are modest, and therefore cannot be completely related to the cardiac benefits of these agents in T2DM patients.

SGLT2i influence ion homeostasis and exert anti-inflammatory and antifibrotic effects.

In the light of ongoing trials evaluating the effects of SGLT2i in patients with HF and preserved ejection fraction, a new chapter of beneficial SGLT2i mechanisms is expected, which might resolve their main underlying action.

Introduction

The management of CVDs becomes even more complicated with the development of diabetes mellitus (DM), and vice versa, considering CVDs are a primary cause of death in nearly 80% of individuals with type 2 DM (T2DM) [11].

Diabetic patients are also at high risk for developing heart failure (HF), even 2–4-fold higher compared with healthy subjects [12], with more than 40% of HF-hospitalized patients having DM [13].

Considering the great risk of CVDs in T2DM individuals, the real challenge among pharmaceutical professionals was to manufacture a convenient antidiabetic medication that is safe for the heart of diabetic patients.

In previous years, sodium-glucose cotransporter (SGLT) 2 inhibitors (SLGT2i) conquered a new domain of CV benefits in diabetic patients [14], mainly by improving CV outcomes, not inducing hypoglycemic events (in the light of the relationship between CV events and hypoglycemia) [15, 16], or by their cardioprotective role, which will be the main focus of this review, and even reducing the onset of diabetes by 32% [17].

The real breakdown happened after reporting that the treatment with Rosiglitazone markedly increased the risk of MI (43%) among patients with DM [18].

Physiological Action and Pharmacological Inhibition

On the apical surface of PRT SGLT membrane proteins responsible for the glucose reabsorption are settled [19], mediating a coupled Na^+-glucose (1:1) cotransport [20].

SGLT1 transporters are located in the S2/S3 segment of PRT and mediate around 10% of glucose reabsorption, while SGLT2 transporters are located in the early S1 segment of PRT and are the major contributor in this process, providing reabsorption of more than 90% of filtered glucose [21].

Previous studies showed that T2DM patients have a higher threshold for glycosuria, as well as increased glucose reabsorption capacity, which might reflect an adaptive mechanism followed by greater SGLT2 expression in kidneys [14].

With their unique insulin-independent mechanism of action based on blocking SGLT2 transporters in PRT, SGLT2i cause a decrease in glucose reabsorption and consequent glycosuria, which results in lowered plasma glucose and HbA1c levels [22].

Insights into Cardioprotective Effects of SGLT2i from Clinical Trials

One meta-analysis showed that SGLT2i consistently reduce the relative risk of HHF by 31% in diabetic patients independently of atherosclerotic CVD or a prior HF [23].

In post hoc analysis of the EMPA-REG OUTCOME trial, Empagliflozin was consistently successful in reducing HHF, all-cause, and CV mortality in T2DM patients with HF at baseline (10.1%) as in those without HF [24].

To prove those assumptions, additional trials with SGLT2i have already revealed promising effects in patients with HF with reduced ejection fraction (HFrEF), irrespectively of diabetes.

Another SGLT2i was rushing towards the same position, in EMPEROR-REDUCED (Empagliflozin Outcome Trial in Patients with Chronic Heart Failure and a Reduced Ejection Fraction) trial, which most recently shared promising results of Empagliflozin in HFrEF patients in comparison to the placebo, reflected through significant relative risk reduction of CV mortality and HHF (25%), irrespectively of diabetes status [25].

SGLT2i: Mechanisms of Cardioprotection

While SGLT2i affect body composition mainly by reducing visceral adipose tissue [26], this metabolic effect might further contribute to improving the cardiometabolic risk profile in T2DM patients.

Beneficial effects of increased ketogenesis with SGLT2i were seen in the non-diabetic porcine model of HF, where Empagliflozin improved LV remodeling and systolic function by turning cardiac fuel utilization into more efficient heart energetics [27].

In doxorubicin-induced HF in mice, increased β-hydroxybutyrate levels due to Empagliflozin treatment, mediated through lowering levels of reactive oxygen species (ROS) production and improving mitochondrial dysfunction in heart cells, lead to reduction of LV mass, perivascular, and interstitial fibrosis [28].

In the BTBR ob/ob diabetic mice model, Dapagliflozin has shown favorable effects on cardiac fibrosis, remodeling, and function of LV, in an AMPK-dependent manner, accompanied with reduced activation of NLRP3 inflammasome and decreased levels of IL1-β, IL-6, tumor necrosis factor-alpha (TNF-α), and caspase-1 [29].

Conclusion

We have highlighted the cardioprotective potential of SGLT2i as well as several most discussed mechanisms responsible for their cardioprotection.

If we assume that possible CV benefits arise from the joint action of systemic and molecular mechanisms, it is still not possible to elucidate which of those mechanisms exert the greatest contribution.

SGLT2i are efficient and safe hypoglycemic drugs that are ready for use in everyday clinical practice and thus convenient for further investigations in patients with different CVDs.

Possible beneficial findings from currently ongoing trials evaluating the effects of SGLT2i in patients with HFpEF might open a new chapter of potential actions and maybe resolve the main underlying cardioprotective mechanism of SGLT2i.

Molecular Mechanisms Underlying the Cardiovascular Benefits of SGLT2i and GLP-1RA

A machine generated summary based on the work of Khat, Dorrin Zarrin; Husain, Mansoor

2018 in Current Diabetes Reports

Abstract-Summary SGLT2i and GLP-1RA exert cardiovascular effects by targeting in both common and distinctive ways (A) several mediators of macro- and microvascular pathophysiology: namely (A1) inflammation and atherogenesis, (A2) oxidative stress-induced endothelial dysfunction, (A3) vascular smooth muscle cell reactive oxygen species (ROS) production and proliferation, and (A4) thrombosis.

This review highlights that while GLP-1RA exert direct effects on vascular (endothelial and smooth muscle) cells, the effects of SGLT2i appear to include the activation of signaling pathways that prevent adverse vascular remodeling.

Both SGLT2i and GLP-1RA confer hemodynamic effects that counter adverse cardiac remodeling.

Introduction

In the Empagliflozin Cardiovascular Outcome Event Trial in Type 2 Diabetes Mellitus Patients–Removing Excess Glucose (EMPA-REG) OUTCOME study, treatment with empagliflozin (SGLT2i) showed a 38% reduction in cardiovascular death, a non-significant (13%) reduction in non-fatal MI, a non-significant (24%) increase non-fatal stroke, and a 35% reduction in hospitalizations for HF as compared to placebo [30].

In the subsequent Liraglutide Effect and Action in Diabetes: Evaluation of Cardiovascular Outcome Results (LEADER) study, patients treated with liraglutide (GLP-1RA) exhibited a 22% reduction in cardiovascular death, a non-significant (12%) reduction in non-fatal MI, a non-significant (11%) reduction non-fatal stroke, and a non-significant (13%) reduction in the rates of hospitalization for HF as compared to placebo [31].

The Exenatide Study of Cardiovascular Event Lowering (EXSCEL) reported a non-significant 9% reduction (HR 0.91, 95% CI 0.83–1.00) in the primary composite outcome (death from cardiovascular causes, non-fatal MI, or non-fatal stroke) in patients treated with exenatide (Ex-4) vs. placebo [32].

Potential Mechanisms of CV Protection with GLP-1RA and SGLT2i

GLP-1RA therapy can also modulate innate immune-mediated inflammation in the setting of T2D and has been associated with significant reductions in the inflammatory cytokines TNF-α, IL-1β, and IL-6, and an increase in adiponectin, an anti-inflammatory adipokine [33].

To protecting against immune-mediated inflammation and oxidative stress, GLP-1 treatment has been shown to suppress oxidized LDL-induced macrophage foam cell formation in a receptor-dependent manner, which was associated with increased acyl-coenzyme A cholesterol acyltransferase-1 and CD36, and decreased ATP-binding cassette transporter A1 [34].

Similar to the experimental animal studies investigating the anti-inflammatory role of GLP-1RA in the progression of atherosclerosis, several studies of SGLT2i therapy have demonstrated therapeutic effect on atherosclerosis by assessing many of the same markers, as well as some distinct mechanisms of inflammatory response.

SGLT2i therapy also reduced immune-mediated inflammation as empagliflozin treatment reduced M1-polarized macrophage accumulation and induced the anti-inflammatory M2 phenotype of macrophages within white adipocyte tissue and liver, and lowered plasma TNF-α levels in diet-induced obese mice [35].

Future Perspectives

The DURATION-8 study has reported significantly greater reductions in glycemic parameters, including HbA1c, fasting, and postprandial glucose as well as greater reductions in weight and BP with combined treatment of dapagliflozin and Ex-4 vs. placebo [36].

The CANVAS study reported significant reductions in HbA1c levels and weight loss in patients receiving canagliflozin on a background of GLP-1RA [37].

Given the greater reductions in glycemic parameters with combination therapy, in addition to the hemodynamic and vascular mechanistic findings we have discussed, there seems to be potential for an additive or synergistic cardioprotective benefit conferred by these two agents.

Conclusion

Some cardiovascular outcome studies have demonstrated that employing combination therapy with both drug classes holds promise for the management of hyperglycemia and possibly also cardioprotection [36].

Preclinical studies have demonstrated mechanisms of action that are shared (metabolic, endocrine, remodeling, and hemodynamic benefits) and unique to each anti-diabetic drug class.

Clinical and preclinical studies reporting glycemic outcomes of combination therapy and either drug class alone have demonstrated the potential for additive or synergistic cardioprotective effects in combining GLP-1RA and SGLT2i therapies [36, 38].

Additional studies comparing, contrasting, and combining the GLP-1RA and SGLT2i in preclinical models of MI will certainly help to delineate their mechanisms of action and determine which of these agents, if not their combination, is best for the treatment and prevention of HF.

SGLT2 Inhibitors: Benefits for CKD and Cardiovascular Disease in Type 2 Diabetes

A machine generated summary based on the work of Singhal, Rohit; Hechanova, Lisa Aimee

2022 in Current Cardiology Reports

Abstract-Summary The purpose of this review is to outline the key findings of the recent major outcome clinical trials on SGLT2 inhibitors, review the indications for their use, and improve adoption of these medications in patients with type 2 diabetes mellitus (T2DM).

Recent studies have shown a benefit for SGLT2 inhibitors in patients with heart failure (HF) and kidney disease both in the presence and absence of T2DM.

Available data suggests that SGLT2 inhibitors should be used in all eligible patients with HFrEF and/or CKD with albuminuria to decrease progression of CKD, hospitalizations for heart failure, major atherosclerotic cardiovascular events, and cardiovascular death, with and without T2DM.

Introduction

In patients with prevalent kidney disease at baseline, empagliflozin reduced the risk of cardiovascular death by 29% compared with placebo (HR, 0.71; 95% CI, 0.52–0.98), the risk of all-cause mortality by 24% (HR, 0.76; 95% CI, 0.59–0.99), the risk of hospitalization for heart failure by 39% (HR, 0.61; 95% CI, 0.42–0.87), and the risk of all-cause hospitalization by 19% (HR, 0.81; 95% CI, 0.72–0.92) [39] The reductions in risk of 3-point MACE, cardiovascular death, all-cause mortality, hospitalization for heart failure, and all-cause hospitalization with empagliflozin versus placebo were consistent between patients with eGFR <60 and ≥ 60 ml per min per 1.73 m^2 of body-surface area [39].

Empagliflozin also significantly reduced the risk for the composite renal end point which included progression to macroalbuminuria, doubling of serum creatinine, initiation of renal replacement therapy, or death resulting from renal disease, versus placebo in the subgroup of patients with prevalent kidney disease at baseline (HR, 0.58; 95% CI, 0.47–0.71) [39].

This trial showed that persons with chronic kidney disease who received dapagliflozin had a significantly lower risk of a composite of a sustained decline in the eGFR of at least 50%, end-stage kidney disease, or death from renal or cardiovascular causes than those who received placebo, independent of the presence or absence of T2DM.

Conclusion

These trials established the superiority of an SGLT2 inhibitor added to the standard of care for CKD in T2DM for a primary outcome of kidney disease end points.

Trials like DAPA-HF also showed cardiorenal endpoint benefits of SGLT2 inhibitors in patients without T2DM.

It was concluded that SGLT2 inhibitors should be used when possible in patients with T2DM to reduce risks for CKD and CVD.

The use of SGLT2 inhibitors should also be considered in all patients with HF and albuminuric kidney disease, even in the absence of T2DM..

Minireview: Are SGLT2 Inhibitors Heart Savers in Diabetes?

A machine generated summary based on the work of Grubić Rotkvić, Petra; Cigrovski Berković, Maja; Bulj, Nikola; Rotkvić, Luka

2019 in Heart Failure Reviews

Abstract-Summary Sodium-glucose cotransporter 2 (SGLT2) inhibitors, a class of drugs that promote urinary glucose excretion in the treatment of diabetes, have provoked large interest of scientific and professional community due to their positive and, somehow, unexpected results in the three major cardiovascular outcome trials (EMPA-REG OUTCOME trial with empagliflozin, CANVAS Program with canagliflozin, and DECLARE-TIMI 58 with dapagliflozin).

It would be of great importance to better understand SGLT2 inhibitor mechanisms of action since they could have a potential to be used in early stages of diabetes as cardioprotective agents.

There are widely available biomarkers as well as echocardiography that are used in everyday clinical practice and could elucidate physiological mechanisms in the heart protection with SGLT2 inhibitors treatment but studies are still lacking.

The purpose of this minireview is to summarize the latest concepts about SGLT2 inhibitors and its benefits regarding diabetic cardiomyopathy especially on its early stage development and to discuss controversies and potential future developments in the field.

Introduction

Before the results of the three major outcome trials with SGLT2 inhibitors (EMPA-REG OUTCOME trial with empagliflozin, CANVAS Program with canagliflozin, and DECLARE-TIMI 58 with dapagliflozin), no one could have predicted that SGLT2 inhibitors, that work to promote urinary glucose excretion in the treatment of hyperglycemia, would notably reduce mortality in patients with type 2 diabetes, possibly driven by a reduction in heart failure as opposed to atherothrombotic events [4–29, 39–85].

The time frame of the effect precludes a glucose- and antiatherosclerotic-mediated effect and while struggling to understand the potential mechanisms responsible for cardioprotective effects of SGLT2 inhibitors and their clinical implications, some questions have come into focus: can SGLT2 inhibitors be used to prevent heart failure in diabetes, do SGLT2 inhibitors reverse pathological cardiac remodeling in subjects with diabetes, and can SGLT2 inhibitors be a treatment for heart failure in patients without type 2 diabetes [86–89]?

Discussion and Future Perspective

The current hypotheses of possible mechanisms of action to explain cardiac protection and effect on cardiac performance regarding heart failure by SGLT2 inhibitors are discussed below: 1.

In the setting of diabetes with heart failure, ketone bodies can act as a "super fuel" by releasing energy more efficiently than glucose or fatty acids and it has been shown that SGLT2 inhibitors can switch metabolism from glucose to fatty acid oxidation with increased synthesis of ketones [90, 91].

Data on CRP and other inflammatory markers are relatively scarce in humans and further studies in diabetes patients with specific assessment of inflammatory markers are still necessary to determine the contribution of the anti-inflammatory action of SGLT2 inhibitors to the reduction of cardiovascular complications [92].

To diabetic cardiomyopathy, there are several ongoing studies at the moment addressing the issue of SGLT2 inhibitors in individuals with chronic heart failure and chronic kidney disease without established diabetes [93].

Mechanisms and Evidence for Heart Failure Benefits from SGLT2 Inhibitors

A machine generated summary based on the work of Wojcik, Cezary; Warden, Bruce A.

2019 in Current Cardiology Reports

Abstract-Summary To review the clinical trial data and underlying mechanistic principles in support of the robust cardiovascular (CV) benefits, in particular, heart failure (HF) outcomes association with sodium-glucose co-transporter-2 (SGLT2) inhibitors.

Several large CV outcome trials in patients with type 2 diabetes mellitus (T2DM) and with either established atherosclerotic CV disease (ASCVD) or at high risk for ASCVD reveal that SGLT2 inhibitors cause reductions in CV and HF endpoints.

Recent evidence has unveiled the irrefutable data that SGLT2 inhibitors reduce CV events in patients with T2DM, with a profound effect on reductions in hospitalization for HF.

The arrival of SGLT2 inhibitors has ushered in a new era of CV risk reductions therapies.

Introduction

A recent meta-analysis of the three CVOT which included almost 35,000 patients (60.2% with established ASCVD) did show that SGLT2 inhibitors reduced major adverse cardiovascular events (MACE) by 11% (95% confidence interval [CI], 0.83–0.96, $p = 0.0014$), with statistically significant benefit seen only in patients with ASCVD (14% relative risk reduction [RRR], 95% CI, 0.80–0.93, $p < 0.001$).

SGLT2 inhibitors reduced the risk of CV death or HF hospitalization by 23% (95% CI, 0.71–0.84, $p < 0{\cdot}0001$) regardless of pre-existing ASCVD or HF.

The results of this meta-analysis contrast with data from a large observational study CVD-REAL (Comparative Effectiveness of Cardiovascular Outcomes in New Users of SGLT2 Inhibitors), which demonstrated benefit in reduction of CV events also in patients without pre-existing ASCVD.

Clinical Trial Evidence

In this high-risk, secondary prevention population, empagliflozin lowered the primary composite outcome of myocardial infarction (MI), stroke, and CV death by 14% (95% CI, 0.74–0.99; $p < 0.001$), CV death by 38% (95% CI, 0.49–0.77; $p < 0.001$), death from any cause by 32% (95% CI, 0.57–0.82, $p < 0.001$), and reduced HF hospitalizations by 35% (95% CI, 0.50–0.85; $p = 0.002$) [94].

To empagliflozin, canagliflozin lowered the primary composite outcome of MI, stroke, and CV death by 14% (95% CI, 0.75–0.97; $P < 0.001$) and reduced HF hospitalizations by 33% (95% CI, 0.52–0.87, $p < 0.001$).

Compared to GLP-1 RA, the hazard ratio (HR) for the composite CV outcome (MI, stroke, mortality, and hospitalization for HF) was 1.10 (95% CI 0.95–1.26) for patients with ASCVD, and 1.23 (95% CI, 1.08–1.41) for patients without ASCVD.

Mechanism of Action—Glucose Reduction

In the absence of diabetes, glucosuria appears when blood glucose levels exceed 180 mg/dL. However, in those with diabetes, SLGT2 is paradoxically upregulated, leading to increased glucose reabsorption in the PCT and therefore shifting the threshold of glycosuria up to ≈ 220 mg/dL. SGLT2 activity requires energy provided by the sodium gradient created by the Na^+/K^+ ATPase located in the basolateral surface of PCT epithelial cells, in contrast to the passive transport of glucose from cytoplasm towards plasma via GLUT2 [95, 96].

Inhibition of SGLT2 causes glucosuria with glucose levels much lower than ≈ 220 mg/dL as long as they are above 40–80 mg/dL (depending on the SGLT2 inhibitor studied).

As blood glucose levels drop, glucosuria caused by SGLT2 inhibitors decreases, preventing the occurrence of hypoglycemia.

SGLT2 inhibitors display a modest efficacy in lowering plasma glucose levels, reducing HbA1C by ≈ 0.5–1%.

Mechanism of Action—Cardiovascular Protection

SGLT2 inhibitors have a more robust and consistent effect on the prevention of HF and renal outcomes than on ASCVD.

Although treatment with SGLT2 inhibitors appears to result in a moderate reduction in the risk of MACE solely in patients with established ASCVD, reductions in the risk of HF and renal outcomes occur regardless of patient characteristics [23].

SGLT2 inhibitors reduce renal afferent nervous activity and suppress associated central reflex mechanisms that contribute to generalized sympathetic activation.

Published studies of SGLT2 inhibitors demonstrated their ability to induce a reduction in epicardial fat and thus providing another possible mechanism for the beneficial CV and HF outcomes [97–99].

SGLT2 inhibitors, by way of inducing glycosuria, reduce the workload of the renal PCT and reverse the downstream consequences, resulting in erythropoiesis and improved oxygen delivery to tissues [100].

Conclusion

The T2DM epidemic is on the rise with associated increases in morbidity and mortality, predominantly associated with CV complications, such as ASCVD events and HF.

Through their unique mechanism of action, SGLT2 inhibitors significantly improve HF-related outcomes, decreasing the frequency of HF-related hospitalizations as well as CV-related death.

The theorized protective CV mechanisms induced by SGLT2 inhibitors are several fold and include optimization of ASCVD risk factors, improvement in hemodynamics, prevention of cardiac and renal remodeling, inhibiting hormone dysregulation, use of a more efficient metabolic substrate, NHE inhibition, anti-inflammatory effects, and anti-oxidant effects.

The future of SGLT2 inhibitors and its role in preventing catastrophic CV events is bright.

Dual SGLT1/SGLT2 inhibitors are theorized to be even more beneficial through additional effects.

Addendum

A recent subanalysis of DECLARE-TIMI 58 has shown that dapagliflozin reduced HF hospitalizations both in those with HFrEF (HR, 0.64 [95% CI, 0.43–0.95]) and in those without HFrEF (HR, 0.76 [95% CI, 0.62–0.92]); however, it reduced CV death (HR, 0.55 [95% CI, 0.34–0.90]) and all-cause mortality (HR, 0.59 [95% CI, 0.40–0.88]) only in patients with HFrEF [101].

Dapagliflozin reduced the relative risk of MACE by 16% (15.2% versus 17.8%; hazard ratio [HR], 0.84; 95% CI, 0.72–0.99; P = 0.039) in patients with previous MI, whereas there was no effect in patients without previous MI including in patients with established ASCVD but no history of MI [102].

Direct Cardiac Effects of SGLT2 Inhibitors

A machine generated summary based on the work of Chen, Sha; Coronel, Ruben; Hollmann, Markus W.; Weber, Nina C.; Zuurbier, Coert J.
2022 in Cardiovascular Diabetology

Abstract-Summary Sodium-glucose-cotransporter 2 inhibitors (SGLT2is) demonstrate large cardiovascular benefit in both diabetic and non-diabetic, acute and chronic heart failure patients.

We review the literature on direct effects of SGLT2is on various cardiac cells and derive at an unifying working hypothesis.

We postulate that cardiac benefit modulated by SGLT2i's can be commonly attributed to their inhibition of sodium-loaders in the plasma membrane (NHE-1, Nav1.5, SGLT) affecting intracellular sodium-homeostasis (the sodium-interactome), thereby providing a unifying view on the various effects reported in separate studies.

The cardiac sodium-interactome provides a unifying testable working hypothesis and a possible, at least partly, explanation to the clinical benefits of SGLT2is observed in the diseased patient.

Introduction

It seems unlikely that these kidney-mediated effects can explain the full spectrum of benefits, since previous trials with similar effects on glucose homeostasis or blood pressure are without such large and acute [103] beneficial effects on cardiac pathology observed with SGLT2is.

These observations have initiated a plethora of studies uncovering direct SGLT2is effects on various cardiac cells, such as cardiomyocytes, endothelial cells, fibroblasts, smooth muscle cells, all of which largely devoid of SGLT2.

It was soon recognized early that many of these off-target effects on cardiac cells target pathogenic mechanisms underlying heart failure (HF) and diabetic cardiomyopathy, and may thus contribute to the reported cardiovascular effects of these drugs [104–106].

We provide an up-to-date literature review summarising the current knowledge of the direct effects of SGLT2is on ion homeostasis, oxidative stress and inflammation, cell proliferation, fibrosis, energetic status and metabolism of cardiomyocytes, endothelial cells, smooth muscle cells, fibroblasts, platelets, and isolated hearts.

Literature Search

Exclusion criteria were studies employing clinically unrealistically high doses of SGLT2is (empagliflozin (EMPA), dapagliflozin (DAPA) and sotagliflozin (SOTA) > 1 μM; canagliflozin (CANA) > 3 μM).

A total of 70 studies were initially retrieved from electronic databases.

Twenty-nine studies were excluded because of non-compliance with the eligibility criteria: direct cardiac effects were not examined (6 articles), [SGLT2is] is overdosed (8 articles), research was not original (15 articles).

Literature Search Results

Low-dose EMPA (100 nM) effects in the presence of albumin on hyperglycaemia-induced senescence of native and freshly isolated porcine coronary artery endothelial cells, show that EMPA reduced high glucose-induced ROS production and restored eNOS expression and NO formation through prevention of the activation of the endogenous angiotensin (Ang) system [107].

In cultured human aortic smooth muscle cells, EMPA (1 μM) in the presence of albumin pre-treatment reduced the pro-inflammatory IL-17α-induced oxidative stress, NLRP3 expression, caspase-1 activation, IL-1β and IL-18 secretion, partly through inhibition of SGLT2 [108].

Direct metabolic effects of SGLT2is on cardiac cells showed that 1 μM EMPA for 24 h in the presence of albumin increased expression of glucose transporter (GLUT) 1, but not GLUT4, in isolated quiescent cardiomyocytes from human end-stage HF transplanted hearts or healthy and transverse aortic constriction (TAC)-induced HF murine hearts [109].

Discussion

The discrepancies between laboratories are possibly due to differences in experimental conditions and/or models that determine whether (1) the suggested SGLT2i-targets (NHE-1, Nav1.5, SGLT1 or 2) are present and active, (2) the suggested outcome variables (NO, AMP, Na^+, Ca^{2+}, ROS) can be modulated, and (3) the applied methods are sensitive enough to detect small changes in the variable.

While there is still much to be understood about the various factors which determine how SGLT2i's affect cardiac cells, most research clearly demonstrates that direct cardiac effects of these SGLT2i can be observed, especially in pathological conditions, and that the effects are mediated by altered intracellular sodium.

This makes these observed cardiac cellular effects highly relevant for the understanding of underlying mechanisms in the clinical condition where SGLT2i's are only used in diseased patients.

Conclusion

SGLT2is can have direct cardiac effects that all seems to be mediated by modulation of intracellular sodium concentration, the sodium-interactome.

Further experiments in various ex vivo and in vivo conditions are needed to test and validate this working hypothesis that SGLT2i have direct cardiac effects through alteration of the sodium-interactome.

The changes are likely an explanation, at least partly, for the clinical benefits of SGLT2i-treatment.

SGLT2 Inhibitors: Cardiovascular Benefits Beyond HbA1c—Translating Evidence into Practice

https://doi.org/10.1007/s13300-019-0657-8

A machine generated summary based on the work of Ali, Amar; Bain, Steve; Hicks, Debbie; Newland Jones, Phillip; Patel, Dipesh C.; Evans, Marc; Fernando, Kevin; James, June; Milne, Nicola; Viljoen, Adie; Wilding, John

2019 in Diabetes Therapy

Abstract-Summary In assessing the cardiovascular (CV) safety profiles of anti-diabetic drugs, sodium-glucose co-transporter-2 inhibitor (SGLT2i) therapies have emerged with robust evidence for reducing the risk of adverse CVD outcomes in people with T2DM who have either established CVD or are at risk of developing CVD.

This paper builds on these findings and presents practical guidance for maximising the pleiotropic benefits of this class of medicines in people with T2DM in terms of reducing adverse CVD outcomes.

The Improving Diabetes Steering Committee aims to offer evidence-based practical guidance for the use of SGLT2i therapies in people with T2DM stratified by CVD risk.

The Improving Diabetes Steering Committee seeks to support healthcare professionals (HCPs) in appropriate treatment selection for people with T2DM who are at risk of developing or have established CVD and examines the role of SGLT2i therapy for these people.

The Role of the Improving Diabetes Steering Committee

The Committee aims to ensure that HCPs who prescribe diabetes medicines have access to balanced and accurate information and evidence concerning type 2 diabetes mellitus (T2DM) medicines, with a specific focus on the sodium–glucose co-transporter-2 inhibitor (SGLT2i) class of treatments.

The group is committed to providing healthcare colleagues with clarity concerning the evidence base supporting SGLT2i agents, highlighting the relative benefits and risks of these therapies.

Educational materials and publications, such as the previous consensus document [40], provided by the panel are intended to increase confidence and understanding regarding the appropriate place of these medicines within the current UK T2DM treatment paradigm.

Taking Type 2 Diabetes Out of Isolation: The Impact of Cardiovascular Disease

People with T2DM commonly live with multiple comorbidities, among which hypertension and cardiovascular disease (CVD) are the most common [41].

A systematic review of global clinical records from over 4.5 million people with T2DM (median duration 10 years) observed that CVD was a comorbidity in approximately one third of people with T2DM; of those, 29.1% had atherosclerosis, 21.2% had coronary heart disease (CHD), 14.9% had heart failure (HF), 14.6% had angina, 10.0% had had a myocardial infarction (MI) and 7.6% had experienced stroke [42].

The burden of CVD in T2DM is considerable, both for people living with comorbid conditions and for the healthcare systems that support them.

Efficacious management of CVD risk and disease in people with T2DM is therefore a priority for both the individuals affected and for healthcare systems more broadly.

The Relationship Between Type 2 Diabetes and Cardiovascular Disease: Common Factors

T2DM and CVD share risk factors for the onset and worsening of disease [43].

The presence of hyperglycaemia, which defines T2DM, is an independent risk factor for CVD [44].

Obesity is recognised as a risk factor for CVD and HF, and contributes to the development of insulin resistance [45–47].

Insulin resistance develops prior to onset of hyperglycaemia in T2DM, and both of these disorders increase the risk of developing CVD [48, 49].

Increasing insulin resistance and consequent dysglycaemia should be recognised as risk factors for CVD; a study in nearly 12,000 patients without a history of diabetes demonstrated that asymptomatic hyperglycaemia was associated with higher risk of CV death compared with patients with low post-load glucose levels [50–52].

Heart Failure: A New Focus for Cardiovascular Disease in Diabetes

The prevalence of people with T2DM with comorbid HF in primary care management is relatively common (>22% of patients) [53]; it has also been recognised that HF may be underdiagnosed in routine care [54, 55].

Insulin resistance and hyperglycaemia are common factors in the development of both T2DM and HF, along with advancing age and inflammation [56–58].

In T2DM, the risk of HF rises by 8–32% per 1% increase in HbA1c [59]; thus HF risk appears to be associated with HbA1c in those with and without diabetes, independent of other risk factors.

Development of HF in people with T2DM is associated with significantly greater mortality than in those with T2DM who do not develop HF [60].

Over 7.7 years of follow-up, T2DM developed across New York Heart Association (NYHA) severities I–III of HF: 17% of patients in class I, 15% in class II and 20% in class III (P for trend = 0.05).

The Role of Glycaemic Control in Managing Cardiovascular Risk in People with Type 2 Diabetes

In a prospective study of 1626 people with T2DM and 1321 people without diabetes, the RR of CHD increased by 1.14 (95% confidence interval [CI] 1.07–1.21) per percentage point increase in HbA1c, across all HbA1c values, and RR increased by 2.36 (95% CI 1.43–3.90) per percentage point in patients without diabetes but with an HbA1c of more than 4.6% [61].

No significant benefits were observed with intensive treatment of hyperglycaemia in the Action to Control Cardiovascular Risk in Diabetes (ACCORD; targeting an HbA1c below 6.0%) study [62], the Action in Diabetes and Vascular Disease: Preterax and Diamicron MR Controlled Evaluation (ADVANCE; targeting an

HbA1c below 6.5%) study [63] or the Veterans Affairs Diabetes Trial (VADT; median HbA1c of 6.9%) [64].

Appropriate, early intervention is needed to improve CV outcomes in people with T2DM, with treatment goals beyond achieving glycaemic control alone.

Recent CV outcomes studies have demonstrated cardiovascular benefits in people receiving an SGLT2i therapy for the management of T2DM [4, 65–70].

Why Might SGLT2I Treatments Influence Cardiovascular Outcomes?

Biomarkers and surrogate endpoints measured in these trials demonstrate that SGLT2 inhibition modifies many risk factors for CVD, beyond glucose levels, including BP, weight, visceral adiposity, hyperinsulinaemia, arterial stiffness, albuminuria, circulating uric acid levels and oxidative stress [71, 72].

In the context of SGLT2 inhibition, there is considerable overlap between these factors; for example, SGLT2i-induced BP lowering may be associated with reduced arterial stiffness, natriuresis and weight loss.

Although SGLT2i treatments have a reduced glucose-lowering effect in people with reduced renal function, the renal benefits of SGLT2i agents appear to be preserved among people both with and without chronic kidney disease (CKD); these benefits include significant reduction in albuminuria and reduced incidence of worsening albuminuria [73, 74].

The efficacy of SGLT2i treatment will be further elucidated in the forthcoming Canagliflozin and Renal Endpoints in Diabetes with Established Nephropathy Clinical Evaluation (CREDENCE) trial (unpublished at time of paper development), which will prospectively assess the efficacy and safety of canagliflozin in clinically important renal and CV outcomes [75].

What Evidence Exists for the Management of CVD Risk in T2DM Treatment with SGLT2i Agents?

EMPA-REG OUTCOME reported a 14% relative risk reduction (RRR) in the 3P-MACE primary outcome versus placebo (HR 0.86; 95.02% CI 0.74–0.99; $P = 0.04$ for superiority), a 38% RRR in CV deaths (HR 0.62; 95% CI 0.49–0.77; $P < 0.001$), a 35% RRR for HHF (HR 0.65; 95% CI 0.50–0.85; $P = 0.002$) and a 32% RRR in all-cause mortality (HR 0.68; 95% CI 0.57–0.82, $P < 0.001$) [65].

A sub-analysis assessing HF reported that, compared with placebo, canagliflozin was associated with a significantly lower risk of composite CV death or HHF (HR 0.78; 95% CI 0.67–0.91), as was fatal or HHF (HR 0.70; 95% CI 0.55–0.89) or HHF alone (HR 0.67; 95% CI 0.52–0.87) [76].

Broadening the Evidence Base: The Role of Real-World Evidence in Informing Treatment Decisions

Real-world studies facilitate the confirmation of RCT findings against observations in routine clinical practice and can therefore help increase the external validity and generalisability of RCT data.

RWE also has limitations: data capture is performed in an uncontrolled setting, which is less robust than in an RCT environment, and real-world studies may be more prone to, and less able to adjust for, confounding data than RCTs [77, 78].

RWE can provide insight into how a drug performs in the real-world treatment of people and these findings, often in large study populations, can support HCPs in making appropriate, evidence-based, therapy choices.

This is of particular relevance when considering benefits beyond glucose control, as the people observed in real-world studies will have typical comorbidities and concomitant treatments that may have resulted in them being excluded from RCTs [79].

SGLT2i Treatments in Routine Practice: Real-World Evidence for Cardiovascular Benefits in People with Type 2 Diabetes

The CVD-REAL study followed a propensity-matched population of 309,056 people with T2DM, newly initiated on either an SGLT2i agent or 'other glucose-lowering drugs' (oGLD) for 374 days in the SGLT2i-treated cohort and 392 days in the oGLD cohort.

CVD-REAL reported that SGLT2i treatment, versus oGLD in people with T2DM either with (13% of the matched population) or without established CVD, was associated with lower risk of HF (HR 0.72; 95% CI 0.62–0.83 and HR 0.61; 95% CI 0.48–0.78, respectively) and composite HF and death (HR 0.63; 95% CI 0.57–0.07 and HR 0.56; 95% CI 0.50–0.62, respectively).

Initial insights from the EMPRISE study, assessing the real-world efficacy in reducing HHF in people with T2DM (with or without existing CVD) with empagliflozin against DPP-4 inhibitors, have shown a 44% reduction in favour of the SGLT2i treatment [80].

Primary and Secondary Prevention: When Might Initiation of an SGLT2i Therapy Provide Benefit?

The benefits of SGLT2i treatment are robustly supported in secondary prevention of CVD and HF, with an increasing wealth of evidence demonstrating significant benefits in people with no established CVD or HF [4, 23, 65–68, 70, 81, 82].

A recent meta-analysis across the three published SGLT2i CVOT trials (EMPA-REG, CANVAS and DECLARE-TIMI 58) provided further support for the benefits of SGLT2i treatment in patients with existing CVD; however, it observed no role in reducing MACE in those without pre-existing CVD, and noted more emphasis on HF outcomes [23].

It is the opinion of the Improving Diabetes Steering Committee that for people with T2DM and risk factors for CVD, regardless of the presence of established CVD or HF, that the early initiation of an SGLT2i treatment provides people with T2DM with an optimum management strategy by reducing hyperglycaemia, aiding weight loss and lowering systolic BP.

How is this Evolving Evidence-Base Being Reflected in Practical Guidelines?

Current NICE guidelines do not yet offer advice on selection of T2DM treatment according to CVD risk [83].

The Committee suggests that in the period before NICE guidelines are updated to reflect the CVD and HF considerations of treatment selection, wider implementation of the ADA/EASD consensus would be of value in improving outcomes.

It would therefore be valuable to have broader and more accessible advice for the use of SGLT2i treatments in people with T2DM at risk of CVD.

This Improving Diabetes Steering Committee consensus paper aims to offer practical advice to HCPs in the selection of treatment as an add-on to metformin and seeks to facilitate personalisation of medicine for people with T2DM and at risk of developing CVD.

Overcoming Treatment Comfort in Type 2 Diabetes Management: And Preparing for New Treatment Approaches

As HCPs look beyond a glucocentric management strategy for people with T2DM at risk of CVD there are several challenges to adopting new treatment approaches, including a lack of familiarity with newer agents, limited prescribing options through local formulary practice and a lack of flexibility within prevailing local guidelines.

Demonstrating the efficacy of SGLT2i therapies in CVD outcomes in the context of other common CVD drugs may help physicians appreciate the magnitude of CVD benefit offered by this class.

Given the comfort with which HCPs consider the prescription of these routine drugs, the Committee notes that early and appropriate intervention with SGLT2i therapies may yield economical and clinically meaningful benefits in people with T2DM at risk of CVD.

Practical Advice: The Use of SGLT2i Treatment in People Receiving Diuretics

There is opinion that SGLT2i agents are broadly appropriate to use alongside diuretics, with routine monitoring of renal function, especially in patients receiving loop diuretics [84].

Although the primary pharmacological action of SGLT2i agents occurs in the proximal convoluted tubule (the location of the SGLT2 transporter), it has been suggested that the diuretic action that they induce could be a secondary downstream effect of altered sodium balance in the loop of Henle, meaning that SGLT2i treatments could be considered to act similarly to loop diuretics [85].

HCPs initiating an SGLT2i therapy in a person receiving a combination antihypertensive therapy that includes a diuretic may choose to reduce or discontinue loop or thiazide diuretic before commencing the SGLT2i treatment; this consideration is of particular importance in the elderly.

Conduct routine electrolyte and renal function measurements, as appropriate for individual circumstances, comorbidities and concomitant medications, checking 1 month after initiation of an SGLT2i in people receiving diuretics.

Maximising Benefits in the Treatment of Type 2 Diabetes: Beyond HbA1c

The SGLT2i class is associated with weight loss and lowering of BP, no increase in hypoglycaemia and, via a number of mechanisms, has increasingly robust evidence for the reduction of CVD, HF hospitalisation and CV death, in people with and without pre-existing CVD [4, 23, 65–70, 82].

SGLT2i treatments are well tolerated and have a favourable risk–benefit profile for many people with T2DM [40].

Treating each condition in isolation may lead to missed opportunities in improving overall outcomes for people with T2DM.

The Improving Diabetes Steering Committee suggests that SGLT2i therapies, for many people with T2DM and at risk of CVD, may represent a logical first escalation from metformin.

It is prudent therefore to consider the CVD risk factors people with T2DM may have and then consider treatment options that take these factors into account.

Summary and Practical Considerations

Recent evidence from CVOTs and real-world studies provides robust support for the initiation of SGLT2i medication in people with T2DM and who either have established CVD or are at risk of developing CVD, and HF in particular, or at risk of renal decline and progression into CKD.

In selecting efficacious treatment for people with T2DM and risk of CVD, the ADA/EASD consensus statement notes that both SGLT2i and GLP-1 RA interventions may be appropriate, and recommend determining the existence of established CVD, or the probable risk of developing CVD or CKD.

The Improving Diabetes Steering Committee provides practical advice on the use of SGLT2i treatment in four major groups of people with T2DM: people with established CVD, people at high risk for developing CVD, people at lower risk of developing CVD and frail people.

Heart Failure in Type 2 Diabetes: Current Perspectives on Screening, Diagnosis and Management

A machine generated summary based on the work of Ceriello, Antonio; Catrinoiu, Doina; Chandramouli, Chanchal; Cosentino, Francesco; Dombrowsky, Annique Cornelia; Itzhak, Baruch; Lalic, Nebojsa Malić; Prattichizzo, Francesco; Schnell, Oliver; Seferović, Petar M.; Valensi, Paul; Standl, Eberhard

2021 in Cardiovascular Diabetology

Abstract-Summary Type 2 diabetes is one of the most relevant risk factors for heart failure, the prevalence of which is increasing worldwide.

The aim of the review is to highlight the current perspectives of the pathophysiology of heart failure as it pertains to type 2 diabetes.

We also discuss the current criteria used for heart failure diagnosis and the gold standard screening tools for individuals with type 2 diabetes.

The influence of the presence of type 2 diabetes as well as heart failure on COVID-19 severity is briefly discussed.

Introduction

Clinically manifest HF is present in 10–30% of all subjects with T2D, especially common at the age of 70 years and older, while 30–40% of all cases of acute or chronic HF have prevalent T2D [110].

T2D and HF are interrelated: T2D increases the risk of HF, HF is highly prevalent in patients with T2D, and HF might increase the risk of developing T2D [111].

While the incidence of HF is increasing in people older than 85 years but also at younger age in recent years [112] and the epidemiologic linkage between T2D and HF is clear [110], recognition of those at risk and/or those with prevalent HF is lagging.

We describe the pathophysiology of the different HF subtypes, focusing on the myocardial alterations induced by T2D in the absence of coronary disease and other risk factors, i.e., cardiomyopathy in diabetes.

Classification of Heart Failure and Epidemiological Aspects

In a setting of chronic, low-grade systemic inflammation, the amount of EFT is elevated, and its role potentially changes from a heart- protecting and supporting structure to a local source of pro-inflammatory cytokines in the heart, which probably worsens endothelial dysfunction and leads to increased cardiac fibrosis and stiffness and thus inducing HF, in particular HFpEF [113].

The presence of subclinical myocardial damage increases the risk for CV events and HF, with the highest CV risk for people with T2D [114].

The SAVOR-TIMI 53 trial reported that diabetic individuals without known CVD but with elevated NT-proBNP levels have a 3-fold increased risk of HF than counterparts with known CVD and normal NT-proBNP levels [115].

The ADVANCE trial and other studies demonstrated that NT-proBNP strongly predicts HF risk, the overall excess mortality, and CV mortality in people with T2D [116, 117].

Detection of Heart Failure in Diabetes

Strategies in people with diabetes to reduce the risk for HF: The 2019 ESC-EASD guidelines recommend routine assessment of microalbuminuria and eGFR in order to identify patients at high risk of renal dysfunction or future CVD [111].

Metformin Metformin monotherapy is the first-line treatment for patients with T2D without CVD and at moderate CV risk according to the 2019 ESC-EASD guidelines on diabetes, and it is recommended for diabetes treatment in patients with HF if the eGFR is stable and $\geq$ 30 mL/min/1.73m^2 (level of evidence: C) [111].

The 2019 ADA/EASD consensus recommends SGLT-2 inhibitors on top of metformin in people with diabetes and HF (especially HFrEF) in order to reduce HHF, MACE, and CV death [118].

To saxagliptin, there is no treatment recommendation for pioglitazone for diabetes management in people at risk for HF because it increases the incidence of HF in T2D patients compared with placebo [111, 119].

Diabetes, HF and COVID-19

To the increased risk of infection, SARS-CoV-2-infected individuals with diabetes are also likely to have serious complications or die, especially in conjunction with CV risk factors such as hypertension, obesity and smoking, especially those who are at poor metabolic control [120].

As serious complications in SARS-CoV-2-infected diabetic people, acute myocarditis (36.6% vs. 15.5%), acute HF (25.3% vs. 5.6%), and acute MI (9.9% vs. 1.4%) have been observed compared to non-diabetics.

If diabetes and SARS-CoV-2 infection are accompanied by the risk factors male sex, a longer duration of diabetes, as well as a history of micro- and macrovascular complications and HF, significantly increased death rates have been detected [121].

Irrespective of the presence of diabetes in SARS-CoV-2 infected subjects, a history of HF alone was also significantly associated with the need for hospitalization for coronavirus disease 2019 (COVID-19) and a higher mortality [122].

Conclusions

Heart failure remains an important issue for life expectancy, especially for people with diabetes.

New therapeutic tools, such as the SGLT-2 inhibitors, are offering the opportunity for better management of this very serious complication of T2D. Using biomarkers such as NT-proBNP can help diagnose HF early to predict prognosis and therapeutic efficacy of medications for HF or/and diabetes.

NT-proBNP measurement should be implemented early in the monitoring of subjects with diabetes at high CV risk.

The importance of screening for HF in diabetes becomes significant, especially during the COVID-19 pandemic in which people with diabetes and concomitant HF are particularly vulnerable to SARS-CoV-2 infection and often have worse disease progression and prognosis than healthy individuals.

Redox-Driven Cardioprotective Effects of Sodium-Glucose Co-transporter-2 Inhibitors: Comparative Review

https://doi.org/10.1186/s12933-023-01822-7

A machine generated summary based on the work of Hoehlschen, Julia; Hofreither, Dominik; Tomin, Tamara; Birner-Gruenberger, Ruth

2023 in Cardiovascular Diabetology

Abstract-Summary Sodium-glucose co-transporter-2 inhibitors are used in the treatment of diabetes but are also emerging as cardioprotective agents in heart diseases even in the absence of type 2 diabetes.

Upon providing a short overview of common pathophysiological features of diabetes, we review the clinically reported cardio- and nephroprotective potential of sodium-glucose co-transporter-2 inhibitors currently available on the market, including Dapagliflozin, Canagliflozin, and Empagliflozin.

Introduction

Reduction of blood glucose has been shown to improve microvascular complications such as nephron- and neuropathy, but to be insufficient to prevent the death from cardiovascular events, the most relevant macrovascular complication of type 2 diabetes [123].

One such emerging drug class are sodium-glucose co-transporter-2 (SGLT-2) inhibitors, a relatively novel anti-diabetic medication.

In diabetes, the renal transport maximum for glucose can be increased by inducing tubular growth or raising the expression of SGLT-1 and 2, contributing to the state of hyperglycemia [96, 124].

It has become increasingly recognized that SGLT-2 inhibitors exhibit tissue-protective effects beyond their systematic, glucose-lowering properties.

We summarize the clinically reported organ-protective potential of SGLT-2 inhibitors currently available on the market, before specifically focusing on their cardioprotective, antioxidative properties, a trait that will most likely propel this drug class from curative to preventive care.

Renal Complications Related to Diabetes and Proposed Protective Mechanisms of Gliflozins

Attempting to cope with hyperglycemia, diabetic patients struggle with renal hyperfiltration (manifested by an increased glomerular filtration rate (GFR)) which results from high glomerular pressure and increased sodium and glucose reabsorption via SGLT-1 and 2.

The diabetes-driven boost in Na^+ reabsorption in the proximal tubule, causes a decreased Na^+ delivery to the macula densa leading to a reduced tubuloglomerular feedback (TGF), accompanied by increasing filtration rates [125].

When inhibiting this process by SGLT-2 inhibitors, sodium delivery to the macula densa is enabled and hyperfiltration rates are reduced [126].

Upon SGLT-2 inhibition, the highly increased sodium cannot be sufficiently cleared by the Na^+/K^+ ATPases of macula cells, resulting in an osmotic gradient leading to macula cell swelling and leakage of adenosine triphosphate (ATP) from the basolateral membrane, which is extracellularly converted to adenosine.

Studies in diabetic mice as well as isolated kidney cells have demonstrated the ability of Empagliflozin to reprogram renal metabolism and to improve mitochondrial function and antioxidative defense [127, 128].

Cardiovascular Complications Related to Diabetes: Focus on Oxidative Stress

To preserve homeostasis and contractile function in response to stress, the heart offers compensation strategies, including cell growth as well as increase in angiogenesis, energy efficiency, autophagy, and antioxidant generation [129, 130].

Essential, these adaptive processes might result in fibrosis, altered sarcomere structure, impaired Ca^{2+} handling, induction of fetal gene programming, mitochondrial dysfunction, disbalance in reactive oxygen species (ROS), metabolic remodeling and cell death, potentially leading to progressive HF in the long term [129–133].

The adaptive increase in glycolysis may not be matched in glucose oxidation and lead to an uncoupling between substrate uptake and oxidation, further impairing cellular metabolic function and redox homeostasis [130, 132, 134, 135].

In the failing heart, oxidative stress is not only linked to dysregulated cardiac metabolism but also to systemic factors such as diabetes, metabolic syndrome and ageing [136, 137].

Restoring metabolic capability, mitochondrial function, and, ultimately, energy output in (diabetic) HF may be essential to ameliorate its progression and facilitate treatment [138, 139].

Cardioprotective Effects of SGLT-2 Inhibitors from Clinical Trials

The aim of the EMPA-REG Outcome™ trial [140] was to determine long-term effects of Empagliflozin on cardiovascular safety in type 2 diabetes patients (≥18 years) with a high risk of cardiovascular events as well as its cardioprotective effects.

Patients suffering from type 2 diabetes, having a glycated hemoglobin value (HbA_{1c}) in a certain range and established cardiovascular diseases were randomly divided into three groups (1:1:1) receiving Empagliflozin (10 mg or 25 mg) or placebo once daily.

Similar results in terms of positive cardiovascular effects were obtained in a long-term study on Canagliflozin (CANVAS) in which 10,142 patients suffering from type 2 diabetes were included and randomized to receive Canagliflozin (100 mg or 300 mg) or placebo (1:1:1) [4].

In 2019 and 2020, two studies were published, investigating whether the positive cardiovascular effects of Dapagliflozin and Empagliflozin would be restricted to type 2 diabetes patients.

Potential Cardioprotective Mechanisms of SGLT-2 Inhibitors beyond Systemic Effects

Treatment of cardiomyocytes from healthy rats and rabbits cultivated in medium containing 5 mM or 10 mM glucose supplemented with Empagliflozin (1 μM) reduced cytoplasmic concentrations of Na^+ and Ca^{2+} and increased mitochondrial Ca^{2+} concentrations, reversing the negative effects of increased glucose concentrations [141].

Treatment of these animal cells with Empagliflozin followed by subsequently NHE inhibitor Cariporide only minimally affected the change in cytoplasmic Na^+ concentration chosen as indicator for NHE inhibition [141].

In silico docking studies on the extracellular Na^+ binding site of NHE proved high binding affinity for all three inhibitors (−34.3 kJ/mol Empagliflozin, −32.2 kJ/mol Dapagliflozin, −37.2 kJ/mol Canagliflozin) compared to negative control glucose (−24.3 kJ/mol) [142].

To Canagliflozin, which significantly activated AMPK in HEK293 cells and murine hepatocytes already at concentrations similar to those in human plasma when treated with the drug, Empa- and Dapagliflozin showed weaker effects even at higher therapeutic doses [143].

SGLT-2 Inhibitors and Oxidative Stress

Markers of oxidative stress (lipid hydroperoxide, glutathione peroxidase (GSH-Px), superoxide dismutase (SOD) and malondialdehyde (MDA)) were also investigated in tissue from diabetic mouse hearts treated and not treated with Empagliflozin.

Their levels were found to be significantly higher (lipid hydroperoxide, MDA) or lower (SOD, GSH-Px) in diabetic untreated mice compared to Empagliflozin treated ones [144].

fibrosis and membrane thickening was further confirmed by treating diabetic cardiac microvascular endothelial cells (CMEC) with Empagliflozin.

Diabetes induced mitochondrial fission was also prevented by Empagliflozin, which brought the ratio of AMP:ATP closer to the one observed in control cells, leading to the activation of AMPK [145].

A study in non-diabetic failing pig hearts also showed that Empagliflozin positively influenced cardiac metabolism typically found in failing hearts by diverting ATP production to beta oxidation and ketogenesis, decreasing the consumption of carbohydrates and thereby approaching the conditions found in healthy hearts [146].

Conclusion

Some of the clinical studies also searched for protein biomarkers in the blood which could tell us more regarding the underlying effects of the drugs.

In case of the EMPEROR study (Empagliflozin), comparing samples taken right before the treatment's start (baseline), after 12 weeks and 52 weeks of treatment, showed no significant differences in protein expression between the two timepoints during the treatment, hinting that the effect of Empagliflozin is time-independent.

A small group of intracellular proteins involved in autophagic flux, weakening of oxidative stress and inflammation processes in the heart as well as promotion of repair and regeneration in heart and kidney were found to be differentially expressed upon treatment with Empagliflozin [147].

Both in vitro and in vivo studies agree in one thing: SGLT-2 inhibitors are able to protect our heart independent of their glucose lowering effects.

Cardiorenal Protection: Potential of SGLT2 Inhibitors and GLP-1 Receptor Agonists in the Treatment of Type 2 Diabetes

https://doi.org/10.1007/s13300-019-00680-5

A machine generated summary based on the work of Nagahisa, Taichi; Saisho, Yoshifumi

2019 in Diabetes Therapy

Abstract-Summary Recent large clinical trials on sodium-glucose cotransporter 2 (SGLT2) inhibitors and glucagon-like peptide-1 (GLP-1) receptor agonists, with the aim of verifying cardiovascular safety, have revealed that these medications have a preventative advantage on adverse cardiovascular outcomes, including worsening of heart failure and deterioration of nephropathy, in patients with type 2 diabetes (T2D).

Given the results from recent studies, the American Diabetes Association (ADA) and the European Association for the Study of Diabetes (EASD) recommend that patients with T2D and clinical cardiovascular disease (CVD) with inadequate glucose control despite treatment with metformin should receive an SGLT2 inhibitor or GLP-1 receptor agonist.

We summarize the results of recent cardiovascular outcome trials and discuss the potential clinical advantage of SGLT2 inhibitors and GLP-1 receptor agonists.

Introduction

Major clinical trials, including those on the cardiovascular safety of dipeptidyl peptidase-4 (DPP-4) inhibitors, glucagon-like peptide-1 (GLP-1) receptor agonists, and sodium-glucose co-transporter-2 (SGLT2) inhibitors, have been published.

Three trials of GLP-1 receptor agonists, namely, the Liraglutide Effect and Action in Diabetes: Evaluation of Cardiovascular Outcome Results (LEADER) trial, the Semaglutide Unabated Sustainability in Treatment of Type 2 Diabetes 6 (SUSTAIN-6) trial, and the Albiglutide and cardiovascular outcomes in patients with type 2 diabetes and cardiovascular disease (Harmony Outcomes) trial, also demonstrated risk reduction in major adverse cardiovascular events [148–150], with a consistent result recently reported on the use of dulaglutide in the Researching Cardiovascular Events with a Weekly Incretin in Diabetes (REWIND) trial [151].

Given the implications of new evidence derived from these cardiovascular outcomes trials (CVOTs), the American Diabetes Association (ADA) and the European Association for the Study of Diabetes (EASD) recently recommended that patients with T2D and clinical cardiovascular disease (CVD) inadequately controlled with metformin therapy and lifestyle intervention should be treated with an SGLT2 inhibitor or GLP-1 receptor agonist and that among those in whom heart failure coexists, an SGLT2 inhibitor should be preferentially prescribed [152].

Methods

The articles cited in this review were retrieved from the literature using Google Scholar with the search terms "SGLT2 inhibitor", "GLP-1 receptor agonist", "cardiovascular", and "outcome".

Related articles were also collected from a personal database.

This review article is based on previously conducted studies and does not contain any studies with human participants or animals performed by any of the authors.

Era Before SGLT2 Inhibitors and GLP-1 Receptor Agonists

In UKPDS 34 [153], in which 1704 overweight patients were randomly assigned to conventional treatment or intensive glycemic control with a sulfonylurea, insulin, or metformin, participants allocated metformin had a significantly reduced risk of any diabetes-related endpoint (HR 0.68, 95% CI 0.53–0.87, p = 0.0023), diabetes-related death (HR 0.58, 95% CI 0.37–0.91p = 0.017), all-cause mortality (HR 0.64, 95% CI 0.45–0.91, p = 0.011), and myocardial infarction (HR 0.61, 95% CI 0.41–0.89, p = 0.01), as opposed to participants who received intensive glycemic control achieved with a sulfonylurea or insulin.

None of three subsequent major trials that examined intensive glycemic control, namely, the Action to Control Cardiovascular Risk in Diabetes (ACCORD) trial, the Action in Diabetes and Vascular Disease: Preterax and Diamicron Modified-Release Controlled Evaluation (ADVANCE) trial, and the Veterans Affairs Diabetes Trial (VADT) [64, 154, 155], exhibited a beneficial effect of intensive control on cardiovascular events, with the exception of the ACCORD trial in which non-fatal myocardial infarction decreased in the intensive control group.

SGLT2 Inhibitors

Although only 27% of patients had established CVD, treatment with SGLT2 inhibitors was also associated with significant risk reduction in hospitalization for heart failure and all-cause death (HR 0.64, 95% CI 0.50–0.82, p = 0.001 and HR 0.51 95% CI 0.37–0.70, p < 0.001, respectively), with a directionally similar trend regardless of the existence of prior CVD [156].

The results of a meta-analysis of 53 trials of SGLT2 inhibitors indicated that only empagliflozin demonstrates a lower risk of acute renal impairment/failure events relative to placebo (OR 0.72; 95% CI 0.59–0.87), compared with canagliflozin (OR 1.82; 95% CI 0.28–11.77) and dapagliflozin (OR 1.93; 95% CI 0.42–8.83) [157].

GLP-1 Receptor Agonists

The Semaglutide Unabated Sustainability in Treatment of Type 2 Diabetes 6 (SUSTAIN-6) trial, which enrolled 3297 patients who were administered semaglutide 0.5 or 1.0 mg per week or placebo, showed a significant 26% reduction in 3-point MACE (HR 0.74, 95% CI 0.58–0.95), a significant reduction in nonfatal stroke (HR 0.61, 95% CI 0.38–0.99), and a directionally concordant result in nonfatal MI (HR 0.74, 95% CI 0.51–1.08).

In the Functional Impact of GLP-1 for Heart Failure Treatment (FIGHT) trial, which involved 300 patients with advanced heart failure, the liraglutide group showed a numerically higher (but not statistically significant) risk of rehospitalization for heart failure (HR 1.30, 95% CI 0.89–1.88, $p = 0.17$) compared with the placebo group [158].

Discussion

A series of cardiovascular outcome trials revealed an unexpected benefit on cardiovascular outcome with SGLT2 inhibitors and GLP-1 receptor agonists, highlighting the advantage of secondary prevention in patients with established CVD.

The efficacy of combination therapy with a GLP-1 receptor agonist and SGLT2 inhibitor has been elucidated [159, 160], with further improvement of glycemic control compared with monotherapy also observed, although the achieved glycemic efficacy was subadditive partially due to stimulatory effects on glucagon and hepatic glucose production correlated with glycosuria derived from SGLT2 inhibitors [161].

Three separately conducted 52-week open-label studies to evaluate the efficacy and safety of SGLT2 inhibitors, involving canagliflozin, ipragliflozin, and luseogliflozin, in combination with a GLP-1 receptor agonist showed a further decrease in HbA1c and body weight without any increase in serious adverse events including severe hypoglycemia [162–164].

This combination is therefore an attractive therapeutic option for patients with obesity refractory to treatment with an SGLT2 inhibitor or GLP-1 receptor agonist alone or in combination with insulin therapy in terms of long-term glycemic control and body weight control.

Conclusion

Recent clinical trials have revealed a novel role of SGLT2 inhibitors and GLP-1 receptor agonists beyond their glucose-lowering effect, and both agents have received more attention as a paradigm shift from "the lower glucose the better" to "how to optimize glycemic control without hypoglycemia and overweight" has been generated by current guidelines.

Full advantage of the pleiotropic benefit of these agents should be taken to prevent secondary adverse cardiovascular events and to mitigate the advance of renal complications without increased risk of hypoglycemia.

A Bioinformatics Investigation into the Pharmacological Mechanisms of Sodium-Glucose Co-transporter 2 Inhibitors in Diabetes Mellitus and Heart Failure Based on Network Pharmacology

https://doi.org/10.1007/s10557-021-07186-y

A machine generated summary based on the work of Mai, Ziling; Li, Huanqiang; Chen, Guanzhong; Chen, Enzhao; Liu, Liwei; Lun, Zhubin; Lai, Wenguang; Zhou, Chunyun; Yu, Sijia; Liu, Jin; Chen, Shiqun; Chen, Jiyan; Liu, Yong

2021 in Cardiovascular Drugs and Therapy

Abstract-Summary Sodium-glucose co-transporter 2 (SGLT2) inhibitors have demonstrated consistent benefits in the reduction of hospitalization for HF in patients with DM.

To investigate the mechanisms of SGLT2 inhibitors in DM with HF, we performed target prediction and network analysis by a network pharmacology method.

We selected targets of SGLT2 inhibitors and DM status with HF from databases and studies.

There were 125 effective targets between SGLT2 inhibitors and DM status with HF.

It was predicted that the Rap1 signaling pathway, MAPK signaling pathway, EGFR tyrosine kinase inhibitor resistance, AGE-RAGE signaling pathway in diabetic complications and other signaling pathways were involved in the treatment of DM with HF by SGLT2 inhibitors.

Our study elucidated the possible mechanisms of SGLT2 inhibitors from a systemic and holistic perspective based on pharmacological networks.

The key targets and pathways will provide new insights for further research on the pharmacological mechanism of SGLT2 inhibitors in the treatment of DM with HF.

Introduction

Some drugs have been recommended for the treatment of DM with HF, such as metformin and sulfonylureas, but they are insufficient in treating diabetes with heart failure.

Clinical trials from many countries, including the EASEL Population-Based Cohort Study [165], the EMPA-REG OUTCOME trial [65] and the CVD-REAL 2 study [166], have proven that SGLT2 inhibitors reduce the risk of non-fatal myocardial infarction, non-fatal stroke, and all-cause death, as well as the risk of hospitalization and death associated with heart failure.

Based on these composite data, SGLT2 inhibitors represent an important new therapeutic approach for the prevention of heart failure in at-risk patients with diabetes mellitus.

The DAPA-HF study is a prospective randomized placebo-controlled trial to determine the effectiveness and safety of dapagliflozin in patients with heart failure with reduced ejection fraction based on conventional treatment.

The therapeutic targets and mechanism of SGLT2 inhibitors acting on HF have not yet been revealed, especially in patients with DM, which needs to be further explored and analyzed.

Methods

We collected disease targets from the studies reporting existing network analysis on actual patients with DM status with HF [167, 168].

The four SGLT2 inhibitors, their corresponding targets and the intersection targets of diseases and drugs were sorted and input into Cytoscape v3.6.1 to construct the following networks: (1) network between four SGLT2 inhibitors (canagliflozin, dapagliflozin, empagliflozin, and ertugliflozin) and their corresponding targets; (2) network between four SGLT2 inhibitors, intersection targets, and diseases (DM status with HF).

The intersection targets of SGLT2 inhibitors and DM status with HF were then imported to construct the protein–protein interaction network.

The STRING online platform was used to build the PPI network of core targets.

After selecting the multiple proteins module, the Gene Name list of target proteins was uploaded to the network, limiting the species to Homo sapiens, and the confidence score was set to >0.9.

Results

The purple nodes are the four SGLT2 inhibitors (dapagliflozin, empagliflozin, canagliflozin and ertugliflozin); the red nodes are HF and DM; the green nodes represent 125 common targets.

There is an interaction between one SGLT2 inhibitor and multiple targets in the treatment of DM with HF.

The STRING database platform was used to construct a network of target protein interactions, and the 33 core targets of SGLT2 inhibitors-HF-DM were imported.

To study the mechanism of SGLT2 inhibitors in DM with HF more systematically, the 33 core target genes of the SGLT2 inhibitors-HF-DM intersection were introduced into R statistical programming language to analyze the GO biological function and KEGG signaling pathway.

The core targets might affect signaling pathways including the Rap1 signaling pathway, MAPK signaling pathway, EGFR tyrosine kinase inhibitor resistance and AGE-RAGE signaling pathway in diabetic complications, which predicts that SGLT2 inhibitors might be effective for treatment of DM with HF by regulating the aforementioned signaling pathways.

Discussion

The key pathways were screened by KEGG analysis, mainly involving the Rap1 signaling pathway, MAPK signaling pathway, EGFR tyrosine kinase inhibitor resistance and AGE-RAGE signaling pathway in diabetic complications.

Our results suggest that the four signaling pathways may be involved in the mechanisms of SGLT2 inhibitors affecting DM status with HF.

Network pharmacology revealed the potential targets of SGLT2 inhibitors, as well as targets of DM with HF, and bioinformatics was used to study the main enrichment pathways.

Based on the network pharmacology, our study predicted the potential therapeutic targets of SGLT2 inhibitors in DM with HF and revealed their action on the main pathways through core genes, which explained the mechanisms of SGLT2 inhibitors in DM with HF and provided scientific evidence for SGLT2 inhibitors to treat DM with HF.

Conclusions

Our study systematically predicted, screened and analyzed the targets and pathways that might play a vital role in the biological process, which elaborated the possible mechanisms of SGLT2 inhibitors in DM status with HF.

These results provide evidence and new insights for further research on the pharmacological mechanism of SGLT2 inhibitors.

Different Effects of SGLT2 Inhibitors According to the Presence and Types of Heart Failure in Type 2 Diabetic Patients

https://doi.org/10.1186/s12933-020-01042-3

A machine generated summary based on the work of Hwang, In-Chang; Cho, Goo-Yeong; Yoon, Yeonyee E.; Park, Jin Joo; Park, Jun-Bean; Lee, Seung-Pyo; Kim, Hyung-Kwan; Kim, Yong-Jin; Sohn, Dae-Won

2020 in Cardiovascular Diabetology

Abstract-Summary We investigated the changes in cardiac function in diabetic patients according to the presence and types of heart failure (HF).

After a median 13 months of follow-up, HF patients with SGLT2i showed a significant decrease in left ventricular end-diastolic dimension (LV-EDD; from 57.4 mm [50.0–64.9] to 53.0 mm [48.0–60.0]; $p < 0.001$) and improvement in LV-EF (from 36.1% [25.6–47.5] to 45.0% [34.8–56.3]; $p < 0.001$).

LV mass index and diastolic parameters also showed improvements in HF patients with SGLT2i.

The SGLT2i-induced improvements in cardiac function were more prominent in HF patients than those without HF, and in HFrEF patients than HFpEF patients.

Use of SGLT2i improved cardiac function in diabetic patients, regardless of the presence of HF.

The improvements were more prominent in HF patients, especially in those with HFrEF.

Background

The SGLT2 inhibitors (SGLT2i) have demonstrated robust benefits in terms of the prevention of heart failure (HF) and the reduction in cardiovascular mortality, which was the first evidence for prevention of major cardiovascular events by anti-diabetic medications.

These hypotheses were further supported by the recently published trial of dapagliflozin, the Dapagliflozin and Prevention of Adverse-outcomes in Heart Failure (DAPA-HF) trial, which extended the benefits of SGLT2i to those with HF with reduced ejection fraction (HFrEF) even in the absence of diabetes.

It is unclear whether the cardiovascular benefits of SGLT2i would be similar between the diabetic patients with versus without HF, and between those with HFrEF versus HFpEF.

We aimed to compare the SGLT2i-induced changes in cardiac function and geometry assessed by echocardiography in type 2 diabetic patients according to the presence and types of HF, using a retrospective cohort.

Methods

For the patients with SGLT2i prescription, those with all echocardiograms performed before, but not after, the initial SGLT2i prescription were excluded.

Patients with all echocardiograms performed after, but not before, the initial SGLT2i prescriptions were also excluded.

Patients with no echocardiography performed 6–24 months after the initial SGLT2i prescription were excluded.

After exclusion, 202 diabetic patients for whom SGLT2i were prescribed, and for whom the baseline echocardiography was performed before the initial SGLT2i prescription and the follow-up echocardiography was performed at 6–24 months after the initial SGLT2i prescription were identified.

As a sensitivity analysis, we compared the changes in echocardiographic parameters according to the use of SGLT2i between patients with HF with reduced EF (LV-EF < 40% at baseline) and those with HF with preserved EF (HFpEF) (LV-EF ≥ 40% at baseline).

Results

Use of angiotensin converting enzyme inhibitors (ACEi), angiotensin receptor blocker (ARB), beta-blockers, mineralocorticoid antagonists (MRA), and diuretics were more frequent in patients with HF (groups 3 and 4) compared to those without HF (groups 1 and 2), but were not different according to the use of SGLT2i (groups 1 vs. 2; groups 3 vs. 4).

In the HF patients, those with SGLT2i treatment (group 4) showed a prominent improvement in LV-EF (from 36.1 [25.6–47.5] to 45.0% [34.8–56.3]; $p < 0.001$) as well as LV-GLS (from 10.3 [7.3–12.5] to 11.4% [8.4–14.3]; $p = 0.001$).

The changes in LV-EF and LV-GLS did not show different according to the SGLT2i treatment in HFpEF patients.

Discussion

Several studies that showed improvements in LV diastolic function and reduction in LV-MI by SGLT2i in diabetic patients without overt HF [169, 170].

Our findings are consistent with these studies that the use of SGLT2i resulted in small but significant improvements in LV geometry and diastolic function in diabetic patients without overt HF.

We observed more prominent improvements in LV function by SGLT2i in diabetic patients with HF compared to those without, which was independent of the use of cardioprotective medications for HF (ACEi, ARB, beta-blockers, and MRA).

Beneficial effect of SGLT2i has also been suggested in patients with HFpEF: in an echocardiographic study by Soga and others the mitral E/e' ratio, LV-MI, and LAVI were decreased with dapagliflozin treatment among diabetic patients with high prevalence of HFpEF (69%) and HFmrEF (17%), whereas the improvement in LV systolic function and the reduction in BNP levels were minimal [171].

Conclusion

In this retrospective cohort study, the use of SGLT2i improved LV systolic and diastolic function, as well as LV geometry, in diabetic patients regardless of the presence of HF.

The improvement in LV function was more prominent in those with HFrEF patients compared to those with HFpEF or those without HF.

These effects of SGLT2i may contribute to the reduction in HF morbidity and mortality in diabetic patients.

Association of SGLT2 Inhibitors with Lower Incidence of Death in Type 2 Diabetes Mellitus and Causes of Death Analysis

https://doi.org/10.1038/s41598-022-13760-7

A machine generated summary based on the work of Chung, Mu-Chi; Hsu, Hui-Tsung; Chang, Chao-Hsiang; Hung, Peir-Haur; Hsiao, Po-Jen; Wu, Laing-You; Wu, Ming-Ju; Shieh, Jeng-Jer; Chung, Chi-Jung

2022 in Scientific Reports

Abstract-Summary Sodium-glucose cotransporter 2 inhibitor (SGLT2i) potentially decrease all-cause and cardiovascular death, however, associations with non-cardiovascular death remain unclear.

We investigated SGLT2i associations with death and the cause of death.

Incident type 2 diabetes mellitus (T2DM) patients and propensity score matched T2DM SGLT2i and Dipeptidyl peptidase 4 inhibitor (DPP4i) users were investigated.

Patients were followed-up until death or December 2018.

The overall incidence of all-cause death was 8.67/1000 patient-years for SGLT2i and 12.41 for DPP4i users during follow-up.

After adjusting for potential risk factors in the propensity score matched population, SGLT2i users were associated with lower risks of all-cause death, cardiovascular death, cancer death, and non-cancer, non-vascular death compared with DPP4i-users.

For specific death causes, significantly lower death risks from heart disease, cerebrovascular disease, and accidents were associated with SGLT2i-use.

Compared with DPP4i-use, SGLT2i-use for T2DM was associated with lower disease and death risk.

Introduction

DM patients have a twofold risk of all-cause death when compared with other non-DM patients [172].

Sodium-glucose Cotransporter 2 Inhibitor (SGLT2i), which reduce blood sugar levels, are highly effective in preventing diabetic kidney disease progression and cardiovascular diseases in type 2 DM (T2DM) patients.

Predominantly due to cardiovascular mechanisms beyond glycemic control, SGLT2i-use facilitates significant risk reductions [173] in all-cause death and cardiovascular death for patients already receiving secondary preventative medication for heart disease in large randomized clinical trials (RCTs).

Survival is the primary standard end-point when investigating SGLT2i effects, however, deaths may be too low to show statistically significant effects or identify specific causes of death other than cardiovascular death in these trials.

Methods

The index study date was defined as the first day of SGLT2i- or DPP4i-use.

After excluding individuals <18 years old and those simultaneously receiving SGLT2i and DPP4i before study entry and undergoing end stage renal disease (ESRD), 53,838 and 207,373 patients were identified as filling SGLT2i or DPP4i prescriptions, respectively, and enrolled.

To avoid the confounding effects of baseline comorbidities and medicine-use, we performed a 1:1 propensity score matching on 53,264 pairs receiving SGLT2i or DPP4i in T2DM patients, based on age, gender, index year, comorbidities, and other medicines.

We compared the distribution of baseline comorbidities, and medicine prescription history between groups receiving SGLT2i or DPP4i.

Patient descriptive data were presented according to SGLT2i or DPP4i groups, and included the mean and standard deviation for continuous as well as number and frequency of categorical variables.

Multiplicative interactions between SGLT2i-use and baseline comorbidities and other medications on all-cause death were calculated by adding cross-product terms in multiple Cox proportional hazard regression models.

Results

When further adjusted by age, gender, hypertension, hyperlipidemia, cerebral vascular disease, coronary artery disease, chronic kidney disease, diabetes medications usage (GLP-1 agonist, insulin, and metformin), and other medication usages (aspirin, ACEI/ARB and statin), SGLT2i users were similarly associated with a lower risk of all-cause death, cardiovascular death, cancer death, and non-cancer, non-vascular death (HR = 0.66 for all-cause death, HR = 0.68 for cardiovascular death, HR = 0.73 for cancer death, and HR = 0.62 for non-cancer, non-vascular death).

SGLT2i users were mostly associated with a lower risk of all-cause death in post hoc subgroup analyses for age, sex, baseline comorbidities, and medication use.

Among characteristics, statistical interactions were identified between SGLT2i-use and patients receiving ACEI/ARB for all-cause death risk (interaction $p = 0.02$).

Discussion

SGLT2i-use in T2DM was significantly associated with a decreased risk of death when compared with DPP4i-use in a national cohort in Taiwan.

To cardiovascular death, SGLT2i-use was also associated with a lower risk for cancer death and non-cancer, non-vascular death.

Our study indicated an association between SGLT2i-use and a lower risk of all-cause death in a real-world database, in agreement with data from RCTs [173].

Other population-based studies [174, 175] also showed a reduced risk of all-cause death for SGLT2i therapy when compared with other glucose-lowering drugs.

We observed a 32% lower risk of cardiovascular death with SGLT2i-use, including a 28% lower risk of death from heart disease and 52% lower risk from cerebrovascular disease.

Our study is the first to indicate associations between SGLT2i-use and a lower risk of non-cancer, non-vascular death.

Conclusions

In T2DM patients, we identified an association between SGLT2i and a lower risk of death when compared with DPP4i-use.

The potential beneficial effects of SGLT2i on cancer death and non-cancer, non-vascular death must be comprehensively investigated in future studies.

Use of Sodium-Glucose Co-transporter-2 Inhibitors in Clinical Practice for Heart Failure Prevention and Treatment: Beyond Type 2 Diabetes. A Narrative Review

https://doi.org/10.1007/s12325-021-01989-z

A machine generated summary based on the work of Rao, Shaline
2021 in Advances in Therapy

Abstract-Summary An established treatment for T2D, sodium-glucose cotransporter-2 inhibitors (SGLT-2is; canagliflozin, dapagliflozin, empagliflozin, and ertugliflozin) have demonstrated beneficial effects on CV outcomes in long-term studies of patients with T2D with established CV disease and/or a broad range of CV risk factors.

Recent studies have extended these findings to patients with HF, with and without T2D, finding that SGLT-2is (particularly dapagliflozin and empagliflozin) are effective therapeutic interventions for the treatment and prevention of HF.

This narrative review article discusses the use of SGLT-2is in the treatment and prevention of HF in patients with and without T2D. Dapagliflozin was the first SGLT-2i to receive US Food and Drug Administration (FDA) approval for treatment of HF, to reduce the risk of CV death and hospitalization for HF in adults with HF with reduced ejection fraction (HFrEF) with and without T2D. Recently, the FDA also approved empagliflozin for this indication.

Given the new HFrEF indications for dapagliflozin and empagliflozin, and the likelihood of similar approvals for other SGLT-2is, cardiology guidelines are beginning to integrate SGLT-2is into a standard-of-care treatment regimen for patients with HFrEF.

Further clinical trial evidence may lead to more widespread use and further integration of SGLT-2is into standard-of-care regimens for the treatment and management of HF in patients with and without T2D.

Introduction

SGLT-2is have been shown to have beneficial effects on both CV and renal outcomes in patients with T2D [4, 65, 66, 176–180], and SGLT-2is are the first class of antidiabetic drugs to have demonstrated beneficial effects on HF outcomes and, thus, may serve as a novel treatment option for patients without T2D with or at risk of HF.

As with general CV and renal effects, the beneficial effects of SGLT-2is on HF outcomes specifically are thought to be due to nonglycemic mechanisms [176, 177].

This narrative review examines the role of SGLT-2is for the prevention and treatment of HF in individuals with T2D but also as a novel approach to HF treatment in patients without T2D. An assessment of important SGLT-2i CV outcome trials (CVOTs) will provide guidance on the use of SGLT-2is in routine clinical practice, specifically their placement in the T2D-specific and general HF treatment paradigm.

Methods

The topic of this narrative review article is the use of SGLT-2is in the prevention and treatment of HF in patients with or without T2D. To identify key studies relevant to this topic, non-systematic literature searches were conducted in the PubMed database using search terms associated with SGLT-2is (i.e., "SGLT-2 inhibitor," "sodium-glucose cotransporter 2 inhibitor," "canagliflozin," "dapagliflozin," "empagliflozin," "ertugliflozin," "sotagliflozin") and heart failure.

The PubMed literature searches were limited to recent publications in English, published between July 2015 and October 2021, and to those reporting clinical trials and meta-analyses of SGLT-2is.

Publications identified through the literature search results were reviewed, and studies reporting CV and/or renal outcomes for SGLT-2is were included in the review.

Although applying a date range to the search excluded studies published before July 2015, it is unlikely to affect the content of this review because HF is a new indication for SGLT-2is.

SGLT-2i Effects on Cardiovascular Outcomes

A meta-analysis of three of these CVOTs (DECLARE-TIMI 58, CANVAS, and EMPA-REG OUTCOME) showed significant reductions in the risk of CV death or HHF by 23% and the risk of HHF by 31% with SGLT-2is across patients, regardless of the presence of CVD or HF at baseline [23].

DAPA-CKD demonstrated a significantly reduced risk of the primary composite outcome (i.e., sustained decline in eGFR ≥50%, end-stage renal disease [ESRD], or death from renal or CV causes; HR, 0.61; $P < 0.001$) with dapagliflozin versus placebo [181].

In the CREDENCE study with a patient population at high risk of kidney failure, canagliflozin was associated with significant reductions in the risk of HHF (39%; $P < 0.001$), the risk of CV death or HHF (31%; $P < 0.001$), and the risk of the composite renal outcome (ESRD, doubling of serum creatinine level, or death from renal or CV causes; 30%; $P = 0.00001$) [179].

SGLT-2is and HF Outcomes

Additional findings pertaining to the beneficial effects of an SGLT-2i in patients with HFrEF were reported by the Empagliflozin Outcome Trial in Patients with Chronic Heart Failure and a Reduced Ejection Fraction (EMPEROR-Reduced) study [25].

Sotagliflozin reduced the risk of the revised primary endpoint of total number of deaths from CV causes and HHF and urgent visits for HF by 33% (HR, 0.67 [95% CI 0.52–0.85]; $P < 0.001$).

A significant reduction in the first hierarchical secondary outcome of the number of HHF/urgent visits for HF was also seen (HR, 0.64; $P < 0.001$), but there were no significant effects on other secondary endpoints, including all-cause deaths.

The primary composite endpoint of death from CV causes or HHF was significantly reduced with empagliflozin compared with placebo by 21% (HR, 0.79 [95% CI 0.69–0.90]; $P < 0.001$) [182].

Knowledge Gaps Regarding the Use of SGLT-2is for HF in Clinical Practice

Despite mounting evidence of the cardioprotective effects of SGLT-2is in patients with and without T2D, there are several knowledge gaps associated with their use in clinical practice for the prevention and treatment of HF [183].

The differential effects of SGLT-2is on HF outcomes in patients with HFpEF versus HFrEF are only just being clarified.

The Dapagliflozin Evaluation to Improve the Lives of Patients with Preserved Ejection Fraction Heart Failure (DELIVER) study is investigating the effects of SGLT-2is on CV and HF outcomes in patients with HFpEF [184].

It is hoped that data from ongoing and future studies will provide additional evidence regarding the beneficial effects of SGLT-2is on outcomes in patients with HF irrespective of T2D status as well as demonstrating that SGLT-2is are safe and effective in both patients with HFpEF and HFrEF and those with acute HF.

Clinical Ramifications of SGLT-2is for HF Prevention and Treatment

In 2019, the European Society of Cardiology (ESC) guidelines recommended SGLT-2is (canagliflozin, dapagliflozin, and empagliflozin) to reduce the risk of HHF in patients with T2D and risk of CKD progression [111].

This was followed by two position papers in 2020 by the Heart Failure Association (HFA) of the ESC recommending the use of SGLT-2is (empagliflozin, canagliflozin, dapagliflozin, and ertugliflozin) to reduce the risk of HHF in patients with T2D with either established CVD or high CV risk [185, 186].

The 2021 ESC guidelines recommended SGLT-2is (canagliflozin, dapagliflozin, empagliflozin, ertugliflozin, and sotagliflozin) for the reduction of HHF, major CV events, end-stage renal dysfunction, and CV death in patients with T2D at risk of CV events [187].

In patients with HFrEF and T2D, the SGLT-2is dapagliflozin, empagliflozin, and sotagliflozin were recommended to reduce HHF and CV death by the 2021 ESC guidelines [188].

Physicians' Perspectives Regarding the Role of SGLT-2is in Treating HF

To optimize CV outcomes, an important consideration may be the use of SGLT-2i therapy as part of the initial therapeutic approach in patients with T2D at risk of CVD [189].

The following serious AEs, although rare, have been associated with SGLT-2i therapy and should be taken into consideration in patients with underlying comorbidities and concomitant medications: diabetic ketoacidosis (DKA), renal injury, volume depletion, and lower-limb amputation [190].

Healthcare professionals can reduce the potential for serious or severe AEs among their patients through risk assessment and identification of patients who are at a lower risk of AEs before initiating SGLT-2i therapy, ongoing monitoring through regular clinic visits, and by being aware of and educating their patients to recognize early signs and symptoms associated with possible development of complications and the need to seek medical attention should these occur.

Conclusions

Additional studies are providing clinical evidence on the role of SGLT-2is in the treatment of patients with HFpEF with or without T2D. The EMPEROR-Preserved study results of empagliflozin in HFpEF are encouraging, and the ongoing DELIVER study will also provide data on dapagliflozin use in HFpEF.

The increasing amount of evidence for SGLT-2i therapy in patients with HF who do not have T2D will likely lead to increased use in cardiology practice.

Given their favorable benefit-risk profile and wide-ranging effects, it is hoped that SGLT-2is will provide a useful treatment option to help reduce the significant disease burden associated with HF in patients without T2D as well as in those with T2D.

Insights into SGLT2 Inhibitor Treatment of Diabetic Cardiomyopathy: Focus on the Mechanisms

https://doi.org/10.1186/s12933-023-01816-5

A machine generated summary based on the work of Huang, Keming; Luo, Xianling; Liao, Bin; Li, Guang; Feng, Jian

2023 in Cardiovascular Diabetology

Abstract-Summary SGLT2i treatment benefits metabolism, microcirculation, mitochondrial function, fibrosis, oxidative stress, endoplasmic reticulum stress, programmed cell death, autophagy, and the intestinal flora, which are involved in diabetic cardiomyopathy.

This review summarizes the current knowledge of the mechanisms of SGLT2i for the treatment of diabetic cardiomyopathy.

Introduction

Diabetes may have been recognized more than 3000 years ago [191], and the incidence and prevalence of this ancient disease have increased with improvements in living and health standards.

The pathology of diabetic cardiomyopathy includes abnormal carbohydrate and fatty acid metabolism, microvascular disease, endothelial dysfunction, mitochondrial dysfunction, myocardial diastolic dysfunction and fibrosis, excessive cardiomyocyte programmed cell death, increased oxidative stress, endoplasmic reticulum (ER) stress, and glycotoxicity [192–194].

Diabetic cardiomyopathy is known to significantly increase the risk of heart failure and can lead to a preserved or reduced ejection fraction [195].

In a randomized controlled trial, dapagliflozin reduced heart failure by 27% in T2DM (type 2 diabetes mellitus) patients with cardiovascular disease.

SGLT2i and Improved Heart Function

The aromatic O-glycoside sergliflozin and the aromatic C-glycoside dapagliflozin officially opened the era of selective SGLT inhibitors [196].

Empagliflozin, dapagliflozin, and canagliflozin are 2600, 1200, and 150 times more selective for SGLT2 than for SGLT1 [197].

SGLT1 is expressed by cardiomyocytes and may be a target of SGLT2i that improves heart failure [198].

Inhibiting SGLT1 with canagliflozin was shown to reduce nicotinamide adenine dinucleotide phosphate (NADPH) oxidase activity in cardiomyocytes, thereby inhibiting the production of superoxide and decreasing inflammation [198].

Dapagliflozin and canagliflozin were reported to directly inhibit Na^+/H^+ exchanger-1 (NHE1) and abrogate the increase in cytosolic Na^+ in cardiomyocytes.

Other studies have shown that the cardiac sodium channel Nav1.5 was a target of SGLT2i and that inhibiting sodium channels ameliorated dysfunctional sodium and calcium homeostasis, improved calcium overload, and decreased the incidence of malignant arrhythmias [199].

SGLT2i and the Regulation of Heart Metabolism

Although each molecule of fatty acid produces more ATP than glucose, complete oxidation requires more oxygen.

Compared with the absence of diabetes, oxidative metabolism in cardiomyocytes under diabetic conditions consumes a higher percentage of fatty acids and a lower percentage of glucose [200], and there is an increase in the use of ketone bodies [201].

Empagliflozin has been shown to increase glucose uptake in the human and murine myocardium that was associated with increased GLUT1 expression [109].

Increased fatty acid utilization increases the oxygen requirements of cardiomyocytes.

The mRNA and protein expression of CPT1b was reduced by subcutaneous injection of empagliflozin [202], which indicates that SGLT2i improved cardiomyocyte energy metabolism by reducing fatty acid utilization.

Adiponectin is a peptide that is secreted by adipocytes, and its effects on lipid metabolism are reflected by a negative correlation with serum TG and association with increased utilization of glucose and fatty acids by muscle tissue [203].

SGLT2i and Myocardial Mitochondria

Mitochondrial biogenesis and the growth and division of preexisting mitochondria are regulated by AMPK, peroxisome-proliferator-activated receptor γ coactivator-1α (PGC-1α), and nuclear respiratory factors (NRF)-1 and -2 [204].

AMPK activation was shown to increase the transcription of the PGC-1α gene in rat cell nuclei, which then induced the expression of the transcription factor NRF-1 [205].

Activation of PGC-1α, NRF-1, and mtTFA increases the transcription and replication of mitochondrial DNA.

Secker and others [206] found that canagliflozin inhibited the activity of mitochondrial respiratory complex I and promoted complex II activity, and empagliflozin and dapagliflozin increased the activity of complex I. Improvements in mitochondrial function by SGLT2i may be related to a decrease in O-GlcNAcylation.

Dapagliflozin and other SGLT2i may improve the function of the mitochondrial respiratory chain by directly reducing O-GlcNAc transferase activity and O-GlcNAcylation [207].

SGLT2i Improve Cardiovascular Disease and Microcirculation

Primary cultures of rat aortic endothelial cells transduced with an adenovirus encoding a dominant-negative Drp1K38A mutant showed significant inhibition of TNF-α-induced NF-κB-driven promoter activity and VCAM-1 induction.

SGLT2i were reported to improve endothelial function in mice with STZ-induced diabetes by inhibiting abnormal mitochondrial fission and endothelial inflammation [208].

Uric acid concentrations higher than physiological levels inhibit NO synthesis, reduce NO activity and induce NF-κB, leading to the induction of monocyte chemoattractant protein 1 and cyclooxygenase 2 (COX-2), which mediate inflammation and atherosclerosis [209].

Uthman and others [210] reported that dapagliflozin and empagliflozin inhibited TNFα-induced ROS generation in human coronary arterial endothelial cells, and the subsequent decrease in NO consumption was responsible for improved blood vessel dilatation.

Canagliflozin also inhibited angiogenesis in the lower limbs of mice with diabetes and lower limb ischaemia by inhibiting the secretion of vascular endothelial growth factor A by bone marrow-derived mesenchymal stem cells and reducing the proliferation and migration of mesenchymal stem cells [211].

SGLT2i Improve Ventricular Compliance and Myocardial Fibrosis

Myocardial fibrosis occurs in cardiomyopathy associated with diabetes, and it involves the accumulation of advanced glycation end products (AGEs) [212] and increased myocardial stiffness that interferes with ventricular diastole.

Activation of the receptor for AGE (RAGE) by AGEs promotes the proliferation, function, and migration of cardiac fibroblasts, which exacerbates myocardial fibrosis and accelerates cardiac ageing [212–214].

In a mouse model of type 2 diabetes, myocardial expression of collagen I and collagen III proteins and connective tissue fraction was increased compared with that in nondiabetic mice and was partially reversed by empagliflozin [215].

The effect of SGLT2i on this pathway was demonstrated by Lee and others [216], who found that dapagliflozin induced macrophage polarization to the M2 phenotype and inhibited the M1 phenotype by stimulating signal transducer and activator of transcription 3 (STAT3) signalling in mice with myocardial infarction and attenuated the increase in collagen after infarction.

SGLT2i Inhibit Oxidative Stress

In an isoprenaline (ISO)-induced oxidative stress model, the phosphorylation of eNOS was significantly inhibited in the heart and kidney and was reversed by canagliflozin [217, 218].

In an ISO-induced oxidative stress model, myocardial expression of iNOS was upregulated more than 3 times, but canagliflozin significantly reduced iNOS levels, which also decreased superoxide and nitrate [217].

Myocardial oxidative stress caused by ISO manifested as increased levels of MDA, advanced protein oxidation products, and myeloperoxidase and decreased levels of catalase, SOD, and GSH in the myocardium and plasma.

SIRT1 could decrease oxidative stress in diabetic cardiomyopathy [219, 220].

SGLT2i activate SIRT1 and its downstream signals [221, 222], which helps to explain how SGLT2i decrease oxidative stress in diabetic cardiomyopathy.

The antioxidant effect induced by the activation of SIRT1 in T1DM diabetic cardiomyopathy mainly includes the SIRT1/Nrf2 signalling pathway [219], while in T2DM, it includes the Sirtl/forkhead box class O1 (FOXO1) signalling pathway [220].

In Diabetes Patients, SGLT2i Rescue Cardiomyocytes from Programmed Cell Death

Recent studies reported that SGLT2i inhibited caspase-1 and that the mechanism involved a pathway including AMPK/NLRP3/apoptosis-associated speck-like protein containing a CARD (ASC) [223–226].

The mRNA expression of NLRP3, ASC, IL-1β, and caspase-1 in cardiomyocytes did not increase significantly in wild-type mice but did so in the myocardia of type 2 diabetic (BTBR ob/ob) mice [29].

Dapagliflozin was not associated with the expression of NLRP3, ASC, IL-1β, or caspase-1 in normal wild-type mice but did reverse these factors in BTBR mice.

LPS increased the mRNA expression of NLRP3 and caspase-1 and decreased the P-AMPK/total-AMPK ratio in cardiac fibroblasts in wild-type and BTBR mice.

Preincubation of cardiac fibroblasts with dapagliflozin attenuated the changes in the mRNA expression of NLRP3 and caspase-1 and the ratio of P-AMPK/total AMPK induced by LPS in wild-type and BTBR mice [29].

SGLT2i and Autophagy in the Myocardium

Empagliflozin has been reported to increase autophagy in the atrial tissue of ZDF rats.

Li and others [227] reported that empagliflozin decreased the protein expression of CD36, which was associated with an increase in p-AMPK, which activated the AMPK/Unc-51-like kinase 1 (Ulk1)/Beclin1 pathway, increased Ulk1 and Beclin1 expression, and promoted autophagy.

The difference might be related to nutritional status in the two models because AMPK activates Ulk1 to promote autophagy during glucose starvation.

Jiang and others [228] reported that in T1DM or T2DM and myocardial infarction, cardiomyocyte survival benefitted from the inhibition of enhanced autophagy by empagliflozin, which depended on the downregulation of NHE1 and NHE1-related genes that induce autophagy, such as Beclin 1 and autophagy-related protein 5.

Empagliflozin was shown to inhibit the increase in autophagy caused by myocardial infarction with acute hyperglycaemia.

Empagliflozin can also reverse the increase in the autophagy-related protein LC3II/I and decrease in P62 in cardiomyocytes induced by Tat-beclin1.

SGLT2i Reverse ER Stress in Diabetic Cardiomyopathy

ER stress involves disturbances in Ca^{2+} or redox balance and the accumulation of misfolded or unfolded proteins that cannot be processed, which initiates an unfolded protein response (UPR) that leads to apoptosis [229].

PERK/eIF2α/ATF4/C/EBP-homologous protein (CHOP) are signalling pathways involved in ER stress.

In these ER stress models induced by heart pressure overload or I/R injury, dapagliflozin and empagliflozin inhibited the increase in p-PERK and its downstream molecules associated with ER stress due to pressure overload by activating SIRT1 and preventing GRP78 detachment [230, 231].

SGLT2i have been shown to inhibit ER stress through similar downstream pathways in various organs.

SGLT2i Improve Diabetic Cardiomyopathy by Regulating the Intestinal Microbiota

Dapagliflozin has been associated with changes in the gut microbiota, the function of extraintestinal blood vessels, and improvements in cardiovascular dysfunction caused by diabetes.

Eight weeks of dapagliflozin treatment significantly increased Akkermansia muciniphila in the gut microbiota and improved generalized vascular dysfunction in mice with T2DM [232].

An increase in the abundance of A. muciniphila and improvements in glucose tolerance and blood glucose levels have been confirmed and correlated with induction of Foxp3-positive regulatory T cells [233].

An increase in A. muciniphila was also shown to reduce endotoxaemia and inflammation and prevent atherosclerosis by inducing the expression of tight junction proteins in the gut [234].

Empagliflozin has been associated with an increase in the population of SCFA-producing bacteria and improvements in diabetes and cardiovascular function [235].

These findings suggest that inhibition of SGLT1 reduces glucose uptake, while unabsorbed glucose temporarily reaches the lower small intestine [236], resulting in an altered glucose load and a possibly altered gut microbiota composition.

SGLT2i in Clinical Treatment

SGLT2i improves myocardial metabolism in diabetic patients.

SGLT2i (dapagliflozin, empagliflozin, canagliflozin) reduce the expression of PPAR-γ in the hearts of patients.

In a clinical randomized controlled trial, the SGLT2i empagliflozin significantly reduced the left ventricular mass relative to body surface area [237].

A randomized controlled trial of dapagliflozin demonstrated a significant reduction in left ventricular mass (LVM) in patients with T2DM and left ventricular hypertrophy (LVH) [238].

In diabetes patients with atherosclerotic disease, endothelial changes occur in the microvasculature and macrovasculature, and 12 weeks of dapagliflozin treatment resulted in a significant increase in FMD [239].

In a 12 week double-blind randomized trial, significant changes in gut microbiota diversity or composition were not observed in T2DM patients after dapagliflozin treatment [240].

In patients with HFpEF, especially those with stage A-B heart failure, the effect of SGLT2i treatment is not significant.

Current Challenges and Future Therapeutic Strategies

The use of SGLT2i has been reported to increase the risk of urinary and genital tract infections by more than 3 times [241].

The use of SGLT2i is strongly recommended in patients with HFrEF and with or without T2DM, patients with T2DM and coronary heart disease, patients with T2DM were over 50 years old who had risk factors associated with coronary heart disease, and patients with albuminuric renal disease with or without T2DM.

For patients with suspected ketoacidosis symptoms such as nausea, vomiting, abdominal pain, and dyspnoea during SGLT2i use, blood and urine ketone body analysis should be performed in time.

For patients with urinary tract infection during medication use, SGLT2i administration should be paused, and anti-infective therapy should be given.

SGLT2i should be discontinued in patients with recurrent urinary tract infections.

Patients taking SGLT2i and diuretics together need to monitor their blood pressure.

Conclusions

We mainly focused on basic studies to elucidate the pharmacological mechanism of SGLT2i and related signalling pathways or targets for the treatment of diabetic cardiomyopathy.

Studies have shown that SGLT2i can improve diabetic cardiomyopathy by improving myocardial metabolism, restoring mitochondrial function, improving microcirculatory disorders, reducing myocardial fibrosis, reducing oxidative stress, inhibiting programmed death, regulating autophagy, inhibiting ER stress and regulating the intestinal flora.

Our aim was to arouse more attention from readers through this review to further explore the potential mechanisms and targets of SGLT2i in the treatment of diabetic cardiomyopathy in the clinic and lay a solid foundation for the reasonable use of SGLT2i; SGLT2i can save more patients with diabetic cardiomyopathy.

Improved Erythrocyte Deformability Induced by Sodium-Glucose Cotransporter 2 Inhibitors in Type 2 Diabetic Patients

https://doi.org/10.1007/s10557-020-07067-w

A machine generated summary based on the work of Son, Minkook; Lee, Ye Sung; Hong, A Ram; Yoon, Jee Hee; Kim, Hee Kyung; Kang, Ho-Cheol; Yang, Sung

2020 in Cardiovascular Drugs and Therapy

Abstract-Summary Sodium-glucose cotransporter 2 (SGLT-2) inhibitors are anti-diabetic drugs that improve cardiovascular outcomes.

Although these factors increase blood viscosity and the risk of cardiovascular disease, SGLT-2 inhibitors have protective effects on the cardiovascular system.

The mechanisms for this paradoxical phenomenon remain unclear, and the effect of SGLT-2 inhibitors on hemorheology has not been studied.

Both blood viscosity and erythrocyte aggregation increased in the SGLT-2 inhibitor group, although erythrocyte deformability was significantly improved compared with that of the DPP-4 inhibitor group (DPP-4 inhibitor 43.71 ± 5.13 nm; SGLT-2 inhibitor 53.88 ± 4.88 nm; $p < 0.001$).

When the two groups were compared after propensity score matching, no differences in blood viscosity at high shear rates and erythrocyte aggregation were observed, although erythrocyte deformability was significantly improved in the SGLT-2 inhibitor group (DPP-4 inhibitor 45.01 ± 5.28 nm; SGLT-2 inhibitor 53.14 ± 4.72 nm; $p = 0.001$).

This study demonstrates that erythrocyte deformability was improved in the SGLT-2 inhibitor group compared with that in the DPP-4 inhibitor group.

Introduction

Although many studies have investigated the effects of conventional antidiabetic drugs on cardiovascular complications, in most cases, no significant improvement in cardiovascular outcomes is observed following treatment with these drugs, regardless of the efficacy of their glucose-lowering activity [242].

Although the mechanisms underlying the effects of SGLT-2 inhibitors on the cardiovascular system remain unclear, it is difficult to reconcile these cardiovascular effects simply with blood glucose control, and several different mechanisms may be responsible [87, 243].

Although a previous study has reported that blood viscosity increases with increased hematocrit following treatment with SGLT-2 inhibitors [244], the effect of this drug on erythrocyte aggregation and deformability in terms of hemorheology has not been reported.

In this study, the hemorheological effects of antidiabetic drugs including SGLT-2 inhibitors were investigated, and the effects of these changes on the cardiovascular system were analyzed.

Materials and Methods

At the outpatient visit, patient weight, height, blood pressure, and heart rate were measured.

A physical examination was performed, and smoking and alcohol drinking habits, comorbidities, medications, and diabetic complications of each patient were recorded.

The venous blood of all patients was then collected after fasting for at least 8 h and transferred to an EDTA tube for blood tests.

Blood glucose, creatinine, total cholesterol, high-density lipoprotein (HDL), low-density lipoprotein (LDL), and triglyceride levels were measured using a Cobas 8000 c702 modular analyzer (Roche, Penzberg, Germany).

Blood viscosity was measured twice per patient at shear rates of 5, 45, 90, 200, 300, 500, and 1000/s at 37 °C, using a rotational cone-and-plate viscometer (HAAKE MARS II, Thermo Scientific, Waltham, USA).

After diluting 2 μL of blood 200-fold in Alsever's solution (Sigma-Aldrich, St. Louis, MO, USA), individual samples were loaded into Tomodish (Tomocube,

Daejeon, Korea), and 40 random erythrocytes were examined per patient using the microscope.

Results

In the erythrocyte aggregation assessment, λ_{ESR} of the DPP-4 inhibitor group was significantly higher in both hematocrit (hematocrit 30%: DPP-4 inhibitor 4.68 ± 1.48, SGLT-2 inhibitor 3.86 ± 1.29, $p = 0.019$; hematocrit 40%: DPP-4 inhibitor 7.76 ± 2.10, SGLT-2 inhibitor 6.74 ± 2.11, $p = 0.047$).

Erythrocyte membrane fluctuation was significantly higher in the SGLT-2 inhibitor group (DPP-4 inhibitor: 43.71 ± 5.13 nm, SGLT-2 inhibitor: 53.88 ± 4.88 nm, $p < 0.001$).

In the erythrocyte aggregation assessment, λ_{ESR} of the DPP-4 inhibitor group tended to be higher, but the result was not significant (hematocrit 30%: DPP-4 inhibitor 4.45 ± 1.55, SGLT-2 inhibitor 3.80 ± 1.19, $p = 0.139$; hematocrit 40%: DPP-4 inhibitor 7.33 ± 1.94, SGLT-2 inhibitor 6.73 ± 1.90, $p = 0.303$).

Discussion

Of previous studies, it can be assumed that the erythrocyte deformability of diabetic patients is already impaired, with a higher possibility of impairment in those using SGLT-2 inhibitors.

The SGLT-2 inhibitor group had elevated levels of hemoglobin and hematocrit compared with the DPP-4 inhibitor group, and blood viscosity was higher at all shear rates.

There was no significant difference in blood viscosity between the groups at shear rates of 200 to 1000/s. At these high shear rates, viscosity is affected by erythrocyte deformability, indirectly indicating that despite the increase in hematocrit, blood viscosity may drop owing to the improvement in membrane deformability in the SGLT-2 inhibitor group.

The average erythrocyte membrane fluctuation in the SGLT-2 inhibitor group was 53.88 nm, which was lower than that observed in healthy subjects, but higher than that in the DPP-4 inhibitor group.

Switch to SGLT2 Inhibitors and Improved Endothelial Function in Diabetic Patients with Chronic Heart Failure

https://doi.org/10.1007/s10557-021-07254-3

A machine generated summary based on the work of Correale, Michele; Mazzeo, Pietro; Mallardi, Adriana; Leopizzi, Alessandra; Tricarico, Lucia; Fortunato,

Martino; Magnesa, Michele; Tucci, Salvatore; Maiellaro, Pasquale; Pastore, Giuseppe; Lamacchia, Olga; Iacoviello, Massimo; Di Biase, Matteo; Brunetti, Natale Daniele

2021 in Cardiovascular Drugs and Therapy

Abstract-Summary We therefore sought to evaluate possible changes in endothelial function assessed by flow-mediated dilation (FMD) in patients with chronic heart failure (CHF) and type-2 diabetes mellitus (T2DM), switching from other oral hypoglycemic agents to SGLT2i in an observational study.

Three months of therapy with SGLT2i were associated with a statistically significant improvement in endothelial function (19.0 ± 5.7% vs 8.5 ± 4.1%, $p < 0.0001$); baseline levels of FMD were comparable between groups (p n.s.).

Therapy with SGLT2i was significantly associated to improved FMD levels even at multivariable stepwise regression analysis ($p < 0.001$).

Switch to SGLT2i in patients with CHF and T2DM was associated in an observational non-randomized study with an improved endothelial function.

Background

The EMPA-REG OUTCOME trial [65] was the first to demonstrate significant cardioprotective benefits in HF patients with empagliflozin, a SGLT2i.

Its impressive 35% reduction in HF hospitalizations supported a possible role for SGLT2i among drugs for HF therapy, either with or without diabetes.

The use of SGLT2i was associated in previous studies with an improved vascular function in non-human experimental models [87, 232–246]; this improvement may represent an important mechanism underlying the cardiovascular benefits of SGLT2i treatment.

We therefore sought to evaluate possible changes in endothelial function assessed by flow-mediated dilation (FMD) in patients with CHF and T2DM switching from other oral hypoglycemic agents to SGLT2i in an observational study.

Methods

In all patients, endothelial function was assessed by FMD at baseline and after 3 months of follow-up.

All patients underwent blood analysis and ECG in an ambulatory setting, under resting conditions at baseline and after 3 months of therapy with SGLT2i.

FMD of the brachial artery was assessed under standardized condition, according to the "Brachial Artery Reactivity Task Force's guidelines" [247].

A high-resolution US device Philips EPIQ 7C ultrasound system with vascular software, a 7.5–12-MHz linear array transducer, and an ECG-gated image capture system for calculating the brachial artery diameter in real time by analyzing B mode US images were used.

After 1 min of flow image baseline acquisition, the artery was occluded by inflating the cuff to a suprasystolic pressure for 5 min (typically at least 50 mmHg above systolic pressure).

FMD was analyzed as the percentage increase in brachial artery diameter after the application of a pressure stimulus, as reported elsewhere [248].

Results

Of 22 patients treated with SGLT2i, 64% (14) received empagliflozin, 18% (4) dapagliflozin, and 18% (4) canagliflozin; 3 were also treated with both insulin and oral antidiabetics (14%), 8 with insulin (36%), and 9 with OAD (41%).

Of 23 patients not receiving SGLT2i, 2 were treated with both insulin and OAD (8.7%), 5 with insulin (21.7%), and 16 with OAD (69.6%).

Treatment with SGLT2i was also associated with statistically significant reductions in glycated hemoglobin levels (7.7 ± 1.0% vs 8.2 ± 1.2%, $p < 0.01$) and non-significant reductions in CRP (2.0 ± 2.2 vs 3.0 ± 3.6 mg/dl, p n.s.) and NTproBNP levels (581.6 ± 564.5 vs 1609.3 ± 2543.3, p 0.09).

Discussion

In the EMBLEM trial [249], a multicenter, placebo-controlled, double-blind, randomized trial designed to evaluate the effect of empagliflozin on endothelial function as assessed by reactive hyperemia-peripheral arterial tonometry (RH-PAT) in patients with T2DM and established CVD, 24 weeks of treatment did not affect endothelial function compared with placebo.

Results from ADDENDA-BHS2 study (a prospective, single-center, active-controlled, open, randomized trial, where 98 participants were randomized to either dapagliflozin 10 mg/day or glibenclamide 5 mg/day on top of metformin) demonstrated that dapagliflozin improved micro- and macrovascular endothelial function compared to glibenclamide (rest FMD changed by +3.3(8.2)% and − 1.2(7.5)% for the dapagliflozin and glibenclamide arms, respectively ($p = 0.0001$)), regardless of glycemic control in patients with T2DM and subclinical carotid atherosclerotic disease [239].

Conclusions

Switch to SGLT2i in patients with CHF and T2DM was associated in an observational non-randomized study with an improved endothelial function.

Main limitation of the study is the small number of patients enrolled and the observational nature of the study; these preliminary results need to be confirmed in properly powered multicentric and randomized studies.

No data are available on plasma levels of nitrite/nitrate and or endothelin, which would be of great interest in order to clarify possible pathways of interaction.

The study is underpowered to consider possible difference between groups of borderline significance (see mineralocorticoids receptor antagonists).

The Enhanced Cardiac Outcome of Conjugated SGLT2 Inhibitors and GLP-1RA Therapy in Diabetic Patients

https://doi.org/10.1007/s11886-021-01619-8

A machine generated summary based on the work of Fadah, Kahtan; Alashi, Alaa; Deoker, Abhizith

2022 in Current Cardiology Reports

Abstract-Summary We assess the most recent findings of synergistic effects of combined glucagon-like peptide 1 receptor agonists (GLP-1RAs) and sodium-glucose cotransporter 2 (SGLT2) inhibitors in lowering cardiac complications in the diabetic population.

SGLT2 inhibitors and GLP-1RAs have gained popularity due to their ability to reduce major adverse cardiovascular events in diabetic patients.

There is emerging evidence of the additional cardiovascular benefit from the combined application of SGLT2 inhibitors and GLP-1RAs therapy demonstrated by a recent real-world cohort study.

Introduction

Cardiovascular disease (CVD) remains the leading cause of death worldwide.

Cardiovascular events are significantly associated with diabetes mellitus type 2 (DM2), which is the primary driver of mortality and morbidity in patients with DM2.

These therapies became an attractive selection, due to their putative mechanisms to reduce the risk of major adverse cardiovascular events (MACE) with the exception of the exenatide, which was not different from placebo [32, 66, 250, 251].

Both the American Diabetes Association and the European Society of Cardiology in 2019 recommend the use of SGLT-2 inhibitors and GLP-1 RAs in diabetic patients with underlying cardiovascular disease who require further glycemic control [111, 252].

Article, we summarize the mechanism of action and cardiovascular benefits of both SGLT2 inhibitors and GLP-1RAs and highlight the enhanced value of combined therapy on major cardiovascular events (MACE).

SGLT2 Inhibitors Mechanism of Action

SGLT2 inhibitors and GLP-1 RAs have repeatedly shown an improvement in cardiovascular outcomes as monotherapy or add-on therapy to other anti-diabetic drugs.

A recent large real-world cohort study of cardiovascular incremental outcome from combined SGLT2 inhibitors and GLP-1 RAs in diabetic patients by Dave and others was published at circulation [253].

This study noted 107 cardiovascular endpoint events with an adjusted pooled hazard ratio (HR) of 0.76 (95% CI: 0.59, 0.98) among patients who had SGLT2 inhibitors on top of GLP-1RAs compared to 129 events among those who had sulfonylurea initiators as an add-on therapy.

The overall outcome of these analyses demonstrated the additional cardiovascular value of combined SGLT2 inhibitors and GLP-1RAs therapy in diabetic patients.

This study provides critical clinical information of expected improved cardiovascular outcomes when SGLT2 inhibitors added to GLP-1 RAs therapy.

Conclusion

GLP-1RAS and SGLT2 inhibitors individually have shown superior effect on improving MACE and CV deaths and are being increasingly used.

While limitation such drug cost, drug side effects such as genital infection and gastrointestinal have restricted the size of diabetic population that could benefit from these two drug classes.

The emerging new evidence of the additional value of dual GLP-1RAS and SGLT2 inhibitors treatment is of major importance to further minimize the number of CV-related deaths annually.

In return, further randomized prospective clinical trials to evaluate potential advantage of GLP-1RAS and SGLT2 inhibitors dual therapy are needed to guide future anti-diabetic treatment with confidence.

Benefits of SGLT2i for the Treatment of Heart Failure Irrespective of Diabetes Diagnosis: A State-of-the-Art Review

https://doi.org/10.1007/s13300-022-01278-0

A machine generated summary based on the work of Delgado, Elías; Jódar, Esteban; Mezquita-Raya, Pedro; Moreno-Pérez, Óscar

2022 in Diabetes Therapy

Abstract-Summary HF-associated risk in patients with type 2 diabetes mellitus (T2D) is even higher than in patients without T2D owing to the strong reciprocal relationship between conditions.

Until recently, no therapy to treat patients with diabetes also reduced cardiovascular risks related to HF.

Recent clinical studies (DAPA-HF, EMPEROR-Reduced and EMPEROR-Preserved, SOLOIST-WHF trial) and meta-analysis have demonstrated that sodium–glucose cotransporter-2 inhibitors (SGLT2i) are among the first antidiabetic drugs capable of reducing cardiovascular risks related to HF and improving the prognosis of patients with and without diabetes.

Introduction

In patients with HF, morbidity and mortality remain high despite advances in therapy.

Patients with type 2 diabetes mellitus (T2D) who had five risk-factor variables within target ranges [glycated hemoglobin level, low-density lipoprotein cholesterol level (LDLc), albuminuria, smoking, and blood pressure] appeared to have little or no excess risk of death, myocardial infarction, or stroke compared with the general population.

The overall hazard ratio for hospitalization for HF among patients with no risk-factor variables outside the target ranges, compared with controls, was 1.45 [95% confidence interval (CI) 1.34–1.57] [254].

Several HF risk scores have been published, and most of them have reported a remarkably consistent list of the principal risk factors, including age, sex, coronary artery disease (CAD), myocardial infarction (MI), hypertension, obesity, and diabetes mellitus (DM), particularly T2D [255].

General Mechanisms of Heart Failure (Preserved and Reduced)

Of worsening LV remodeling and cardiac decompensation, patients transition from asymptomatic to symptomatic HF [256].

HF with reduced ejection fraction (HFrEF) is considered in patients with an LVEF ≤40%, with or without signs of clinical HF.

Those patients with an LVEF between 41% and 49% have HF with mildly reduced EF (HFmrEF), and those with an LVEF ≥50% and symptoms and signs of HF, with evidence of structural and/or functional cardiac abnormalities and/or raised natriuretic peptides (NPs), have HF with preserved ejection fraction (HFpEF).

The definition of pre-HFpEF is taking shape as presenting in an asymptomatic patient (absence of signs or symptoms of HF) with preserved LVEF, structural heart abnormalities (similar to those reported for HFpEF), and elevated biomarker surrogates of cardiac dysfunction (mainly natriuretic peptides, with cut-point values similar to those reported for HFpEF).

Heart Failure in Patients With and Without T2DM, Current Understanding and Clinical Practice Consequences

T2D is an independent risk factor for HF in many hospital-based and population-based cardiovascular studies, and in particular, it has been estimated that, compared with patients without diabetes, the risk of HF is fivefold and twofold higher in women and men with diabetes, respectively [257].

The presence of diabetes markedly increases the risk of 1-year adverse clinical outcomes in outpatients with HF independent of multiple common risk factors.

Patients with T2D have an increased risk of developing HF, but also those with HF are at higher risk for the development of T2D and a worse prognosis when both pathologies are present [258].

The development of HF in these patients produces an increased mortality risk and worse evolution.

Description of the Pathological Mechanisms that Link T2D with Heart Failure: Direct and Indirect Effects of SGLT2i on Myocardial Function

T2D can lead to the development of HFrEF and HFpEF through diverse mechanisms.

The available evidence suggests that T2D can promote the development of HFrEF by two main mechanisms: (1) by activating the sodium–hydrogen exchanger and undermining cardiomyocyte survival [259] and (2) by suppressing nutrient deprivation signaling autophagy and thereby promoting cardiomyocyte stress and dysfunction [259].

T2D can promote the development of HFpEF by enhancing the expansion of visceral (and especially epicardial) adipose tissue depots, which can promote cardiac inflammation, fibrosis, and microcirculatory dysfunction.

SGLT2i in Clinical Trials and Meta-Analyses in Heart Failure

The main outcome (cardiovascular death or hospitalization for heart failure) event was significantly reduced in the empagliflozin (19.4%) group compared with the placebo (24.7%) group (HR 0.75, 95% CI 0.65–0.86, $P < 0.001$; NNT 19), and this reduction was consistent in patients regardless of their diabetes status.

In the EMPEROR-Preserved Trial carried out in 5988 patients with HF and EF > 40%, empagliflozin was also demonstrated to reduce the combined risk of cardiovascular death or hospitalization for HF in patients with HFpEF (HR 0.79, 95% CI 0.69–0.90, $P < 0.001$), regardless of the presence or absence of diabetes, with an NNT of 31.

In these patients with T2D with newly diagnosed, worsening heart failure, sotagliflozin therapy started before or shortly after discharge resulted in a significantly lower total number of deaths from cardiovascular causes and hospitalizations and urgent visits for HF than placebo (HR 0.67, 95% CI 0.52–0.85, $P < 0.001$).

New Guidelines: Moving towards an Intensive and Multidimensional Approach for HF Treatment

On the basis of this clinical evidence, several HF guidelines have introduced SGLT2i as a first-line HF treatment [187, 260, 261].

The Canadian guidelines [261] recommend that, in the absence of contraindications, patients with HFrEF be treated with combination therapy from the beginning, including one evidenced-based medication from each of the categories (ARNI, B-blocker, MRA, and SGLT2i) (strong recommendation; moderate level of evidence).

Future Perspectives in the Treatment of HF for Patients with and Without T2D

On the basis of these promising findings in patients with chronic HF, it would be interesting to develop studies that assess the early use of SGLT2i in the acute phase of admission for HF and personalize treatment for the most significant benefit.

The EMPULSE-HF study has shown that, among patients with acute decompensated HF, empagliflozin versus placebo is associated with significant clinical benefits at 90 days.

Some authors suggest the importance of evaluating the clinical efficacy and safety of the SGLT2i in nondiabetic patients with acute decompensated HF [262].

In the DARE-19 trial, treatment with dapagliflozin did not result in a statistically significant risk reduction in organ dysfunction, death, or improvement in clinical recovery in patients with coronavirus disease 2019 (COVID-19) [263].

Conclusions

In HF, morbidity and mortality remain high despite advances in therapy, and new therapies are needed to improve the prognosis of these patients, mainly when T2D is also present.

Several recent clinical studies (DAPA-HF, EMPEROR-Reduced, EMPEROR-Preserved, SOLOIST-WHF trial) and meta-analyses have demonstrated that SGLT2i reduce the risk of HF hospitalization, improve QOL, and increase survival in HF across the whole LVEF spectrum.

In light of the favorable results obtained in the studies as mentioned above, SGLT2i are among the first antidiabetic drugs capable of reducing cardiovascular risks related to HF and consistently improving the prognosis in different populations and settings.

On the basis of this clinical evidence, several HF guidelines have introduced SGLT2i as a first-line treatment for HF from the start, and several studies are underway to specify the role of SGLT2i with regard to HF outcomes in different vulnerable populations, including the hospital setting.

Emerging Horizons in Heart Failure with Preserved Ejection Fraction: The Role of SGLT2 Inhibitors

https://doi.org/10.1007/s13300-022-01204-4

A machine generated summary based on the work of Heath, Rebecca; Johnsen, Håkon; Strain, W. David; Evans, Marc

2022 in Diabetes Therapy

Abstract-Summary Heart failure with preserved ejection fraction (HFpEF) is a condition with increasing disease burden.

Prevalence of HFpEF is increasing, reflecting an increasingly elderly and comorbid population, as well as reinforcing the need for more treatments for this disease.

These results indicate a promising future for sodium-glucose co-transporter 2 (SGLT2) inhibitors in HFpEF.

The ongoing DELIVER trial (investigating the use of dapagliflozin in HFpEF) is awaited but could provide further evidence of support for SGLT2 inhibitors in HFpEF.

With hospital admissions for HFpEF increasing in the UK, the economic impact of treatments that reduce HHF is vast.

The European Society of Cardiology (ESC) recently added SGLT2 inhibitors to their guidelines for treatment of heart failure with reduced ejection fraction (HFrEF) following DAPA-HF and EMPEROR-Reduced trials and we suggest that similar changes be made to guidelines to support the use of SGLT2 inhibitors in the management of HFpEF in upcoming months.

Introduction

The European Society of Cardiology (ESC) recommends a simplified approach to diagnosis: signs and symptoms of HF, an LVEF of more than or equal to 50%, and objective evidence of cardiac structural and/or functional abnormalities consistent with presence of left ventricular (LV) diastolic dysfunction/raised LV filling pressures (such as LV hypertrophy, left atrial enlargement or raised natriuretic peptides) [264, 265].

The recognition of LV diastolic dysfunction and a normal ejection fraction with the clinical syndrome of HF has been around for decades, although the underlying pathophysiology in HFpEF is perhaps poorly understood when compared with HFrEF [266].

Slow LV relaxation is seen in HFpEF, especially at higher heart rates, which, along with myocardial stiffness and impaired ventricular-arterial coupling all leading to reduced stroke volume, may explain the abnormal systolic function seen in patients under stress in HFpEF despite normal systolic function at rest [265, 267].

Current Treatment Strategies in HFpEF

Unlike HFrEF, there are no treatments for HFpEF (as a unifying diagnosis) that have been proven to reduce morbidity and mortality [264, 266, 267], despite the worrying trend of increasing prevalence of this condition.

Treatment should be individually based, with treatment focusing on underlying comorbidities (this may of course mean patients are on treatments such as ACE inhibitors and beta blockers anyway).

Sodium-glucose co-transporter 2 (SGLT2) inhibitors were very recently added to the ESC guidelines for treatment of HFrEF after EMPEROR-Reduced and DAPA-HF trials showed reduced risk of cardiovascular death or hospitalisation for HF in patients with HFrEF [25, 103].

The purpose of this review is to highlight and discuss data from the recently published EMPEROR-Preserved study, as well as review previously published data on SGLT2 inhibitors and its effect on HFpEF in the context of the EMPEROR-Preserved study.

SGLT2 Inhibitors in HFrEF

The Dapagliflozin in Patients with HF and reduced Ejection Fraction (DAPA-HF) study from 2019 investigated the efficacy of SGLT2 inhibitors in patients with established HF and reduced ejection fraction, regardless of the patient being diagnosed with T2DM.

The DAPA-HF study found that death from cardiovascular causes reduced from 11.5% in the placebo group to 9.6% in the group being commenced on dapagliflozin [103].

The benefits of dapagliflozin in HFrEF were found to be consistent regardless of the patient being diagnosed with T2DM or not [103].

SGLT2 Inhibitors in HFpEF

The Empagliflozin in HF with a Preserved Ejection Fraction (EMPEROR-Preserved) study from 2021 investigated the efficacy of an SGLT2 inhibitor in patients with HF and preserved ejection fraction.

The EMPEROR-Preserved study found that treatment with empagliflozin reduced the occurrence of HHF and cardiovascular death as a combined primary outcome.

Whereas several studies investigating sacubitril/valsartan, spironolactone and candesartan in HFpEF have been unable to provide undisputable proof for their effectiveness in patients with an EF of 50% or more [268–272], subgroup analysis of the EMPEROR-Preserved patient cohort showed that empagliflozin reduced the number of primary outcome events (cardiovascular death or HHF) in patients with an EF ranging between 50% and 60% and more than 60%, when compared with placebo.

The results from the EMPEROR-Preserved study suggest that empagliflozin is beneficial for patients with HFpEF.

Potential Mechanisms Improved by SGLT2 Inhibitors on HFpEF

Recent studies suggest that empagliflozin and SGLT2 inhibitors exert their pleiotropic effect in HFpEF through various mechanisms.

A study published in 2018 where cardiomyocytes from humans and rats were exposed to empagliflozin and then investigated with the aim of discovering the mechanism of empagliflozin on cardiomyocytes concluded with empagliflozin exerting a direct effect on the cardiomyocytes [273].

Kolijn and others obtained results suggesting a further mechanism reducing myocardial stiffness: exposure to empagliflozin resulted in a significant reduction in oxidative stress and inflammation in HFpEF cardiomyocytes, and also improved endothelial vasorelaxation [274], in turn improving ventricular relaxation.

The evidence is now suggesting that SGLT2 inhibitors improve HF by exerting their effect on various mechanisms: reducing myocardial stiffness, improving the intracellular electrolyte balance, reducing oxidative inflammation, enhanced erythropoiesis and improved kidney function.

Practical Implications

A study investigating the addition of an SGLT2 inhibitor to patients with an acute myocardial infarction and a preserved ejection fraction could be very interesting regarding future management.

Subgroup analysis of the SOLOIST-WHF study suggests that an SGLT2 inhibitor is beneficial in acute decompensation of HFpEF; this study included 1222 patients who were randomised to either sotagliflozin or placebo groups, but only 20.9% of the sotagliflozin group and 21% of the placebo group had an LVEF >50% [275].

To the SOLOIST-WHF study, a future investigation should aim to include both patients with diabetes and patients without diabetes and aim to include more patients suffering from an acute decompensation of HFpEF, increasing the degree of evidence supporting the beneficial effects of an SGLT2 inhibitor in the management of HFpEF.

A pilot trial of polydiuretic therapy, including an SGLT2 inhibitor, in a small number of patients with HFpEF is ongoing with results due next year [276].

Conclusion

Their benefits in HF, but particularly in HFpEF cannot be ignored and we excitedly await further results from ongoing studies as mentioned in this review article.

The ESC recently added SGLT2 inhibitors to the management guidelines for HFrEF following good outcomes from DAPA-HF [103] and EMPEROR-Reduced [25] over the last 2 years.

We hope that further supporting evidence for SGLT2 inhibitors in the management of HFpEF follows with the results of the ongoing DELIVER trial expected soon, and that as a result similar changes to guidelines may be added to support the use of SGLT2 inhibitors in the management of HFpEF.

Efficacy and Safety of Sodium-Glucose Cotransporter 2 Inhibitors Initiation in Patients with Acute Heart Failure, with and Without Type 2 Diabetes: A Systematic Review and Meta-Analysis

https://doi.org/10.1186/s12933-022-01455-2

A machine generated summary based on the work of Salah, Husam M.; Al'Aref, Subhi J.; Khan, Muhammad Shahzeb; Al-Hawwas, Malek; Vallurupalli, Srikanth; Mehta, Jawahar L.; Mounsey, J. Paul; Greene, Stephen J.; McGuire, Darren K.; Lopes, Renato D.; Fudim, Marat

2022 in Cardiovascular Diabetology

Abstract-Summary There is uncertainty and limited data regarding initiation of sodium-glucose cotransporter 2 (SGLT2) inhibitors among patients hospitalized with acute heart failure (AHF).

This systematic review and meta-analysis aim to establish the efficacy and safety of SGLT2 inhibitors initiated in patients hospitalized for AHF.

PubMed/Medline, Embase, and Cochrane library were searched using the following terms: ("sglt2" and "acute heart failure") and ("sglt2" and "worsening heart failure") from inception till November 15th, 2021 for randomized controlled trials (RCTs) comparing the efficacy and safety of initiating an SGLT2 inhibitor compared with placebo in patients with AHF.

Initiation of SGLT2 inhibitors in patients with AHF reduced the risk of rehospitalization for heart failure (OR 0.52; 95% CI [0.42, 0.65]) and improved Kansas City Cardiomyopathy Questionnaire scores (mean difference 4.12; 95% CI [0.1.89, 6.53]).

There was no statistically significant effect for initiation of SGLT2 inhibitors in patients with AHF on all-cause mortality (OR 0.70; 95% CI [0.46, 1.08]).

Initiation of SGLT2 inhibitors in patients with AHF did not increase the acute kidney injury (OR 0.76; 95% CI [0.50, 1.16]), hypotension (OR 1.17; 95% CI [0.80, 1.71]), or hypoglycemia (OR 1.51; 95% CI [0.86, 2.65]).

Initiation of SGLT2 inhibitors in patients hospitalized for AHF during hospitalization or early post-discharge (within 3 days) reduces the risk of rehospitalization for heart failure and improves patient-reported outcomes with no excess risk of adverse effects.

Background

In a meta-analysis of the EMPEROR-Reduced and DAPA-HF trials, both of which investigated SGLT2 inhibitors in patients with chronic HF with reduced ejection fraction (HFrEF), SGLT2 inhibitors resulted in a 13% reduction in all-cause death, 14% reduction in cardiovascular death, 31% reduction in first hospitalization for HF, and 38% reduction in adverse renal outcomes in these patients [277].

This underscores the importance of evaluating the efficacy and safety of SGLT2 inhibitor initiation in patients hospitalized for AHF.

The aim of this meta-analysis is to derive more reliable estimate of the efficacy and safety of SGLT2 inhibitors initiated in patients hospitalized for AHF.

Method

The prespecified selection criteria were: (1) randomized placebo-controlled clinical trials (RCTs); (2) the active arm of the trial included an SGLT2 inhibitor that was initiated in patients hospitalized with AHF; (3) trials reported selected prespecified efficacy and safety outcomes.

Prespecified efficacy outcomes were all-cause mortality, rehospitalization for heart failure, and improvement in Kansas City Cardiomyopathy Questionnaire (KCCQ) scale score [278, 279].

The efficacy outcomes were chosen based on prior studies showing reduction in the risk of all-cause mortality and hospitalization for HF and improvement in KCCQ scale score in patients receiving SGLT2 inhibitors outside of the context of AHF [280, 281].

A random effects model meta-analysis was conducted using Mantel–Haenszel odds ratios (ORs) and the associated 95% confidence intervals (CIs) to assess all-cause mortality, rehospitalization for HF, worsening HF, AKI, hypotension, and hypoglycemia, and the inverse variance of weighted mean difference and associated 95% CIs were used to assess changes in KCCQ.

Results

The initial search yielded 106 studies (94 from databases and 12 from scientific meetings).

Follow-up periods differed between the included studies (60 days in the EMPA-RESPONSE-AHF, 90 days in the EMPULSE trial, and a median of 9 months in the SOLOIST-WHF trial).

Risk of bias and certainty of evidence for the unpublished EMPULSE trial were assessed based on the published study design and the AHA Scientific Sessions 2021 presentation [262].

Discussion

The main findings of this systematic review and meta-analysis are that initiation of SGLT2 inhibitors in patients with AHF during hospitalization or early post-discharge carries 48% lower odds of rehospitalization for HF and significant improvements in patient-reported outcomes (as measured by KCCQ), without excess risk of AKI, hypotension, or hypoglycemia.

The present meta-analysis demonstrates that initiating GDMT with SGLT2 inhibitor in patients with AHF during their hospitalizations or shortly thereafter (within 3 days of discharge) is safe and significantly reduces the risk of rehospitalization following discharge.

While both EMPA-RESPONSE-AHF and EMPULSE initiated treatment with SGLT2 prior to discharge in all patients hospitalized for AHF, the SOLOIST-WHF allowed inclusion of patients receiving the first dose of SGLT2 inhibitor up to 3 days after discharge.

Association of Sodium-Glucose Cotransporter 2 Inhibitors with Post-Discharge Outcomes in Patients with Acute Heart Failure with Type 2 Diabetes: A Cohort Study

https://doi.org/10.1186/s12933-023-01896-3

A machine generated summary based on the work of Park, Sohee; Jeong, Han Eol; Lee, Hyesung; You, Seng Chan; Shin, Ju-Young

2023 in Cardiovascular Diabetology

Abstract-Summary We investigated whether initiating treatment with SGLT2is after an episode of acute heart failure reduces the risks of post-discharge heart failure readmission or cardiovascular mortality among patients with type 2 diabetes.

A retrospective cohort study was conducted in a cohort of patients with type 2 diabetes who hospitalized for heart failure, using Korean Health Insurance Review & Assessment database (2015–2020).

We assessed hazards of post-discharge heart failure readmission and cardiovascular death at 1-year, and 30-, 60-, and 90-day from the date of discharge in the SGLT2is users and non-users.

Among 56,343 patients with type 2 diabetes hospitalized for heart failure, 29,290 patients were included in the study cohort (mean [SD] age, 74.1 [10.8] years; 56.1% women); 818 patients (2.8%) were prescribed SGLT2is during index hospitalization or at discharge.

Patients with a prescription for SGLT2i vs. those without prescription had lower rates of heart failure readmission or cardiovascular death at 1 year (22.4% vs. 25.3%; adjusted hazard ratio, 0.90 [95% confidence interval, 0.87–0.93]), and also at 30 days (7.0% vs. 7.7%; 0.74 [0.69–0.79]).

Among patients with type 2 diabetes, initiating SGLT2i treatment after an episode of acute heart failure was significantly associated with a reduced combined risk of heart failure readmission and cardiovascular mortality in a nationwide cohort reflecting routine clinical practice.

Background

Since three pivotal trials initially showed the benefit of the SGLT2i on reducing HF hospitalization in patients with T2D [4–29, 39–171, 187, 254–276, 282–290], their effects on HF have been intensively investigated and there have been substantial changes in the role of SGLT2is in clinical practice and guidelines.

Although trials with empagliflozin and sotagliflozin have individually shown meaningful clinical benefits in patients hospitalized for acute HF [275, 291], whether these observed benefits can be extended to the class of SGLT2is remains elusive as there is no available data on dapagliflozin.

Awaiting the results of ongoing trials with dapagliflozin on acute HF, we conducted a retrospective cohort study using real-world data from claims database to assess whether initiating SGLT2is after an episode of acute HF reduce combined risk of post-discharge HF readmission and cardiovascular death among patients with T2D.

Methods

We applied asymmetric propensity score trimming to exclude patients who were treated most contrary to prediction to reduce bias due to unmeasured confounders in this situation [292]; thresholds were 1st and 99th percentiles of the propensity score distribution in the SGLT2i and non-use groups, respectively.

The log-rank test and Cox proportional hazards regression models were used to evaluate the association between SGLT2i versus non-uses and the primary outcome and secondary outcome of cardiovascular death in the crude and weighted populations [293].

To assess confounding by indication, we applied two alternative comparator groups of: (1) any second-line antidiabetic agents prescribed during hospitalization or at discharge, but excluded those prescribed metformin, sulfonylurea, or insulin as monotherapy, and (2) dipeptidyl peptidase-4 inhibitor alone or in combination with other non-use antidiabetics prescribed during hospitalization or at discharge.

Results

The SGLT2i treated patients were younger (mean [SD] age, 69.1 [12.1] years), and more likely to be female (50.4%) and hospitalized for decompensated HF (27.5%) compared with the non-use group.

The SGLT2i group generally had a fewer history of comorbidities (e.g., coronary artery disease) and medication use (e.g., calcium channel blockers), despite having a higher proportion of use of HF medications at discharge such as, RASi, mineralocorticoid receptor antagonist, and angiotensin receptor/neprilysin inhibitor.

The absolute IR in the SGLT2i group was lower than the non-use group at 365 days after discharge: 26.9 versus 31.7 cases per 100 person-years.

The risk of HF readmission or cardiovascular death was lower with SGLT2is than non-use (crude HR 0.87, 95% CI 0.75–1.00; weighted HR 0.90, 95% CI 0.87–0.93) although the crude analysis did not show the statistical significance.

Discussion

After the introduction of SGLT2is as a potential therapeutic option for chronic HF, several observational studies have assessed the effectiveness of SGLT2is on acute HF and findings consistently suggested clinical benefit of SGLT2is [294–297].

Due to the nature of the retrospective database study, our study cohort was patients hospitalized for HF among T2D. As SGLT2is were exclusively prescribed for the treatment of T2D during our study period given the local reimbursement criteria in South Korea, we couldn't define a study population without restriction to diabetic patients for comparability, even though current need for evidence of the effectiveness of SGLT2is is at the patients hospitalized for HF regardless of T2D. This led to relatively small sample size in this study and findings from this study are not likely to be generalizable to patients with HF without T2D. Future studies with larger sample size and a broader population should examine the effect of SGLT2i on post-discharge outcome of acute HF addressing the additional HF-related confounding.

Conclusions

Initiating SGLT2i treatment after an episode of acute HF was significantly associated with a reduced risk of composite outcome of HF readmission and cardiovascular mortality when compared with non-use among patients with T2D. These findings suggest that potential clinical benefit of SGLT2is in the care of patients hospitalized for acute HF.

While results from ongoing trials addressing this clinical question are expected to be shared soon, our findings based on real-world data provide valuable evidence for the current context of SGLT2is.

Potential Impact of SGLT2 Inhibitors on Left Ventricular Diastolic Function in Patients with Diabetes Mellitus

https://doi.org/10.1007/s10741-018-9668-1

A machine generated summary based on the work of Tanaka, Hidekazu; Hirata, Ken-ichi

2018 in Heart Failure Reviews

Abstract-Summary The pathogenesis of diabetes mellitus (DM)-related cardiac dysfunction is thought to be multifactorial, and possibly a key factor for the development of heart failure with preserved ejection fraction (HFpEF) in patients with DM and preserved left ventricular (LV) ejection fraction.

To reduction of glycated hemoglobin levels in patients with type 2 DM, SGLT2 inhibitors are associated with weight loss and reductions in blood pressure.

Despite such intriguing results, it remains uncertain whether SGLT2 inhibitors are beneficial for LV diastolic function in patients with DM.

This review deals with the impact of SGLT2 inhibitors on LV diastolic function in patients with DM and their current potential for prevention of the future development of HFpEF in such patients.

Introduction

SGLT2 inhibitors have the potential to result in improvements in cardiovascular risk profiles, including lower blood pressure and weight loss, in addition to reducing glycated hemoglobin levels in patients with type 2 DM [65, 298, 299].

Despite such promising results, however, it remains uncertain whether SGLT2 inhibitors are beneficial for LV diastolic function in patients with DM.

This article reviews the impact of SGLT2 inhibitors on LV diastolic function in patients with DM and their current potential for prevention of the future development of HFpEF in such patients.

Association of DM with HFpEF

HFrEF evolved into a distinct therapeutic entity partly because large outcome trials demonstrated the efficacy of neurohumoral inhibition.

No similar evolution has occurred in the case of HFpEF, where large trials testing neurohumoral inhibition consistently failed to attain a positive primary outcome [300, 301].

The failure of the large HFpEF outcome trials to demonstrate neurohumoral inhibition led some investigators to challenge the notion of HFpEF as a distinct HF phenotype [302, 303].

More recent views have attributed this failure to differences in the systemic and myocardial signaling in HFpEF and HFrEF or to differences in phenotypes within the HFpEF patient population [304–306].

DM-Related Cardiac Dysfunction

LV longitudinal myocardial systolic dysfunction, known as global longitudinal strain (GLS), has been identified in DM patients with preserved LVEF without overt coronary artery disease or HF [307–316].

Some investigators have maintained that LV longitudinal myocardial systolic dysfunction, rather than LV diastolic dysfunction, should be considered the first marker of a preclinical form of DM-related cardiac dysfunction in DM patients with preserved LVEF without overt HF [307, 317].

Ernande and others showed that LV longitudinal myocardial systolic dysfunction detected as GLS < 18% was present even in DM patients with preserved LVEF and normal LV diastolic function [307].

It has thus been suggested that progression of uncontrolled DM led to LV myocardial systolic dysfunction as well as LV diastolic dysfunction, that GLS is associated with LV diastolic function, and that reduced GLS can coexist with LV diastolic dysfunction in DM patients with preserved LVEF, leading to HFpEF.

Potential Impact of SGLT2 Inhibitors on LV Diastolic Function in DM

To reducing glycated hemoglobin levels in patients with type 2 DM, SGLT2 inhibitors are associated with weight loss and reductions in blood pressure without an increase in heart rate [65, 298, 299].

A small degree of weight loss may also result from mild osmotic diuresis, but body composition studies have shown that weight loss accompanying the use of SGLT2 inhibitors principally resulted from reduction in body fat mass [318, 319]. Therefore, SGLT2 inhibitors have favorable effects on DM, hypertension, and overweight/obesity, which in turn have a significant impact on LV diastolic function, so that they may ultimately have a potential beneficial effect on LV diastolic function in patients with DM.

SGLT2 inhibitors may therefore have a positive impact on LV diastolic function in asymptomatic patients with DM and preserved LVEF, and can prevent the future development of HFpEF in such patients.

Effects of Treatment with SGLT-2 Inhibitors on Arginine-Related Cardiovascular and Renal Biomarkers

https://doi.org/10.1186/s12933-021-01436-x

A machine generated summary based on the work of Gessner, Arne; Gemeinhardt, Anna; Bosch, Agnes; Kannenkeril, Dennis; Staerk, Christian; Mayr, Andreas; Fromm, Martin F.; Schmieder, Roland E.; Maas, Renke

2022 in Cardiovascular Diabetology

Abstract-Summary Their effects on l-arginine (Arg) related risk markers asymmetric and symmetric dimethylarginine (ADMA and SDMA) and the protective biomarker L-homoarginine (hArg) linking T2D to cardiovascular and renal disease have not yet been reported.

Treatment with empagliflozin and dapagliflozin was associated with a reduction of plasma hArg by 17.5% and 13.7% (both $p < 0.001$), respectively, and increase in plasma SDMA concentration of 6.7% and 3.6%, respectively ($p < 0.001$ and $p < 0.05$), while plasma Arg and ADMA concentrations were not significantly altered.

24-h urinary excretion of ADMA was reduced by 15.2% after treatment with empagliflozin ($p < 0.001$) but not after dapagliflozin treatment, while excretion of the other markers was not significantly altered.

A reduction in ADMA clearance was observable after empagliflozin treatment only (− 15.5%, $p < 0.001$), but not after dapagliflozin.

Treatment effects on l-arginine related biomarkers were not constantly correlated with effects on glycated hemoglobin, fasting plasma glucose, body mass index, and systolic blood pressure.

Treatment with SGLT-2 inhibitors has divergent effects on Arg-related biomarkers and could affect risk estimates associated with these markers.

The observed effects are unlikely to explain the known cardiovascular and renal benefits of treatment with empagliflozin or dapagliflozin but still may indicate new therapeutic approaches in patients treated with SGLT-2 inhibitors.

Background

Inhibition of the sodium-glucose cotransporter 2 (SGLT-2), e.g. via drugs like empagliflozin and dapagliflozin, has been shown to be a very effective treatment option in T2D. SGLT-2 inhibitors not only improved glycaemic control by increased renal excretion of glucose, but also protected from cardiovascular events and decline of renal function [23, 25, 65, 66, 320–322].

As these markers are structurally and functionally interrelated, but also differ in their metabolism and/or renal handling, we hypothesised that an investigation of the effects of SGLT-2 inhibition with empagliflozin or dapagliflozin on the plasma concentration and renal excretion of Arg-related biomarkers may offer new mechanistic insights beyond the blood glucose lowering effect of the drugs.

We evaluated the effects of SGLT-2 inhibition with empagliflozin and dapagliflozin on plasma concentrations and renal excretion of Arg and its derivatives hArg, ADMA and SDMA in plasma and 24-h-urine samples from two recently completed randomized double-blind, placebo-controlled, cross-over trials [323, 324].

Methods

This study combines data and samples from two prospective, randomized, double-blind, placebo-controlled, cross-over trials of empagliflozin and dapagliflozin in patients with T2D (NCT02471963 and NCT02383238).

Blood and 24-h urine samples were collected at baseline, after 6 weeks with placebo, and after 6 weeks with empagliflozin or dapagliflozin.

In sensitivity analyses linear mixed effects models were used to investigate differences in post-baseline concentrations of biomarkers (after verum and after placebo), adjusting for concentrations at baseline and the ordering in the cross-over design.

Effect estimates of linear mixed models refer to adjusted differences in (log) concentrations between verum and placebo, which are reported with corresponding two-sided 95% confidence intervals and p-values.

In a further exploratory analysis, Pearson correlations were calculated between, on the one hand, the absolute changes in the plasma concentration from baseline to after verum treatment for hArg, Arg, ADMA, and SDMA, and on the other hand, changes in glycated haemoglobin (HbA1c), fasting plasma glucose (FPG), body mass index (BMI), and systolic blood pressure (SBP), respectively.

Results

Mean intraindividual percentage changes in comparison to baseline were −13.9% after empagliflozin treatment and +1.2% after placebo, with a p-value of $p < 0.001$.

Mean intraindividual changes compared to baseline were −10.0% after dapagliflozin and +2.2% after placebo, with a p-value of 0.003.

Mean intraindividual changes compared to baseline were +8.0% after empagliflozin and −2.8% after placebo, with a p-value of $p < 0.001$.

Intraindividual changes in comparison to baseline were −10.5% for empagliflozin and +4.1% for placebo ($p < 0.001$).

The corresponding mean intraindividual changes were −4.6% for empagliflozin and +6.3% for placebo ($p = 0.008$).

Mean intraindividual changes were −9.6% for empagliflozin and +3.0% for placebo ($p = 0.001$).

Discussion

In plasma hArg was significantly reduced and SDMA increased after treatment with both SGLT-2 inhibitors.

The Cl_R for SDMA, ADMA, and creatinine was significantly reduced (for ADMA in the empagliflozin trial only), whereas Cl_R for hArg and Arg was not significantly altered.

The main findings in changes of the biomarkers, namely increase of SDMA and reduction of hArg in plasma, show a high degree of similarity in responses to treatment for both empagliflozin and dapagliflozin.

In our studies the numerical decrease of Arg plasma concentration is not significant but we found a highly significant reduction of hArg concentrations.

The plasma concentration of ADMA was not altered by SGLT-2 inhibition, while Cl_R of ADMA was significantly reduced in the empagliflozin study.

Future studies may investigate if these correlations are coincidental or if non-reduction of SBP correlates with changes in plasma concentrations of hArg or Arg in a similar way.

Conclusions

The SGLT-2 inhibitors empagliflozin and dapagliflozin affect plasma concentrations and/or renal handling of Arg-related risk-markers, which may also affect risk estimates based on these factors.

The pattern of the observed effects on the different biomarkers was unexpected and does not provide a direct explanation (i.e. causal links) for beneficial effects of the SGLT-2 inhibitors on CVD and CKD, as the protective marker hArg was reduced and the deleterious marker SDMA was increased in plasma.

The observed effects may guide future investigations such as an exploration of a potential beneficial impact of hArg supplementation for T2D patients under therapy with an SGLT-2 inhibitor.

Comparison of SGLT2 Inhibitors with DPP-4 Inhibitors Combined with Metformin in Patients with Acute Myocardial Infarction and Diabetes Mellitus

https://doi.org/10.1186/s12933-023-01914-4

A machine generated summary based on the work of Lyu, Young Sang; Oh, Seok; Kim, Jin Hwa; Kim, Sang Yong; Jeong, Myung Ho

2023 in Cardiovascular Diabetology

Abstract-Summary This study evaluated cardiovascular outcomes by comparing SGLT2i with dipeptidyl peptidase-4 inhibitors (DPP-4i) in combination with metformin in diabetic patients with AMI.

This study involved 779 diabetic participants with AMI from a Korean nationwide multicenter observational cohort, who were divided into two groups: (1) metformin plus SGLT2i group (SGLT2i group, n = 186) and (2) metformin plus DPP-4i (DPP-4i group, n = 593).

After IPTW, the rate of MACEs in the SGLT2i group was not significantly lower than that in the DPP-4i group (hazard ratio [HR], 0.99; 95% confidence interval [Cl], 0.46 to 2.14, p = 0.983).

In our exploratory analysis, the left ventricular ejection fraction showed a significant improvement in the SGLT2i group than in the DPP-4i group before achieving statistical balancing (6.10 ± 8.30 versus 2.95 ± 10.34, p = 0.007) and after IPTW adjustment (6.91 ± 8.91 versus 3.13 ± 10.41, p = 0.027).

Our findings demonstrated that SGLT2i did not influence the rate of MACEs compared with DPP-4i in combination with metformin in diabetic patients with AMI but did improve left ventricular ejection fraction.

Background

Cardiovascular disease is the leading cause of mortality in patients with DM [325].

Many clinicians use sodium-glucose cotransporter 2 inhibitors (SGLT2i) or dipeptidyl peptidase-4 inhibitors (DPP-4i) in patients with DM as a second-line therapy in combination with metformin (MET) monotherapy.

In recently published cardiovascular outcome trials (CVOTs), SGLT2i have proven cardiovascular benefits in patients with DM in both primary and secondary prevention [4, 23, 25, 65, 66, 94–122, 166–171, 174, 187, 254–281, 283–290, 320–335], which is driven by a low incidence of cardiovascular death and hospitalization for heart failure (HF).

In patients with AMI, the combination of OHAs appears to be an important strategy for achieving glycemic goals and long-term cardiovascular benefits.

Determining the optimal combination of OHAs is important for the desired clinical outcomes of AMI.

This study aimed to evaluate cardiovascular outcomes by comparing the use of SGLT2i versus DPP-4i in combination with MET in patients with AMI and concomitant DM.

Methods

According to the international guidelines [336], AMI is defined as myocardial injury characterized by a rise or fall in cardiac markers and related clinical manifestations as follows: (1) myocardial ischemia-related symptoms and/or signs; (2) new-onset changes in the 12-lead electrocardiogram (ECG), including deviated ST-segments (either elevation or depression), inverted T-waves, or the development of pathological Q-waves; (3) imaging evidence for loss of viable myocardium or regional wall motion abnormalities; or (4) existence of intracoronary thrombi during coronary angiography.

In IPTW, the propensity score was constructed using multiple logistic regression analysis with the following baseline covariates: age, sex, use of emergency medical services, BMI, Killip classification, medical history, smoking history, family history of CAD, use of thrombolysis, LMCA disease, multivessel CAD, PCI, final diagnosis (STEMI or non-STEMI), initial HbA1c level, post-discharge medications, vascular approach (femoral or non-femoral), use of glycoprotein IIb/IIIa inhibitors, thrombus aspiration, intracoronary imaging guidance, preprocedural TIMI flow grade, ACC/AHA lesion characteristics, treatment strategies, and IRA.

Results

Prior CAD was more frequent in the DPP-4i group than in the SGLT2i group.

The SGLT2i group had more instances of STEMI as a final diagnosis than the DPP-4i group.

Initial HbA1c levels were higher in the SGLT2i group than in the DPP-4i group.

Among discharge medications, beta-blockers were more frequently prescribed to individuals in the SGLT2i group compared to those in the DPP-4i group.

Discussion

This study aimed to compare the cardiovascular outcomes of SGLT2i and DPP-4i as add-on therapies in patients with AMI and concomitant DM receiving MET.

Our study demonstrated the potential benefit of SGLT2i over DPP-4i in improving LVEF, implying that the use of SGLT2i may exert beneficial effects in the clinical setting of AMI, although it did not reduce MACE.

Only one retrospective observational study evaluated patients with AMI and concomitant type 2 DM, revealing that the use of SGLT2i was related with a reduced risk of adverse cardiovascular events [337].

The results of our study were significantly different from those of previous observational [334, 338] and network meta-analyses comparing SGLT2i and DPP-4i [339], demonstrating that SGLT2i have a beneficial effect on cardiovascular disease compared with DPP-4i.

In our study, LVEF was significantly improved in patients treated with SGLT2i than in patients treated with DPP-4i before achieving statistical balancing and after IPTW adjustment.

Conclusions

The use of SGLT2i compared with DPP-4i over one year did not demonstrate a statistically significant difference in composite cardiovascular outcomes in patients with AMI and concomitant DM.

The use of SGLT2i appeared to improve left ventricular systolic function compared with the use of DPP-4i.

Comparison of SGLT2 Inhibitors with DPP-4 Inhibitors Combined with Metformin in Patients with Acute Myocardial Infarction and Diabetes Mellitus

https://doi.org/10.1186/s12933-023-01914-4

A machine generated summary based on the work of Lyu, Young Sang; Oh, Seok; Kim, Jin Hwa; Kim, Sang Yong; Jeong, Myung Ho

2023 in Cardiovascular Diabetology

Abstract-Summary This study evaluated cardiovascular outcomes by comparing SGLT2i with dipeptidyl peptidase-4 inhibitors (DPP-4i) in combination with metformin in diabetic patients with AMI.

This study involved 779 diabetic participants with AMI from a Korean nationwide multicenter observational cohort, who were divided into two groups: (1) metformin plus SGLT2i group (SGLT2i group, n = 186) and (2) metformin plus DPP-4i (DPP-4i group, n = 593).

After IPTW, the rate of MACEs in the SGLT2i group was not significantly lower than that in the DPP-4i group (hazard ratio [HR], 0.99; 95% confidence interval [CI], 0.46 to 2.14, p = 0.983).

In our exploratory analysis, the left ventricular ejection fraction showed a significant improvement in the SGLT2i group than in the DPP-4i group before achieving statistical balancing (6.10 ± 8.30 versus 2.95 ± 10.34, p = 0.007) and after IPTW adjustment (6.91 ± 8.91 versus 3.13 ± 10.41, p = 0.027).

Our findings demonstrated that SGLT2i did not influence the rate of MACEs compared with DPP-4i in combination with metformin in diabetic patients with AMI but did improve left ventricular ejection fraction.

Background

Cardiovascular disease is the leading cause of mortality in patients with DM [325].

Many clinicians use sodium-glucose cotransporter 2 inhibitors (SGLT2i) or dipeptidyl peptidase-4 inhibitors (DPP-4i) in patients with DM as a second-line therapy in combination with metformin (MET) monotherapy.

In recently published cardiovascular outcome trials (CVOTs), SGLT2i have proven cardiovascular benefits in patients with DM in both primary and secondary prevention [4, 23, 25, 65, 66, 94–122, 166–171, 174, 187, 254–281, 283–290, 320–335], which is driven by a low incidence of cardiovascular death and hospitalization for heart failure (HF).

In patients with AMI, the combination of OHAs appears to be an important strategy for achieving glycemic goals and long-term cardiovascular benefits.

Determining the optimal combination of OHAs is important for the desired clinical outcomes of AMI.

This study aimed to evaluate cardiovascular outcomes by comparing the use of SGLT2i versus DPP-4i in combination with MET in patients with AMI and concomitant DM.

Methods

According to the international guidelines [336], AMI is defined as myocardial injury characterized by a rise or fall in cardiac markers and related clinical manifestations as follows: (1) myocardial ischemia-related symptoms and/or signs; (2) new-onset changes in the 12-lead electrocardiogram (ECG), including deviated ST-segments (either elevation or depression), inverted T-waves, or the development of pathological Q-waves; (3) imaging evidence for loss of viable myocardium or regional wall motion abnormalities; or (4) existence of intracoronary thrombi during coronary angiography.

In IPTW, the propensity score was constructed using multiple logistic regression analysis with the following baseline covariates: age, sex, use of emergency medical services, BMI, Killip classification, medical history, smoking history, family history of CAD, use of thrombolysis, LMCA disease, multivessel CAD, PCI, final diagnosis (STEMI or non-STEMI), initial HbA1c level, post-discharge medications, vascular approach (femoral or non-femoral), use of glycoprotein IIb/IIIa inhibitors, thrombus aspiration, intracoronary imaging guidance, preprocedural TIMI flow grade, ACC/AHA lesion characteristics, treatment strategies, and IRA.

Results

Prior CAD was more frequent in the DPP-4i group than in the SGLT2i group.

The SGLT2i group had more instances of STEMI as a final diagnosis than the DPP-4i group.

Initial HbA1c levels were higher in the SGLT2i group than in the DPP-4i group.

Among discharge medications, beta-blockers were more frequently prescribed to individuals in the SGLT2i group compared to those in the DPP-4i group.

Discussion

This study aimed to compare the cardiovascular outcomes of SGLT2i and DPP-4i as add-on therapies in patients with AMI and concomitant DM receiving MET.

Our study demonstrated the potential benefit of SGLT2i over DPP-4i in improving LVEF, implying that the use of SGLT2i may exert beneficial effects in the clinical setting of AMI, although it did not reduce MACE.

Only one retrospective observational study evaluated patients with AMI and concomitant type 2 DM, revealing that the use of SGLT2i was related with a reduced risk of adverse cardiovascular events [337].

The results of our study were significantly different from those of previous observational [334, 338] and network meta-analyses comparing SGLT2i and DPP-4i [339], demonstrating that SGLT2i have a beneficial effect on cardiovascular disease compared with DPP-4i.

In our study, LVEF was significantly improved in patients treated with SGLT2i than in patients treated with DPP-4i before achieving statistical balancing and after IPTW adjustment.

Conclusions

The use of SGLT2i compared with DPP-4i over one year did not demonstrate a statistically significant difference in composite cardiovascular outcomes in patients with AMI and concomitant DM.

The use of SGLT2i appeared to improve left ventricular systolic function compared with the use of DPP-4i.

Effect of SGLT2 Inhibitors on Body Composition, Fluid Status and Renin–Angiotensin–Aldosterone System in Type 2 Diabetes: A Prospective Study Using Bioimpedance Spectroscopy

https://doi.org/10.1186/s12933-019-0852-y

A machine generated summary based on the work of Schork, Anja; Saynisch, Janine; Vosseler, Andreas; Jaghutriz, Benjamin Assad; Heyne, Nils; Peter, Andreas; Häring, Hans-Ulrich; Stefan, Norbert; Fritsche, Andreas; Artunc, Ferruh

2019 in Cardiovascular Diabetology

Abstract-Summary SGLT2-inhibitors are potent antihyperglycemic drugs for patients with type 2 diabetes and have been shown to reduce body weight.

In this longitudinal observational study, we analyzed the body composition of 27 outpatients with type 2 diabetes mellitus during the first week and up to 6 months after initiation of treatment with SGLT2-inhibitors (n = 18 empagliflozin, n = 9 dapagliflozin) using bioimpedance spectroscopy (BCM, Fresenius).

At 6 months, HbA1c decreased by 0.8% (IQR 2.3; 0.4), body weight and BMI by 2.6 kg (1.5; 9.3) and 0.9 kg/m^2 (0.4; 3.3), respectively.

Overhydration (OH) and extracellular water (ECW) decreased by − 0.5 L/1.73 m^2 (− 0.1; − 0.9) and − 0.4 L/1.73 m^2 (− 0.1; − 0.8) at day 3, respectively, and returned to the initial value after 3 and 6 months.

Fluid status of patients with SGLT2 inhibitors after 6 months showed no difference from that of hypertensive patients taking hydrochlorothiazide or healthy persons.

Body weight reduction under the treatment with SGLT2-inhibitors is caused by reduction of adipose tissue mass and transient loss of extracellular fluid, which is accompanied by upregulation of renin–angiotensin–aldosterone system (RAAS).

Background

Previous investigations of changes in body composition under SGLT2 inhibitors mainly relied on calculated indices or x-ray absorptiometry [340–342].

Bioimpedance spectroscopy analysis as a quantitative measurement method can contribute to further define changes of body composition under treatment with SGLT2 inhibitors and to identify changes in fluid status that could be responsible for these favorable effects in heart failure.

We analyzed the course of body composition and fluid status as measured by bioimpedance spectroscopy in a cohort of patients with type 2 diabetes after initiation of therapy with SGLT2 inhibitors empagliflozin or dapagliflozin during the first week and a follow up period of 6 months.

Body composition and fluid status of patients with arterial hypertension and established diuretic therapy with hydrochlorothiazide, and control groups without SGLT2 inhibitors or diuretic medication were analyzed.

Methods

Patients with type 2 diabetes starting medication with a SGLT2 inhibitor due to indication were included after they provided written informed consent (n = 27).

To further compare the fluid status under SGLT2 inhibition with that of healthy individuals, patients with type 2 diabetes without SGLT2 inhibition and hypertensive patients, data obtained from a former study of our group, involving patients with chronic kidney disease of all stages and hypertension, [343] were re-assessed.

For parameters obtained at baseline and follow up measurements of patients with type 2 diabetes starting medication with a SGLT2 inhibitor, Friedman test was used to test for significant changes during the whole period of follow up.

ANOVA and t-test for each pair as post-test was used to test for in between group differences of healthy controls, patients with type 2 diabetes with and without

SGLT2 inhibitor and patients with hypertension with and without hydrochlorothiazide treatment.

Results

The study included consecutively n = 27 patients with type 2 diabetes starting medication with an SGLT2 inhibitor (n = 1 empagliflozin 5 mg; n = 5 empagliflozin 10 mg; n = 12 empagliflozin 25 mg; n = 1 dapagliflozin 5 mg; n = 8 dapagliflozin 10 mg).

Median age was 58 years (interquartile range 52; 68), n = 12 (43%) patients were male and median BMI was 36.3 kg/m^2 (32.6; 46.1) at baseline, respectively.

N = 17 patients were lost to follow up because they had stopped medication with the SGLT2 inhibitor (n = 2) or because they declined or were unable to participate in follow up (n = 15).

Bioimpedance spectroscopy to assess fluid status and body composition was performed at baseline and after 3, 30, 90 and 180 days of medication with an SGLT2 inhibitor, respectively.

Discussion

We found that the reduction of body weight during treatment with the SGLT2 inhibitors empagliflozin and dapagliflozin is caused by changes in volume status with decrease of extracellular water during the first days of intake, and by decrease of adipose tissue mass during the following weeks and months.

In Japanese patients treated with ipragliflozin, Iizuka and others [344] found a reduction of total body water by −0.43 kg at 4 weeks, and a rising tendency at 12 weeks (− 0.37 kg), compared to baseline, respectively, with changes of body fluid mainly caused by extracellular water and no significant changes of intracellular water; however, changes of volume status during the first days of SGLT2 inhibition were not measured and follow up period was shorter, thus missing data on initial as well as long term changes in body fluid status.

Conclusions

Our study shows that body weight reduction under the intake of SGLT2 inhibitors is caused by a decrease of adipose tissue mass after 6 months of intake and by a transient decrease of extracellular water after 3 days and 1 month, which is counterbalanced by upregulation of renin–angiotensin–aldosterone system.

Our data argue against an ongoing fluid loss under treatment with SGLT2 inhibitors, which is also not seen in chronic thiazide treatment.

Observational Study on Unhealthy Eating Behavior and the Effect of Sodium-Glucose Cotransporter 2 Inhibitors: The Luseogliflozin Ehime Diabetes Study

https://doi.org/10.1007/s13300-022-01261-9

A machine generated summary based on the work of Furukawa, Shinya; Miyake, Teruki; Miyaoka, Hiroaki; Matsuura, Bunzo; Hiasa, Yoichi

2022 in Diabetes Therapy

Abstract-Summary Unhealthy eating behavior is associated with diabetes, hypertension, and obesity.

Evidence regarding the effect of medications, including SGLT2 inhibitors, on unhealthy eating behavior is limited.

This study investigated the association between unhealthy eating behavior and the laboratory and physical findings of Japanese patients with type 2 diabetes given luseogliflozin once daily for 24 weeks.

The information regarding unhealthy eating behaviors (eating fast, late dinner, nighttime snack, skipping breakfast, and eating until full) was obtained using self-reported questionnaires.

In the healthy eating behavior group, the improvements of fasting plasma glucose and ALT, but not other variables, were attenuated.

HbA1c level was significantly improved in patients with eating fast, while other unhealthy eating behaviors attenuated the effect of luseogliflozin for HbA1c.

Luseogliflozin might be more effective for controlling plasma glucose in patients with type 2 diabetes who have a tendency to eat fast, but it might have less effect on those with other unhealthy eating habits.

Introduction

These findings suggest that unhealthy eating habits may weaken the therapeutic effects of oral anti-hypoglycemic agents in patients with type 2 diabetes mellitus.

Regarding the relationship of unhealthy eating habits and sodium-glucose cotransporter 2 (SGLT2) inhibitors, an inverse correlation between the amount of visceral fat and the number of unhealthy eating habits has been shown in patients with Japanese type 2 diabetes receiving SGLT2 inhibitors [283].

Although eating habits are considered to be changeable by appropriate interventions, evidence on the relationship between eating behaviors and the effects of anti-hypoglycemic agents is limited.

Unhealthy eating habits might attenuate the effects of SGLT2 inhibitors, including plasma glucose and weight loss.

We explored the relationship between eating habits and the effects of luseogliflozin (an SGLT2 inhibitor) on plasma glucose and weight loss in patients with type 2 diabetes mellitus.

Methods

The primary endpoint was improvement of HbA1c and to investigate the association between eating behavior and the change of HbA1c from baseline to 24 weeks.

Secondary endpoints in this study were weight loss and to investigate to association between eating behavior and weight change from baseline to 24 weeks.

Information regarding eating behaviors were determined from a self-administered questionnaire.

Subjects were considered to have skipped breakfast, engaged in bedtime snacking, eaten a late-night dinner, and eating until full if they answered "Yes" to the questions "Do you skip breakfast at least three times per week?", ".

Do you eat snacks after dinner at least three times per week?", ".

Fast eating was identified if they answered "fast" to the question "Do you think your meal-eating speed is usually rapid compared with other people's?" (from among three response options [slow, normal, and fast]).

Results

The change of fasting plasma glucose and ALT was not significant in the healthy eating behavior group, while fasting plasma glucose and ALT were significantly improved in the unhealthy eating behavior group.

In patients with fast eating behavior, HbA1c was improved significantly.

Significant weight reduction was found regardless of fast eating behavior, nighttime snack, and eating until full.

No relationship between HbA1c improvement and weight reduction was found regardless of eating fast or skipping breakfast.

Discussion

Significant improvement in HbA1c levels was observed in subjects with fast eating behavior, while in subjects with unhealthy behaviors the effect of luseogliflozin was attenuated.

This is the first study to explore the association between eating behaviors and SGLT2 inhibitor effects in patients with type 2 diabetes mellitus.

In two Japanese and one US longitudinal study, fast eating rate was associated with weight gain [284–286].

Eating rate was not correlated with fasting plasma glucose level, while an inverse association between eating rate and HbA1c was found [284].

After administration of leseogliflozin, a significant improvement of HbA1c in patients with fast eating behavior was observed, while other unhealthy eating behaviors attenuated the effect of luseogliflozin for HbA1c.

In patients with fast eating behavior, luseogliflozin might be effective for controlling plasma glucose and weight via urinary glucose excretion, improved hyperglycemia, and enhanced GLP-1 response.

Effects of the SGLT2 Inhibitor Dapagliflozin on Cardiac Function Evaluated by Impedance Cardiography in Patients with Type 2 Diabetes. Secondary Analysis of a Randomized Placebo-Controlled Trial

https://doi.org/10.1186/s12933-019-0910-5

A machine generated summary based on the work of Bonora, Benedetta Maria; Vigili de Kreutzenberg, Saula; Avogaro, Angelo; Fadini, Gian Paolo

2019 in Cardiovascular Diabetology

Abstract-Summary Cardiovascular outcome trials have documented a strong benefit of sodium glucose cotransporter-2 inhibitors (SGLT2i) on the risk of hospitalization for heart failure (HF) in patients with type 2 diabetes (T2D) with or without established cardiovascular disease or prior history of HF.

We aimed to evaluate whether treatment with SGLT2i affected cardiac function using impedance cardiography (ICG) in a randomized placebo-controlled trial.

Thirty-three patients with T2D were randomized to receive blind dapagliflozin 10 mg or matching placebo for 12-week on top of their ongoing glucose lowering medication regimen.

Cardiac function was evaluated by resting ICG at baseline and at the end of the 12-week treatment period.

ICG is a non-invasive technology based on the continuous measurement of thoracic electrical conductivity to process a cardiodynamic parameters related to fluid content, blood flow, cardiac function, and circulatory function.

After 12 weeks, patients randomized to dapagliflozin, as compared to those randomized to placebo, showed improvements in HbA1c (− 1.2%; 13 mmol/mol), systolic blood pressure (− 3.7 mmHg), and body weight (− 3.3 kg).

Based on ICG, in both groups, we detected no significant change in parameters of blood flow (stroke volume, cardiac output, cardiac index), systolic function (ejection fraction, acceleration and velocity indexes, systolic time ratio), circulatory function (systemic vascular resistance index), and fluid status (thoracic fluid content) after treatment.

This is the first study exploring cardiac effects of SGLT2i using ICG in T2D. We observed no change in cardiac function parameters estimated by ICG in T2D patients who received dapagliflozin versus placebo for 12 weeks.

Background

Patients with type 2 diabetes (T2D) have a two-to-fivefold increased risk of developing heart failure (HF) compare to non-diabetic patients [287].

Patients with T2D are more likely to be hospitalized for HF [288], to be re-hospitalized for HF [289], and to experience a longer hospital stay [290] compared to patients without diabetes.

Patients with T2D and HF have a higher risk of cardiovascular and all-cause mortality than HF patients without T2D [288].

The recent results of the four cardiovascular outcome trials (CVOTs) with SGLT2i have shown remarkable benefits in reducing HF hospitalization by about 30% in patients with T2D with or without established cardiovascular disease and also in patient with or without history of heart failure [4, 23, 39, 64–66, 86–171, 187, 254–276, 282–290].

Large retrospective studies confirmed that treatment with SGLT2i, when compared with other glucose-lowering medications (GLMs), was associated with lower rates of hospitalization for HF among patients with and without history of cardiovascular disease [174, 326, 327].

Materials and Methods

The Medis Niccomo ICG device processed these changes with a dedicated algorithm (physiologic adaptive signal analysis) coupling impedance signal and waveform with ECG, noninvasively and continuously provided the following hemodynamic variables: heart rate (HR); systolic blood pressure (SBP), diastolic blood pressure (DBP); SV, stroke index [SI (SV normalized for body surface area)]; CO (SV × HR); cardiac index [CI (CO normalized for body surface area)]; ejection fraction (EF); acceleration index [AI (the maximum acceleration of blood flow in the aorta during systole)]; velocity index [VI (the peak velocity of blood flow in the aorta during systole)]; systolic time ratio (STR); LVET [the time interval between the opening and the closing of the aortic valve (i.e., mechanical systole)]; left cardiac work (LCW) and LCW index (LCWI), which reflected the myocardial oxygen demand; systemic vascular resistance [SVR (estimate of "afterload)] and SVR index [SVRI (SVR normalised to body size); TFC (indicator of chest fluid status); TFC Index [TFCI (TFC, normalized for body surface area)]; total arterial compliance [TAC (indicator of the degree of peripheral arterial stiffness/compliance)], TAC index, [TACI (TAC normalised to body size)]; ICG variables were calculated by using the mean of 2-min beat-to-beat values for 20 min.

Results

In the placebo group, HbA1c increased non-significantly by 0.4% and body weight remained stable (+ 0.2 kg).

Compared with baseline, SBP declined by 4.7 ± 1.3 mmHg in the dapagliflozin group and by 1.0 ± 2.3 mmHg in the placebo group ($p = 0.035$).

Diastolic dysfunction based on the STR cut-off of 0.31 was present in 63.3% of patients (66.7% in the dapagliflozin group and 60% in the placebo group).

At follow-up, the prevalence of diastolic dysfunction based on STR declined by 6.7% in the dapagliflozin group and remained stable in the placebo group ($p = 0.325$).

No significant correlation was detected between change in HbA1c or body weight from baseline to the end of follow-up and change in ICG parameters (not shown).

Discussion

We found no significant effect of the SGLT2i dapagliflozin on measures of cardiac function evaluated by ICG.

A small observational study showed that in patients with T2D and established cardiovascular disease, a short-term empagliflozin treatment was associated with a significant reduction in LV mass index and improved diastolic function measured by 2D echocardiography.

This is the first study exploring the cardiac effects of SGLT2i using ICG in T2D. This study suggests that, in T2D patients without a history of HF, a 12-week treatment with dapagliflozin exerted no overt effect on haemodynamic and cardiac function parameters compared to placebo.

Previous observational studies documented effects of SGLT2i on diastolic cardiac function in T2D, but a recent re-analysis of the DECLARE-TIMI58 study reported that dapagliflozin prevented HF in patients with a normal or reduced EF and improved survival especially in patients with reduced EF [101].

Conclusions

Despite strong evidence that SGLT2i prevent HF in T2D with or without prior HF episodes, we found no effects of dapagliflozin on parameters of cardiac function measured by ICG.

Short duration of treatment, small sample size, lack or specific diastolic function measures, limited correlation of ICG parameters with gold standard examination of cardiac function, and the masking diuretic effects of SGLT2i are all possible explanations of these negative results.

We also speculate that SGLT2i exert no effects on cardiac function parameters in patients with normal cardiac function but may play a major role at the very early onset of cardiac disfunction, preventing hospitalization and mortality.

Further studies are needed to address this hypothesis.

Heart Failure in Type 2 Diabetes: Current Perspectives on Screening, Diagnosis and Management

https://doi.org/10.1186/s12933-021-01408-1

A machine generated summary based on the work of Ceriello, Antonio; Catrinoiu, Doina; Chandramouli, Chanchal; Cosentino, Francesco; Dombrowsky, Annique Cornelia; Itzhak, Baruch; Lalic, Nebojsa Malić; Prattichizzo, Francesco; Schnell, Oliver; Seferović, Petar M.; Valensi, Paul; Standl, Eberhard

2021 in Cardiovascular Diabetology

Abstract-Summary Type 2 diabetes is one of the most relevant risk factors for heart failure, the prevalence of which is increasing worldwide.

The aim of the review is to highlight the current perspectives of the pathophysiology of heart failure as it pertains to type 2 diabetes.

We also discuss the current criteria used for heart failure diagnosis and the gold standard screening tools for individuals with type 2 diabetes.

The influence of the presence of type 2 diabetes as well as heart failure on COVID-19 severity is briefly discussed.

Introduction

Clinically manifest HF is present in 10–30% of all subjects with T2D, especially common at the age of 70 years and older, while 30–40% of all cases of acute or chronic HF have prevalent T2D [110].

T2D and HF are interrelated: T2D increases the risk of HF, HF is highly prevalent in patients with T2D, and HF might increase the risk of developing T2D [111].

While the incidence of HF is increasing in people older than 85 years but also at younger age in recent years [112] and the epidemiologic linkage between T2D and HF is clear [110], recognition of those at risk and/or those with prevalent HF is lagging.

We describe the pathophysiology of the different HF subtypes, focusing on the myocardial alterations induced by T2D in the absence of coronary disease and other risk factors, i.e., cardiomyopathy in diabetes.

Classification of Heart Failure and Epidemiological Aspects

In a setting of chronic, low-grade systemic inflammation, the amount of EFT is elevated, and its role potentially changes from a heart- protecting and supporting structure to a local source of pro-inflammatory cytokines in the heart, which probably worsens endothelial dysfunction and leads to increased cardiac fibrosis and stiffness and thus inducing HF, in particular HFpEF [113].

The presence of subclinical myocardial damage increases the risk for CV events and HF, with the highest CV risk for people with T2D [114].

The SAVOR-TIMI 53 trial reported that diabetic individuals without known CVD but with elevated NT-proBNP levels have a three-fold increased risk of HF than counterparts with known CVD and normal NT-proBNP levels [115].

The ADVANCE trial and other studies demonstrated that NT-proBNP strongly predicts HF risk, the overall excess mortality, and CV mortality in people with T2D [116, 117].

Detection of Heart Failure in Diabetes

Strategies in people with diabetes to reduce the risk for HF: The 2019 ESC-EASD guidelines recommend routine assessment of microalbuminuria and eGFR in order to identify patients at high risk of renal dysfunction or future CVD [111].

Metformin Metformin monotherapy is the first-line treatment for patients with T2D without CVD and at moderate CV risk according to the 2019 ESC-EASD guidelines on diabetes, and it is recommended for diabetes treatment in patients with HF if the eGFR is stable and $\geq$ 30 mL/min/1.73m^2 (level of evidence: C) [111].

The 2019 ADA/EASD consensus recommends SGLT-2 inhibitors on top of metformin in people with diabetes and HF (especially HFrEF) in order to reduce HHF, MACE, and CV death [118].

To saxagliptin, there is no treatment recommendation for pioglitazone for diabetes management in people at risk for HF because it increases the incidence of HF in T2D patients compared with placebo [111, 119].

Diabetes, HF and COVID-19

To the increased risk of infection, SARS-CoV-2-infected individuals with diabetes are also likely to have serious complications or die, especially in conjunction with CV risk factors such as hypertension, obesity and smoking, especially those who are at poor metabolic control [120].

As serious complications in SARS-CoV-2-infected diabetic people, acute myocarditis (36.6% vs. 15.5%), acute HF (25.3% vs. 5.6%), and acute MI (9.9% vs. 1.4%) have been observed compared to non-diabetics.

If diabetes and SARS-CoV-2 infection are accompanied by the risk factors male sex, a longer duration of diabetes, as well as a history of micro- and macrovascular complications and HF, significantly increased death rates have been detected [121].

Irrespective of the presence of diabetes in SARS-CoV-2 infected subjects, a history of HF alone was also significantly associated with the need for hospitalization for coronavirus disease 2019 (COVID-19) and a higher mortality [122].

Conclusions

Heart failure remains an important issue for life expectancy, especially for people with diabetes.

New therapeutic tools, such as the SGLT-2 inhibitors, are offering the opportunity for better management of this very serious complication of T2D. Using biomarkers such as NT-proBNP can help diagnose HF early to predict prognosis and therapeutic efficacy of medications for HF or/and diabetes.

NT-proBNP measurement should be implemented early in the monitoring of subjects with diabetes at high CV risk.

The importance of screening for HF in diabetes becomes significant, especially during the COVID-19 pandemic in which people with diabetes and concomitant HF are particularly vulnerable to SARS-CoV-2 infection and often have worse disease progression and prognosis than healthy individuals.

Observational Study on Unhealthy Eating Behavior and the Effect of Sodium-Glucose Cotransporter 2 Inhibitors: The Luseogliflozin Ehime Diabetes Study

https://doi.org/10.1007/s13300-022-01261-9

A machine generated summary based on the work of Furukawa, Shinya; Miyake, Teruki; Miyaoka, Hiroaki; Matsuura, Bunzo; Hiasa, Yoichi

2022 in Diabetes Therapy

Abstract-Summary Unhealthy eating behavior is associated with diabetes, hypertension, and obesity.

Evidence regarding the effect of medications, including SGLT2 inhibitors, on unhealthy eating behavior is limited.

This study investigated the association between unhealthy eating behavior and the laboratory and physical findings of Japanese patients with type 2 diabetes given luseogliflozin once daily for 24 weeks.

The information regarding unhealthy eating behaviors (eating fast, late dinner, nighttime snack, skipping breakfast, and eating until full) was obtained using self-reported questionnaires.

In the healthy eating behavior group, the improvements of fasting plasma glucose and ALT, but not other variables, were attenuated.

HbA1c level was significantly improved in patients with eating fast, while other unhealthy eating behaviors attenuated the effect of luseogliflozin for HbA1c.

Luseogliflozin might be more effective for controlling plasma glucose in patients with type 2 diabetes who have a tendency to eat fast, but it might have less effect on those with other unhealthy eating habits.

Introduction

These findings suggest that unhealthy eating habits may weaken the therapeutic effects of oral anti-hypoglycemic agents in patients with type 2 diabetes mellitus.

Regarding the relationship of unhealthy eating habits and sodium-glucose cotransporter 2 (SGLT2) inhibitors, an inverse correlation between the amount of visceral fat and the number of unhealthy eating habits has been shown in patients with Japanese type 2 diabetes receiving SGLT2 inhibitors [283].

Although eating habits are considered to be changeable by appropriate interventions, evidence on the relationship between eating behaviors and the effects of anti-hypoglycemic agents is limited.

Unhealthy eating habits might attenuate the effects of SGLT2 inhibitors, including plasma glucose and weight loss.

We explored the relationship between eating habits and the effects of luseogliflozin (an SGLT2 inhibitor) on plasma glucose and weight loss in patients with type 2 diabetes mellitus.

Methods

The primary endpoint was improvement of HbA1c and to investigate the association between eating behavior and the change of HbA1c from baseline to 24 weeks.

Secondary endpoints in this study were weight loss and to investigate to association between eating behavior and weight change from baseline to 24 weeks.

Information regarding eating behaviors were determined from a self-administered questionnaire.

Subjects were considered to have skipped breakfast, engaged in bedtime snacking, eaten a late-night dinner, and eating until full if they answered "Yes" to the questions "Do you skip breakfast at least three times per week?", ".

Do you eat snacks after dinner at least three times per week?", ".

Fast eating was identified if they answered "fast" to the question "Do you think your meal-eating speed is usually rapid compared with other people's?" (from among three response options [slow, normal, and fast]).

Results

The change of fasting plasma glucose and ALT was not significant in the healthy eating behavior group, while fasting plasma glucose and ALT were significantly improved in the unhealthy eating behavior group.

In patients with fast eating behavior, HbA1c was improved significantly.

Significant weight reduction was found regardless of fast eating behavior, nighttime snack, and eating until full.

No relationship between HbA1c improvement and weight reduction was found regardless of eating fast or skipping breakfast.

Discussion

Significant improvement in HbA1c levels was observed in subjects with fast eating behavior, while in subjects with unhealthy behaviors the effect of luseogliflozin was attenuated.

This is the first study to explore the association between eating behaviors and SGLT2 inhibitor effects in patients with type 2 diabetes mellitus.

In two Japanese and one US longitudinal study, fast eating rate was associated with weight gain [284–286].

Eating rate was not correlated with fasting plasma glucose level, while an inverse association between eating rate and HbA1c was found [284].

After administration of leseogliflozin, a significant improvement of HbA1c in patients with fast eating behavior was observed, while other unhealthy eating behaviors attenuated the effect of luseogliflozin for HbA1c.

In patients with fast eating behavior, luseogliflozin might be effective for controlling plasma glucose and weight via urinary glucose excretion, improved hyperglycemia, and enhanced GLP-1 response.

Effects of the SGLT2 Inhibitor Dapagliflozin on Cardiac Function Evaluated by Impedance Cardiography in Patients with Type 2 Diabetes. Secondary Analysis of a Randomized Placebo-Controlled Trial

https://doi.org/10.1186/s12933-019-0910-5

A machine generated summary based on the work of Bonora, Benedetta Maria; Vigili de Kreutzenberg, Saula; Avogaro, Angelo; Fadini, Gian Paolo

2019 in Cardiovascular Diabetology

Abstract-Summary Cardiovascular outcome trials have documented a strong benefit of sodium glucose cotransporter-2 inhibitors (SGLT2i) on the risk of hospitalization for heart failure (HF) in patients with type 2 diabetes (T2D) with or without established cardiovascular disease or prior history of HF.

We aimed to evaluate whether treatment with SGLT2i affected cardiac function using impedance cardiography (ICG) in a randomized placebo-controlled trial.

Thirty-three patients with T2D were randomized to receive blind dapagliflozin 10 mg or matching placebo for 12-week on top of their ongoing glucose lowering medication regimen.

Cardiac function was evaluated by resting ICG at baseline and at the end of the 12-week treatment period.

ICG is a non-invasive technology based on the continuous measurement of thoracic electrical conductivity to process a cardiodynamic parameters related to fluid content, blood flow, cardiac function, and circulatory function.

After 12 weeks, patients randomized to dapagliflozin, as compared to those randomized to placebo, showed improvements in HbA1c (− 1.2%; 13 mmol/mol), systolic blood pressure (− 3.7 mmHg), and body weight (− 3.3 kg).

Based on ICG, in both groups, we detected no significant change in parameters of blood flow (stroke volume, cardiac output, cardiac index), systolic function (ejection fraction, acceleration and velocity indexes, systolic time ratio), circulatory function (systemic vascular resistance index), and fluid status (thoracic fluid content) after treatment.

This is the first study exploring cardiac effects of SGLT2i using ICG in T2D. We observed no change in cardiac function parameters estimated by ICG in T2D patients who received dapagliflozin versus placebo for 12 weeks.

Background

Patients with type 2 diabetes (T2D) have a two-to-fivefold increased risk of developing heart failure (HF) compare to non-diabetic patients [287].

Patients with T2D are more likely to be hospitalized for HF [288], to be rehospitalized for HF [289], and to experience a longer hospital stay [290] compared to patients without diabetes.

Patients with T2D and HF have a higher risk of cardiovascular and all-cause mortality than HF patients without T2D [288].

The recent results of the four cardiovascular outcome trials (CVOTs) with SGLT2i have shown remarkable benefits in reducing HF hospitalization by about 30% in patients with T2D with or without established cardiovascular disease and also in patient with or without history of heart failure [4, 23, 39, 64–66, 86–171, 187, 254–276, 282–290].

Large retrospective studies confirmed that treatment with SGLT2i, when compared with other glucose-lowering medications (GLMs), was associated with lower rates of hospitalization for HF among patients with and without history of cardiovascular disease [174, 326, 327].

Materials and Methods

The Medis Niccomo ICG device processed these changes with a dedicated algorithm (physiologic adaptive signal analysis) coupling impedance signal and waveform with ECG, noninvasively and continuously provided the following hemodynamic variables: heart rate (HR); systolic blood pressure (SBP), diastolic blood pressure (DBP); SV, stroke index [SI (SV normalized for body surface area)]; CO (SV × HR); cardiac index [CI (CO normalized for body surface area)]; ejection fraction (EF); acceleration index [AI (the maximum acceleration of blood flow in the aorta during systole)]; velocity index [VI (the peak velocity of blood flow in the aorta during systole)]; systolic time ratio (STR); LVET [the time interval between the opening and the closing of the aortic valve (i.e., mechanical systole)]; left cardiac work (LCW) and LCW index (LCWI), which reflected the myocardial oxygen demand; systemic vascular resistance [SVR (estimate of "afterload)] and SVR index [SVRI (SVR normalised to body size); TFC (indicator of chest fluid status); TFC Index [TFCI (TFC, normalized for body surface area)]; total arterial compliance [TAC (indicator of the degree of peripheral arterial stiffness/compliance)], TAC index, [TACI (TAC normalised to body size)]; ICG variables were calculated by using the mean of 2-min beat-to-beat values for 20 min.

Results

In the placebo group, HbA1c increased non-significantly by 0.4% and body weight remained stable (+ 0.2 kg).

Compared with baseline, SBP declined by 4.7 ± 1.3 mmHg in the dapagliflozin group and by 1.0 ± 2.3 mmHg in the placebo group ($p = 0.035$).

Diastolic dysfunction based on the STR cut-off of 0.31 was present in 63.3% of patients (66.7% in the dapagliflozin group and 60% in the placebo group).

At follow-up, the prevalence of diastolic dysfunction based on STR declined by 6.7% in the dapagliflozin group and remained stable in the placebo group ($p = 0.325$).

No significant correlation was detected between change in HbA1c or body weight from baseline to the end of follow-up and change in ICG parameters (not shown).

Discussion

We found no significant effect of the SGLT2i dapagliflozin on measures of cardiac function evaluated by ICG.

A small observational study showed that in patients with T2D and established cardiovascular disease, a short-term empagliflozin treatment was associated with a significant reduction in LV mass index and improved diastolic function measured by 2D echocardiography.

This is the first study exploring the cardiac effects of SGLT2i using ICG in T2D. This study suggests that, in T2D patients without a history of HF, a 12-week treatment with dapagliflozin exerted no overt effect on haemodynamic and cardiac function parameters compared to placebo.

Previous observational studies documented effects of SGLT2i on diastolic cardiac function in T2D, but a recent re-analysis of the DECLARE-TIMI58 study reported that dapagliflozin prevented HF in patients with a normal or reduced EF and improved survival especially in patients with reduced EF [101].

Conclusions

Despite strong evidence that SGLT2i prevent HF in T2D with or without prior HF episodes, we found no effects of dapagliflozin on parameters of cardiac function measured by ICG.

Short duration of treatment, small sample size, lack or specific diastolic function measures, limited correlation of ICG parameters with gold standard examination of cardiac function, and the masking diuretic effects of SGLT2i are all possible explanations of these negative results.

We also speculate that SGLT2i exert no effects on cardiac function parameters in patients with normal cardiac function but may play a major role at the very early onset of cardiac disfunction, preventing hospitalization and mortality.

Further studies are needed to address this hypothesis.

Effect of SGLT2 Inhibitors on Body Composition, Fluid Status and Renin–Angiotensin–Aldosterone System in Type 2 Diabetes: A Prospective Study Using Bioimpedance Spectroscopy

https://doi.org/10.1186/s12933-019-0852-y

A machine generated summary based on the work of Schork, Anja; Saynisch, Janine; Vosseler, Andreas; Jaghutriz, Benjamin Assad; Heyne, Nils; Peter, Andreas; Häring, Hans-Ulrich; Stefan, Norbert; Fritsche, Andreas; Artunc, Ferruh

2019 in Cardiovascular Diabetology

Abstract-Summary SGLT2-inhibitors are potent antihyperglycemic drugs for patients with type 2 diabetes and have been shown to reduce body weight.

In this longitudinal observational study, we analyzed the body composition of 27 outpatients with type 2 diabetes mellitus during the first week and up to 6 months after initiation of treatment with SGLT2-inhibitors (n = 18 empagliflozin, n = 9 dapagliflozin) using bioimpedance spectroscopy (BCM, Fresenius).

At 6 months, HbA1c decreased by 0.8% (IQR 2.3; 0.4), body weight and BMI by 2.6 kg (1.5; 9.3) and 0.9 kg/m^2 (0.4; 3.3), respectively.

Overhydration (OH) and extracellular water (ECW) decreased by −0.5 L/1.73 m^2 (−0.1; −0.9) and − 0.4 L/1.73 m^2 (−0.1; −0.8) at day 3, respectively, and returned to the initial value after 3 and 6 months.

Fluid status of patients with SGLT2 inhibitors after 6 months showed no difference from that of hypertensive patients taking hydrochlorothiazide or healthy persons.

Body weight reduction under the treatment with SGLT2-inhibitors is caused by reduction of adipose tissue mass and transient loss of extracellular fluid, which is accompanied by upregulation of renin–angiotensin–aldosterone system (RAAS).

Background

Previous investigations of changes in body composition under SGLT2 inhibitors mainly relied on calculated indices or x-ray absorptiometry [340–342].

Bioimpedance spectroscopy analysis as a quantitative measurement method can contribute to further define changes of body composition under treatment with SGLT2 inhibitors and to identify changes in fluid status that could be responsible for these favorable effects in heart failure.

We analyzed the course of body composition and fluid status as measured by bioimpedance spectroscopy in a cohort of patients with type 2 diabetes after initiation of therapy with SGLT2 inhibitors empagliflozin or dapagliflozin during the first week and a follow up period of 6 months.

Body composition and fluid status of patients with arterial hypertension and established diuretic therapy with hydrochlorothiazide, and control groups without SGLT2 inhibitors or diuretic medication were analyzed.

Methods

Patients with type 2 diabetes starting medication with a SGLT2 inhibitor due to indication were included after they provided written informed consent (n = 27).

To further compare the fluid status under SGLT2 inhibition with that of healthy individuals, patients with type 2 diabetes without SGLT2 inhibition and hypertensive patients, data obtained from a former study of our group, involving patients with chronic kidney disease of all stages and hypertension, [343] were re-assessed.

For parameters obtained at baseline and follow up measurements of patients with type 2 diabetes starting medication with a SGLT2 inhibitor, Friedman test was used to test for significant changes during the whole period of follow up.

ANOVA and t-test for each pair as post-test was used to test for in between group differences of healthy controls, patients with type 2 diabetes with and without SGLT2 inhibitor and patients with hypertension with and without hydrochlorothiazide treatment.

Results

The study included consecutively n = 27 patients with type 2 diabetes starting medication with an SGLT2 inhibitor (n = 1 empagliflozin 5 mg; n = 5 empagliflozin 10 mg; n = 12 empagliflozin 25 mg; n = 1 dapagliflozin 5 mg; n = 8 dapagliflozin 10 mg).

Median age was 58 years (interquartile range 52; 68), n = 12 (43%) patients were male and median BMI was 36.3 kg/m^2 (32.6; 46.1) at baseline, respectively.

N = 17 patients were lost to follow up because they had stopped medication with the SGLT2 inhibitor (n = 2) or because they declined or were unable to participate in follow up (n = 15).

Bioimpedance spectroscopy to assess fluid status and body composition was performed at baseline and after 3, 30, 90 and 180 days of medication with an SGLT2 inhibitor, respectively.

Discussion

We found that the reduction of body weight during treatment with the SGLT2 inhibitors empagliflozin and dapagliflozin is caused by changes in volume status with decrease of extracellular water during the first days of intake, and by decrease of adipose tissue mass during the following weeks and months.

In Japanese patients treated with ipragliflozin, Iizuka and others [344] found a reduction of total body water by −0.43 kg at 4 weeks, and a rising tendency at 12 weeks (− 0.37 kg), compared to baseline, respectively, with changes of body fluid mainly caused by extracellular water and no significant changes of intracellular water; however, changes of volume status during the first days of SGLT2 inhibition were not measured and follow up period was shorter, thus missing data on initial as well as long term changes in body fluid status.

Conclusions

Our study shows that body weight reduction under the intake of SGLT2 inhibitors is caused by a decrease of adipose tissue mass after 6 months of intake and by a transient decrease of extracellular water after 3 days and 1 month, which is counterbalanced by upregulation of renin–angiotensin–aldosterone system.

Our data argue against an ongoing fluid loss under treatment with SGLT2 inhibitors, which is also not seen in chronic thiazide treatment.

Bibliography

1. Frąk W, Hajdys J, Radzioch E, Szlagor M, Młynarska E, Rysz J, Franczyk B (2023) Cardiovascular diseases: therapeutic potential of SGLT-2 inhibitors. Biomedicines 11(7):2085
2. Hou YC, Zheng CM, Yen TH, Lu KC (2020) Molecular mechanisms of SGLT2 inhibitor on cardiorenal protection. Int J Mol Sci 21(21):7833
3. Cersosimo A, Salerno N, Sabatino J, Scatteia A, Bisaccia G, De Rosa S, Dellegrottaglie S, Bucciarelli-Ducci C, Torella D, Leo I (2024 Mar 11) Underlying mechanisms and cardioprotective effects of SGLT2i and GLP-1Ra: insights from cardiovascular magnetic resonance. Cardiovasc Diabetol 23(1):94
4. Neal B, Perkovic V, Mahaffey KW, de Zeeuw D, Fulcher G, Erondu N et al (2017) Canagliflozin and cardiovascular and renal events in type 2 diabetes. N Engl J Med 377:644–657. http://www.nejm.org/doi/10.1056/NEJMoa1611925. Accessed 1 Dec 2017
5. Karg MV, Bosch A, Kannenkeril D et al (2018) SGLT-2-inhibition with dapagliflozin reduces tissue sodium content: a randomised controlled trial. Cardiovasc Diabetol 17:5

6. Wilcox CS, Shen W, Boulton DW, Leslie BR, Griffen SC (2018) Interaction between the sodium-glucose-linked transporter 2 inhibitor dapagliflozin and the loop diuretic bumetanide in normal human subjects. J Am Heart Assoc 7:e007046
7. Baartscheer A, Schumacher CA, Wust RC et al (2017) Empagliflozin decreases myocardial cytoplasmic Na+ through inhibition of the cardiac Na+/H+ exchanger in rats and rabbits. Diabetologia 60:568–573
8. Packer M (2018) Do sodium-glucose co-transporter-2 inhibitors prevent heart failure with a preserved ejection fraction by counterbalancing the effects of leptin? A novel hypothesis. Diabetes Obes Metab. https://doi.org/10.1111/dom.13229
9. Verma S, Bhatt DL, Bain SC et al (2018) Effects of liraglutide on cardiovascular events in patients with type 2 diabetes and polyvascular disease: results of the LEADER trial. Circulation 137:2179–2183
10. Wiviott SD, Raz I, Bonaca MP et al (2018) The design and rationale for the dapagliflozin effect on cardiovascular events (DECLARE)—TIMI 58 trial. Am Heart J 200:83–89
11. Katsiki N, Banach M, Mikhailidis DP (2019) Is type 2 diabetes mellitus a coronary heart disease equivalent or not? Do not just enjoy the debate and forget the patient! Arch Med Sci 15:1357–1364. https://doi.org/10.5114/aoms.2019.89449
12. Dunlay SM, Givertz MM, Aguilar D et al (2019) Type 2 diabetes mellitus and heart failure: a scientific statement from the American Heart Association and the Heart Failure Society of America: this statement does not represent an update of the 2017 ACC/AHA/HFSA heart failure guideline update. Circulation 140:e294–e324. https://doi.org/10.1161/CIR.0000000000000691
13. Echouffo-Tcheugui JB, Xu H, DeVore AD et al (2016) Temporal trends and factors associated with diabetes mellitus among patients hospitalized with heart failure: findings from get with the guidelines-heart failure registry. Am Heart J 182:9–20. https://doi.org/10.1016/j.ahj.2016.07.025
14. Tentolouris A, Vlachakis P, Tzeravini E, Eleftheriadou I, Tentolouris N (2019) SGLT2 inhibitors: a review of their antidiabetic and cardioprotective effects. Int J Environ Res Public Health 16:2965. https://doi.org/10.3390/ijerph16162965
15. Ferrannini E, Solini A (2012) SGLT2 inhibition in diabetes mellitus: rationale and clinical prospects. Nat Rev Endocrinol 8:495–502. https://doi.org/10.1038/nrendo.2011.243
16. Khunti K, Davies M, Majeed A, Thorsted BL, Wolden ML, Paul SK (2015) Hypoglycemia and risk of cardiovascular disease and all-cause mortality in insulin-treated people with type 1 and type 2 diabetes: a cohort study. Diabetes Care 38:316–322. https://doi.org/10.2337/dc14-0920
17. Inzucchi SE, Docherty K, Kober L et al (2020) 271-OR: ADA presidents' select abstract: effect of dapagliflozin on the incidence of diabetes: a prespecified exploratory analysis from DAPA-HF. Diabetes 69:271-OR. https://doi.org/10.2337/db20-271-OR
18. Diamond GA, Bax L, Kaul S et al (2007) Uncertain effects of rosiglitazone on the risk for myocardial infarction and cardiovascular death. Ann Intern Med 147:578–581. https://doi.org/10.7326/0003-4819-147-8-200710160-00182
19. Mather A, Pollock C (2011) Glucose handling by the kidney. Kidney Int Suppl 120:S1–S6. https://doi.org/10.1038/ki.2010.509
20. Kanai Y, Lee WS, You G, Brown D, Hediger MA (1994) The human kidney low affinity Na+/glucose cotransporter SGLT2. Delineation of the major renal reabsorptive mechanism for D-glucose. J Clin Invest 93:397–404. https://doi.org/10.1172/JCI116972
21. Mosley JF 2nd, Smith L, Everton E, Fellner C (2015) Sodium-glucose linked transporter 2 (SGLT2) inhibitors in the management of type-2 diabetes: a drug class overview. P T 40:451–462
22. Vallon V, Thomson SC (2017) Targeting renal glucose reabsorption to treat hyperglycaemia: the pleiotropic effects of SGLT2 inhibition. Diabetologia 60:215–225. https://doi.org/10.1007/s00125-016-4157-3

23. Zelniker TA, Wiviott SD, Raz I, Im K, Goodrich EL, Bonaca MP, Mosenzon O, Kato ET, Cahn A, Furtado RHM et al (2019) SGLT2 inhibitors for primary and secondary prevention of cardiovascular and renal outcomes in type 2 diabetes: a systematic review and meta-analysis of cardiovascular outcome trials. Lancet 393(10166):31–39. https://doi.org/10.1016/S0140-6736(18)32590-X
24. Fitchett D, Zinman B, Wanner C et al (2016) Heart failure outcomes with empagliflozin in patients with type 2 diabetes at high cardiovascular risk: results of the EMPA-REG OUTCOME® trial. Eur Heart J 37:1526–1534
25. Packer M, Anker SD, Butler J, Filippatos G, Pocock SJ, Carson P, Januzzi J, Verma S, Tsutsui H, Brueckmann M et al (2020) Cardiovascular and renal outcomes with empagliflozin in heart failure. N Engl J Med 383(15):1413–1424
26. Schork A, Saynisch J, Vosseler A et al (2019) Effect of SGLT2 inhibitors on body composition, fluid status and renin-angiotensin-aldosterone system in type 2 diabetes: a prospective study using bioimpedance spectroscopy. Cardiovasc Diabetol 18:46. https://doi.org/10.1186/s12933-019-0852-y
27. Santos-Gallego CG, Requena-Ibanez JA, San Antonio R et al (2019) Empagliflozin ameliorates adverse left ventricular remodeling in nondiabetic heart failure by enhancing myocardial energetics. J Am Coll Cardiol 73:1931–1944. https://doi.org/10.1016/j.jacc.2019.01.056
28. Oh CM, Cho S, Jang JY et al (2019) Cardioprotective potential of an SGLT2 inhibitor against doxorubicin-induced heart failure. Korean Circ J 49:1183–1195. https://doi.org/10.4070/kcj.2019.0180
29. Ye Y, Bajaj M, Yang HC, Perez-Polo JR, Birnbaum Y (2017) SGLT-2 inhibition with dapagliflozin reduces the activation of the Nlrp3/ASC inflammasome and attenuates the development of diabetic cardiomyopathy in mice with type 2 diabetes. Further augmentation of the effects with Saxagliptin, a DPP4 inhibitor. Cardiovasc Drugs Ther 31:119–132. https://doi.org/10.1007/s10557-017-6725-2
30. Zinman B, Wanner C, Lachin JM et al (2015) Empagliflozin, cardiovascular outcomes, and mortality in type 2 diabetes. N Engl J Med 373:2117–2128. This study was the first to demonstrate SGLT2i (namely empagliflozin) to lower the rates of death from cardiovascular causes, nonfatal myocardial infarction, or nonfatal stroke in patients with type 2 diabetes at high cardiovascular risk, when added to standard care
31. Marso SP, Daniels GH, Brown-Frandsen K, Kristensen P, Mann JFE, Nauck MA et al (2016) Liraglutide and cardiovascular outcomes in type 2 diabetes. N Engl J Med 375:311–322. This study elucidated the cardiovascular effect of the GLP-1RA, liraglutide, when added to standard care in patients with type 2 diabetes, which was otherwise unknown
32. Holman RR, Bethel MA, Mentz RJ, Thompson VP, Lokhnygina Y, Buse JB et al (2017) Effects of once-weekly exenatide on cardiovascular outcomes in type 2 diabetes. N Engl J Med 377:1228–1239. http://www.ncbi.nlm.nih.gov/pubmed/28910237; http://www.nejm.org/doi/10.1056/NEJMoa1612917. Accessed 15 Jan 2018
33. Hogan AE, Gaoatswe G, Lynch L, Corrigan MA, Woods C, O'Connell J et al (2014) Glucagon-like peptide 1 analogue therapy directly modulates innate immune-mediated inflammation in individuals with type 2 diabetes mellitus. Diabetologia 57:781–784. Available: http://link.springer.com/10.1007/s00125-013-3145-0. Accessed 10 Dec 2017
34. Hirano T, Mori Y (2016) Anti-atherogenic and anti-inflammatory properties of glucagon-like peptide-1, glucose-dependent insulinotropic polypepide, and dipeptidyl peptidase-4 inhibitors in experimental animals. J Diabetes Invest 7:80–86
35. Xu L, Nagata N, Nagashimada M, Zhuge F, Ni Y, Chen G et al (2017) SGLT2 inhibition by empagliflozin promotes fat utilization and browning and attenuates inflammation and insulin resistance by polarizing M2 macrophages in diet-induced obese mice. EBioMedicine 20:137–149. https://doi.org/10.1016/j.ebiom.2017.05.028
36. Frías J, Guja C, Hardy E, Ahmed A, Dong F et al (2016) Exenatide once weekly plus dapagliflozin once daily versus exenatide or dapagliflozin alone in patients with type 2 diabetes inadequately controlled with metformin monotherapy (DURATION-8): a 28 week,

multicentre, double-blind, phase 3, randomised control. Lancet Diabetes Endocrinol. 4:1004–1016. This study exemplies the notion of combination therapy with GLP-1RA and SGLT2i. The study not only evaluates efficacy and safety of co-initiation of the GLP-1 receptor agonist exenatide and the SGLT2 inhibitor dapagliflozin but also compares it to exenatide or dapagliflozin monotherapy in patients with type 2 diabetes inadequately controlled by metformin
37. Fulcher G, Matthews DR, Perkovic V, de Zeeuw D, Mahaffey KW, Mathieu C et al (2016) Efficacy and safety of canagliflozin when used in conjunction with incretin-mimetic therapy in patients with type 2 diabetes. Diabetes Obes Metab 18:82–91. http://doi.wiley.com/10.1111/dom.12589. Accessed 1 Dec 2017
38. Tatarkiewicz K, Polizzi C, Villescaz C, D'Souza LJ, Wang Y, Janssen S et al (2014) Combined antidiabetic benefits of exenatide and dapagliflozin in diabetic mice. Diabetes Obes Metab 16:376–380
39. Perkovic V, Jardine MJ, Neal B, Bompoint S, Heerspink HJ, Charytan DM, Edwards R, Agarwal R, Bakris G, Bull S, Cannon CP (2019) Canagliflozin and renal outcomes in type 2 diabetes and nephropathy. N Engl J Med 380(24):2295–2306. https://doi.org/10.1056/NEJMoa1811744. This is the first double-blind randomized controlled trial showing decreased relative risk of ESRD, while continuing to show decreased risk of cardiovascular death, myocardial infarction, or stroke, decreased hospitalization for heart failure, and no significant difference in amputations or fractures
40. Wilding J, Fernando K, Milne N et al (2018) SGLT2 inhibitors in type 2 diabetes management: key evidence and implications for clinical practice. Diabetes Ther 9:1757–1773
41. Pantalone KM, Hobbs TM, Wells BJ et al (2015) Clinical characteristics, complications, comorbidities and treatment patterns among patients with type 2 diabetes mellitus in a large integrated health system. BMJ Open Diabetes Res Care 3:e000093
42. Einarson TR, Acs A, Ludwig C, Panton UH (2018) Prevalence of cardiovascular disease in type 2 diabetes: a systematic literature review of scientific evidence from across the world in 2007–2017. Cardiovasc Diabetol 17:83
43. De Rosa S, Arcidiacono B, Chiefari E, Brunetti A, Indolfi C, Foti DP (2018) Type 2 diabetes mellitus and cardiovascular disease: genetic and epigenetic links. Front Endocrinol (Lausanne) 9:2
44. Leon BM, Maddox TM (2015) Diabetes and cardiovascular disease: epidemiology, biological mechanisms, treatment recommendations and future research. World J Diabetes 6:1246–1258
45. Gonzalez N, Moreno-Villegas Z, Gonzalez-Bris A, Egido J, Lorenzo O (2017) Regulation of visceral and epicardial adipose tissue for preventing cardiovascular injuries associated to obesity and diabetes. Cardiovasc Diabetol 16:44
46. Ortega FB, Lavie CJ, Blair SN (2016) Obesity and cardiovascular disease. Circ Res 118:1752–1770
47. Lalia AZ, Dasari S, Johnson ML et al (2016) Predictors of whole-body insulin sensitivity across ages and adiposity in adult humans. J Clin Endocrinol Metab 101:626–634
48. Laakso M, Kuusisto J (2014) Insulin resistance and hyperglycaemia in cardiovascular disease development. Nat Rev Endocrinol 10:293–302
49. Ormazabal V, Nair S, Elfeky O, Aguayo C, Salomon C, Zuniga FA (2018) Association between insulin resistance and the development of cardiovascular disease. Cardiovasc Diabetol 17:122
50. Brannick B, Dagogo-Jack S (2018) Prediabetes and cardiovascular disease: pathophysiology and interventions for prevention and risk reduction. Endocrinol Metab Clin N Am 47:33–50
51. DeFronzo RA, Abdul-Ghani M (2011) Assessment and treatment of cardiovascular risk in prediabetes: impaired glucose tolerance and impaired fasting glucose. Am J Cardiol 108:3B–24B
52. Ryden L, Standl E, Bartnik M et al (2007) Guidelines on diabetes, pre-diabetes, and cardiovascular diseases: executive summary. The task force on diabetes and cardiovascular diseases of the European Society of Cardiology (ESC) and of the European Association for the Study of Diabetes (EASD). Eur Heart J 28:88–136

53. Rungby J, Schou M, Warrer P, Ytte L, Andersen GS (2017) Prevalence of cardiovascular disease and evaluation of standard of care in type 2 diabetes: a nationwide study in primary care. Cardiovasc Endocrinol 6:145–151
54. Hancock HC, Close H, Mason JM et al (2013) High prevalence of undetected heart failure in long-term care residents: findings from the Heart Failure in Care Homes (HFinCH) study. Eur J Heart Fail 15:158–165
55. Di Lenarda A, Stellato K, Radini D (2019) The challenge of heart failure diagnosis and management in primary care in elderly population: mere illusion or concrete opportunity? Int J Cardiol 274:248–249
56. Packer M (2018) Heart failure: the most important, preventable, and treatable cardiovascular complication of type 2 diabetes. Diabetes Care 41:11–13
57. Van Linthout S, Tschope C (2017) Inflammation—cause or consequence of heart failure or both? Curr Heart Fail Rep 14:251–265
58. Thomas MC (2016) Type 2 diabetes and heart failure: challenges and solutions. Curr Cardiol Rev 12:249–255
59. Matsushita K, Blecker S, Pazin-Filho A et al (2010) The association of hemoglobin A1c with incident heart failure among people without diabetes: the atherosclerosis risk in communities study. Diabetes 59:2020–2026
60. Carr AA, Kowey PR, Devereux RB et al (2005) Hospitalizations for new heart failure among subjects with diabetes mellitus in the RENAAL and LIFE studies. Am J Cardiol 96:1530–1536
61. Selvin E, Coresh J, Golden SH, Brancati FL, Folsom AR, Steffes MW (2005) Glycemic control and coronary heart disease risk in persons with and without diabetes: the atherosclerosis risk in communities study. Arch Intern Med 165:1910–1916
62. Action to Control Cardiovascular Risk in Diabetes Study Group, Gerstein HC, Miller ME et al (2008) Effects of intensive glucose lowering in type 2 diabetes. N Engl J Med 358:2545–2559
63. Group A, Patel A, MacMahon S et al (2008) Intensive blood glucose control and vascular outcomes in patients with type 2 diabetes. N Engl J Med 358:2560–2572
64. Duckworth W, Abraira C, Moritz T et al (2009) Glucose control and vascular complications in veterans with type 2 diabetes. N Engl J Med 360:129–139
65. Zinman B, Wanner C, Lachin JM, Fitchett D, Bluhmki E, Hantel S, Mattheus M, Devins T, Johansen OE, Woerle HJ, Broedl UC, Inzucchi SE (2015) Empagliflozin, cardiovascular outcomes, and mortality in type 2 diabetes. N Engl J Med 373:2117–2128. https://doi.org/10.1056/NEJMc1600827
66. Wiviott SD, Raz I, Bonaca MP, Mosenzon O, Kato ET, Cahn A, Silverman MG, Zelniker TA, Kuder JF, Murphy SA, Bhatt DL, Leiter LA, McGuire DK, Wilding JPH, Ruff CT, Gause-Nilsson IAM, Fredriksson M, Johansson PA, Langkilde AM, Sabatine MS (2019) Dapagliflozin and cardiovascular outcomes in type 2 diabetes. N Engl J Med 380(4):347–357. https://doi.org/10.1056/NEJMoa1812389. http://www.ncbi.nlm.nih.gov/pubmed/30415602
67. Cavender MA, Norhammar A, Birkeland KI et al (2018) SGLT-2 inhibitors and cardiovascular risk: an analysis of CVD-REAL. J Am Coll Cardiol 71:2497–2506
68. Kosiborod M, Cavender MA, Fu AZ et al (2017) Lower risk of heart failure and death in patients initiated on sodium-glucose cotransporter-2 inhibitors versus other glucose-lowering drugs: the CVD-REAL study (comparative effectiveness of cardiovascular outcomes in new users of sodium-glucose cotransporter-2 inhibitors). Circulation 136:249–259
69. Ryan PB, Buse JB, Schuemie MJ et al (2018) Comparative effectiveness of canagliflozin, SGLT2 inhibitors and non-SGLT2 inhibitors on the risk of hospitalization for heart failure and amputation in patients with type 2 diabetes mellitus: a real-world meta-analysis of 4 observational databases (OBSERVE-4D). Diabetes Obes Metab 20:2585–2597
70. Udell JA, Yuan Z, Rush T, Sicignano NM, Galitz M, Rosenthal N (2018) Cardiovascular outcomes and risks after initiation of a sodium glucose cotransporter 2 inhibitor: results from the EASEL population-based cohort study (evidence for cardiovascular outcomes with sodium glucose cotransporter 2 inhibitors in the real world). Circulation 137:1450–1459
71. Inzucchi SE, Zinman B, Wanner C et al (2015) SGLT-2 inhibitors and cardiovascular risk: proposed pathways and review of ongoing outcome trials. Diab Vasc Dis Res 12:90–100

72. Heerspink HJ, Perkins BA, Fitchett DH, Husain M, Cherney DZ (2016) Sodium glucose cotransporter 2 inhibitors in the treatment of diabetes mellitus: cardiovascular and kidney effects, potential mechanisms, and clinical applications. Circulation 134:752–772
73. Kelly MS, Lewis J, Huntsberry AM, Dea L, Portillo I (2019) Efficacy and renal outcomes of SGLT2 inhibitors in patients with type 2 diabetes and chronic kidney disease. Postgrad Med 131:31–42
74. Seidu S, Kunutsor SK, Cos X et al (2018) SGLT2 inhibitors and renal outcomes in type 2 diabetes with or without renal impairment: a systematic review and meta-analysis. Prim Care Diabetes 12:265–283
75. Jardine MJ, Mahaffey KW, Neal B et al (2017) The Canagliflozin and Rrenal Endpoints in Diabetes with Established Nephropathy Clinical Evaluation (CREDENCE) study rationale, design, and baseline characteristics. Am J Nephrol 46:462–472
76. Radholm K, Figtree G, Perkovic V et al (2018) Canagliflozin and heart failure in type 2 diabetes mellitus. Circulation 138:458–468
77. Suvarna VR (2018) Real world evidence (RWE)—are we (RWE) ready? Perspect Clin Res 9:61–63
78. Camm AJ, Fox KAA (2018) Strengths and weaknesses of 'real-world' studies involving non-vitamin K antagonist oral anticoagulants. Open Heart 5:e000788
79. Roche N, Reddel H, Martin R, et al (2014) Quality standards for real-world research. Focus on observational database studies of comparative effectiveness. Ann Am Thorac Soc 11(Suppl 2):S99–S104
80. Boehringer Ingelheim (2018) Initial results from EMPRISE real-world evidence study shows empagliflozin was associated with reduced risk for hospitalisation for heart failure compared with DPP-4 inhibitors in people with type 2 diabetes with and without cardiovascular disease. https://www.boehringer-ingelheim.com/press-release/initial-results-emprise-real-world-evidence-study
81. Verma S, McMurray JJV (2018) SGLT2 inhibitors and mechanisms of cardiovascular benefit: a state-of-the-art review. Diabetologia 61:2108–2117
82. Fitchett D, Butler J, van de Borne P et al (2018) Effects of empagliflozin on risk for cardiovascular death and heart failure hospitalization across the spectrum of heart failure risk in the EMPA-REG OUTCOME® trial. Eur Heart J 39:363–370
83. Barnett AH, O'Hare P, Halcox J (2017) Guidelines for type 2 diabetes: keeping a finger on the pulse. Lancet Diabetes Endocrinol 5:420
84. Opingari E, Partridge ACR, Verma S, Bajaj HS (2018) SGLT2 inhibitors: practical considerations and recommendations for cardiologists. Curr Opin Cardiol 33:676–682
85. Kimura G (2016) Diuretic action of sodium-glucose cotransporter 2 inhibitors and its importance in the management of heart failure. Circ J 80:2277–2281
86. Verma S, McMurray JJV, Cherney DZI (2017) The metabolodiuretic promise of sodium-dependent glucose cotransporter 2 inhibition: the search for the sweet spot in heart failure. JAMA Cardiol 2(9):939–940
87. Staels B (2017) Cardiovascular protection by sodium glucose cotransporter 2 inhibitors: potential mechanisms. Am J Med 130(6S):S30–S39
88. Byrne NJ, Parajuli N, Levasseur JL et al (2017) Empagliflozin prevents worsening of cardiac function in an experimental model of pressure overload-induced heart failure. JACC: Basic Transl Sci 2(4):347–354
89. Verma S, McMurray JJV (2018) SGLT2 inhibitors and mechanisms of cardiovascular benefit: a state-of-the-art review. Diabetologia 61(10):2108–2117
90. Mudaliar S, Alloju S, Henry RR (2016) Can a shift in fuel energetics explain the beneficial cardiorenal outcomes in the EMPA-REG OUTCOME study? A unifying hypothesis. Diabetes Care 39:1115–1122
91. Daniele G, Xiong J, Solis-Herrera C, Merovci A, Eldor R, Tripathy D, DeFronzo RA, Norton L, Abdul-Ghani M (2016) Dapagliflozin enhances fat oxidation and ketone production in patients with type 2 diabetes. Diabetes Care 39:2036–2041

92. Bonnet F, Scheen AJ (2018) Effects of SGLT2 inhibitors on systemic and tissue low-grade inflammation: the potential diabetes complications and cardiovascular disease. Diabetes Metab 44(6):457–464
93. https://clinicaltrials.gov/. Accessed 5 Jul 2019
94. Zinman B, Wanner C, Lachin JM et al (2015) Empagliflozin, cardiovascular outcomes, and mortality in type 2 diabetes. N Engl J Med 373:2117–2128. EMPAREG-OUTCOMES trial reporting the CV outcomes of empagliflozin
95. Mather A, Pollock C (2011) Glucose handling by the kidney. Kidney Int Suppl 79:S1–S6
96. Rieg T, Vallon V (2018) Development of SGLT1 and SGLT2 inhibitors. Diabetologia 61:2079–2086
97. Sato T, Aizawa Y, Yuasa S, Kishi S, Fuse K, Fujita S et al (2018) The effect of dapagliflozin treatment on epicardial adipose tissue volume. Cardiovasc Diabetol 17:6
98. Bouchi R, Terashima M, Sasahara Y, Asakawa M, Fukuda T, Takeuchi T et al (2017) Luseogliflozin reduces epicardial fat accumulation in patients with type 2 diabetes: a pilot study. Cardiovasc Diabetol 16:32
99. Yagi S, Hirata Y, Ise T, Kusunose K, Yamada H, Fukuda D et al (2017) Canagliflozin reduces epicardial fat in patients with type 2 diabetes mellitus. Diabetol Metab Syndr 9:78
100. Sano M, Takei M, Shiraishi Y, Suzuki Y (2016) Increased hematocrit during sodium-glucose cotransporter 2 inhibitor therapy indicates recovery of tubulointerstitial function in diabetic kidneys. J Clin Med Res 8:844–847
101. Kato ET, Silverman MG, Mosenzon O et al (2019) Effect of dapagliflozin on heart failure and mortality in type 2 diabetes mellitus. Circulation 139:2528–2536
102. Furtado HM, Bonaca MP, Raz I et al (2019) Dapagliflozin and cardiovascular outcomes in patients with type 2 diabetes mellitus and previous myocardial infarction. Circulation 139:2516–2527
103. McMurray JJV, Solomon SD, Inzucchi SE et al (2019) Dapagliflozin in patients with heart failure and reduced ejection fraction. N Engl J Med 381:1995–2008. https://doi.org/10.1056/NEJMoa1911303
104. Uthman L, Baartscheer A, Schumacher CA et al (2018) Direct cardiac actions of sodium glucose cotransporter 2 inhibitors target pathogenic mechanisms underlying heart failure in diabetic patients. Front Physiol 9:1575. https://doi.org/10.3389/fphys.2018.01575
105. Zelniker TA, Braunwald E (2020) Mechanisms of cardiorenal effects of sodium-glucose cotransporter 2 inhibitors: JACC state-of-the-art review. J Am Coll Cardiol 75(4):422–434. https://doi.org/10.1016/j.jacc.2019.11.031
106. Lopaschuk GD, Verma S (2020) Mechanisms of cardiovascular benefits of sodium glucose co-transporter 2 (SGLT2) inhibitors: a state-of-the-art review. JACC Basic Transl Sci 5:632–644. https://doi.org/10.1016/j.jacbts.2020.02.004
107. Khemais-Benkhiat S, Belcastro E, Idris-Khodja N et al (2020) Angiotensin II-induced redox-sensitive SGLT1 and 2 expression promotes high glucose-induced endothelial cell senescence. J Cell Mol Med 24(3):2109–2122. https://doi.org/10.1111/jcmm.14233
108. Sukhanov S, Higashi Y, Yoshida T et al (2021) The SGLT2 inhibitor Empagliflozin attenuates interleukin-17A-induced human aortic smooth muscle cell proliferation and migration by targeting TRAF3IP2/ROS/NLRP3/Caspase-1-dependent IL-1beta and IL-18 secretion. Cell Signal 77:109825. https://doi.org/10.1016/j.cellsig.2020.109825
109. Mustroph J, Lucht CM, Wagemann O et al (2019) Empagliflozin enhances human and murine cardiomyocyte glucose uptake by increased expression of GLUT1. Diabetologia 62(4):726–729. https://doi.org/10.1007/s00125-019-4819-z
110. Seferović PM, Petrie MC, Filippatos GS, Anker SD, Rosano G, Bauersachs J et al (2018) Type 2 diabetes mellitus and heart failure: a position statement from the Heart Failure Association of the European Society of Cardiology. Eur J Heart Fail 20(5):853–872
111. Cosentino F, Grant PJ, Aboyans V, Bailey CJ, Ceriello A, Delgado V et al (2020) 2019 ESC guidelines on diabetes, pre-diabetes, and cardiovascular diseases developed in collaboration with the EASD. Eur Heart J 41(2):255–323. http://www.ncbi.nlm.nih.gov/pubmed/31497854

112. Zannad F (2018) Rising incidence of heart failure demands action. Lancet 391(10120):518–519
113. Packer M (2018) Epicardial adipose tissue may mediate deleterious effects of obesity and inflammation on the myocardium. J Am Coll Cardiol 71(20):2360–2372
114. Kenny HC, Abel ED (2019) Heart failure in type 2 diabetes mellitus. Circ Res 124(1):121–141
115. Scirica BM, Bhatt DL, Braunwald E, Steg PG, Davidson J, Hirshberg B et al (2013) Saxagliptin and cardiovascular outcomes in patients with type 2 diabetes mellitus. N Engl J Med 369(14):1317–1326
116. Ohkuma T, Jun M, Woodward M, Zoungas S, Cooper ME, Grobbee DE et al (2017) Cardiac stress and inflammatory markers as predictors of heart failure in patients with type 2 diabetes: the ADVANCE trial. Diabetes Care 40(9):1203–1209
117. Tarnow L, Gall MA, Hansen BV, Hovind P, Parving HH (2006) Plasma N-terminal pro-B-type natriuretic peptide and mortality in type 2 diabetes. Diabetologia 49(10):2256–2262
118. Buse JB, Wexler DJ, Tsapas A, Rossing P, Mingrone G, Mathieu C et al (2020) 2019 update to: management of hyperglycemia in type 2 diabetes, 2018. A consensus report by the American Diabetes Association (ADA) and the European Association for the Study of Diabetes (EASD). Diabetes Care 43(2):487–493
119. Erdmann E, Charbonnel B, Wilcox RG, Skene AM, Massi-Benedetti M, Yates J et al (2007) Pioglitazone use and heart failure in patients with type 2 diabetes and preexisting cardiovascular disease. Data from the PROactive Study. Diabetes Care 30(11):2773–2778
120. Ceriello A, Standl E, Catrinoiu D, Itzhak B, Lalic NM, Rahelic D et al (2020) Issues of cardiovascular risk management in people with diabetes in the COVID-19 era. Diabetes Care 8:200941
121. Wargny M, Potier L, Gourdy P, Pichelin M, Amadou C, Benhamou P-Y et al (2021) Predictors of hospital discharge and mortality in patients with diabetes and COVID-19: updated results from the nationwide CORONADO study. Diabetologia 64(4):778–794
122. Standl E, Schnell O (2021) Heart failure outcomes and Covid-19. Diabetes Res Clin Pract 175:108794
123. Chatterjee S, Khunti K, Davies MJ (2017) Type 2 diabetes. Lancet 389(10085):2239–2251
124. Aguillón AR, Mascarello A, Segretti ND, de Azevedo HFZ, Guimaraes CRW, Miranda LSM et al (2018) Synthetic strategies toward SGLT2 inhibitors. Org Process Res Dev 22(4):467–488
125. Hallow KM, Gebremichael Y, Helmlinger G, Vallon V (2017) Primary proximal tubule hyperreabsorption and impaired tubular transport counterregulation determine glomerular hyperfiltration in diabetes: a modeling analysis. Am J Physiol-Renal Physiol 312(5):F819–F835
126. Wilcox CS (2020 Apr) Antihypertensive and renal mechanisms of SGLT2 (sodium-glucose linked transporter 2) inhibitors. Hypertension 75(4):894–901
127. Jo HA, Seo JH, Lee S, Yu M-y, Bae E, Kim DK et al (2023) Metabolomic profiling in kidney cells treated with a sodium glucose-cotransporter 2 inhibitor. Sci Rep 4(1):2026
128. Lu YP, Zhang ZY, Wu HW, Fang LJ, Hu B, Tang C et al (2022) SGLT2 inhibitors improve kidney function and morphology by regulating renal metabolic reprogramming in mice with diabetic kidney disease. J Transl Med 14(1):420
129. Nakamura M, Sadoshima J (2018) Mechanisms of physiological and pathological cardiac hypertrophy. Nat Rev Cardiol. 15(7):387–407
130. Tran DH, Wang Z v (2019) Glucose metabolism in cardiac hypertrophy and heart failure. J Am Heart Assoc 8(12):e012673
131. Pereira RO, Wende AR, Olsen C, Soto J, Rawlings T, Zhu Y et al (2013) Inducible overexpression of GLUT1 prevents mitochondrial dysfunction and attenuates structural remodeling in pressure overload but does not prevent left ventricular dysfunction. J Am Heart Assoc 2(5):e000301
132. Zhang L, Jaswal JS, Ussher JR, Sankaralingam S, Wagg C, Zaugg M et al (2013) Cardiac insulin-resistance and decreased mitochondrial energy production precede the development of systolic heart failure after pressure-overload hypertrophy. Circ Heart Fail 6(5):1039–1048

133. Makarewich CA, Zhang H, Davis J, Correll RN, Trappanese DM, Hoffman NE et al (2014) Transient receptor potential channels contribute to pathological structural and functional remodeling after myocardial infarction. Circ Res 115(6):567–580
134. Ritterhoff J, Tian R (2017) Metabolism in cardiomyopathy: every substrate matters. Cardiovasc Res 113(4):411–421
135. Makrecka-Kuka M, Liepinsh E, Murray AJ, Lemieux H, Dambrova M, Tepp K et al (2020) Altered mitochondrial metabolism in the insulin-resistant heart. Acta Physiol 228(3):e13430
136. Giordano FJ (2005) Oxygen, oxidative stress, hypoxia, and heart failure. J Clin Invest 115(3):500–508
137. Izzo C, Vitillo P, di Pietro P, Visco V, Strianese A, Virtuoso N et al (2021) The role of oxidative stress in cardiovascular aging and cardiovascular diseases. Life 11(1):60
138. Kiyuna LA, Albuquerque RP, Chen CH, Mochly-Rosen D, Ferreira JCB (2018) Targeting mitochondrial dysfunction and oxidative stress in heart failure: challenges and opportunities. Free Radic Biol Med 129:155–168
139. Noordali H, Loudon BL, Frenneaux MP, Madhani M (2018) Cardiac metabolism—a promising therapeutic target for heart failure. Pharmacol Ther 182:95–114
140. Zinman B, Inzucchi SE, Lachin JM, Wanner C, Ferrari R, Fitchett D et al (2014) Rationale, design, and baseline characteristics of a randomized, placebo-controlled cardiovascular outcome trial of empagliflozin (EMPA-REG OUTCOME™). Cardiovasc Diabetol 13(1):102
141. Baartscheer A, Schumacher CA, Wüst RCI, Fiolet JWT, Stienen GJM, Coronel R et al (2017) Empagliflozin decreases myocardial cytoplasmic Na + through inhibition of the cardiac Na+/H + exchanger in rats and rabbits. Diabetologia 60(3):568–573
142. Uthman L, Baartscheer A, Bleijlevens B, Schumacher CA, Fiolet JWT, Koeman A et al (2018 Mar 2) Class effects of SGLT2 inhibitors in mouse cardiomyocytes and hearts: inhibition of Na+/H + exchanger, lowering of cytosolic Na + and vasodilation. Diabetologia 61(3):722–726
143. Hawley SA, Ford RJ, Smith BK, Gowans GJ, Mancini SJ, Pitt RD et al (2016) The Na+/glucose cotransporter inhibitor Canagliflozin activates AMPK by inhibiting mitochondrial function and increasing cellular AMP levels. Diabetes 65(9):2784–2794
144. Li C, Zhang J, Xue M, Li X, Han F, Liu X et al (2019) SGLT2 inhibition with empagliflozin attenuates myocardial oxidative stress and fibrosis in diabetic mice heart. Cardiovasc Diabetol 2(1):15
145. Zhou H, Wang S, Zhu P, Hu S, Chen Y, Ren J (2018) Empagliflozin rescues diabetic myocardial microvascular injury via AMPK-mediated inhibition of mitochondrial fission. Redox Biol 15:335–346
146. Zelniker TA, Braunwald E (2020) Mechanisms of cardiorenal effects of sodium-glucose cotransporter 2 inhibitors. J Am Coll Cardiol 75(4):422–434
147. Zannad F, Ferreira JP, Butler J, Filippatos G, Januzzi JL, Sumin M et al (2022) Effect of empagliflozin on circulating proteomics in heart failure: mechanistic insights into the EMPEROR programme. Eur Heart J 43(48):4991–5002
148. Hernandez AF, Green JB, Janmohamed S et al (2018) Albiglutide and cardiovascular outcomes in patients with type 2 diabetes and cardiovascular disease (harmony outcomes): a double-blind, randomised placebo-controlled trial. Lancet 392:1519–1529
149. Marso SP, Daniels GH, Brown-Frandsen K et al (2016) Liraglutide and cardiovascular outcomes in type 2 diabetes. N Engl J Med 375:311–322
150. Marso SP, Bain SC, Consoli A et al (2016) Semaglutide and cardiovascular outcomes in patients with type 2 diabetes. N Engl J Med 375:1834–1844
151. Gerstein HC, Colhoun HM, Dagenais GR et al (2019) Dulaglutide and cardiovascular outcomes in type 2 diabetes (REWIND): a double-blind, randomised placebo-controlled trial. Lancet 394:121–130
152. Davies MJ, D'Alessio DA, Fradkin J et al (2018) Management of hyperglycemia in type 2 diabetes, 2018. A consensus report by the American Diabetes Association (ADA) and the European Association for the Study of Diabetes (EASD). Diabetes Care 2018(41):2669–2701

153. UK Prospective Diabetes Study (UKPDS) Group (1998) Effect of intensive blood-glucose control with metformin on complications in overweight patients with type 2 diabetes (UKPDS 34). UK Prospective Diabetes Study (UKPDS) Group. Lancet 352:854–865
154. Gerstein HC, Miller ME, Byington RP et al (2008) Effects of intensive glucose lowering in type 2 diabetes. N Engl J Med 358:2545–2559
155. Patel A, MacMahon S, Chalmers J et al (2008) Intensive blood glucose control and vascular outcomes in patients with type 2 diabetes. N Engl J Med 24:2560–2572
156. Kosiborod M, Lam CSP, Kohsaka S et al (2018) Cardiovascular events associated with SGLT-2 inhibitors versus other glucose-lowering drugs: the CVD-REAL 2 study. J Am Coll Cardiol 71:2628–2639
157. Tang H, Li D, Zhang J et al (2017) Sodium-glucose co-transporter-2 inhibitors and risk of adverse renal outcomes among patients with type 2 diabetes: a network and cumulative meta-analysis of randomized controlled trials. Diabetes Obes Metab 19:1106–1115
158. Margulies KB, Hernandez AF, Redfield MM et al (2016) Effects of liraglutide on clinical stability among patients with advanced heart failure and reduced ejection fraction: a randomized clinical trial. JAMA 316:500–508
159. Frias JP, Guja C, Hardy E et al (2016) Exenatide once weekly plus dapagliflozin once daily versus exenatide or dapagliflozin alone in patients with type 2 diabetes inadequately controlled with metformin monotherapy (DURATION-8): a 28 week, multicentre, double-blind, phase 3, randomised controlled trial. Lancet Diabetes Endocrinol 4:1004–1016
160. Ludvik B, Frias JP, Tinahones FJ et al (2018) Dulaglutide as add-on therapy to SGLT2 inhibitors in patients with inadequately controlled type 2 diabetes (AWARD-10): a 24-week, randomised, double-blind, placebo-controlled trial. Lancet Diabetes Endocrinol 6:370–381
161. DeFronzo RA (2017) Combination therapy with GLP-1 receptor agonist and SGLT2 inhibitor. Diabetes Obes Metab 19:1353–1362
162. Harashima SI, Inagaki N, Kondo K et al (2018) Efficacy and safety of canagliflozin as add-on therapy to a glucagon-like peptide-1 receptor agonist in Japanese patients with type 2 diabetes mellitus: a 52-week, open-label, phase IV study. Diabetes Obes Metab 20:1770–1775
163. Ishihara H, Yamaguchi S, Nakao I et al (2018) Ipragliflozin add-on therapy to a GLP-1 receptor agonist in Japanese patients with type 2 diabetes (AGATE): a 52-week open-label study. Diabetes Ther Res Treat Educ Diabetes Rel Disord 9:1549–1567
164. Seino Y, Yabe D, Sasaki T et al (2018) Sodium-glucose cotransporter-2 inhibitor luseogliflozin added to glucagon-like peptide 1 receptor agonist liraglutide improves glycemic control with bodyweight and fat mass reductions in Japanese patients with type 2 diabetes: a 52-week, open-label, single-arm study. J Diabetes Invest. 9:332–340
165. Udell JA et al (2018) Cardiovascular outcomes and risks after initiation of a sodium glucose cotransporter 2 inhibitor: results from the EASEL population-based cohort study (evidence for cardiovascular outcomes with sodium glucose cotransporter 2 inhibitors in the real world). Circulation 137(14):1450–1459
166. Kosiborod M, Lam CSP, Kohsaka S et al (2018) Lower cardiovascular risk associated with SGLT-2i in >400,000 patients: the CVD-REAL 2 study. J Am Coll Cardiol 71:2628. https://doi.org/10.1016/j.jacc.2018.03.009
167. Sharma A et al (2017) A network analysis to compare biomarker profiles in patients with and without diabetes mellitus in acute heart failure. Eur J Heart Fail 19(10):1310–1320
168. Tromp J et al (2020) Distinct pathological pathways in patients with heart failure and diabetes. JACC Heart Fail 8(3):234–242
169. Matsutani D, Sakamoto M, Kayama Y, Takeda N, Horiuchi R, Utsunomiya K (2018) Effect of canagliflozin on left ventricular diastolic function in patients with type 2 diabetes. Cardiovasc Diabetol 17(1):73
170. Otagaki M, Matsumura K, Kin H, Fujii K, Shibutani H, Matsumoto H, Takahashi H, Park H, Yamamoto Y, Sugiura T et al (2019) Effect of tofogliflozin on systolic and diastolic cardiac function in type 2 diabetic patients. Cardiovasc Drugs Ther 33(4):435–442

171. Soga F, Tanaka H, Tatsumi K, Mochizuki Y, Sano H, Toki H, Matsumoto K, Shite J, Takaoka H, Doi T et al (2018) Impact of dapagliflozin on left ventricular diastolic function of patients with type 2 diabetic mellitus with chronic heart failure. Cardiovasc Diabetol 17(1):132
172. Yang JJ et al (2019) Association of diabetes with all-cause and cause-specific mortality in asia: a pooled analysis of more than 1 million participants. JAMA Netw Open 2:e192696
173. Heerspink JL, Stefánsson BV, Correa-Rotter R, Chertow GM, Greene T, Hou F-F et al (2020) Dapagliflozin in patients with chronic kidney disease. N Engl J Med 383(15):1436–1446. Accession Number: 32970396. https://doi.org/10.1056/NEJMoa2024816
174. Kosiborod M, Cavender MA, Fu AZ, Wilding JP, Khunti K, Holl RW et al (2017) Lower risk of heart failure and death in patients initiated on sodium-glucose cotransporter-2 inhibitors versus other glucose-lowering drugs: the CVD-REAL study (comparative effectiveness of cardiovascular outcomes in new users of sodium-glucose cotransporter-2 inhibitors). Circulation 136:249–259. http://www.ncbi.nlm.nih.gov/pubmed/28522450. Accessed 15 Jan 2018
175. Koh ES et al (2021) Renal outcomes and all-cause death associated with sodium-glucose co-transporter-2 inhibitors versus other glucose-lowering drugs (CVD-REAL 3 Korea). Diabetes Obes Metab 23:455–466
176. Fitchett D, Zinman B, Wanner C et al (2016) Heart failure outcomes with empagliflozin in patients with type 2 diabetes at high cardiovascular risk: results of the EMPA-REG OUTCOME® trial. Eur Heart J 37:1526–1534. https://doi.org/10.1093/eurheartj/ehv728
177. Rådholm K, Figtree G, Perkovic V et al (2018) Canagliflozin and heart failure in type 2 diabetes mellitus: results from the CANVAS program. Circulation 138:458–468
178. Verma S, Wanner C, Zwiener I et al (2019) Influence of microvascular disease on cardiovascular events in type 2 diabetes. J Am Coll Cardiol 73:2780–2782
179. Perkovic V, Jardine MJ, Neal B et al (2019) Canagliflozin and renal outcomes in type 2 diabetes and nephropathy. N Engl J Med 380:2295–2306
180. Furtado RHM, Bonaca MP, Raz I et al (2019) Dapagliflozin and cardiovascular outcomes in patients with type 2 diabetes mellitus and previous myocardial infarction. Circulation 139:2516–2527
181. Heerspink HJL, Stefansson BV, Correa-Rotter R et al (2020) Dapagliflozin in patients with chronic kidney disease. N Engl J Med 383:1436–1446
182. Anker SD, Butler J, Filippatos G et al (2021) Empagliflozin in heart failure with a preserved ejection fraction. N Engl J Med 385:1451–1461
183. O'Meara E, McDonald M, Chan M et al (2020) CCS/CHFS heart failure guidelines: clinical trial update on functional mitral regurgitation, SGLT2 inhibitors, ARNI in HFpEF, and tafamidis in amyloidosis. Can J Cardiol 36:159–169
184. Butler J, Handelsman Y, Bakris G, Verma S (2020) Use of sodium-glucose co-transporter-2 inhibitors in patients with and without type 2 diabetes: implications for incident and prevalent heart failure. Eur J Heart Fail 22:604–617
185. Seferovic PM, Fragasso G, Petrie M et al (2020) Heart Failure Association of the European Society of Cardiology update on sodium-glucose co-transporter 2 inhibitors in heart failure. Eur J Heart Fail 22:1984–1986
186. Seferovic PM, Fragasso G, Petrie M et al (2020) Sodium glucose co-transporter-2 inhibitors in heart failure: beyond glycaemic control. A position paper of the Heart Failure Association of the European Society of Cardiology. Eur J Heart Fail 22:1495–1503
187. McDonagh TA, Metra M, Adamo M et al (2021) 2021 ESC guidelines for the diagnosis and treatment of acute and chronic heart failure. Eur Heart J 42(36):3599–3726
188. Ali A, Bain S, Hicks D et al (2019) SGLT2 inhibitors: cardiovascular benefits beyond HbA1c-translating evidence into practice. Diabetes Ther 10:1595–1622
189. Gonzalez DE, Foresto RD, Ribeiro AB (1992) SGLT-2 inhibitors in diabetes: a focus on renoprotection. Rev Assoc Med Bras 2020(66):s17–s24
190. Vardeny O, Vaduganathan M (2019) Practical guide to prescribing sodium-glucose cotransporter 2 inhibitors for cardiologists. JACC Heart Fail 7:169–172

191. Ahmed AM (2002) History of diabetes mellitus. Saudi Med J 23:373–378
192. Jia G, Whaley-Connell A, Sowers JR (2018) Diabetic cardiomyopathy: a hyperglycaemia- and insulin-resistance-induced heart disease. Diabetologia 61:21–28
193. Isfort M, Stevens SC, Schaffer S, Jong CJ, Wold LE (2014) Metabolic dysfunction in diabetic cardiomyopathy. Heart Fail Rev 19:35–48
194. Bugger H, Abel ED (2014) Molecular mechanisms of diabetic cardiomyopathy. Diabetologia 57:660–671
195. Holscher ME, Bode C, Bugger H (2016) Diabetic cardiomyopathy: does the type of diabetes matter? Int J Mol Sci 17:2136
196. Isaji M (2011) SGLT2 inhibitors: molecular design and potential differences in effect. Kidney Int Suppl 79:S14. https://doi.org/10.1038/ki.2010.511.S14-9
197. Saisho Y (2020) SGLT2 inhibitors: the star in the treatment of type 2 diabetes? Diseases 8:14
198. Kondo H, Akoumianakis I, Badi I et al (2021) Effects of canagliflozin on human myocardial redox signalling: clinical implications. Eur Heart J 42:4947. https://doi.org/10.1093/eurheartj/ehab420
199. Philippaert K, Kalyaanamoorthy S, Fatehi M et al (2021) Cardiac late sodium channel current is a molecular target for the sodium/glucose cotransporter 2 inhibitor empagliflozin. Circulation 143(22):2188–2204. https://doi.org/10.1161/CIRCULATIONAHA.121.053350
200. Dakhili SAT, Greenwell AA, Ussher JR (2023) Pyruvate dehydrogenase complex and glucose oxidation as a therapeutic target in diabetic heart disease. J Lipid Atheroscler 12:47–57
201. Mizuno Y, Harada E, Nakagawa H et al (2017) The diabetic heart utilizes ketone bodies as an energy source. Metabolism 77:65–72
202. Oshima H, Miki T, Kuno A, Mizuno M, Sato T, Tanno M et al (2019) Empagliflozin, an SGLT2 inhibitor, reduced the mortality rate after acute myocardial infarction with modification of cardiac metabolomes and antioxidants in diabetic rats. J Pharmacol Exp Ther 368:524–534
203. Yanai H, Yoshida H (2019) Beneficial effects of adiponectin on glucose and lipid metabolism and atherosclerotic progression: mechanisms and perspectives. Int J Mol Sci 20:1190
204. Jornayvaz FR, Shulman GI (2010) Regulation of mitochondrial biogenesis. Essays Biochem 47:69–84
205. Scarpulla RC (2011) Metabolic control of mitochondrial biogenesis through the PGC-1 family regulatory network. Biochim Biophys Acta 1813:1269–1278
206. Secker PF, Beneke S, Schlichenmaier N, Delp J, Gutbier S, Leist M et al (2018) Canagliflozin mediated dual inhibition of mitochondrial glutamate dehydrogenase and complex I: an off-target adverse effect. Cell Death Dis 9:226
207. Hodrea J, Balogh DB, Hosszu A, Lenart L, Besztercei B, Koszegi S et al (2020) Reduced O-GlcNAcylation and tubular hypoxia contribute to the antifibrotic effect of SGLT2 inhibitor dapagliflozin in the diabetic kidney. Am J Physiol Renal Physiol 318:F1017–F1029
208. Zhou H, Wang S, Zhu P, Hu S, Chen Y, Ren J (2018) Empagliflozin rescues diabetic myocardial microvascular injury via AMPK-mediated inhibition of mitochondrial fission. Redox Biol 15:335–346. https://doi.org/10.1016/j.redox.2017.12.019
209. Albu A, Para I, Porojan M (2020) Uric acid and arterial stiffness. Ther Clin Risk Manag 16:39–54
210. Uthman L, Homayr A, Juni RP et al (2019) Empagliflozin and dapagliflozin reduce ROS generation and restore NO bioavailability in tumor necrosis factor alpha-stimulated human coronary arterial endothelial cells. Cell Physiol Biochem 53(5):865–886. https://doi.org/10.33594/000000178
211. Lin Y, Nan J, Shen J, Lv X, Chen X, Lu X et al (2020) Canagliflozin impairs blood reperfusion of ischaemic lower limb partially by inhibiting the retention and paracrine function of bone marrow derived mesenchymal stem cells. EBioMedicine 52:102637
212. Zhao J, Randive R, Stewart JA (2014) Molecular mechanisms of AGE/RAGE-mediated fibrosis in the diabetic heart. World J Diabetes 5:860–867

213. Shamhart PE, Luther DJ, Adapala RK, Bryant JE, Petersen KA, Meszaros JG et al (2014) Hyperglycemia enhances function and differentiation of adult rat cardiac fibroblasts. Can J Physiol Pharmacol 92:598–604
214. Fang M, Wang J, Li S, Guo Y (2016) Advanced glycation end-products accelerate the cardiac aging process through the receptor for advanced glycation end-products/transforming growth factor-β-Smad signaling pathway in cardiac fibroblasts. Geriatr Gerontol Int 16:522–527
215. Li C, Zhang J, Xue M et al (2019) SGLT2 inhibition with empagliflozin attenuates myocardial oxidative stress and fibrosis in diabetic mice heart. Cardiovasc Diabetol 18:15. https://doi.org/10.1186/s12933-019-0816-2
216. Lee TM, Chang NC, Lin SZ (2017) Dapagliflozin, a selective SGLT2 inhibitor, attenuated cardiac fibrosis by regulating the macrophage polarization via STAT3 signaling in infarcted rat hearts. Free Radic Biol Med 104:298–310
217. Hasan R, Lasker S, Hasan A, Zerin F, Zamila M, Chowdhury FI et al (2020) Canagliflozin attenuates isoprenaline-induced cardiac oxidative stress by stimulating multiple antioxidant and anti-inflammatory signaling pathways. Sci Rep 10:14459
218. Hasan R, Lasker S, Hasan A, Zerin F, Zamila M, Parvez F et al (2020) Canagliflozin ameliorates renal oxidative stress and inflammation by stimulating AMPK-Akt-eNOS pathway in the isoprenaline-induced oxidative stress model. Sci Rep 10:14659
219. Zhang B, Zhai M, Li B, Liu Z, Li K, Jiang L et al (2018) Honokiol ameliorates myocardial ischemia/reperfusion injury in type 1 diabetic rats by reducing oxidative stress and apoptosis through activating the SIRT1-Nrf2 signaling pathway. Oxidative Med Cell Longev 2018:3159801
220. Ren BC, Zhang YF, Liu SS, Cheng XJ, Yang X, Cui XG et al (2020) Curcumin alleviates oxidative stress and inhibits apoptosis in diabetic cardiomyopathy via Sirt1-Foxo1 and PI3K-Akt signalling pathways. J Cell Mol Med 24:12355–12367
221. Kim JW, Lee YJ, You YH, Moon MK, Yoon KH, Ahn YB et al (2019) Effect of sodium-glucose cotransporter 2 inhibitor, empagliflozin, and α-glucosidase inhibitor, voglibose, on hepatic steatosis in an animal model of type 2 diabetes. J Cell Biochem 120:8534–8546
222. Mohamed HE, Asker ME, Keshawy MM, Hasan RA, Mahmoud YK (2020) Inhibition of tumor necrosis factor-α enhanced the antifibrotic effect of empagliflozin in an animal model with renal insulin resistance. Mol Cell Biochem 466:45–54
223. Zhang J, Huang L, Shi X, Yang L, Hua F, Ma J et al (2020) Metformin protects against myocardial ischemia-reperfusion injury and cell pyroptosis via AMPK/NLRP3 inflammasome pathway. Aging 12:24270–24287
224. Hu R, Wang MQ, Ni SH, Wang M, Liu LY, You HY et al (2020) Salidroside ameliorates endothelial inflammation and oxidative stress by regulating the AMPK/NF-kappaB/NLRP3 signaling pathway in AGEs-induced HUVECs. Eur J Pharmacol 867:172797
225. Ma C, Wang X, Xu T, Yu X, Zhang S, Liu S et al (2019) Qingkailing injection ameliorates cerebral ischemia-reperfusion injury and modulates the AMPK/NLRP3 inflammasome signalling pathway. BMC Complement Altern Med 19:320
226. Yue RC, Lu SZ, Luo Y, Wang T, Liang H, Zeng J et al (2019) Calpain silencing alleviates myocardial ischemia-reperfusion injury through the NLRP3/ASC/Caspase-1 axis in mice. Life Sci 233:116631
227. Li Y, Yang P, Zhao L, Chen Y, Zhang X, Zeng S et al (2019) CD36 plays a negative role in the regulation of lipophagy in hepatocytes through an AMPK-dependent pathway. J Lipid Res 60:844–855
228. Jiang K, Xu Y, Wang D, Chen F, Tu Z, Qian J et al (2022) Cardioprotective mechanism of SGLT2 inhibitor against myocardial infarction is through reduction of autosis. Protein Cell 13:336–359
229. Lee WS, Yoo WH, Chae HJ (2015) ER stress and autophagy. Curr Mol Med 15:735–745
230. Ren FF, Xie ZY, Jiang YN, Guan X, Chen QY, Lai TF et al (2022) Dapagliflozin attenuates pressure overload-induced myocardial remodeling in mice via activating SIRT1 and inhibiting endoplasmic reticulum stress. Acta Pharmacol Sin 43:1721–1732

231. Wang CC, Li Y, Qian XQ, Zhao H, Wang D, Zuo GX et al (2022) Empagliflozin alleviates myocardial I/R injury and cardiomyocyte apoptosis via inhibiting ER stress-induced autophagy and the PERK/ATF4/Beclin1 pathway. J Drug Target 30:858–872
232. Lee DM, Battson ML, Jarrell DK, Hou S, Ecton KE, Weir TL et al (2018) SGLT2 inhibition via dapagliflozin improves generalized vascular dysfunction and alters the gut microbiota in type 2 diabetic mice. Cardiovasc Diabetol 17:62
233. Shin NR, Lee JC, Lee HY, Kim MS, Whon TW, Lee MS et al (2014) An increase in the Akkermansia spp. population induced by metformin treatment improves glucose homeostasis in diet-induced obese mice. Gut 63:727–735
234. Li J, Lin S, Vanhoutte PM, Woo CW, Xu A (2016) Akkermansia muciniphila protects against atherosclerosis by preventing metabolic endotoxemia-induced inflammation in Apoe−/− mice. Circulation 133:2434–2446
235. Deng X, Zhang C, Wang P, Wei W, Shi X, Wang P et al (2022) Cardiovascular benefits of empagliflozin are associated with gut microbiota and plasma metabolites in type 2 diabetes. J Clin Endocrinol Metab 107:1888–1896
236. Röder PV, Geillinger KE, Zietek TS, Thorens B, Koepsell H, Daniel H (2014) The role of SGLT1 and GLUT2 in intestinal glucose transport and sensing. PLoS One 9:e89977
237. Verma S, Mazer CD, Yan AT et al (2019) Effect of empagliflozin on left ventricular mass in patients with type 2 diabetes mellitus and coronary artery disease: the EMPA-HEART CardioLink-6 randomized clinical trial. Circulation 140:1693–1702. https://doi.org/10.1161/CIRCULATIONAHA.119.042375
238. Brown AJM, Gandy S, McCrimmon R, Houston JG, Struthers AD, Lang CC (2020) A randomized controlled trial of dapagliflozin on left ventricular hypertrophy in people with type two diabetes: the DAPA-LVH trial. Eur Heart J 41:3421. https://doi.org/10.1093/eurheartj/ehaa419
239. Sposito AC, Breder I, Soares AAS, Kimura-Medorima ST, Munhoz DB, Cintra RMR et al (2021) Dapagliflozin effect on endothelial dysfunction in diabetic patients with atherosclerotic disease: a randomized active-controlled trial. Cardiovasc Diabetol 20:74
240. van Bommel EJM, Herrema H, Davids M, Kramer MHH, Nieuwdorp M, van Raalte DH (2020) Effects of 12-week treatment with dapagliflozin and gliclazide on faecal microbiome: results of a double-blind randomized trial in patients with type 2 diabetes. Diabetes Metab 46:164–168
241. Dave CV, Schneeweiss S, Patorno E (2019) Comparative risk of genital infections associated with sodium-glucose co-transporter-2 inhibitors. Diabetes Obes Metab 21:434–438
242. Abdul-Ghani M, DeFronzo RA, Del Prato S, Chilton R, Singh R, Ryder REJ (2017) Cardiovascular disease and type 2 diabetes: has the dawn of a new era arrived? Diabetes Care 40(7):813–820. https://doi.org/10.2337/dc16-2736
243. Brown E, Rajeev SP, Cuthbertson DJ, Wilding JPH (2019) A review of the mechanism of action, metabolic profile and haemodynamic effects of sodium-glucose co-transporter-2 inhibitors. Diabetes Obes Metab 21(Suppl 2):9–18. https://doi.org/10.1111/dom.13650
244. Irace C, Casciaro F, Scavelli FB, Oliverio R, Cutruzzola A, Cortese C et al (2018) Empagliflozin influences blood viscosity and wall shear stress in subjects with type 2 diabetes mellitus compared with incretin-based therapy. Cardiovasc Diabetol 17(1):52. https://doi.org/10.1186/s12933-018-0695-y
245. Ganbaatar B, Fukuda D, Shinohara M, Yagi S, Kusunose K, Yamada H, Soeki T, Hirata KI, Sata M (2020) Empagliflozin ameliorates endothelial dysfunction and suppresses atherogenesis in diabetic apolipoprotein E-deficient mice. Eur J Pharmacol 875:173040
246. Gaspari T, Spizzo I, Liu H et al (2018) Dapagliflozin attenuates human vascular endothelial cell activation and induces vasorelaxation: a potential mechanism for inhibition of atherogenesis. Diab Vasc Dis Res 15(1):64–73. https://doi.org/10.1177/1479164117733626
247. Corretti MC, Anderson TJ, Benjamin EJ, Celermajer D, Charbonneau F, Creager MA, Deanfield J, Drexler H, Gerhard-Herman M, Herrington D, Vallance P, Vita J, Vogel R, International Brachial Artery Reactivity Task Force (2002) Guidelines for the ultrasound

assessment of endothelial-dependent flow-mediated vasodilation of the brachial artery: a report of the International Brachial Artery Reactivity Task Force. J Am Coll Cardiol 39:257–265
248. Correale M, Leopizzi A, Mallardi A, Ranieri A, Suriano MP, D'Alessandro D, Tricarico L, Mazzeo P, Tucci S, Pastore G, Maulucci G, Di Biase M, Brunetti ND (2020) Switch to direct anticoagulants and improved endothelial function in patients with chronic heart failure and atrial fibrillation. Thromb Res 195:16–20
249. Tanaka A et al (2017) Rationale and design of a multicenter placebo-controlled double-blind randomized trial to evaluate the effect of empagliflozin on endothelial function: the EMBLEM trial. Cardiovasc Diabetol 16:48
250. Gerstein HC, Colhoun HM, Dagenais GR, Diaz R, Lakshmanan M, Pais P et al (2019) Dulaglutide and cardiovascular outcomes in type 2 diabetes (REWIND): a double-blind, randomised placebo-controlled trial. Lancet 394(10193):121–130. http://www.ncbi.nlm.nih.gov/pubmed/31189511
251. Hernandez AFF, Green JBB, Janmohamed S, D'Agostino RBB, Granger CBB, Jones NPP et al (2018) Albiglutide and cardiovascular outcomes in patients with type 2 diabetes and cardiovascular disease (harmony outcomes): a double-blind, randomised placebo-controlled trial. Lancet 392(10157):1519–1529. http://www.ncbi.nlm.nih.gov/pubmed/30291013
252. American Diabetes Association (2019) 10. Cardiovascular disease and risk management: standards of medical care in diabetes-2019. Diabetes Care 42(Suppl 1):S103–S123. http://www.ncbi.nlm.nih.gov/pubmed/30559236
253. Dave CV, Kim SC, Goldfine AB, Glynn RJ, Tong A, Patorno E (2021) Risk of Cardiovascular outcomes in patients with type 2 diabetes after addition of SGLT2 inhibitors versus sulfonylureas to baseline GLP-1RA therapy. Circulation 143:770–779. Finding from this real-world cohort study suggests the additional value of combined GLP-1RA and SGLT2 inhibitors on reducing cardiovascular risk. Cardiovascular benefits seen here are comparable with several trials of SGLT2 inhibitors or GLP-1RA
254. Rawshani A, Rawshani A, Franzén S et al (2018) Risk factors, mortality, and cardiovascular outcomes in patients with type 2 diabetes. N Engl J Med 379(7):633–644
255. Echouffo-Tcheugui JB, Greene SJ, Papadimitriou L et al (2015) Population risk prediction models for incident heart failure. Circ Heart Fail 8:438–447
256. Kemp CD, John V, Conte JV (2012) The pathophysiology of heart failure. Cardiovasc Pathol 21(5):365–371
257. American Diabetes Association (2018) Pharmacologic approaches to glycemic treatment: standards of medical care in diabetes-2018. Diabetes Care 41:S73–S85
258. De Couto G, Ouzounian M, Liu PP (2010) Early detection of myocardial dysfunction and heart failure. Nat Rev Cardiol 7(6):334–344
259. Packer M (2021) Critical examination of mechanisms underlying the reduction in heart failure events with SGLT2 inhibitors: identification of a molecular link between their actions to stimulate erythrocytosis and to alleviate cellular stress. Cardiovasc Res 117(1):74–84
260. Maddox TM, Januzzi JL Jr et al (2021) Update to the 2017 ACC expert consensus decision pathway for optimization of heart failure treatment: answers to 10 pivotal issues about heart failure with reduced ejection fraction: a report of the American College of Cardiology solution set oversight committee. J Am Coll Cardiol 77(6):772–810
261. McDonald M, Virani S, Chan M et al (2021) CCS/CHFS heart failure guidelines update: defining a new pharmacologic standard of care for heart failure with reduced ejection fraction. Can J Cardiol 37(4):531–546
262. Tromp J, Ponikowski P, Salsali A et al (2021) Sodium–glucose co-transporter 2 inhibition in patients hospitalized for acute decompensated heart failure: rationale for and design of the EMPULSE trial. Eur J Heart Fail 23:826–834
263. Kosiborod MN, Esterline R, Furtado RHM et al (2021) Dapagliflozin in patients with cardiometabolic risk factors hospitalised with COVID-19 (DARE-19): a randomised, double-blind, placebo-controlled, phase 3 trial. Lancet Diabetes Endocrinol 9(9):586–594

264. McDonagh TA, Metra M, Adamo M et al (2021) 2021 ESC guidelines for the diagnosis and treatment of acute and chronic heart failure: developed by the Task Force for the diagnosis and treatment of acute and chronic heart failure of the European Society of Cardiology (ESC) with the special contribution of the Heart Failure Association (HFA) of the ESC. Eur Heart J 42(36):3599–3726. https://doi.org/10.1093/eurheartj/ehab368
265. Borlaug BA, Paulus WJ (2011) Heart failure with preserved ejection fraction: pathophysiology, diagnosis, and treatment. Eur Heart J 32(6):670–679
266. Davidson A, Raviendran N, Murali CN, Myint PK (2020) Managing heart failure with preserved ejection fraction. Ann Transl Med 8(6):395
267. Borlaug BA (2014) The pathophysiology of heart failure with preserved ejection fraction. Nat Rev Cardiol 11:507–515
268. Yusuf S, Pfeffer MA, Swedberg K et al (2003) Effects of candesartan in patients with chronic heart failure and preserved left-ventricular ejection fraction: the CHARM-Preserved trial. Lancet 362:777–781
269. Pitt B, Pfeffer MA, Assmann SF et al (2014) Spironolactone for heart failure with preserved ejection fraction. N Engl J Med 370:1383–1392
270. Solomon SD, McMurray JJV, Anand IS et al (2019) Angiotensin-neprilysin inhibition in heart failure with preserved ejection fraction. N Engl J Med 381:1609–1620
271. Solomon S, Claggett B, Lewis E et al (2015) Influence of ejection fraction on outcomes and efficacy of spironolactone in patients with heart failure with preserved ejection fraction. Eur Heart J 37(5):455–462
272. Lund L, Claggett B, Liu J et al (2018) Heart failure with mid-range ejection fraction in CHARM: characteristics, outcomes and effect of candesartan across the entire ejection fraction spectrum. Eur J Heart Fail 20(8):1230–1239
273. Pabel S, Wagner S, Bollenberg H et al (2018) Empagliflozin directly improves diastolic function in human heart failure. Eur J Heart Fail 20(12):1690–1700. https://doi.org/10.1002/ejhf.1328
274. Kolijn D, Pabel S, Tian Y et al (2021) Empagliflozin improves endothelial and cardiomyocyte function in human heart failure with preserved ejection fraction via reduced pro-inflammatory-oxidative pathways and protein kinase Galpha oxidation. Cardiovasc Res 117(2):495–507. https://doi.org/10.1093/cvr/cvaa123
275. Bhatt D, Szarek M, Steg P et al (2021) Sotagliflozin in patients with diabetes and recent worsening heart failure. N Engl J Med 384(2):117–128
276. Polydiuretic therapy for heart failure with preserved ejection fraction and diabetes mellitus. N=20. NCT04697485. 2021. https://clinicaltrials.gov/ct2/show/NCT04697485 Accessed 8 Nov 2021
277. Zannad F, Ferreira JP, Pocock SJ et al (2020) SGLT2 inhibitors in patients with heart failure with reduced ejection fraction: a meta-analysis of the EMPEROR-Reduced and DAPA-HF trials. Lancet 396(10254):819–829. https://doi.org/10.1016/s0140-6736(20)31824-9
278. Green CP, Porter CB, Bresnahan DR, Spertus JA (2000) Development and evaluation of the Kansas City Cardiomyopathy Questionnaire: a new health status measure for heart failure. J Am Coll Cardiol 35(5):1245–1255
279. Spertus JA, Jones PG (2015) Development and validation of a short version of the Kansas City Cardiomyopathy Questionnaire. Circ Cardiovasc Qual Outcomes 8(5):469–476
280. Salah HM, Al'Aref SJ, Khan MS et al (2021) Effect of sodium-glucose cotransporter 2 inhibitors on cardiovascular and kidney outcomes—systematic review and meta-analysis of randomized placebo-controlled trials. Am Heart J 232:10–22
281. Butler J, Anker SD, Filippatos G et al (2021) Empagliflozin and health-related quality of life outcomes in patients with heart failure with reduced ejection fraction: the EMPEROR-Reduced trial. Eur Heart J 42(13):1203–1212
282. Vaduganathan M, Januzzi JL Jr (2019) Preventing and treating heart failure with sodium-glucose co-transporter 2 inhibitors. Am J Cardiol 124(Suppl 1):S20–s27

283. Tajiri Y, Tsuruta M, Ohki T et al (2012) Long-term efficacy of sitagliptin for the treatment of type 2 diabetic patients in Japan. Endocr J 59:197–204
284. Ohkuma T, Fujii H, Iwase M et al (2013) Impact of eating rate on obesity and cardiovascular risk factors according to glucose tolerance status: the Fukuoka Diabetes Registry and the Hisayama Study. Diabetologia 56:70–77
285. Gerace TA, George VA (1996) Predictors of weight increases over 7 years in fire fighters and paramedics. Prev Med 25:593–600
286. Otsuka R, Tamakoshi K, Yatsuya H et al (2006) Eating fast leads to obesity: findings based on self-administered questionnaires among middle-aged Japanese men and women. J Epidemiol 16:117–124
287. Kannel WB, Hjortland M, Castelli WP (1974) Role of diabetes in congestive heart failure: the Framingham Study. Am J Cardiol 34:29–34
288. MacDonald MR, Petrie MC, Varyani F, Östergren J, Michelson EL, Young JB et al (2008) Impact of diabetes on outcomes in patients with low and preserved ejection fraction heart failure: an analysis of the Candesartan in Heart failure: Assessment of Reduction in Mortality and morbidity (CHARM) programme. Eur Heart J 29:1377–1385
289. Targher G, Dauriz M, Laroche C, Temporelli PL, Hassanein M, Seferovic PM et al (2017) In-hospital and 1-year mortality associated with diabetes in patients with acute heart failure: results from the ESC-HFA Heart Failure Long-Term Registry. Eur J Heart Fail 19:54–65
290. Kapoor JR, Fonarow GC, Zhao X, Kapoor R, Hernandez AF, Heidenreich PA (2011) Diabetes, quality of care, and in-hospital outcomes in patients hospitalized with heart failure. Am Heart J 162(480–486):e3
291. Voors AA, Angermann CE, Teerlink JR, Collins SP, Kosiborod M, Biegus J et al (2022) The SGLT2 inhibitor empagliflozin in patients hospitalized for acute heart failure: a multinational randomized trial. Nat Med 28(3):568–574
292. Stürmer T, Rothman KJ, Avorn J, Glynn RJ (2010) Treatment effects in the presence of unmeasured confounding: dealing with observations in the tails of the propensity score distribution—a simulation study. Am J Epidemiol 172(7):843–854
293. Cox DR (1972) Regression models and life-tables. J R Stat Soc Ser B Stat Methodol 34(2):187–202
294. Griffin M, Riello R, Rao VS, Ivey-Miranda J, Fleming J, Maulion C et al (2020) Sodium glucose cotransporter 2 inhibitors as diuretic adjuvants in acute decompensated heart failure: a case series. ESC Heart Fail 7(4):1966–1971
295. Savarese G, Sattar N, Januzzi J, Verma S, Lund LH, Fitchett D et al (2019) Empagliflozin is associated with a lower risk of post-acute heart failure rehospitalization and mortality. Circulation 139(11):1458–1460
296. Martín E, López-Aguilera J, González-Manzanares R, Anguita M, Gutiérrez G, Luque A et al (2021) Impact of Canagliflozin in patients with type 2 diabetes after hospitalization for acute heart failure: a Cohort study. J Clin Med 10(3)
297. Pérez-Belmonte LM, Sanz-Cánovas J, Millán-Gómez M, Osuna-Sánchez J, López-Sampalo A, Ricci M et al (2022) Clinical benefits of empagliflozin in very old patients with type 2 diabetes hospitalized for acute heart failure. J Am Geriatr Soc 70(3):862–871
298. Haring HU, Merker L, Seewaldt-Becker E, Weimer M, Meinicke T, Woerle HJ, Broedl UC, Investigators E-RMT (2013) Empagliflozin as add-on to metformin plus sulfonylurea in patients with type 2 diabetes: a 24-week, randomized, double-blind, placebo-controlled trial. Diabetes Care 36(11):3396–3404. https://doi.org/10.2337/dc12-2673
299. Rosenstock J, Jelaska A, Frappin G, Salsali A, Kim G, Woerle HJ, Broedl UC, Investigators E-RMT (2014) Improved glucose control with weight loss, lower insulin doses, and no increased hypoglycemia with empagliflozin added to titrated multiple daily injections of insulin in obese inadequately controlled type 2 diabetes. Diabetes Care 37(7):1815–1823. https://doi.org/10.2337/dc13-3055

300. Paulus WJ, van Ballegoij JJ (2010) Treatment of heart failure with normal ejection fraction: an inconvenient truth. J Am Coll Cardiol 55(6):526–537. https://doi.org/10.1016/j.jacc.2009.06.067
301. Holland DJ, Kumbhani DJ, Ahmed SH, Marwick TH (2011) Effects of treatment on exercise tolerance, cardiac function, and mortality in heart failure with preserved ejection fraction. A meta-analysis. J Am Coll Cardiol 57(16):1676–1686. https://doi.org/10.1016/j.jacc.2010.10.057
302. Sanderson JE (2007) Heart failure with a normal ejection fraction. Heart 93(2):155–158. https://doi.org/10.1136/hrt.2005.074187
303. Packer M (2011) Can brain natriuretic peptide be used to guide the management of patients with heart failure and a preserved ejection fraction? The wrong way to identify new treatments for a nonexistent disease. Circ Heart Fail 4(5):538–540. https://doi.org/10.1161/CIRCHEARTFAILURE.111.963710
304. Shah AM, Solomon SD (2012) Phenotypic and pathophysiological heterogeneity in heart failure with preserved ejection fraction. Eur Heart J 33(14):1716–1717. https://doi.org/10.1093/eurheartj/ehs124
305. Shah AM, Pfeffer MA (2012) The many faces of heart failure with preserved ejection fraction. Nat Rev Cardiol 9(10):555–556. https://doi.org/10.1038/nrcardio.2012.123
306. Ferrari R, Bohm M, Cleland JG, Paulus WJ, Pieske B, Rapezzi C, Tavazzi L (2015) Heart failure with preserved ejection fraction: uncertainties and dilemmas. Eur J Heart Fail 17(7):665–671. https://doi.org/10.1002/ejhf.304
307. Ernande L, Bergerot C, Rietzschel ER, De Buyzere ML, Thibault H, Pignonblanc PG, Croisille P, Ovize M, Groisne L, Moulin P et al (2011) Diastolic dysfunction in patients with type 2 diabetes mellitus: is it really the first marker of diabetic cardiomyopathy? J Am Soc Echocardiogr 24(11):1268–1275
308. Nakai H, Takeuchi M, Nishikage T, Lang RM, Otsuji Y (2009) Subclinical left ventricular dysfunction in asymptomatic diabetic patients assessed by two-dimensional speckle tracking echocardiography: correlation with diabetic duration. Eur J Echocardiogr 10(8):926–932. https://doi.org/10.1093/ejechocard/jep097
309. Ng AC, Delgado V, Bertini M, van der Meer RW, Rijzewijk LJ, Shanks M, Nucifora G, Smit JW, Diamant M, Romijn JA, de Roos A, Leung DY, Lamb HJ, Bax JJ (2009) Findings from left ventricular strain and strain rate imaging in asymptomatic patients with type 2 diabetes mellitus. Am J Cardiol 104(10):1398–1401. https://doi.org/10.1016/j.amjcard.2009.06.063
310. Zoroufian A, Razmi T, Taghavi-Shavazi M, Lotfi-Tokaldany M, Jalali A (2014) Evaluation of subclinical left ventricular dysfunction in diabetic patients: longitudinal strain velocities and left ventricular dyssynchrony by two-dimensional speckle tracking echocardiography study. Echocardiography 31(4):456–463. https://doi.org/10.1111/echo.12389
311. Ernande L, Bergerot C, Girerd N, Thibault H, Davidsen ES, Gautier Pignon-Blanc P, Amaz C, Croisille P, De Buyzere ML, Rietzschel ER et al (2014) Longitudinal myocardial strain alteration is associated with left ventricular remodeling in asymptomatic patients with type 2 diabetes mellitus. J Am Soc Echocardiogr 27(5):479–488
312. Ernande L, Rietzschel ER, Bergerot C, De Buyzere ML, Schnell F, Groisne L, Ovize M, Croisille P, Moulin P, Gillebert TC, Derumeaux G (2010) Impaired myocardial radial function in asymptomatic patients with type 2 diabetes mellitus: a speckle-tracking imaging study. J Am Soc Echocardiogr 23(12):1266–1272. https://doi.org/10.1016/j.echo.2010.09.007
313. Tadic M, Ilic S, Cuspidi C, Stojcevski B, Ivanovic B, Bukarica L, Jozika L, Celic V (2015) Left ventricular mechanics in untreated normotensive patients with type 2 diabetes mellitus: a two- and three-dimensional speckle tracking study. Echocardiography 6:947–955
314. Mochizuki Y, Tanaka H, Matsumoto K, Sano H, Toki H, Shimoura H, Ooka J, Sawa T, Motoji Y, Ryo K et al (2015) Clinical features of subclinical left ventricular systolic dysfunction in patients with diabetes mellitus. Cardiovasc Diabetol 14:37
315. Mochizuki Y, Tanaka H, Matsumoto K, Sano H, Toki H, Shimoura H, Ooka J, Sawa T, Motoji Y, Ryo K, Hirota Y, Ogawa W, Hirata KI (2015) Association of peripheral nerve conduction in diabetic neuropathy with subclinical left ventricular systolic dysfunction. Cardiovasc Diabetol 14(1):47. https://doi.org/10.1186/s12933-015-0213-4

316. Mochizuki Y, Tanaka H, Tatsumi K, Matsumoto K, Imanishi J, Yoshida A, Yokoyama M, Kawai H, Hirata K (2014) Easy-to-use comprehensive speckle-tracking approach for cardiac resynchronization therapy. Circ J 78(9):2250–2258. https://doi.org/10.1253/circj.CJ-14-0114
317. Cognet T, Vervueren PL, Dercle L, Bastie D, Richaud R, Berry M, Marchal P, Gautier M, Fouilloux A, Galinier M, Carrie D, Massabuau P, Berry I, Lairez O (2013) New concept of myocardial longitudinal strain reserve assessed by a dipyridamole infusion using 2D-strain echocardiography: the impact of diabetes and age, and the prognostic value. Cardiovasc Diabetol 12(1):84. https://doi.org/10.1186/1475-2840-12-84
318. Ridderstrale M, Andersen KR, Zeller C, Kim G, Woerle HJ, Broedl UC, investigators E-RHHSt (2014) Comparison of empagliflozin and glimepiride as add-on to metformin in patients with type 2 diabetes: a 104-week randomised, active-controlled, double-blind, phase 3 trial. Lancet Diabetes Endocrinol 2(9):691–700. doi:https://doi.org/10.1016/S2213-8587(14)70120-2
319. Matthaei S, Bowering K, Rohwedder K, Grohl A, Parikh S, Study G (2015) Dapagliflozin improves glycemic control and reduces body weight as add-on therapy to metformin plus sulfonylurea: a 24-week randomized, double-blind clinical trial. Diabetes Care 38(3):365–372. https://doi.org/10.2337/dc14-0666
320. McMurray JJV, Solomon SD, Inzucchi SE, Kober L, Kosiborod MN, Martinez FA, Ponikowski P, Sabatine MS, Anand IS, Belohlavek J et al (2019) Dapagliflozin in patients with heart failure and reduced ejection fraction. N Engl J Med 381(21):1995–2008
321. Bhattarai M, Salih M, Regmi M, Al-akchar M, Koester C, Ibrahim A, Parajuli P, Garcia OL, Bhandari B, Rehman A et al (2021) Comprehensive evaluation of cardiovascular efficacy and safety outcomes of SGLT2 inhibitors in high risk patients of cardiovascular disease: systematic review and meta-analysis. Cardiovasc Endocrinol Metab 10(2):89–98
322. Mosenzon O, Wiviott SD, Cahn A, Rozenberg A, Yanuv I, Goodrich EL, Murphy SA, Heerspink HJL, Zelniker TA, Dwyer JP et al (2019) Effects of dapagliflozin on development and progression of kidney disease in patients with type 2 diabetes: an analysis from the DECLARE-TIMI 58 randomised trial. Lancet Diabetes Endocrinol 7(8):606–617
323. Ott C, Jumar A, Striepe K, Friedrich S, Karg MV, Bramlage P, Schmieder RE (2017) A randomised study of the impact of the SGLT2 inhibitor dapagliflozin on microvascular and macrovascular circulation. Cardiovasc Diabetol 16(1):26–35
324. Bosch A, Ott C, Jung S, Striepe K, Karg MV, Kannenkeril D, Dienemann T, Schmieder RE (2019) How does empagliflozin improve arterial stiffness in patients with type 2 diabetes mellitus? Sub analysis of a clinical trial. Cardiovasc Diabetol 18(1):44–56
325. International Diabetes Federation (2016) Diabetes and cardiovascular disease report. IDF, Brussels
326. Birkeland KI, Jørgensen ME, Carstensen B, Persson F, Gulseth HL, Thuresson M et al (2017) Cardiovascular mortality and morbidity in patients with type 2 diabetes following initiation of sodium-glucose co-transporter-2 inhibitors versus other glucose-lowering drugs (CVD-REAL Nordic): a multinational observational analysis. Lancet Diabetes Endocrinol 5:709–717
327. Patorno E, Pawar A, Franklin JM et al (2019) Empagliflozin and the risk of heart failure hospitalization in routine clinical care. Circulation 139:2822–2830. https://doi.org/10.1161/CIRCULATIONAHA.118.039177
328. Martinez FA, Serenelli M, Nicolau JC, Petrie MC, Chiang CE, Tereshchenko S, Solomon SD, Inzucchi SE, Køber L, Kosiborod MN, Ponikowski P, Sabatine MS, DeMets DL, Dutkiewicz-Piasecka M, Bengtsson O, Sjöstrand M, Langkilde AM, Jhund PS, McMurray JJV (2020) Efficacy and safety of dapagliflozin in heart failure with reduced ejection fraction according to age: insights from DAPA-HF. Circulation 141:100–111
329. Petrie MC, Verma S, Docherty KF, Inzucchi SE, Anand I, Belohlávek J, Böhm M, Chiang CE, Chopra VK, de Boer RA, Desai AS, Diez M, Drozdz J, Dukát A, Ge J, Howlett J, Katova T, Kitakaze M, Ljungman CEA, Merkely B, Nicolau JC, O'Meara E, Vinh PN, Schou M, Tereshchenko S, Køber L, Kosiborod MN, Langkilde AM, Martinez FA, Ponikowski P, Sabatine MS, Sjöstrand M, Solomon SD, Johanson P, Greasley PJ, Boulton D, Bengtsson O, Jhund PS, McMurray JJV (2020) Effect of dapagliflozin on worsening heart failure

and cardiovascular death in patients with heart failure with and without diabetes. JAMA 323:1353–1368
330. Kaku K, Lee J, Mattheus M, Kaspers S, George J, Woerle HJ, EMPA-REG OUTCOME® Investigators (2017) Empagliflozin and cardiovascular outcomes in Asian patients with type 2 diabetes and established cardiovascular disease–results from EMPA-REG OUTCOME®. Circ J 81:227–234
331. Giugliano D, Longo M, Maiorino MI, Bellastella G, Chiodini P, Solerte SB, Esposito K (2020) Efficacy of SGLT-2 inhibitors in older adults with diabetes: systematic review with meta-analysis of cardiovascular outcome trials. Diabetes Res Clin Pract 162:108114
332. Kubo S, Noda T, Myojin T, Nishioka Y, Higashino T, Matsui H, Kato G, Imamura T (2018) National database of health insurance claims and specific health checkups of Japan (NDB): outline and patient-matching technique. Rxiv 10:8
333. Sciacqua A, Succurro E, Armentaro G, Miceli S, Pastori D, Rengo G, Sesti G (2021) Pharmacological treatment of type 2 diabetes in elderly patients with heart failure: randomized trials and beyond. Heart Fail Rev 28:667. https://doi.org/10.1007/s10741-021-10182-x
334. Kohsaka S, Lam CSP, Kim DJ, Cavender MA, Norhammar A, Jørgensen ME, Birkeland KI, Holl RW, Franch-Nadal J, Tangri N, Shaw JE, Ilomäki J, Karasik A, Goh SY, Chiang CE, Thuresson M, Chen H, Wittbrodt E, Bodegård J, Surmont F, Fenici P, Kosiborod M, CVD-REAL 2 Investigators and Study Group (2020) Risk of cardiovascular events and death associated with initiation of SGLT2 inhibitors compared with DPP-4 inhibitors: an analysis from the CVD-REAL 2 multinational cohort study. Lancet Diabetes Endocrinol 8:606–615
335. Cannon CP, Pratley R, Dagogo-Jack S, Mancuso J, Huyck S, Masiukiewicz U, Charbonnel B, Frederich R, Gallo S, Cosentino F (2020) Cardiovascular outcomes with ertugliflozin in type 2 diabetes. N Engl J Med 383(15):1425–1435
336. Thygesen K, Alpert JS, Jaffe AS, Simoons ML, Chaitman BR, White HD, Joint ESCAAHAWHFTFfUDoMI, Authors/Task Force, Members C, Thygesen K, Alpert JS et al (2012) Third universal definition of myocardial infarction. J Am Coll Cardiol 60(16):1581–1598
337. Chang T-Y, Lu C-T, Huang H-L, Chou R-H, Chang C-C, Liu C-T, Huang P-H, Lin S-J (2022) Association of Sodium-Glucose cotransporter 2 (SGLT2) inhibitor use with cardiovascular and renal outcomes in type 2 diabetes mellitus patients with stabilized acute myocardial infarction: a propensity score matching study. Front Cardiovasc Med 9
338. Persson F, Nyström T, Jørgensen ME, Carstensen B, Gulseth HL, Thuresson M, Fenici P, Nathanson D, Eriksson JW, Norhammar A (2018) Dapagliflozin is associated with lower risk of cardiovascular events and all-cause mortality in people with type 2 diabetes (CVD-REAL Nordic) when compared with dipeptidyl peptidase-4 inhibitor therapy: a multinational observational study. Diabetes Obes Metab 20(2):344–351
339. Zheng SL, Roddick AJ, Aghar-Jaffar R, Shun-Shin MJ, Francis D, Oliver N, Meeran K (2018) Association between use of sodium-glucose cotransporter 2 inhibitors, glucagon-like peptide 1 agonists, and dipeptidyl peptidase 4 inhibitors with all-cause mortality in patients with type 2 diabetes: a systematic review and meta-analysis. JAMA 319(15):1580–1591
340. Bolinder J, Ljunggren Ö, Kullberg J, Johansson L, Wilding J, Langkilde AM, Sugg J, Parikh S (2012) Effects of dapagliflozin on body weight, total fat mass, and regional adipose tissue distribution in patients with type 2 diabetes mellitus with inadequate glycemic control on metformin. J Clin Endocrinol Metab 97:1020–1031. https://doi.org/10.1210/jc.2011-2260
341. Neeland IJ, McGuire DK, Chilton R, Crowe S, Lund SS, Woerle HJ, Broedl UC, Johansen OE (2016) Empagliflozin reduces body weight and indices of adipose distribution in patients with type 2 diabetes mellitus. Diabetes Vasc Dis Res. 13(2):119–126
342. Neeland IJ, McGuire DK, Eliasson B, Ridderstrale M, Zeller C, Woerle HJ, Broedl UC, Johansen OE (2015) Comparison of adipose distribution indices with gold standard body composition assessments in the EMPA-REG H2H SU trial: a body composition sub-study. Diabetes Ther. 6(4):635–642

343. Schork A, Woern M, Kalbacher H, Voelter W, Nacken R, Bertog M, Haerteis S, Korbmacher C, Heyne N, Peter A et al (2016) Association of plasminuria with overhydration in patients with CKD. Clin J Am Soc Nephrol 11(5):761–769
344. Iizuka T, Iemitsu K, Takihata M, Takai M, Nakajima S, Minami N, Umezawa S, Kanamori A, Takeda H, Kawata T et al (2016) Efficacy and safety of ipragliflozin in japanese patients with type 2 diabetes: interim outcome of the ASSIGN-K study. J Clin Med Res 8(2):116–125

Chapter 3
SGLT2 Inhibitors for Primary and Secondary Protection from Cardiovascular and Renal Diseases in Type 2 Diabetes

Mukesh Nandave

Introduction by the Editor

Chronic Kidney disease (CKD) is mainly caused by diabetes which results in kidney failure and the need for replacement therapy. Proposed pathways involved in the cardiorenal role of SGLT2i are shown in Fig. 3.1. The major root of death in people with diabetes and CKD is cardiovascular disease (CVD). By limiting the reabsorption of glucose in the proximal tubule, SGLT2i was developed to lower blood glucose levels. Clinical trials designed to validate the CVD efficacy of SGLT2 inhibitors in T2D observed consistent declines in the risks for supplementary renal disease endpoints (albuminuria and an aggregate of increasing serum creatinine or 40% predicted failure in glomerular filtration rate, kidney failure, or death), as well as declines within CVD events.

SGLT2i drugs lessen the main hyper-reabsorption characteristic of PCT that is linked to diabetes. By enhancing salt transport to the macula densa, SGLT2i improve glycosuria and natriuresis, reinstate tubuloglomerular feedback (TGF), and encourage the dilatation of efferent and constriction of afferent arterioles [1]. SGLT2i alters renal hemodynamics to reduce glomerular hypertension, excessive filtration, traumatic brain injury, and albuminuria. These early warning indicators are critical for preventing diabetic kidney disease (DKD), as SGLT2i slows down the disease's progression over time. Table 3.1 provides an overview of clinical trials investigating the impact of SGLT2i, such as canagliflozin, dapagliflozin, and empagliflozin, on renal protection that covers the SGLT2i clinical studies protect against renal diseases. Using the search terms "RCTs," "Renal diseases," and "SGLT2i AND Renal diseases," clinical trial studies was extracted. Five studies were chosen from a total

M. Nandave (✉)
Department of Pharmacology and Pharmaceutical Biotechnology, Delhi Pharmaceutical Sciences and Research University (DPSRU), New Delhi, Delhi, India

M. Nandave (ed.), *Sodium-glucose Cotransporter-2 (SGLT2) Inhibitors in Heart Failure*, https://doi.org/10.1007/978-981-97-7568-2_3

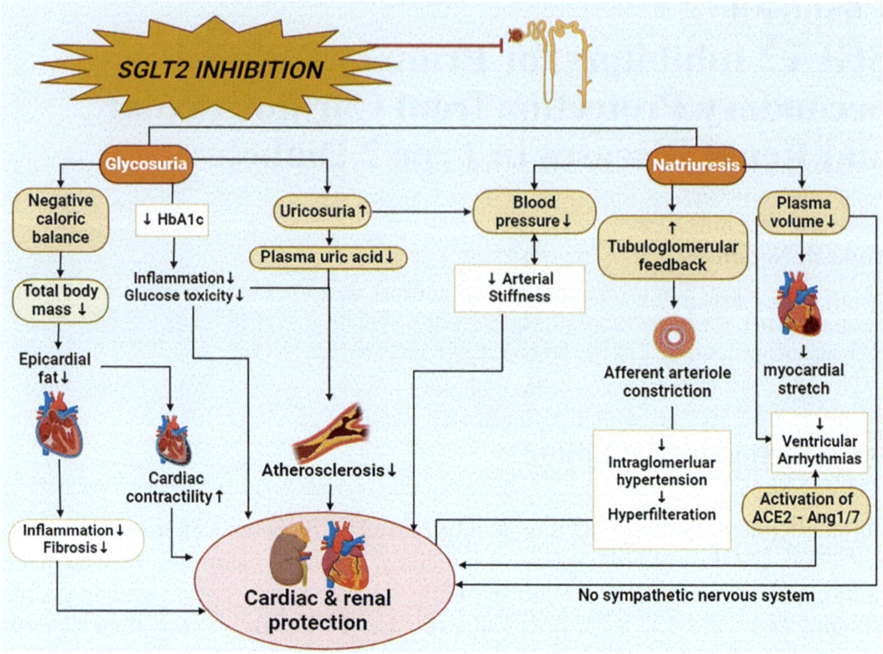

Fig. 3.1 Multiple physiologic mechanisms related to cardiorenal outcomes are modulated with SGLT2i treatments

of about 117 trials based on the drug's protective effect against renal illnesses, its phase III, and its early phase.

The CREDENCE (Canagliflozin and Renal Events in Diabetes with Established Nephropathy Clinical Evaluation) trial, which included T2D patients with a urinary albumin-creatinine ratio > 300 mg/g and an estimated glomerular filtration rate of 30–90 mL/min/1.73 m^2, established the benefits of canagliflozin for patients with CKD in terms of their kidney and cardiovascular systems. The National Kidney Foundation organized a systematic meeting with a global panel of more than 80 specialists to explain and promote the use of SGLT2i for the treatment of T2DM and CKD. They examined the present level of knowledge and open issues to suggest treatment strategies and outline potential areas for future study. SGLT2i are expected to enhance various regional and systemic pathways implicated in the etiology of CKD and CVD in addition to improving glomerular hemodynamic function. According to the criteria for clinical trial admission, patients with T2DM should use SGLT2i as often as feasible to lower their risk of CKD and CVD. Euglycemic ketoacidosis, vaginal mycotic infections, and volume depletion are serious side effects of SGLT2i. The balance between the advantages and disadvantages of SGLT2i and risk-reduction techniques should be carefully considered. To get these life-saving drugs widely used, efficient implementation procedures are required.

Table 3.1 Summary of all current and early phase trials detail of SGLT2i used for the treatment of renal disease

Aim	Identifier	Intervention	Phase	Outcome
Based on safety and efficacy of Canagliflozin adverse events in cardiac patients with diabetes and CKD				
When ACE1 and ARB are administered at the highest permissible labeled daily dose to patients with T2D, stage II or III CKD, renal impairment, and macroalbuminuria, the goal is to ascertain the protective impact of canagliflozin	NCT02065791	Canagliflozin + placebo	III	Canagliflozin reduces the risk of renal disease and cardiac events in those with type 2 diabetes
Based on to determine the probable benefits and adverse effects of Dapagliflozin in T2D with mild/chronic kidney dysfunction				
To assess the impact of dapagliflozin on heart disease mortality and renal outcomes in individuals with long-term renal illness	NCT03036150	Dapagliflozin + Placebo	III	Dapagliflozin significantly reduces the mortality from renal or CV-related causes or on a continuing reduction in assessed GFR of at least 50% towards people with CKD
To evaluate the reduction of proteinuria in chronic renal illness via dapagliflozin	NCT03190694	Dapagliflozin	II	Dabagliflozin treatment for 6 weeks resulted in a decrease in body weight and an immediate and transitory decline in mGFR in individuals with chronic renal failure
To investigate the possible benefits and side effects of dapagliflozin in individuals with acute renal dysfunction due to T2D	NCT02413398	Dapagliflozin + Placebo	III	Dapagliflozin reduced eGFR from baseline more than the placebo did at week 24. However, in week 27, eGFR went back to normal

(continued)

Table 3.1 (continued)

Aim	Identifier	Intervention	Phase	Outcome
It is hypothesized that the administration of SGLT2i might reduce or eliminate the nephrotoxic effects of contrast media, hence decreasing the occurrence of nephropathy during cardiac catheterization and percutaneous coronary intervention	NCT04806633	Dapagliflozin + Placebo	Early phase I	Not provided

Machine Generated Summaries

Disclaimer: The summaries in this chapter were generated from Springer Nature publications using extractive AI auto-summarization: An extraction-based summarizer aims to identify the most important sentences of a text using an algorithm and uses those original sentences to create the auto-summary (unlike generative AI). As the constituted sentences are machine selected, they may not fully reflect the body of the work, so we strongly advise that the original content is read and cited. The auto generated summaries were curated by the editor to meet Springer Nature publication standards. To cite this content, please refer to the original papers.

Machine generated keywords: sglti, dkd, kidney disease, cardiorenal, egfr, ckd, progression, hhf, dka, disease dkd, cardiorenal outcome, metaanalysis, renoprotective, individual tdm, network.

Cardiorenal Protection: Potential of SGLT2 Inhibitors and GLP-1 Receptor Agonists in the Treatment of Type 2 Diabetes [2]

This is a machine-generated summary of:

Nagahisa, Taichi; Saisho, Yoshifumi: Cardiorenal Protection: Potential of SGLT2 Inhibitors and GLP-1 Receptor Agonists in the Treatment of Type 2 Diabetes [2].

Published in: Diabetes Therapy (2019).

Link to original: https://doi.org/10.1007/s13300-019-00680-5

If you want to cite the papers, please refer to the original.

For technical reasons we could not place the page where the original quote is coming from.

Abstract-Summary "Recent large clinical trials on sodium-glucose cotransporter 2 (SGLT2) inhibitors and glucagon-like peptide-1 (GLP-1) receptor agonists, with the aim of verifying cardiovascular safety, have revealed that these medications have a preventative advantage on adverse cardiovascular outcomes, including worsening of heart failure and deterioration of nephropathy, in patients with type 2 diabetes (T2D)."

"Given the results from recent studies, the American Diabetes Association (ADA) and the European Association for the Study of Diabetes (EASD) recommend that patients with T2D and clinical cardiovascular disease (CVD) with inadequate glucose control despite treatment with metformin should receive an SGLT2 inhibitor or GLP-1 receptor agonist."

"We summarize the results of recent cardiovascular outcome trials and discuss the potential clinical advantage of SGLT2 inhibitors and GLP-1 receptor agonists."

Introduction

"Major clinical trials, including those on the cardiovascular safety of dipeptidyl peptidase-4 (DPP-4) inhibitors, glucagon-like peptide-1 (GLP-1) receptor agonists, and sodium-glucose co-transporter-2 (SGLT2) inhibitors, have been published."

"Three trials of GLP-1 receptor agonists, namely, the Liraglutide Effect and Action in Diabetes: Evaluation of Cardiovascular Outcome Results (LEADER) trial, the Semaglutide Unabated Sustainability in Treatment of Type 2 Diabetes 6 (SUSTAIN-6) trial, and the Albiglutide and cardiovascular outcomes in patients with type 2 diabetes and cardiovascular disease (Harmony Outcomes) trial, also demonstrated risk reduction in major adverse cardiovascular events [3–5], with a consistent result recently reported on the use of dulaglutide in the Researching Cardiovascular Events with a Weekly Incretin in Diabetes (REWIND) trial [6]."

"Given the implications of new evidence derived from these cardiovascular outcomes trials (CVOTs), the American Diabetes Association (ADA) and the European Association for the Study of Diabetes (EASD) recently recommended that patients with T2D and clinical cardiovascular disease (CVD) inadequately controlled with metformin therapy and lifestyle intervention should be treated with an SGLT2 inhibitor or GLP-1 receptor agonist and that among those in whom heart failure coexists, an SGLT2 inhibitor should be preferentially prescribed [7]."

Methods

"The articles cited in this review were retrieved from the literature using Google Scholar with the search terms "SGLT2 inhibitor", "GLP-1 receptor agonist", "cardiovascular", and "outcome"."

"Related articles were also collected from a personal database."

"This review article is based on previously conducted studies and does not contain any studies with human participants or animals performed by any of the authors."

Era Before SGLT2 Inhibitors and GLP-1 Receptor Agonists

"In UKPDS 34 [8], in which 1704 overweight patients were randomly assigned to conventional treatment or intensive glycemic control with a sulfonylurea, insulin, or metformin, participants allocated metformin had a significantly reduced risk of any diabetes-related endpoint (HR 0.68, 95% CI 0.53–0.87, $p = 0.0023$), diabetes-related death (HR 0.58, 95% CI 0.37–0.91p = 0.017), all-cause mortality (HR 0.64, 95% CI 0.45–0.91, $p = 0.011$), and myocardial infarction (HR 0.61, 95% CI 0.41–0.89, $p = 0.01$), as opposed to participants who received intensive glycemic control achieved with a sulfonylurea or insulin."

"None of three subsequent major trials that examined intensive glycemic control, namely, the Action to Control Cardiovascular Risk in Diabetes (ACCORD) trial, the Action in Diabetes and Vascular Disease: Preterax and Diamicron Modified-Release Controlled Evaluation (ADVANCE) trial, and the Veterans Affairs Diabetes Trial (VADT) [9–11], exhibited a beneficial effect of intensive control on cardiovascular events, with the exception of the ACCORD trial in which non-fatal myocardial infarction decreased in the intensive control group."

SGLT2 Inhibitors

"Although only 27% of patients had established CVD, treatment with SGLT2 inhibitors was also associated with significant risk reduction in hospitalization for heart failure and all-cause death (HR 0.64, 95% CI 0.50–0.82, $p = 0.001$ and HR 0.51 95% CI 0.37–0.70, $p < 0.001$, respectively), with a directionally similar trend regardless of the existence of prior CVD [12]."

"The results of a meta-analysis of 53 trials of SGLT2 inhibitors indicated that only empagliflozin demonstrates a lower risk of acute renal impairment/failure events relative to placebo (OR 0.72; 95% CI 0.59–0.87), compared with canagliflozin (OR 1.82; 95% CI 0.28–11.77) and dapagliflozin (OR 1.93; 95% CI 0.42–8.83) [13]."

GLP-1 Receptor Agonists

"The Semaglutide Unabated Sustainability in Treatment of Type 2 Diabetes 6 (SUSTAIN-6) trial, which enrolled 3297 patients who were administered semaglutide 0.5 or 1.0 mg per week or placebo, showed a significant 26% reduction in

3-point MACE (HR 0.74, 95% CI 0.58–0.95), a significant reduction in nonfatal stroke (HR 0.61, 95% CI 0.38–0.99), and a directionally concordant result in non-fatal MI (HR 0.74, 95% CI 0.51–1.08)."

"In the Functional Impact of GLP-1 for Heart Failure Treatment (FIGHT) trial, which involved 300 patients with advanced heart failure, the liraglutide group showed a numerically higher (but not statistically significant) risk of rehospitalization for heart failure (HR 1.30, 95% CI 0.89–1.88, p = 0.17) compared with the placebo group [14]."

Discussion

"A series of cardiovascular outcome trials revealed an unexpected benefit on cardiovascular outcome with SGLT2 inhibitors and GLP-1 receptor agonists, highlighting the advantage of secondary prevention in patients with established CVD."

"The efficacy of combination therapy with a GLP-1 receptor agonist and SGLT2 inhibitor has been elucidated [15, 16], with further improvement of glycemic control compared with monotherapy also observed, although the achieved glycemic efficacy was subadditive partially due to stimulatory effects on glucagon and hepatic glucose production correlated with glycosuria derived from SGLT2 inhibitors [17]."

"Three separately conducted 52-week open-label studies to evaluate the efficacy and safety of SGLT2 inhibitors, involving canagliflozin, ipragliflozin, and luseogliflozin, in combination with a GLP-1 receptor agonist showed a further decrease in HbA1c and body weight without any increase in serious adverse events including severe hypoglycemia [18–20]."

"This combination is therefore an attractive therapeutic option for patients with obesity refractory to treatment with an SGLT2 inhibitor or GLP-1 receptor agonist alone or in combination with insulin therapy in terms of long-term glycemic control and body weight control."

Conclusion

"Recent clinical trials have revealed a novel role of SGLT2 inhibitors and GLP-1 receptor agonists beyond their glucose-lowering effect, and both agents have received more attention as a paradigm shift from "the lower glucose the better" to "how to optimize glycemic control without hypoglycemia and overweight" has been generated by current guidelines."

"Full advantage of the pleiotropic benefit of these agents should be taken to prevent secondary adverse cardiovascular events and to mitigate the advance of renal complications without increased risk of hypoglycemia."

SGLT2 Inhibition in Type 1 Diabetes with Diabetic Kidney Disease: Potential Cardiorenal Benefits Can Outweigh Preventable Risk of Diabetic Ketoacidosis [21]

This is a machine-generated summary of:

Liu, Hongyan; Sridhar, Vikas S.; Perkins, Bruce A.; Rosenstock, Julio; Cherney, David Z. I.: SGLT2 Inhibition in Type 1 Diabetes with Diabetic Kidney Disease: Potential Cardiorenal Benefits Can Outweigh Preventable Risk of Diabetic Ketoacidosis [21].

Published in: Current Diabetes Reports (2022).

Link to original: https://doi.org/10.1007/s11892-022-01471-2

If you want to cite the papers, please refer to the original.

For technical reasons we could not place the page where the original quote is coming from.

Abstract-Summary "The aim of this review is to summarize existing research investigating the use of sodium glucose cotransporter-2 (SGLT2) inhibitors in patients with type 1 diabetes mellitus (T1DM) while highlighting potential strategies to mitigate the risk of diabetic ketoacidosis (DKA)."

"Trials in patients with type 2 diabetes mellitus (T2DM) have found an increased risk of DKA with SGLT2 inhibitors, a serious concern in patients with T1DM."

"SGLT2 inhibitors increase the risk of DKA, and there is currently a lack of research investigating the beneficial effects of SGLT2 inhibitors in patients with T1DM."

"Additional research will also be required to determine the kidney protective effects of SGLT2 inhibitors in patients with T1DM and diabetic kidney disease and to quantify the risk of DKA after the implementation of preventative measures, proper patient education, and ketone monitoring."

Introduction

"Thanks to these therapeutic approaches, less patients are progressing towards end-stake kidney disease (ESKD), but little progress has been made to delay the onset or progression of stage 2 and 3 DKD in T1DM [22, 23]."

"Since the cardiorenal protective effects of SGLT2 inhibitors are independent of insulin and glycemic control, there is likely overlap between the mechanisms underlying end-organ protection in patients with T2DM compared to those with T1DM."

"There is a strong theoretical basis for SGLT2 inhibitors as a much-needed option to prevent the progression of DKD in individuals with T1DM."

"SGLT2 inhibitors increase ketogenesis and the risk of diabetic ketoacidosis (DKA), which is of particular concern as a serious adverse event in patients with T1DM [24–26]."

"The objective of this review is to evaluate the potential benefits of SGLT2 inhibitors in patients with T1DM in preventing the development and progression of DKD."

SGLT2 Inhibitors and Diabetic Kidney Disease

"Favorable effects, CV outcome trials (CVOTs) such as the EMPA-REG OUTCOME [27], DECLARE-TIMI 58 [28], CANVAS [29], VERTIS CV [30, 31], and SCORED [32] trials found that SGLT2 inhibitors also reduced CV and kidney outcomes in patients with T2DM."

"Dedicated kidney outcome trials have shown that SGLT2 inhibitors reduce progression of chronic kidney disease (CKD) in both patients with and without T2DM [33, 34]."

"The subsequent DAPA-CKD trial expanded the kidney protective findings and made them more generalizable by involving participants both with and without T2DM, with lower eGFR (25–75 mL/min/1.73 m^2) and UACR (200–5000 mg/g)."

"The ongoing EMPA-KIDNEY trial (NCT03594110) has a similar goal of evaluating the kidney protective effects of the SGLT2 inhibitor, empagliflozin, in patients with CKD and includes individuals with eGFR 20–45 ml/min/1.73 m^2 regardless of albuminuria level—a clinically advanced stage that was excluded from previous SGLT2 inhibitor trials."

Kidney Protective Mechanisms of SGLT2 Inhibitors in T1DM

"Supportive evidence in favor of a reduction in intraglomerular pressure and GFR with SGLT2 inhibition exists in individuals with T1DM and T2DM, though the specific renal hemodynamic effects mediating these reductions may vary between the two groups."

"While the impact of SGLT2 inhibition on kidney function in people with T1DM and DKD is not known, it is anticipated that effects will be similar compared to people with T2DM and DKD since the natriuretic effects are analogous [31, 35–37]."

"In patients with T1DM and preserved eGFR recruited into glycemia-focused trials, SGLT2 inhibition induced an eGFR "dip" and lowered UACR in patients with mild baseline UACR elevation—an effect linked with kidney protection [38]."

"To local hemodynamic effects in the kidney, SGLT2 inhibitors impact systemic hemodynamic function in ways that may improve CV, HF and kidney outcomes in patients with and without T2DM [39]."

Existing Clinical Evidence for SGLT2 Inhibition in T1DM

"In a pooled post hoc analysis of the inTandem 1 and 2 trials, 1575 adults with T1DM were randomized to sotagliflozin (a dual SGLT1 and SGLT2 inhibitor) 200 mg, 400 mg or placebo over a 52-week period [38]."

"In keeping with expected reductions in glomerular pressure with SGLT2 inhibition and in line with effects in T2DM, participants receiving either dose of sotagliflozin experienced significant initial reductions in eGFR compared to placebo by week 4 (sotagliflozin 200 mg: –2.5 mL/min/1.73 m^2 (SE 0.63), $P < 0.0001$; sotagliflozin 400 mg: –2.8 mL/min/1.73 m^2 (SE 0.63), $P < 0.0001$) and these effects persisted in the lower dose sotagliflozin group at 52 weeks."

"As in previous T1DM trials, an initial decline in eGFR was observed, consistent with an acute lowering of glomerular pressures, but the reduction in eGFR from baseline compared to placebo did not reach significance at the end of the trial."

Overall Risks of SGLT2 Inhibitors and Diabetic Ketoacidosis

"The EASE trials reported that with physician mediated reductions in both basal and post-prandial insulin, SGLT2 inhibitors were not associated with increased hypoglycemia risk in participants with T1DM [40]."

"A meta-analysis of 14 studies investigating the effects of SGLT2 inhibitors as add-on therapy to insulin for T1DM found that the odds of DKA was increased by threefold in participants treated with SGLT2 inhibitors [41]."

"RCTs involving SGLT2 inhibitors in patients with T1DM have found a significant increase in DKA risk in participants treated with SGLT2 inhibitors (3.0–4.3%) when compared to placebo (0.5–1.2%) [40, 42, 43]."

"While DKA is a major concern in the use of SGLT2 inhibitors in T1DM, patient reported outcome studies have shown that after receiving education about the benefits and risks of SGLT2 inhibitors, patients with T1DM preferred use of SGLT2 inhibitors as an adjunct-to-insulin therapy, even when DKA risk was identified as the most important safety and efficacy attribute for these patients [26]."

Mitigating Risk of DKA in Patients with T1DM

"The risk of DKA is a major limitation in preventing widespread uptake and use of SGLT2 inhibitors in patients with T1DM."

"The problem of DKA must addressed for all patients with T1DM, not just those at a higher risk such as those receiving SGLT2 inhibitors."

"Balancing risks and benefits of SGLT2 inhibitors will require consideration of patient risk factors for hypoglycemia versus DKA, patient lifestyle and glycemic targets [44]."

"In patients with good glycemic control (HbA1c < 7.0%), a 10–20% reduction in bolus insulins, accompanied by continuous glucose monitoring (or frequent blood glucose tests) and rapid insulin readjustments with input from a health care provider, may be required in those with preserved eGFR but not in those with significant eGFR impairment [45]."

"Patients with T1DM have the greatest potential benefits from these novel technologies, especially those at high risk of DKA, which may include those using adjunct-to-insulin SGLT2 inhibition."

Conclusion

"With the completion of SGLT2 inhibitor CVOTs, dedicated kidney outcome trials, and HF trials, tremendous progress has been made for people with T2DM."

"While SGLT2 inhibitors may offer a therapeutic option to select patients, demonstration of efficacy and safety in patients with established complications is urgently needed in dedicated and properly designed cardiorenal outcome trials."

"We urgently need a Cardiovascular-Kidney Outcome Trial in patients with long-standing T1DM and high cardiorenal risk with established CVD ± eGFR < 90 mL/min/1.73 m^2 or patients with an eGFR < 60 mL/min/1.73 m^2 and microalbuminuria and/or hypertension to MACE, HF and CKD progression."

Renal Protection with SGLT2 Inhibitors: Effects in Acute and Chronic Kidney Disease [46]

This is a machine-generated summary of:

Bailey, Clifford J.; Day, Caroline; Bellary, Srikanth: Renal Protection with SGLT2 Inhibitors: Effects in Acute and Chronic Kidney Disease [46].

Published in: Current Diabetes Reports (2022).

Link to original: https://doi.org/10.1007/s11892-021-01442-z

If you want to cite the papers, please refer to the original.

For technical reasons we could not place the page where the original quote is coming from.

Abstract-Summary "This review offers a critical narrative evaluation of emerging evidence that sodium-glucose co-transporter-2 (SGLT2) inhibitors exert nephroprotective effects in people with type 2 diabetes."

"The SGLT2 inhibitor class of glucose-lowering agents has recently shown beneficial effects to reduce the onset and progression of renal complications in people with and without diabetes."

"Randomised clinical trials and 'real world' observational studies, mostly involving type 2 diabetes patients, have noted that use of an SGLT2 inhibitor can slow the decline in glomerular filtration rate (GFR), reduce the onset of microalbuminuria and slow or reverse the progression of proteinuria."

"The nephroprotective effects of SGLT2 inhibitors are class effects observed with each of the approved agents in people with a normal or impaired GFR."

"Other effects of SGLT2 inhibitors improve tubular oxygenation and metabolism and reduce renal inflammation and fibrosis."

Introduction

"Sodium-glucose co-transporter-2 (SGLT2) inhibitors are glucose-lowering agents that eliminate excess glucose through a glucosuric effect by reducing glucose reabsorption from the renal filtrate [47, 48]."

"Initial concerns about SGLT2 inhibitors focussed on possible detrimental effects on the renal system, particularly to increase genito-urinary infections, compromise bladder health and aggravate acute kidney injury [49]."

"Observations during cardiovascular outcome trials and 'real world' studies have identified potentially advantageous effects of SGLT2 inhibitors to reduce the risk of onset and progression of several cardiovascular conditions and to preserve kidney function."

"MEDLINE, PubMed, and Google Scholar were searched for articles published between January 2010 and March 2021 using the terms 'sodium glucose transporter inhibitor', 'SGLT2 inhibitor' and the generic names of individual SGLT2 inhibitors in combination with the term 'kidney disease', 'acute kidney injury', 'chronic kidney disease', 'renal function', 'diabetes' and 'type 2 diabetes'."

SGLT2 Inhibition

"Canagliflozin exerts some suppression of SGLT1, and sotagliflozin is an SGLT1/2 inhibitor: both of these agents can delay the intestinal absorption of glucose before being absorbed or degraded, which assists prandial glycaemic control."

"The renal threshold for glucose is often breached, and the glucosuria is enhanced by SGLT2 inhibitors which act by reversible competitive inhibition without being transported themselves [48]."

"A trivial (therapeutic) concentration of an SGLT inhibitor in the filtrate can prevent the reabsorption of a large (up to about 100 g/day) amount of filtered glucose."

"Although SGLT2 inhibitors lower the renal threshold for glucose, their glucosuric effect is self-limiting such that they do not incur the risk of clinically significant hypoglycaemia."

Glucose Lowering and Weight Lowering

"The activity of SGLT2 inhibitors is independent of insulin status, i.e. undiminished by insulin resistance or absolute insulin lack, enabling glucose lowering in type 2 and type 1 diabetes."

"Meta-analyses of the reduction in HbA1c with SGLT2 inhibitors in type 2 diabetes have consistently noted reductions of about 0.5 to 1% (6–11 mmol/mol) from a baseline of around 8% (64 mmol/mol) [50–52]."

"Because SGLT2 inhibitors have a different mechanism of action to other glucose-lowering agents, they can be used in combination with other agents including insulin and can often reduce the amount of insulin required in type 2 and type 1 diabetes [53, 54]."

"In clinical trials with type 2 diabetes patients, the weight reducing effect of SGLT2 inhibitors has typically been around 3 kg, levelling out by 6–12 months, although 'real world' observational studies have often noted reductions >6 kg that continue beyond a year."

Cardiovascular Effects

"Beyond glucose lowering and weight lowering, SGLT2 inhibitors have consistently reduced blood pressure (systolic by 3–5 mmHg and diastolic by 2–3 mmHg) during clinical trials without causing hypotension [55]."

"The benefit is evident within a few weeks of starting an SGLT2 inhibitor, occurs in people with and without diabetes and is independent of the extent of effects on glucose, weight or blood pressure [56–58]."

"Studies in which ejection fraction was quantified have mostly involved patients with reduced ejection fraction (HFrEF), but there is emerging evidence that SGLT2 inhibitors can also benefit those with preserved and mid-range ejection fraction. [59–62]."

Diabetic Kidney Disease

"All types of diabetes are associated with increased risk of impaired kidney function (referred to as diabetic nephropathy or diabetic kidney disease (DKD))."

"This is typically recognised by a progressive chronic kidney disease (CKD) with an estimated glomerular filtration rate (eGFR) < 60 ml/min/1.73 m^2 that can be attributed to diabetes [63]."

"The normal age-related rate of decline in eGFR (~ 1 ml/min/1.73 m^2 per year when eGFR > 60 ml/min/1.73 m^2) is typically doubled in type 2 diabetes with CKD and may exceed 3 ml/min/1.73 m^2 per year in individuals with macroalbuminuria [64]."

"Observational studies suggest that 20–40% of people with type 2 diabetes incur an eGFR < 60 ml/min/1.73 m^2, mostly amongst older patients and those with poor glycaemic control."

Kidney Disease and Use of SGLT2 Inhibitors

"Because a reduction in GFR reduces the amount of glucose delivered into the proximal tubules, the glucosuric efficacy (and thereby antihyperglycaemic efficacy) of SGLT2 inhibitors declines approximately in line with a decline in GFR."

"The product labels for SGLT2 inhibitors define GFR values below which it is recommended to not initiate or continue treatment [65–68]."

Renal Endpoints

"Recognition that SGLT2 inhibitors could alter the course of diabetic kidney disease was initially clouded by short-term observations focussed on the initial dip in eGFR."

"Evidence from long-term trials in type 2 diabetes, notably the post-marketing cardiovascular outcome trials (CVOTs) described below, indicated that eGFR subsequently declined at a slower rate with use of an SGLT2 inhibitor than in placebo-treated patients and that albuminuria was less severe."

"Prespecified secondary endpoints in the CVOTs assessed various individual and composite measures of renal function that included progression of albuminuria (indicated by UACR), doubling of serum creatinine, decrease in eGFR (to either <45 or <60 ml/min/1.73 m^2), end-stage kidney disease, kidney-related death or renal replacement therapy (dialysis or transplantation)."

Large Randomised Trials in Type 2 Diabetes

"In the EMPA-REG OUTCOME trial, the renal composite (doubling of serum creatinine, eGFR ≤45 ml/min/1.73 m^2, initiation of renal replacement therapy or death from kidney disease) was reduced by 46% in the groups receiving empagliflozin [27, 69]."

"Progression to macroalbuminuria (UACR > 300 mg/g) was reduced by 38% with use of empagliflozin, and there were also significant reductions in the number of patients with a doubling of serum creatinine, decline in eGFR to ≤ 45 ml/min/1.73 m^2, and starting renal replacement therapy."

"The DECLARE-TIMI 58 trial found that use of dapagliflozin was associated with a 47% reduction in a renal composite of a sustained decrease of eGFR by ≥ 40% to < 60 ml/min/1.73 m^2, new ESKD or death from a renal cause [28]."

Trials in People with Impaired Renal Status

"This was addressed in the CREDENCE study in which type 2 diabetes patients were recruited with an eGFR range of 30–90 ml/min/1.73 m^2, macroalbuminuria (UACR > 300 to < 5,000 mg/g) and RAAS blockade [33]."

"Of particular note, the effectiveness of the SGLT2 inhibitor to slow the decline in eGFR and reduce progression of albuminuria was similar for patients with a baseline eGFR > or < 45 ml/min/1.73 m^2 and a UACR > or <1,000 mg/g, and the SGLT2 inhibitor also slowed the decline in eGFR for patients with a baseline eGFR <30 ml/min/1.73 m^2."

"The DAPA-CKD trial examined the effect of dapagliflozin in people with (67%) and without (33%) type 2 diabetes who had renal impairment (eGFR 25–75 ml/min/1.73 m^2, mean 43.1 ml/min/1.73 m^2; and UACR 200–5000 mg/g, median ~ 950 mg/g with 48.3% of patients having a UACR > 1000 mg/g) [32]."

Additional Evidence from Populations With and Without Diabetes

"DAPA-HF included patients with an eGFR down to 30 ml/min/1.73 m^2 (mean 66 ml/min/1.73 m^2) and noted that the renal composite (≥ 50% sustained decline in eGFR, ESKD or renal death) was numerically lower (by 39%, not statistically significant) with use of dapagliflozin [70]."

"The rate of decline in eGFR was significantly slower with dapagliflozin than placebo (mean –1.09 versus –2.85 ml/min/1.73 m^2/year)."

"The decline in eGFR was significantly slower with empagliflozin than placebo (mean –0.55 versus –2.28 ml/min/1.73 m^2/year)."

Renal Mechanisms of SGLT2 Inhibitors

"Although reduced glucotoxicity associated with sustained improvements in glucose homeostasis lessens the risks and severity of renal complications in type 2 diabetes irrespective of the glucose-lowering medication [71], the renal benefits offered by SGLT2 inhibitors appear to be somewhat greater and faster in onset than with intensified glucose lowering and show little association with their glycaemic effect."

"This then causes cell damage and fibrosis through an accumulation of intracellular lipid, whereas SGLT2 inhibition reduces reliance on energy production from glucose, increases fatty acid utilisation and reduces lipotoxic cell damage [72]."

"SGLT2 inhibitors suppress the activity of the sodium-hydrogen exchanger-3 (NHE-3) which has the potential to influence renal sodium handling, acid–base and metabolic activities at least partly independently of the inhibition of glucose reabsorption [73, 74]."

"Hyperuricaemia is associated with increased renal interstitial fibrosis, and SGLT2 inhibitors reduce plasma uric acid, probably through increased renal urate elimination due to competition of extra glucose for the urate transporter GLUT9b [75]."

Acute Kidney Injury

"Given the alterations of renal function associated with the use of SGLT2 inhibitors, there has been ongoing caution regarding possible detrimental effects of these agents on the risk and prognosis of AKI."

"Clinical trial data have consistently found no increase in risk of AKI or adverse outcomes of AKI with use of an SGLT2 inhibitor."

"Several meta-analyses of clinical trial data have concluded that use of an SGLT2 inhibitor in T2DM reduces the risk of AKI by 30–40%, and analyses of data from 'real world' observational studies have indicated reductions in risk of AKI by >40% [76–78]."

"The reduced risk and severity of heart failure associated with use of an SGLT2 inhibitor, particularly HFrEF, provides a potentially important contribution to the reduced occurrence and better prognosis of AKI with this class of glucose-lowering agents [79, 80]."

Conclusion

"Damage to the glomerulus often starts with the hyperfiltration that accompanies hyperinsulinaemic insulin resistance in prediabetes and early stages of type 2 diabetes."

"This sets in train the profibrotic changes, faster decline in GFR and functional disturbances of diabetic kidney disease."

"SGLT2 inhibitors exert a variety of effects on the kidney, directly and indirectly linked to reduced glucose reabsorption, providing acute and chronic nephroprotective effects that reduce progression and may partially reverse the characteristic markers of diabetic kidney disease."

The Na/K-ATPase Signaling and SGLT2 Inhibitor-Mediated Cardiorenal Protection: A Crossed Road? [81]

This is a machine-generated summary of:

Liu, Jiang; Tian, Jiang; Sodhi, Komal; Shapiro, Joseph I.: The Na/K-ATPase Signaling and SGLT2 Inhibitor-Mediated Cardiorenal Protection: A Crossed Road? [81].

Published in: The Journal of Membrane Biology (2021).

Link to original: https://doi.org/10.1007/s00232-021-00192-z

If you want to cite the papers, please refer to the original.

For technical reasons we could not place the page where the original quote is coming from.

Abstract-Summary "In different large-scale clinic outcome trials, sodium (Na^+)/glucose co-transporter 2 (SGLT2) inhibitors showed profound cardiac- and renal-protective effects, making them revolutionary treatments for heart failure and kidney disease."

Introduction

"More and more insightful theories are proposed to explain the "off-target" but incredible effects of SGLT2 inhibitors other than the designed glucose-lowering property initially, as reviewed in more detail elsewhere."

"The molecular mechanism(s) to delineate the cardiorenal protection of SGLT2 inhibitors are still not fully understood."

"The protection of SGLT2 inhibitors could not be fully explained by a single mechanism since different clinic treatment strategies targeting different conditions are short of the overall effect of the SGLT2 inhibitors."

"This review explores the possible role of Na/K-ATPase and its signaling function that might affect SGLT2 and SGLT2 inhibitors."

The Biology of the Na/K-ATPase

"Cardiotonic steroids (CTS, also known as digitalis-like substances) are specific Na/K-ATPase inhibitors and ligands."

"CTS has been used to treat heart failure for over 200 years through its inotropic effect due to partial inhibition of Na/K-ATPase induced intracellular Na^+ change coupled with increases in intracellular calcium (Ca^{2+}) through Na^+/Ca^{2+} exchanger (NCX)."

"CTS also stimulates the signaling function of the Na/K-ATPase, which has been contributed to cardiac hypertrophy and fibrosis, Na^+ reabsorption in renal proximal tubule cells (RPTs), systemic oxidative stress, and release of inflammatory cytokines. """.

"Identification of ouabain-like substance in human plasma and in vivo studies with genetically modified mouse models (humanized ouabain-sensitive Na/K--ATPase α1) have unequivocally demonstrated that endogenous CTS regulates renal Na^+ excretion and blood pressure through the Na/K-ATPase (Dostanic-Larson and others 81; Dostanic and others 82; Hamlyn and others 83; Loreaux and others 84)."

"CTS has been classified as a new class of hormones, making Na/K-ATPase a potential therapeutic target for cardiac and renal diseases (Aperia 85; Bagrov and Shapiro, 86; Bagrov and others 87; Schoner 88; Yatime and others 89)."

The Biology of SGLTs

"The glucose reabsorption from glomerular filtrate in RPTs is an energy-requiring process that reabsorbs ~ 180 g per day through SGLTs."

"In RPTs, SGLTs at the apical membrane mediate the entry of glucose, and glucose transporters (GLUTs) at the basolateral membrane mediate the extrusion of glucose into the circulation."

"SGLT2 is a high-capacity, low-affinity transporter (co-transport Na^+ and glucose at 1:1 stoichiometry) located on the S1 and S2 segments, reabsorbing ~ 90% filtered glucose."

"SGLT1 is a high-affinity, low-capacity transporter (co-transport Na^+ and glucose at 2:1 stoichiometry) located on the S3 segment, reabsorbing the ~ 10% filtered glucose (unabsorbed glucose by SGLT2) (Brown 90; Hediger and Rhoads 91; Lee and others 92; Wright and others 93, 94)."

"Changes in glucose or Na^+ filtered rate modulates the glucose transporter's (SGLT1/2 and GLUT1/2) gene expression (Vestri and others 95)."

Protection Effects of SGLT2 Inhibitor on Renal Disease

"Data from CV outcome trials showed that SGLT2 inhibitors slow the progression of kidney function decline and reduce the risks of kidney outcomes in T2DM patients with preserved kidney function (Mosenzon and others 96; Neal and others 97; Wiviott and others 98; Zinman and others 99)."

"The DAPA-CKD trial demonstrated that dapagliflozin reduces the risks of major adverse kidney and CV events and all-cause mortality in diabetic and non-diabetic CKD patients with or without T2DM (Heerspink and others 100; Wheeler and others 101)."

"In patients with heart failure and reduced ejection fraction with and without T2DM, the DAPA-HF trial (Dapagliflozin and Prevention of Adverse Outcomes in Heart Failure) demonstrated that the SGLT2 inhibitor reduces the risk of heart failure hospitalizations or CV death and slow the progression of kidney function decline (Jhund and others 102; Packer and others 103)."

"In the CREDENCE trial, SGLT2 inhibitor canagliflozin reduces blood pressure independent of starting blood pressure levels and other concomitant blood pressure-lowering agents in patients with T2DM and CKD (Ye and others 104)."

Protection Effects of SGLT2 Inhibitor on Cardiovascular Disease (CVD)

"Inhibition of SGLT2 has been shown to improve CV outcomes in patients with diabetic kidney disease and patients without diabetics."

"The EMPA-REG OUTCOME study (Zinman and others 105) was the first clinical trial to mark success for secondary and tertiary CVD prevention with an SGLT2 inhibitor."

"Results from the CANVAS trial further substantiated the preventive effect of SGLT2 inhibitors in CV outcomes."

"In a recent meta-analysis using data from 27 clinical studies with over 7000 patients with diabetes or chronic kidney disease, SGLT2 inhibitors were found to reduce the risk of the composite CV outcome, hospitalized or fatal heart failure, and myocardial infarction."

"Since SGLT2 is dominantly expressed in the kidney proximal tubules, the beneficial effect of SGLT2 inhibitors on CV outcomes was mostly considered as a secondary effect of the renal function improvement and systematic glucose-lowering effect."

Mechanistic Perception of SGLT2 Inhibitor and Na/K-ATPase

"Activation of the Na/K-ATPase signaling function induces coordinated endocytosis of the Na/K-ATPase and NHE3 that leads to reduced Na^+ reabsorption and natriuresis to cause volume contraction and blood pressure-lowering (Cai and others 106; Liu and others 107, 108, 109; Liu and Shapiro 110; Periyasamy and others 111)."

"SGLT2 inhibitors reduce SGLT2-mediated Na^+ uptake into RPTs, which favors an E2(P) conformation of the Na/K-ATPase that tends to activate the signaling function."

"A culprit is that the Na/K-ATPase signaling may increase ROS generation, whereas the SGLT2 inhibitor reduces oxidative stress."

"The Na/K-ATPase signaling and its amplification loop play an essential role in the regulation of cardiac hypertrophy, salt-sensitive hypertension in both Dahl salt-sensitive rats and polygenic obese TALLYHO/JngJ mice (a mouse model mimics the state of obesity in humans with a polygenic background of type 2 diabetes), RPT Na^+ reabsorption, systemic redox status, experimental CKD-induced cardiomyopathy (including left ventricle hypertrophy and cardiac/renal fibrosis) and anemia (Liu and others 112, 113, 109, 114; Pratt and others 115; Sodhi and others 116; Wang and Shapiro 117; Yan and others 118)."

"Disrupting the Na/K-ATPase-related signaling and inhibition of Src activation by pNaKtide increased miR-29b-3p expression in heart tissue and thus attenuated cardiac fibrosis in these animals (Drummond and others 119)."

Conclusion

"The Na/K-ATPase is the driving force for the reabsorption of Na^+ and glucose as the primary ion transporter, also affects other cellular processes as a signal transducer."

"Compared with SGLT2 inhibitor's beneficial effects, the Na/K-ATPase and its signaling function exert some similar effects mainly through the kidney, such as natriuresis, blood pressure-lowering, and through the heart, such as reduction of cardiac hypertrophy and fibrosis."

"Since the signaling function of the Na/K-ATPase is redox-sensitive, a balanced ROS environment would be more beneficial."

"The possibility that the Na/K-ATPase and its signaling affect SGLT2 function, and vice versa, worth exploring."

Renal Protection: A Leading Mechanism for Cardiovascular Benefit in Patients Treated with SGLT2 Inhibitors [82]

This is a machine-generated summary of:

Margonato, Davide; Galati, Giuseppe; Mazzetti, Simone; Cannistraci, Rosa; Perseghin, Gianluca; Margonato, Alberto; Mortara, Andrea: Renal protection: a leading mechanism for cardiovascular benefit in patients treated with SGLT2 inhibitors [82].

Published in: Heart Failure Reviews (2020).

Link to original: https://doi.org/10.1007/s10741-020-10024-2

If you want to cite the papers, please refer to the original.

For technical reasons we could not place the page where the original quote is coming from.

Abstract-Summary "Developed as glucose-lowering drugs, sodium-glucose co-transporter type 2 inhibitors (SGLT2i) have demonstrated to be effective agents for the risk reduction of cardiovascular (CV) events in patients with type 2 diabetes mellitus (T2DM)."

"Data has emerged showing a significant CV benefit in patients treated with SGLT2i regardless of diabetes status."

"As clinical guidelines rapidly evolve and the role of SGLT2i appears to become pivotal for CV, T2DM, and kidney disease management, in this review, we analyze the renal effects of SGLT2, the benefits derived from its inhibition, and how this may result in the multiple CV and renal benefits evidenced in recent clinical trials."

Introduction

"Sodium-glucose co-transporter type 2 inhibitors (SGLT2i) were originally developed to reduce hyperglycemia in diabetic patients via an insulin-independent mechanism, through their glycosuric effect."

"Chronic kidney disease (CKD) occurs in approximately 40% type 2 diabetes mellitus (T2DM) patients [83] and is associated with a very high risk of CV diseases [84]."

"The growing evidence from many RCTs on SGLT2i as a CV protective class of drugs led to a class 1 level A recommendation for their use in patients with T2DM and established atherosclerotic CV disease (ACVD), or in patients with T2DM and multiple risk factors but without an ACVD [85]."

"SGLT2i showed to significantly reduce morbidity and mortality even in HF irrespective of diabetes status [60, 85]· Specific nephroprotection as a primary adjusted outcome has been evaluated only recently in the CREDENCE trial [33]; however, the mechanisms leading to renal benefit in patients treated with SGLT2i are still under debate."

The Role of SGLTs in the Kidney

"SGLT2 is a high-capacity low-affinity transporter located in the first segment of the proximal tubule and is responsible for the reabsorption of about 90% of filtered glucose."

"Residual glucose is reabsorbed by the high-affinity low-capacity transporter SGLT1 in the distal segment of the proximal tubule [47]."

"In an individual with preserved glomerular filtration rate (GFR) and normoglycemia, all the glucose filtered in the proximal tubules is reabsorbed; conversely, an increase in the concentration of plasma glucose leads to a constant increase in filtered glucose, until the threshold of reabsorption is reached (normally for values of glycemia around 180–215 mg/dl) and glycosuria begins [86]."

"Diabetes mellitus is associated with an improved capacity of renal glucose reabsorption probably through an increased activity of SGLT2 in the proximal tubules, sustaining hyperglycemia in a sort of vicious cycle [87]."

Direct Renal Benefits

"Osmotic diuresis induced by SGLT2i is particularly relevant in the situation of interstitial volume overload working in synergy with the other diuretics, in particular loop diuretics [88]."

"It has been demonstrated that SGLT2i primarily reduces interstitial volume, with a minor effect on intravascular volume [88, 89], while loop diuretics mostly reduce intravascular volume."

"This synergistic effect of SGLT2i and loop diuretics on both intravascular and interstitial volumes is very useful in states of volume overload by also limiting adverse effects of other diuretics such as inappropriate reflex neurohormonal stimulation, a response to intravascular volume depletion, and uric acid levels increase [90, 91]."

"SGLT2i give a significant advantage particularly in HF because they reduce the need for the first introduction of a loop diuretic—as shown in EMPA-REG-Outcome—limiting the renin-angiotensin-aldosterone system (RAAS) activation [92, 93]· SGLT2i also mitigates the direct kidney damage with a suppression of numerous pathways linked to tubular hypoxia and fibrosis, such as oxidative stress, and inflammasome activity [94–96] regardless of diabetes [97] together with a proven significant reduction of urinary excretion of inflammatory markers [98]."

Indirect Renal Benefits

"The cross-talk between the sympathetic nervous system and SGLT2 has been proved with compelling evidence in animal models: in fact, it has been demonstrated that chemical sympathetic denervation in neurogenic hypertensive mice resulted in reduced renal SGLT2 expression, and that dapagliflozin-treated mice showed a significant decrease in the expression of markers of sympathetic activity and a reduction in blood pressure [99, 100]."

"Small reduction of blood pressure seems to be associated with minor renal benefit in the literature: in particular, as a reduction in albuminuria has been showed, favorable data on hard renal outcomes are controversial [101] but more recently emerging in the literature [102, 103]."

"It is important to underline that the direct benefit of SGLT2i on the myocardium, especially in patients with HF or with an established cardiac disease, has beneficial effects also on kidney function and on renal outcomes."

Renal Outcomes in RCTs on SGLT2 Inhibitors: State of the Art

"In the 7020 patients with T2DM and established ACVD of the EMPA-REG OUTCOME [27], empagliflozin showed a significant 14% relative risk reduction (RRR) of the primary composite outcome (CV death, non-fatal myocardial infarction, or non-fatal stroke) driven by a 38% RR reduction of CV mortality (3.7% vs. 5.9%; hazard ratio [HR] 0.62; 95% confidence interval [CI] 0.49–0.77, $p < 0.001$) and a 35% RR reduction of hospitalizations for HF (2.7% vs. 4.1%, HR 0.65; 95% CI 0.5–0.85, $p = 0.002$) which was consistent across predefined subgroups, including patients with and without a previous history of HF."

"Despite a neutral effect on the MACE outcome, dapagliflozin was significantly superior to placebo in reducing CV death or HF hospitalization with a 17% reduction of the RR (4.7% vs. 5.8%; HR 0.83; 95%, CI 0.73–0.95, $p = 0.005$) [28]."

The Credence Trial

"This trial randomized 4401 patients with TD2M and albuminuric CKD, defined as values of eGFR ≥ 30 and < 90 ml/min/1.73 m^2 and UAC between 300 and 5000 mg/g, to receive either 100 mg daily of canagliflozin or placebo; all patients were treated with RAAS blockade and 50% had a history of CV disease."

"The primary outcome was a composite endpoint of ESRD (defined as dialysis, transplantation, or a sustained eGFR less than 15 ml/min/1.73 m^2), a doubling of the serum creatinine level, or death from renal or cardiovascular cause."

"The event rate of the primary endpoint was significantly reduced in the canagliflozin group compared with placebo, with a RR reduction of 30% (HR 0.70; 95% CI 0.59–0.82, $p = 0.00001$) [33]."

"Patients randomized to canagliflozin presented a significant RRR of 34% (HR 0.66; 95% CI 0.53–0.8, $p < 0.001$) for the renal composite outcome of ESRD, doubling of the serum creatinine level, or renal death [33]; the nephroprotective role of canagliflozin was consistent also for the single components of composite endpoint ESRD (HR 0.68; 95% CI 0.54–0.86, $p = 0.002$) and for the exploratory outcome of dialysis, kidney transplantation, or renal death (HR 0.72; 95% CI 0.54 to 0.97) [33]."

Conclusions

"In line with the CREDENCE trial, in patients with T2DM post hoc analysis [104] of two registration trials with ertugliflozin, a new drug in the class with high selectivity for SGLT2, confirmed that over 104 weeks of treatment, eGFR values were higher and UAC reduced compared with non-SGLT2i treatment, even though changes in HbA1c did not differ between the groups; with respect to this drug, data from the CV safety VERTIS trial, recently presented at the American Diabetes Association, including secondary composite renal endpoints are eagerly awaited."

"Additional studies will clarify the potential clinical role of SGLT2i on kidney function in patients without T2DM: at this stage, we have data generated following a very short period of time (6 weeks) of treatment with dapagliflozin, the DIAMOND trial [36], in which patients with non-diabetes-related CKD did not show a beneficial effect on proteinuria when compared with the placebo group."

Renoprotection with SGLT2 Inhibitors in Type 2 Diabetes over a Spectrum of Cardiovascular and Renal Risk [105]

This is a machine-generated summary of:

Giorgino, Francesco; Vora, Jiten; Fenici, Peter; Solini, Anna: Renoprotection with SGLT2 inhibitors in type 2 diabetes over a spectrum of cardiovascular and renal risk [105].

Published in: Cardiovascular Diabetology (2020).
Link to original: https://doi.org/10.1186/s12933-020-01163-9

If you want to cite the papers, please refer to the original.

For technical reasons we could not place the page where the original quote is coming from.

Abstract-Summary "Although patients in most cardiovascular outcomes trials had higher prevalence of existing cardiovascular disease compared with those normally seen in clinical practice, the proportion of patients with renal impairment was similar to that observed in a real-world context."

"Patient cardiovascular risk profiles did not relevantly impact the renoprotective benefits observed in these studies."

"Benefits were observed in patients across a spectrum of renal risk, but were evident also in those without renal damage, suggesting a role for SGLT2 inhibition in the prevention of CKD in people with T2D. In addition, recent studies such as CREDENCE and DAPA-CKD offer a greater insight into the renoprotective effects of SGLT2 inhibitors in patients with moderate-to-severe CKD."

"This review outlines the evidence that SGLT2 inhibitors may prevent the development of CKD and prevent and delay the worsening of CKD in people with T2D at different levels of renal risk."

Introduction

"Renal disorders are common in type 2 diabetes (T2D), with approximately 50% of patients developing some degree of renal impairment and an increasing prevalence of both conditions over time [106]."

"An analysis of the US Diabetes Collaborative Registry revealed that 94% of people with T2D presented with at least one cardiovascular (CV), metabolic, or renal comorbidity, including 20% with chronic kidney disease (CKD) [107]."

"In large outcomes trials evaluating angiotensin receptor blockers in people with T2D, progression of nephropathy occurred in approximately 15–27% of placebo-treated patients over 2 years, depending on the level of baseline risk [108–110]."

"Progressive renal impairment increases the risk of patients experiencing not only renal but also CV morbidity and mortality."

"SGLT2 inhibitors have shown clear CV and renal benefits in people with T2D [27–29, 111–113]."

"The renoprotective effects of SGLT2 inhibitors across the spectrum of both CV and renal risk are reviewed here."

Renal Benefits of SGLT2 Inhibitors in People with T2D

"Unlike EMPA-REG OUTCOME and the CANVAS program, the recent VERTIS CV study investigating ertugliflozin in 8246 people with T2D and established CVD did not show a statistically significant reduction in the secondary composite renal outcome (death from renal causes, RRT, or doubling of serum creatinine levels) in the ertugliflozin group compared with placebo (HR: 0.81; 95% CI 0.63, 1.04) [114]."

"Two independent meta-analyses of the EMPA-REG OUTCOME, CANVAS program, DECLARE-TIMI 58, and CREDENCE trials found that SGLT2 inhibitors significantly reduced the risk of a renal composite including worsening renal function, ESKD, or death from renal causes compared with placebo (relative risk [RR]: 0.67; 95% CI 0.52, 0.86 [115] and RR: 0.63; 95% CI 0.56, 0.71; number needed to treat [NNT] = 67) [116]."

"These findings were also consistent with those of a meta-analysis of 27 studies involving 7363 patients treated with SGLT2 inhibitors (empagliflozin, dapagliflozin, canagliflozin, and ertugliflozin) [117], which revealed a significantly reduced risk of doubling of serum creatinine (or 40% decline in eGFR, in the case of DECLARE-TIMI 58), ESKD, or renal death (HR: 0.71; 95% CI 0.53, 0.95)."

Renoprotective Effects of SGLT2 Inhibitors According to Baseline Risk

"Studies investigating SGLT2 inhibitors in patients with heart failure with reduced ejection fraction (with and without T2D) have also recently reported numerical and substantial reductions in renal composite outcomes compared with placebo [dapagliflozin: HR: 0.71; 95% CI 0.44, 1.16 (eGFR < 50%, ESKD, or renal death) [60]; empagliflozin: HR: 0.50; 95% CI 0.32, 0.77 (eGFR < 50% or ESKD)] [118]."

"In a population with relatively less renal impairment, DECLARE-TIMI 58 did not report a significant difference in the efficacy of dapagliflozin as measured by the renal composite outcome based on patient baseline eGFR or UACR, although there were some numeric differences suggesting that the renoprotective effects of dapagliflozin may be slightly larger in patients with normal renal function (eGFR ≥ 90 mL/min/1.73 m^2: HR: 0.50; 95% CI 0.34, 0.73; and eGFR 60 to < 90 mL/min/1.73 m^2: HR: 0.54; 95% CI 0.40, 0.73; eGFR < 60 mL/min/1.73 m^2: HR: 0.60; 95% CI 0.35, 1.02) and those with macroalbuminuria (UACR > 300 mg/g: HR: 0.38; 95% CI 0.25, 0.58; UACR < 30 mg/g: HR: 0.52; 95% CI 0.37, 0.74; and UACR 30–300 mg/g: HR: 0.59; 95% CI 0.39, 0.87) [119]."

Safety of SGLT2 Inhibitors in T2D and Renal Impairment

"CVOT analyses actually show that there may be fewer AKI events in patients on SGLT2 inhibitor therapy compared with placebo [115]."

"Meta-analyses also confirmed no overall increase in amputation or fracture risk with SGLT2 inhibitors, but did highlight significant heterogeneity between trials [117, 120–122]."

"In a meta-analysis of 27 studies, including approximately 7300 patients, treatment with SGLT2 inhibitors in people with T2D and CKD was not associated with increased risks of adverse renal events (HR: 1.04; 95% CI 0.68, 1.61), AKI (HR: 0.69; 95% CI 0.45, 1.06), or hyperkalemia (HR: 0.63; 95% CI 0.48, 0.83), compared with controls [117]."

"The adverse event profiles of SGLT2 inhibitors may be slightly more pronounced in elderly patients."

"The available evidence suggests that SGLT2 inhibitors are not associated with dehydration in elderly patients [123, 124]."

Conclusions

"In the EMPA-REG OUTCOME trial, the impact of empagliflozin treatment on the rates of acute renal failure and AKI was greatest in patients with baseline eGFR < 60 mL/min/1.73 m^2 [27]."

"In a meta-analyses of these CV and renal outcome trials, the renoprotective effects of SGLT2 inhibitors were seen across all levels of baseline eGFR, although the largest benefits were apparent in patients with preserved renal function at baseline [115]."

"The outcomes of these trials demonstrate how the benefits of SGLT2 inhibitors, used in combination with RAS inhibitors, span the renal risk continuum, from patients with mild/moderate CKD (as seen in the EMPA-REG OUTCOME, CANVAS program, and DECLARE-TIMI 58 trials) to those with moderate/severe CKD (as observed in CREDENCE and DAPA-CKD)."

"Further insights into the potential benefits of SGLT2 inhibitors in patients at different stages on the renal and CV risk continuum are likely to come from the EMPA-KIDNEY (NCT03594110) trial in patients with diabetic as well as nondiabetic CKD."

Potential Mechanisms Responsible for Cardioprotective Effects of Sodium–Glucose Co-transporter 2 Inhibitors [125]

This is a machine-generated summary of:

Lahnwong, Sarayut; Chattipakorn, Siriporn C.; Chattipakorn, Nipon: Potential mechanisms responsible for cardioprotective effects of sodium–glucose co-transporter 2 inhibitors [125].

Published in: Cardiovascular Diabetology (2018).

Link to original: https://doi.org/10.1186/s12933-018-0745-5

If you want to cite the papers, please refer to the original.

For technical reasons we could not place the page where the original quote is coming from.

Abstract-Summary "Sodium–glucose co-transporter 2 (SGLT-2) inhibitors are a novel class of antidiabetic drugs with cardiovascular benefits beyond other antidiabetic drugs."

"The possible mechanisms of SGLT-2 inhibitors are proposed to be systemic effects by hemodynamic and metabolic actions."

"Reports concerning the effects of SGLT-2 inhibitors in models of diabetic cardiomyopathy, heart failure and myocardial ischemia from in vitro, in vivo as well as clinical reports are comprehensively summarized and discussed."

"By current evidences, it may be concluded that the direct effects of SGLT-2 inhibitors are potentially mediated through their ability to reduce cardiac inflammation, oxidative stress, apoptosis, mitochondrial dysfunction and ionic dyshomeostasis."

Background

"The EMPA-REG OUTCOME trial (2010–2015) showed the cardioprotective effect of empagliflozin by significantly lowering the rate of death from cardiovascular causes [38% relative risk reduction (RRR)], all-cause death (32% RRR) and heart failure hospitalization (HHF) (35% RRR) in T2DM patients with established cardiovascular diseases (CVD) [27]."

"The CVD-REAL study which reported the cardiovascular effect of SGLT-2 inhibitors compared to other glucose-lowering drugs showed that SGLT-2 inhibitors could significantly decrease the rate of HHF (HR 0.49, 95% CI 0.41–0.57) and all-cause death (HR 0.61, 95% CI 0.51–0.73) [126]."

"Both hemodynamic and metabolic actions of SGLT-2 inhibitors potentially work together for improving diabetic cardiomyopathy and finally resulting in cardioprotection as shown in the EMPA-REG OUTCOME trial."

"Only systemic mechanisms may be not enough to explain much better cardiovascular benefits of SGLT-2 inhibitors when compared to other glucose-lowering drugs."

Effects of SGLT-2 Inhibitors on Cardiac Structure

"SGLT-2 inhibitors have been shown to improve cardiac histopathologic changes in the diabetic cardiomyopathy models of mice and rats, the heart failure model of zebrafish embryos and also the myocardial ischemic model of rats."

"After 10 weeks of treatment, empagliflozin significantly reduced left ventricular weight, cardiomyocyte size, cardiac interstitial fibrosis and cardiac interstitial macrophage infiltration."

"Several reports that studied the effect of empagliflozin in genetic diabetic mouse models also suggested the improvement of cardiac morphologic changes by decreasing the cardiomyocyte cross sectional area, interstitial collagen I and III depositions, interstitial fibrosis and interstitial macrophage infiltration [127, 128]."

"Ye and others showed that the treatment of dapagliflozin for 8 weeks decreased myocardial collagen-1 and collagen-3 mRNA levels and percentage of fibrosis in genetic diabetic mice [129]."

"Empagliflozin could attenuate the expression of heart failure markers including atrial natriuretic peptide and brain natriuretic peptide."

Effects of SGLT-2 Inhibitors on Cardiac Function

"These reports indicated that dapagliflozin could improve both systolic and diastolic LV function in diabetic mice."

"In genetic diabetic mice, empagliflozin improved diastolic function as seen by increased septal wall motion and decreased LV filling pressure [128]."

"In a diabetic cardiomyopathy rat model, empagliflozin also improved LV function by the increase of end-systolic pressure (ESP), + dp/dt and − dp/dt (the maximal ascending rate and the maximal descending rate of left ventricular pressure, respectively) and the decrease of end-diastolic pressure (EDP) [130]."

"Before I/R injury operation, 4-week dapagliflozin treatment already showed the improvement of E/A ratio, EF, IVRT, DT and EDWT which referred to both systolic and diastolic LV function."

"Similar results were found in Wistar rats with MI treated with dapagliflozin for 4 weeks in which the improvement of cardiac function as evidenced by increasing the maximal rate of LV + dP/dt and − dP/dt were observed [131]."

Potential Mechanisms of SGLT-2 Inhibitors Responsible for Cardioprotection

"Ye and others tested the effect of 8-week dapagliflozin treatment on cardiac inflammation in genetic diabetic mice and found that dapagliflozin decreased the levels of myocardial mRNA associated with NLRP3 inflammasome and pro-inflammatory cytokines including NALP-3, ASC, caspase-1, IL-1β, IL-6 and TNFα [129]."

"By current evidences, SGLT-2 inhibitors seem to attenuate apoptotic myocardial cells in diabetic cardiomyopathy and MI, however more studies are required to explore their roles on cardiac apoptosis."

"We have demonstrated that a 4-week treatment with dapagliflozin attenuated the increase of cardiac mitochondrial fission and the decrease of mitochondrial fusion as evidenced by decreased DRP1 and increased MFN2 and OPA1 expressions in obese-insulin resistant rats undergoing cardiac I/R injury [132]."

"Despite no SGLT-2 expression in the heart [133–135], empagliflozin could have cardiac effects by decreasing myocardial $[Na^+]_c$ and $[Ca^{2+}]_c$ and increasing $[Ca^{2+}]_m$ through the inhibition of NHE directly."

Conclusions and Perspectives

"The cardioprotection of SGLT-2 inhibitors has been demonstrated in models of diabetic cardiomyopathy, heart failure and myocardial ischemia."

"The direct effects of SGLT-2 inhibitors could potentially mediate through their abilities to attenuate cardiac inflammation, oxidative stress, apoptosis, mitochondrial dysfunction and ionic dyshomeostasis."

"The mechanisms of SGLT-2 inhibitors responsible for these benefits could be due to their systemic as well as direct cardiac effects."

"For reducing HHF, natriuretic effect of SGLT-2 inhibitors results in lowering plasma volume and blood pressure, which are subsequently decreasing cardiac preload and afterload [136–138]."

"SGLT-2 inhibitors also directly improve cardiac calcium handling via inhibiting myocardial NHE which subsequently decrease intracellular Na^+ and Ca^{2+} loading mostly found in heart failure [139]."

"Despite these growing number of reports, the cardioprotective effects in some respects such as cardiac apoptosis and mitochondrial dysfunctions are still unclear whether they are the direct effects or systemic effects of SGLT-2 inhibitors."

SGLT2i and GLP-1 RA Therapy in Type 1 Diabetes and Reno-Vascular Outcomes: A Real-World Study [140]

This is a machine-generated summary of:

Anson, Matthew; Zhao, Sizheng S.; Austin, Philip; Ibarburu, Gema H.; Malik, Rayaz A.; Alam, Uazman: SGLT2i and GLP-1 RA therapy in type 1 diabetes and reno-vascular outcomes: a real-world study [140].

Published in: Diabetologia (2023).

Link to original: https://doi.org/10.1007/s00125-023-05975-8

If you want to cite the papers, please refer to the original.

For technical reasons we could not place the page where the original quote is coming from.

Abstract-Summary "We sought to investigate the real-world impact of sodium–glucose cotransporter 2 inhibitor (SGLT2i) and glucagon-like peptide-1 receptor agonist (GLP-1 RA) therapy in individuals with type 1 diabetes in relation to effect on blood glucose levels, adverse events and cardio-renal outcomes."

"We included patients who had been treated with an SGLT2i or GLP-1 RA for at least 6 months and analysed the efficacy, safety and cardio-renal outcomes 5 years after initiation of therapy."

"We identified 196,691 individuals with type 1 diabetes, 13% of whom were treated with adjunctive glucose-lowering therapy in addition to insulin."

"Included in the core analysis were 1822 patients treated with a GLP-1 RA and 992 individuals treated with an SGLT2i."

"The SGLT2i treated cohort showed preservation of eGFR over a 5-year period compared with the GLP-1 RA treated cohort (+ 3.5 ml/min per 1.73 m^2 vs −7.2 ml/min per 1.73 m^2, respectively), including patients with established chronic kidney disease (CKD)."

"The SGLT2i treated cohort experienced higher rates of diabetic ketoacidosis (DKA) (RR 2.08 [95% CI 1.05, 4.12] $p = 0.0309$) and urinary tract infection/

pyelonephritis (RR 2.27 [95% CI 1.12, 4.55] p = 0.019) compared with the GLP-1 RA treated cohort."

"SGLT2is provide cardio-renal benefits, despite an increase in the risk of DKA and urinary tract infection compared with GLP-1 RA therapy."

"Long-term evaluation of the efficacy and safety of these adjunctive therapies is required to guide their use in individuals with type 1 diabetes."

Introduction

"The incidence and prevalence of type 1 diabetes is increasing."

"Intensification of glucose-lowering therapy in type 1 diabetes includes multiple daily insulin injections, continuous subcutaneous insulin infusion, alongside continuous glucose monitoring and increasingly closed-loop insulin delivery [141]."

"SGLT2is, and GLP-1 RAs in particular promote weight loss, and therefore especially may be of benefit, given that overweight and obesity is increasingly prevalent (62%) in individuals with type 1 diabetes [142]."

"Both SGLT2i and GLP-1 RA demonstrate robust and consistent cardio-renal benefits [143], both agents seem to be an attractive option to fulfil an unmet therapeutic need in type 1 diabetes."

"All adjuvant glucose-lowering therapies in type 1 diabetes are used off-label and contrary to local and national guidance [144]."

"This study has investigated the real-world impact of SGLT2i and GLP-1 RA therapy on individuals with type 1 diabetes in relation to efficacy, safety and cardio-renal outcomes."

Methods

"We performed a retrospective cohort study of all patients aged 18 or over with type 1 diabetes using the TriNetX platform."

"For this retrospective cohort analysis, ~200,000 patients from 90 HCOs were identified."

"This initial group of participants were then divided into two cohorts, 'SGLT2i' and 'GLP-1 RA'."

"The analyses were conducted on the above cohorts: (1) SGLT2i and (2) GLP-1 RA with each analysis propensity score matched (PSM) for age, sex, BMI, presence of heart failure (ICD-10-CM-I50), hypertension (ICD-10-CM-I10), ischaemic heart disease (IHD) (ICD-10-CM-I20–25), chronic kidney disease (CKD) (ICD-10-CM-N18) and HbA_{1c} value so as to balance the analysis (1:1 matching) being undertaken."

"The analysis on the respective cohorts was based on the following safety outcomes over 5 years from drug initiation: DKA, hypoglycaemia requiring admission to secondary care, urinary tract infection (UTI), pyelonephritis, candidiasis of the lower genital tract, acute pancreatitis and gastrointestinal upset."

Results

"Participants in the SGLT2i group demonstrated improvement in renal function with an increase in mean eGFR over the 5-year follow-up period (+ 3.5 ml/min per 1.73 m^2), compared with an overall reduction in eGFR in the GLP-1 RA cohort (−7.2 ml/min per 1.73 m^2)."

"Over 5 years, 28 participants from the SGLT2i group developed DKA, compared with 11 in the GLP-1 RA group."

"Patients treated with SGLT2i were less likely to be diagnosed with new CKD over a 5-year period post initiation compared with the GLP-1 RA cohort (RR 0.49 [95% CI 0.28, 0.86] p = 0.0118)."

"We identified individuals within the SGLT2i and GLP-1 RA cohort who had a pre-existing diagnosis of CKD and conducted further subgroup analysis on this group over 5 years."

Discussion

"We have conducted the largest real-world retrospective cohort study to date investigating the safety and outcomes of individuals with type 1 diabetes using SGLT2i and GLP-1 RA therapy, and the first to report cardio-renal benefits."

"These data suggest that physicians may be preferentially selecting patients with type 1 diabetes thought to benefit most from either cardio-renal benefits of SGLT2i therapy or the weight reduction associated with GLP-1 RA, established in type 2 diabetes [145]."

"Given the relatively positive safety profile of GLP-1 RA with a reduction in weight and HbA_{1c}, without an increased risk of DKA, they are an appealing adjunctive therapy for people with type 1 diabetes."

"We report that individuals with type 1 diabetes treated with SGLT2i therapy demonstrate preservation of renal function, reduced rates of hospitalisation and reduced risk of heart failure when compared with patients receiving GLP-1 RA."

SGLT2 Inhibitors: Slowing of Chronic Kidney Disease Progression in Type 2 Diabetes [146]

This is a machine-generated summary of:

Wheeler, David C.; James, June; Patel, Dipesh; Viljoen, Adie; Ali, Amar; Evans, Marc; Fernando, Kevin; Hicks, Debbie; Milne, Nicola; Newland-Jones, Philip; Wilding, John: SGLT2 Inhibitors: Slowing of Chronic Kidney Disease Progression in Type 2 Diabetes [146].

Published in: Diabetes Therapy (2020).

Link to original: https://doi.org/10.1007/s13300-020-00930-x

Copyright of the summarized publication:

If you want to cite the papers, please refer to the original.

For technical reasons we could not place the page where the original quote is coming from.

Abstract-Summary "It is a progressive and costly complication associated with increased risk of adverse cardiovascular (CV) and renal outcomes and mortality."

"Ongoing monitoring of the estimated glomerular filtration (eGFR) rate alongside the urine albumin:creatinine ratio (ACR) is recommended during regular T2DM reviews to enable a prompt DKD diagnosis or to assess disease progression, providing an understanding of adverse risk for each individual."

"Many people with DKD will progress to end-stage kidney disease (ESKD), requiring renal replacement therapy (RRT), typically haemodialysis or kidney transplantation."

"Improvements in renal end points observed in SGLT2i CV outcome trials (CVOTs) highlighted the possible impact of these agents in the management of DKD."

"Data from the canagliflozin CREDENCE trial (Canagliflozin and Renal Events in Diabetes with Established Nephropathy Clinical Evaluation) have since demonstrated the effectiveness of this medicine in reducing the risk of kidney failure and CV events in a population comprising individuals with T2DM and renal disease."

"CREDENCE was the first SGLT2i study to examine renal outcomes as the primary end point."

"This article summarises the evidence regarding the use of SGLT2i medicines in slowing the progression of DKD and examines the possible mechanisms underpinning the renoprotective effects of these agents."

Role of the Improving Diabetes Steering Committee

"The Committee aims to ensure that healthcare professionals (HCPs) who prescribe diabetes medicines have access to balanced and accurate information and evidence concerning type 2 diabetes mellitus (T2DM) medicines, with a specific focus on the sodium-glucose co-transporter-2 inhibitor (SGLT2i) class of treatments."

"The group is committed to providing healthcare colleagues with clarity regarding the evidence base supporting SGLT2i agents, highlighting the relative benefits and risks of these therapies."

"Educational materials and publications, such as the previously published consensus documents, provided by the panel are intended to increase confidence and understanding regarding the appropriate place of these medicines within the current UK T2DM treatment paradigm [147, 148]."

Digital Features

"This article is published with digital features to facilitate understanding of the article."

"You can access the digital features on the article's associated Figshare page."

"To view digital features for this article, go to https://doi.org/10.6084/m9.figshare.12937334 ."

Introduction

"Diabetic kidney disease (DKD) is a widely recognised and growing concern among clinicians involved in the management of type 2 diabetes mellitus (T2DM)."

"As the T2DM treatment pathway continues to evolve, an emerging role has been highlighted for SGLT2i therapies in slowing DKD progression to end-stage kidney disease (ESKD) [33, 149]."

"The Improving Diabetes Steering Committee discusses current data and the proposed mechanisms that may underpin renoprotective effects of these agents, as well as the potential value that SGLT2i therapies offer in delaying the onset and progression of chronic kidney disease (CKD)."

"The Tool is included as a supplementary item alongside this article and can also be accessed online via the Diabetes Therapy website."

The Burden of Kidney Disease in T2DM

"Approximately 40% of people with T2DM have kidney disease, and this is predicted to rise to around 50% by 2025 [150, 151]."

"There have been significant increases in the number of people living with T2DM and DKD, as well as the proportion of this population requiring renal replacement therapy (RRT); dialysis and/or kidney transplantation [152]."

"Increased mortality rates associated with T2DM are believed to be predominantly due to kidney disease, and global disease burden data show that the number of deaths due to DKD rose by 94% between the years 1990–2012 [63, 153]."

"The rising number of people with DKD requiring RRT has significant implications for health resource use and costs of care for people with T2DM."

Evaluation and Classification of DKD Disease Markers

"Although much debate exists regarding the most appropriate and accurate markers for progression of DKD, a moderately increased urinary albumin:creatinine ratio (ACR) (albuminuria) and declining estimated glomerular filtration rate (eGFR) are currently regarded as the most acceptable and widely used early indicators of kidney disease in the absence of specific biomarkers and diagnostic tools [33, 154]."

"Decreasing eGFR and increasing ACR are each considered to be independent risk factors for adverse outcomes and mortality [153, 155]."

"Elevated ACR and declining eGFR, in combination, multiply the risk of adverse outcomes [155]."

Slowing or Preventing DKD Progression

"Recommendations on the use of aspirin and other anti-platelet medications in people with T2DM and kidney disease are unclear [155, 156]."

"NICE guidelines for the management of T2DM do not recommend aspirin for people without CV disease and the NICE CKD guidelines highlight the need for additional evidence on the benefits of aspirin as a primary prevention measure for people with CKD at the highest risk of CV disease [155, 156]."

"The Steno-2 trial showed the benefit of intensive multifactorial treatment approaches (e.g. lifestyle changes, glycaemic control, RAAS inhibitors) on CV and renal outcomes in people with T2DM and severely increased ACR [157]."

"Published evidence from large-scale randomised trials and real-world studies supports the use of SGLT2i treatments in reducing the overall rate of kidney function decline and adverse renal risk among those with T2DM [27, 28, 33, 112, 116, 119, 158, 159]."

SGLT2i Treatments: Renal Outcomes Data

"The primary outcome event rate was significantly lower in the canagliflozin group compared with the placebo group: 43.2 versus 61.2 per 1000 patient-years, providing a 30% relative risk reduction (HR 0.70; 95% CI 0.59–0.82; $P = 0.00001$) [33]."

"Pooled relative risk (RR) among people with T2DM and CV disease or CV risk factors was lower for those treated with an SGLT2i compared with placebo for the composite renal outcome of doubling of serum creatinine or 40% decrease in eGFR, initiation of RRT or death due to renal disease (RR 0.63; 95% CI 0.56–0.71) [116]."

"The pooled RR for the same composite renal outcome among those with CV disease or CV risk factors and eGFR < 60 ml/min/1.73 m^2 was also lower for those treated with an SGLT2i versus placebo (RR 0.67; 95% CI 0.59–0.76) [116]."

Potential Mechanisms Underpinning the Renoprotective Action of SGLT2I Treatments

"In the presence of hyperglycaemia due to diabetes, hyperfiltration occurs; SGLT2 co-transporters are upregulated in the proximal tubule and glucose and Na^+ reabsorption increases."

"Adenosine levels drop due to reduced Na^+/K^+ ATPase activity and the afferent arteriole dilates, enabling increased blood flow through the glomerulus [149, 160, 161]."

"The SGLT2i class of drugs reduces reabsorption of glucose and Na^+ via inhibition of SGLT2 co-transporters within the proximal tubule, which re-establishes Na^+ delivery to the macula densa [149, 160, 161]."

"Current models suggest that the afferent arteriole may constrict in response to raised adenosine levels, driven by increased membrane Na^+/K^+ ATPase activity, to regulate and reduce glomerular blood flow [149, 160, 161]."

"As SGLT2i agents block uptake of glucose within proximal tubular cells, it is possible that their renoprotective effect may be partly due to a reduced local inflammatory response and fibrosis [149]."

Implications for Clinical Practice

"It is important that people with T2DM receive education to help them understand the importance of their annual eGFR and urine ACR test in evaluating their current level of risk concerning CV complications and renal failure."

"These medicines should be considered for those with increased risk of renal and CV disease (with hypertension and/or microalbuminuria), where appropriate, and in accordance with NICE and local prescribing guidelines [155, 162–164]."

"Although, as mentioned previously, clinicians should keep in mind the residual risk for people with T2DM and monitor regularly for disease progression [108, 109]."

"The ADA/EASD guidelines already reflect the growing evidence base for SGT2i medicines in the treatment of people with T2DM who may be at risk of DKD, and the latest KDIGO guidelines are aligned with these recommendations [163, 165]."

"CREDENCE was the first published SGLT2i study specifically examining renal outcomes in a high-risk population, providing confirmatory and robust data on the effects of canagliflozin on patient-relevant renal end points [33, 166]."

Conclusion

"Looking to the future, clinicians working across primary care, diabetes services and renal services will need to collaborate effectively with commissioners to ensure that the diagnosis and ongoing management of DKD are prioritised and that colleagues are appropriately supported to implement this work."

"Equitable access to testing and monitoring services, alongside the medications that have been shown to be effective in slowing the progression of DKD, will be critical in protecting this vulnerable group and stemming the ever-increasing costs and HRQoL implications of kidney failure and RRT."

Renoprotective Effect of SGLT-2 Inhibitors among Type 2 Diabetes Patients with Different Baseline Kidney Function: A Multi-Center Study [167]

This is a machine-generated summary of:

Lin, Fang-Ju; Wang, Chi-Chuan; Hsu, Chien-Ning; Yang, Chen-Yi; Wang, Chih-Yuan; Ou, Huang-Tz: Renoprotective effect of SGLT-2 inhibitors among type 2 diabetes patients with different baseline kidney function: a multi-center study [167].

Published in: Cardiovascular Diabetology (2021).

Link to original: https://doi.org/10.1186/s12933-021-01396-2

If you want to cite the papers, please refer to the original.

For technical reasons we could not place the page where the original quote is coming from.

Abstract-Summary "To assess the effect of sodium glucose cotransporter-2 inhibitors (SGLT-2is) for type 2 diabetes on kidney outcomes stratified by patient baseline estimated glomerular filtration rate (eGFR) levels (i.e., eGFR $\leq$ 60, 60 < eGFR $\leq$ 90, and eGFR > 90 mL/min/1.73 m^2)."

"One-to-one propensity score matching in the overall study cohort and in each eGFR subgroup between SGLT-2i and oGLD users was applied to ensure between-group comparability in baseline characteristics."

"While a sustained eGFR decline was revealed in oGLD-treated patients (mean values [standard errors] from 85.61 [0.43] to 82.49 [0.44] mL/min/1.73 m^2 during the 12 months after treatment initiation), the mean eGFR values of SGLT-2i users decreased in the first 3 months (85.68 [0.37] to 79.71 [0.41] mL/min/1.73 m^2) but then improved and sustained until the end of follow-up."

"There were 2300, 5705, and 5509 matched SGLT-2i and oGLD users in the eGFR ≤ 60, 60 < eGFR ≤ 90, and eGFR > 90 subgroups, respectively."

"Using SGLT-2is versus oGLDs was significantly associated with slower eGFR declines; hazard ratios (HRs) were 0.51 (95% CI 0.37–0.69), 0.51 (0.37–0.70), and 0.47 (0.31–0.71) for 40% eGFR reduction in the eGFR ≤ 60, 60 < eGFR ≤ 90, and eGFR > 90 subgroups, respectively."

"The renoprotective effect of SGLT-2is versus oGLDs was confirmed in the outcomes of 30% and 50% eGFR reduction across the three eGFR subgroups."

Background

"Studies that include a large, broad type 2 diabetes patient population treated in routine practice are essential for determining whether the renal benefits of SGLT-2is found in trial settings can be translated to clinical practice and quantifying the magnitude of SGLT-2i effectiveness."

"One such study is Comparative Effectiveness of Cardiovascular Outcomes in New Users of SGLT2 Inhibitors 3 (CVD-REAL 3) [158], which included more than 71,000 type 2 diabetes patients across five countries."

"It provided supporting evidence for the real-world kidney outcomes of SGLT-2i use and suggested that the kidney benefits reported in clinical trials can be extended to clinical practice settings [158]."

"The present study includes a large number of type 2 diabetes patients from three large healthcare delivery systems in Taiwan to extend existing real-world evidence to a larger Asian population and provide further evidence from patient subgroups with different baseline eGFR levels (i.e., eGFR ≤ 60, 60 < eGFR ≤ 90, and eGFR > 90 mL/min/1.73 m^2)."

Methods

"Using the alternative on-treatment (OT) approach (sensitivity analysis), patients were followed up from the index date until the occurrence of study outcomes, discontinuation of index medication, switch to or addition of other type of oGLD, last encounter date in the EHR database, last date of the study period, or death, whichever came first."

"The following study covariates were measured at the baseline and treated as potential confounders to be adjusted in the analyses: age, gender, body mass index, smoking, HbA1c, eGFR, eGFR change (slope), frailty status, prior use of oGLDs and other medications (e.g., antihypertensive drugs, aldosterone antagonists, antiplatelets, and statins), which were measured in the year before the index date, and history of microvascular diseases and CVDs (i.e., myocardial infarction, unstable angina, heart failure, atrial fibrillation, stroke, and peripheral artery disease), which were based on all available diagnosis records in the EHR databases before the index date."

Results

"These differences between SGLT-2i and oGLD users in the overall study cohort are similar to those in the eGFR subgroups, except that the baseline eGFR of oGLD users was slightly higher than that of SGLT-2i users in the eGFR > 90 subgroup (114.7 versus 112.6 mL/min/1.73 m^2)."

"Regarding the three eGFR subgroups, the patients in the eGFR > 90 subgroup were the youngest and had the fewest comorbidities (i.e., average age of 55 years, and 39% and 26% of patients having microvascular diseases and CVDs, respectively)."

"Although the patterns of these changes between the two drug groups were slightly different across the three eGFR subgroups, in general, the use of SGLT-2is attenuated the decline of eGFR levels in all subgroups."

"The eGFR change of SGLT-2i versus oGLD use seems more profound in the eGFR > 90 subgroup (in terms of lower HR values) but with wider CIs."

Discussion

"This is the largest real-world study (more than 25,000 patients) of an Asian population to examine the renoprotective effect of SGLT-2i in a cohort of type 2 diabetes patients and patient subgroups with different baseline kidney functions."

"It is noteworthy that despite the differences in patient characteristics and study designs across studies, the benefit of restoring kidney function associated with SGLT-2i versus oGLD use was similar; i.e., HR (95% CI) for 40% eGFR reduction was 0.46 (0.38–0.56) in our study, 0.56 (0.45–0.70) in CVD-REAL 3 [158], and 0.54 (0.43–0.67) in the DECLARE-TIMI 58 trial [119]."

"Our study results further support that the renoprotective effect of SGLT-2i use is consistent across different eGFR subgroups, even in patients without CKD."

"The pattern of eGFR response to SGLT-2i use was consistent across patient groups with different baseline eGFR levels, further suggesting that this effect may be independent of the severity of kidney damage of type 2 diabetes patients."

Conclusions

"The use of SGLT-2is versus oGLDs yielded a favorable effect in slowing eGFR declines, regardless of patient baseline renal function, in a real-world type 2 diabetes population."

"Our results extend the evidence from existing trials and real-world studies on the renoprotective effect of SGLT-2i to a large Asian population."

Kidney Disease in Type 2 Diabetes Mellitus and Benefits of Sodium-Glucose Cotransporter 2 Inhibitors: A Consensus Statement [168]

This is a machine-generated summary of:

Roy, Ajitesh; Maiti, Animesh; Sinha, Anirban; Baidya, Arjun; Basu, Asish Kumar; Sarkar, Dasarathi; Sanyal, Debmalya; Biswas, Dibakar; Maisnam, Indira; Pandit, Kaushik; Raychaudhuri, Moutusi; Sengupta, Nilanjan; Chakraborty, Partha Pratim; Mukhopadhyay, Pradip; Raychaudhuri, Pradip; Sahana, Pranab Kumar; Chatterjee, Purushottam; Bhattacharjee, Rana; Dasgupta, Ranen; Saraogi, Ravi Kant; Pal, Salil Kumar; Mukhopadhyay, Sarmishtha; Mukhopadhyay, Satinath; Goswami, Soumik; Chowdhury, Subhankar; Ghosh, Sujoy: Kidney Disease in Type 2 Diabetes Mellitus and Benefits of Sodium-Glucose Cotransporter 2 Inhibitors: A Consensus Statement [168].

Published in: Diabetes Therapy (2020).

Link to original: https://doi.org/10.1007/s13300-020-00921-y

If you want to cite the papers, please refer to the original.

For technical reasons we could not place the page where the original quote is coming from.

Abstract-Summary "Sodium-glucose cotransporter 2 inhibitors (SGLT2i) control hyperglycemia by blocking renal glucose reabsorption in addition to preventing inflammation, thereby improving endothelial function and reducing oxidative stress; consequently, this class of prescription medicines is emerging as an important addition to the therapeutic armamentarium."

"The EMPA-REG OUTCOME, DECLARE TIMI 58, and CANVAS trials demonstrated the renoprotective effects of SGLT2i, such as restricting decline in glomerular filtration rate, in the progression of albuminuria, and in death due to renal causes."

"The renoprotection provided by SGLT2i was further confirmed in the CREDENCE study, which showed a 30% reduction in progression of chronic kidney disease, and in the DELIGHT study, which demonstrated a reduction in albuminuria with dapagliflozin compared with placebo (−21.0%, confidence interval [CI] −34.1 to −5.2, $p = 0.011$)."

"A meta-analysis demonstrated a reduced risk of dialysis, transplantation, or death due to kidney disease (relative risk 0.67; 95% CI 0.52–0.86; $p = 0.0019$) and a 45% risk reduction in worsening of renal function, end-stage renal disease, or renal death (hazard ratio 0.55, CI 0.48–0.64, $p < 0.0001$) with SGLT2i, irrespective of baseline estimated glomerular filtration rate."

"There is emerging evidence that SGLT2i may be used to curb the mortality and improve the quality of life in patients with DKD."

"In this consensus statement, we have qualitatively synthesized evidence demonstrating the renal effects of SGLT2i and proposed recommendations for optimal use of SGLT2i to effectively manage and delay progression of DKD."

Digital Features

"This article is published with digital features to facilitate understanding of the article."

"To view digital features for this article go to https://doi.org/10.6084/m9.figshare.12871889".

Introduction

"In the third National Health and Nutrition Examination Survey conducted in the USA, 42.3% of the individuals with diabetes had chronic kidney disease (CKD) ($N = 15{,}046$), and the 10-year cumulative mortality, standardized to population age, sex, and race, in this patient population was 31.1% (95% confidence interval [CI] 24.7–37.5%) [153]."

"Based on data from the Screening and Early Evaluation of Kidney Disease (SEEK)-India community-based cohort, hypertension and diabetes are the most common risk factors for CKD."

"A study of US electronic medical records demonstrated that CKD was associated with the highest incremental risk of all-cause mortality (ACM) in people newly diagnosed with T2DM [169]."

"CKD contributes to a 1.4- to 2.9-fold increase in cardiovascular (CV) mortality in individuals with diabetes."

Methodology

"The therapeutic strategies for managing CKD in people with T2DM using SGLT2i are presented in this consensus statement in the form of recommendations."

"In order to generate these recommendations, we performed a literature search of the MEDLINE and EMBASE databases using combinations of the following key terms: "SGLT2i," "composite renal outcomes," "T2DM," "chronic kidney disease," "CKD," "Diabetes," "renoprotection," "eGFR," "ACR," "creatinine," "death," "mortality," and "nephropathy"."

"Key experts in the field of endocrinology and nephrology critically reviewed the results presented in the literature, and the recommendations were developed."

"The recommendations were reviewed once again and modified to incorporate the clinical practice experience to generate the consensus recommendations presented here."

Diagnosis and Prognosis of Chronic Kidney Disease

"The National Kidney Foundation-Kidney Disease Outcomes Quality Initiative (NKF-KDOQI) guideline defines CKD as the presence of either one or both of the following two criteria for at least 3 months: (1) GFR < 60 mL/min/1.73 m^2; (2) markers of kidney damage (≥1), such as albuminuria (albumin: creatinine ratio [ACR] ≥ 30 mg/g), urinary sediment abnormality, electrolyte, or other abnormality due to tubular disorder, abnormalities on histology, structural abnormalities detected by imaging, or history of kidney transplantation [170–172]."

"The prognosis of CKD is determined by assessing the GFR category together with the albuminuria category."

Pathophysiology and Therapeutic Targets of DKD

"The Diabetes Control and Complications Trial was the first to demonstrate the renoprotective effects of intensive glycemic control through a reduction in the incident micro- and macro-albuminuria in persons with insulin-dependent diabetes mellitus by 39 and 54%, respectively [173]."

"Similar results with significant reductions in the risk of ESRD by 65%, microalbuminuria by 9%, and macroalbuminuria by 30% were obtained with intensive glycemic control in the Action in Diabetes and Vascular Disease: Preterax and Diamicron MR Controlled Evaluation (ADVANCE) trial with gliclazide [174]."

"These were the earliest two landmark trials in type 1 DM and T2DM, respectively, that demonstrated the renoprotective effects of good glycemic control."

"The Aliskiren Trial in Type 2 Diabetes Using Cardiorenal Endpoints (ALTITUDE), which studied the addition of aliskiren (direct renin inhibitor) to RAAS blockade in people with T2DM with high CV and renal risk, was prematurely halted because of an increase in adverse events (AEs), with no reduction in CV or renal outcomes [175]."

Role of SGLT2i in DKD

"Osmotic effects of high luminal glucose concentration due to SGLT2i action increase distal tubular fluid delivery and lower GFR by increasing hydrostatic pressure in Bowman's space."

"The SGLT2i have demonstrated glycemic efficacy as well as other benefits such as weight reduction, reduction in blood pressure, and an increase in high-density lipoprotein-cholesterol."

"Several meta-analyses and RCTs have demonstrated the glycemic efficacy of SGLT2i (empagliflozin [176, 177], canagliflozin [178, 179], and dapagliflozin [180]) to be comparable to that of other antihyperglycemic agents, with the additional benefits of reduction in body weight and blood pressure."

"Dapagliflozin resulted in a lower rate of CV death or HHF compared with placebo (4.9 vs. 5.8%; HR 0.83, 95% CI 0.73–0.95, $p = 0.005$)."

"Empagliflozin, compared with placebo, demonstrated significantly lower rates of death from CV causes (3.7 vs. 5.9%; HR 0.62, 95% CI 0.49–0.77) and death from any cause (5.7 and 8.3%; HR 0.68, 95% CI 0.57–0.82)."

Clinical Evidence of Renoprotective Effect with SGLT2i

"The DECLARE-TIMI 58 trial in people with T2DM with and without established CVD found that patients treated with dapagliflozin were at a lower risk of composite renal outcomes compared with patients receiving placebo (3.7 vs. 7.0 events/1000 patient-years; HR 0.53, 95% CI 0.43–0.66) [28]."

"A significant risk reduction in terms of composite renal events (sustained decrease in eGFR by at least 40% to < 60 mL/min/1.73 m^2, ESRD, or renal death) was achieved with dapagliflozin compared with placebo in people with T2DM with multiple risk factors and without established ASCVD (HR 0.51, CI 0.37–0.69), as well as in those with established ASCVD (HR 0.55, CI 0.41–0.75)."

Recommendations for Optimal Use of SGLT2 Inhibitors

"Sodium-glucose cotransporter 2 inhibitors reduce the risk of progression to DKD and renal death by approximately 40–50% in people with T2DM who are at risk of CV events and are on ACE-Is and ARBs."

"SGLT2i have emerged as the new drugs that must be included in the armamentarium for the management for people with T2DM having CVD or mild-to-moderate DKD to curb morbidity and mortality."

"The recommendations for optimal use of SGLT2i, generated on the basis of evidence from RCTs and meta-analyses, is summarized below."

Comparative Efficacy of Five SGLT2i on Cardiorenal Events: A Network Meta-Analysis Based on Ten CVOTs [181]

This is a machine-generated summary of:

Qiu, Mei; Ding, Liang-Liang; Zhou, Hai-Rong: Comparative Efficacy of Five SGLT2i on Cardiorenal Events: A Network Meta-analysis Based on Ten CVOTs [181].

Published in: American Journal of Cardiovascular Drugs (2021).

Link to original: https://doi.org/10.1007/s40256-021-00484-8

If you want to cite the papers, please refer to the original.

For technical reasons we could not place the page where the original quote is coming from.

Abstract-Summary "The eight endpoints of interest were major adverse cardiovascular events (MACE), myocardial infarction (MI), stroke, cardiovascular death (CVD), CVD or hospitalization for heart failure (HHF), HHF, kidney function progression (KFP), and all-cause death (ACD)."

"Canagliflozin (hazard ratio [HR] 0.64; 95% confidence interval [CI] 0.53–0.77), dapagliflozin (HR 0.70; 95% CI 0.62–0.79), empagliflozin (HR 0.68; 95% CI 0.59–0.78), ertugliflozin (HR 0.70; 95% CI 0.54–0.90), and sotagliflozin (HR 0.66; 95% CI 0.56–0.77) versus placebo reduced HHF, whereas none reduced MI and stroke."

"Empagliflozin reduced CVD or HHF (HR 0.81; 95% CI 0.67–0.99) and KFP (HR 0.65; 95% CI 0.45–0.93), and dapagliflozin reduced KFP (HR 0.69; 95% CI 0.52–0.92), versus ertugliflozin."

"Canagliflozin had the greatest SUCRA values for the reduction of MACE, stroke, and HHF, whereas empagliflozin had the greatest SUCRA values for the reduction of MI, CVD, CVD or HHF, KFP, and ACD."

"Canagliflozin, dapagliflozin, empagliflozin, ertugliflozin, and sotagliflozin versus placebo reduce HHF but none reduces MI and stroke."

"Canagliflozin is most effective in reducing MACE and HHF, and empagliflozin is most effective in reducing CVD, CVD or HHF, KFP, and ACD."

Introduction

"The relative efficacy of different SGLT2i on cardiorenal outcomes is unclear because randomized trials comparing all SGLT2i in the reduction of cardiorenal events are lacking."

"SGLT2i CVOTs [27–45, 47–66, 68–80, 83–104, 106–124, 126–139, 141–145, 147–166, 169–180, 182–215] have evaluated their effects on cardiorenal and mortality outcomes in three different underlying diseases: type 2 diabetes mellitus (T2D), heart failure (HF), and chronic kidney disease (CKD)."

"It remains unclear whether the efficacy of SGLT2i differs for cardiorenal and mortality endpoints in different underlying diseases."

"We conducted this meta-analysis to assess the relative efficacy of different SGLT2i on cardiorenal outcomes and to assess the impact of the type of underlying disorder (T2D, HF, CKD) on the efficacy of SGLT2i on cardiorenal outcomes."

Methods

"This network meta-analysis was conducted according to the Preferred Reporting Items for Systematic Reviews and Meta-Analyses (PRISMA) extension statement for network meta-analyses [216]."

"The study protocol for this network meta-analysis was published before data extraction began and is available at https://inplasy.com/inplasy-2020-12-0105 ."

"Studies included in this network meta-analysis were randomized controlled trials (RCTs) assessing the efficacy of any SGLT2i treatment versus placebo control or active drug control on cardiorenal outcomes in patients with T2D, HF, or CKD."

"We used hazard ratios (HRs) and 95% confidence intervals (CIs) as reported in the included original studies to perform fixed-effects traditional and network meta-analyses."

"Traditional meta-analysis within the frequentist framework was conducted stratified by type of underlying disorder to assess the effects of underlying disorders on the efficacy of SGLT2i."

"Network meta-analysis within the Bayesian framework was conducted to produce estimators of the relative efficacy of different SGLT2i."

Results

"In terms of the comparisons between active drugs and placebo, compared with placebo, canagliflozin (HR 0.84; 95% CI 0.76–0.93), empagliflozin (HR 0.86; 95% CI 0.74–1.00), and sotagliflozin (HR 0.84; 95% CI 0.72–0.99) significantly reduced MACE; canagliflozin, dapagliflozin, empagliflozin, and ertugliflozin had a neutral effect on the occurrence of MI and stroke; canagliflozin (HR 0.83; 95% CI 0.72–0.97), dapagliflozin (HR 0.88; 95% CI 0.79–0.99), and empagliflozin (HR 0.77; 95% CI 0.67–0.90) significantly reduced CVD; canagliflozin (HR 0.74; 95% CI 0.66–0.84), dapagliflozin (HR 0.78; 95% CI 0.71–0.85), empagliflozin (HR 0.72; 95% CI 0.64–0.80), and sotagliflozin (HR 0.75; 95% CI 0.66–0.85) significantly reduced CVD or HHF; canagliflozin (HR 0.64; 95% CI 0.53–0.77), dapagliflozin (HR 0.70; 95% CI 0.62–0.79), empagliflozin (HR 0.68; 95% CI 0.59–0.78), ertugliflozin (HR 0.70; 95% CI 0.54–0.90), and sotagliflozin (HR 0.66; 95% CI 0.56–0.77) significantly reduced HHF; canagliflozin (HR 0.63; 95% CI 0.54–0.75), dapagliflozin (HR 0.56; 95% CI 0.48–0.64), and empagliflozin (HR 0.53; 95% CI

0.41–0.68) significantly reduced KFP; and canagliflozin (HR 0.85; 95% CI 0.76–0.97), dapagliflozin (HR 0.86; 95% CI 0.79–0.94), and empagliflozin (HR 0.79; 95% CI 0.70–0.90) significantly reduced ACD."

Discussion

"This network meta-analysis is the first study to assess the comparative efficacy of five SGLT2i (canagliflozin, dapagliflozin, empagliflozin, ertugliflozin, and sotagliflozin) on the cardiorenal outcomes MACE, MI, stroke, CVD, CVD or HHF, HHF, KFP, and ACD."

"Compared with placebo, incorporating an SGLT2i significantly reduced MACE and MI but did not significantly reduce stroke in patients with T2D, whereas incorporating SGLT2i significantly reduced CVD, CVD or HHF, HHF, KFP, and ACD regardless of the type of underlying disorder (T2D, HF, CKD)."

"These published network meta-analyses [217–222] did not evaluate the impact of type of underlying disease on the efficacy of SGLT2i, whereas our network meta-analysis revealed that type of underlying disease (T2D, HF, CKD) had no significant effects on the efficacy of SGLT2i on CVD, CVD or HHF, HHF, KFP, and ACD."

Conclusion

"When compared with placebo, all five of the assessed SGLT2i (i.e., canagliflozin, dapagliflozin, empagliflozin, ertugliflozin, and sotagliflozin) reduced HHF, but none reduced MI and stroke."

"Canagliflozin and empagliflozin versus placebo reduced MACE, CVD, CVD or HHF, HHF, KFP and ACD; dapagliflozin and sotagliflozin reduced some of them; and ertugliflozin only reduced HHF."

"Compared with ertugliflozin, empagliflozin reduced CVD or HHF and KFP, and dapagliflozin reduced KFP."

Redox-Driven Cardioprotective Effects of Sodium-Glucose Co-transporter-2 Inhibitors: Comparative Review [223]

This is a machine-generated summary of:

Hoehlschen, Julia; Hofreither, Dominik; Tomin, Tamara; Birner-Gruenberger, Ruth: Redox-driven cardioprotective effects of sodium-glucose co-transporter-2 inhibitors: comparative review [223].

Published in: Cardiovascular Diabetology (2023).

Link to original: https://doi.org/10.1186/s12933-023-01822-7

Copyright of the summarized publication:

If you want to cite the papers, please refer to the original.

For technical reasons we could not place the page where the original quote is coming from.

Abstract-Summary "Sodium-glucose co-transporter-2 inhibitors are used in the treatment of diabetes but are also emerging as cardioprotective agents in heart diseases even in the absence of type 2 diabetes."

"Upon providing a short overview of common pathophysiological features of diabetes, we review the clinically reported cardio- and nephroprotective potential of sodium-glucose co-transporter-2 inhibitors currently available on the market, including Dapagliflozin, Canagliflozin, and Empagliflozin."

Introduction

"Reduction of blood glucose has been shown to improve microvascular complications such as nephron- and neuropathy, but to be insufficient to prevent the death from cardiovascular events, the most relevant macrovascular complication of type 2 diabetes [224]."

"One such emerging drug class are sodium-glucose co-transporter-2 (SGLT-2) inhibitors, a relatively novel anti-diabetic medication."

"In diabetes, the renal transport maximum for glucose can be increased by inducing tubular growth or raising the expression of SGLT-1 and 2, contributing to the state of hyperglycemia [225, 226]."

"It has become increasingly recognized that SGLT-2 inhibitors exhibit tissue-protective effects beyond their systematic, glucose-lowering properties."

"We summarize the clinically reported organ-protective potential of SGLT-2 inhibitors currently available on the market, before specifically focusing on their cardioprotective, antioxidative properties, a trait that will most likely propel this drug class from curative to preventive care."

Renal Complications Related to Diabetes and Proposed Protective Mechanisms of Gliflozins

"Attempting to cope with hyperglycemia, diabetic patients struggle with renal hyperfiltration (manifested by an increased glomerular filtration rate (GFR)) which results from high glomerular pressure and increased sodium and glucose reabsorption via SGLT-1 and 2."

"The diabetes-driven boost in Na^+ reabsorption in the proximal tubule, causes a decreased Na^+ delivery to the macula densa leading to a reduced tubuloglomerular feedback (TGF), accompanied by increasing filtration rates [227]."

"When inhibiting this process by SGLT-2 inhibitors, sodium delivery to the macula densa is enabled and hyperfiltration rates are reduced [73]."

"Upon SGLT-2 inhibition, the highly increased sodium cannot be sufficiently cleared by the Na^+/K^+ ATPases of macula cells, resulting in an osmotic gradient leading to macula cell swelling and leakage of adenosine triphosphate (ATP) from the basolateral membrane, which is extracellularly converted to adenosine."

"Studies in diabetic mice as well as isolated kidney cells have demonstrated the ability of Empagliflozin to reprogram renal metabolism and to improve mitochondrial function and antioxidative defense [228, 229]."

Cardiovascular Complications Related to Diabetes: Focus on Oxidative Stress

"To preserve homeostasis and contractile function in response to stress, the heart offers compensation strategies, including cell growth as well as increase in angiogenesis, energy efficiency, autophagy, and antioxidant generation [230, 231]."

"Essential, these adaptive processes might result in fibrosis, altered sarcomere structure, impaired Ca^{2+} handling, induction of fetal gene programming, mitochondrial dysfunction, disbalance in reactive oxygen species (ROS), metabolic remodeling and cell death, potentially leading to progressive HF in the long term [230–234]."

"The adaptive increase in glycolysis may not be matched in glucose oxidation and lead to an uncoupling between substrate uptake and oxidation, further impairing cellular metabolic function and redox homeostasis [231, 233, 235, 236]."

"In the failing heart, oxidative stress is not only linked to dysregulated cardiac metabolism but also to systemic factors such as diabetes, metabolic syndrome and ageing [237, 238]."

"Restoring metabolic capability, mitochondrial function, and, ultimately, energy output in (diabetic) HF may be essential to ameliorate its progression and facilitate treatment [239, 240]."

Cardioprotective Effects of SGLT-2 Inhibitors from Clinical Trials

"The aim of the EMPA-REG Outcome™ trial [241] was to determine long-term effects of Empagliflozin on cardiovascular safety in type 2 diabetes patients (≥18 years) with a high risk of cardiovascular events as well as its cardioprotective effects."

"Patients suffering from type 2 diabetes, having a glycated hemoglobin value (HbA_{1c}) in a certain range and established cardiovascular diseases were randomly divided into three groups (1:1:1) receiving Empagliflozin (10 mg or 25 mg) or placebo once daily."

"Similar results in terms of positive cardiovascular effects were obtained in a long-term study on Canagliflozin (CANVAS) in which 10,142 patients suffering from type 2 diabetes were included and randomized to receive Canagliflozin (100 mg or 300 mg) or placebo (1:1:1) [29]."

"In 2019 and 2020, two studies were published, investigating whether the positive cardiovascular effects of Dapagliflozin and Empagliflozin would be restricted to type 2 diabetes patients."

Potential Cardioprotective Mechanisms of SGLT-2 Inhibitors beyond Systemic Effects

"Treatment of cardiomyocytes from healthy rats and rabbits cultivated in medium containing 5 mM or 10 mM glucose supplemented with Empagliflozin (1 μM) reduced cytoplasmic concentrations of Na^+ and Ca^{2+} and increased mitochondrial Ca^{2+} concentrations, reversing the negative effects of increased glucose concentrations [139]."

"Treatment of these animal cells with Empagliflozin followed by subsequently NHE inhibitor Cariporide only minimally affected the change in cytoplasmic Na^+ concentration chosen as indicator for NHE inhibition [139]."

"In silico docking studies on the extracellular Na^+ binding site of NHE proved high binding affinity for all three inhibitors (−34.3 kJ/mol Empagliflozin, −32.2 kJ/mol Dapagliflozin, −37.2 kJ/mol Canagliflozin) compared to negative control glucose (−24.3 kJ/mol) [242]."

"To Canagliflozin, which significantly activated AMPK in HEK293 cells and murine hepatocytes already at concentrations similar to those in human plasma when treated with the drug, Empa- and Dapagliflozin showed weaker effects even at higher therapeutic doses [243]."

SGLT-2 Inhibitors and Oxidative Stress

"Markers of oxidative stress (lipid hydroperoxide, glutathione peroxidase (GSH-Px), superoxide dismutase (SOD) and malondialdehyde (MDA)) were also investigated in tissue from diabetic mouse hearts treated and not treated with Empagliflozin."

"Their levels were found to be significantly higher (lipid hydroperoxide, MDA) or lower (SOD, GSH-Px) in diabetic untreated mice compared to Empagliflozin treated ones [244]."

"fibrosis and membrane thickening was further confirmed by treating diabetic cardiac microvascular endothelial cells (CMEC) with Empagliflozin."

"Diabetes induced mitochondrial fission was also prevented by Empagliflozin, which brought the ratio of AMP:ATP closer to the one observed in control cells, leading to the activation of AMPK [245]."

"A study in non-diabetic failing pig hearts also showed that Empagliflozin positively influenced cardiac metabolism typically found in failing hearts by diverting ATP production to beta oxidation and ketogenesis, decreasing the consumption of carbohydrates and thereby approaching the conditions found in healthy hearts [246]."

Conclusion

"Some of the clinical studies also searched for protein biomarkers in the blood which could tell us more regarding the underlying effects of the drugs."

"In case of the EMPEROR study (Empagliflozin), comparing samples taken right before the treatment's start (baseline), after 12 weeks and 52 weeks of treatment, showed no significant differences in protein expression between the two timepoints during the treatment, hinting that the effect of Empagliflozin is time-independent."

"A small group of intracellular proteins involved in autophagic flux, weakening of oxidative stress and inflammation processes in the heart as well as promotion of repair and regeneration in heart and kidney were found to be differentially expressed upon treatment with Empagliflozin [247]."

"Both in vitro and in vivo studies agree in one thing: SGLT-2 inhibitors are able to protect our heart independent of their glucose lowering effects."

Dose-Dependent Renoprotection Efficacy of sglt2 Inhibitors in Type 2 Diabetes: Systematic Review and Network Meta-Analysis [248]

This is a machine-generated summary of:

Hegde, Naveen C.; Kumar, Ankit; Patil, Amol N.; Bhattacharjee, Samiksha; Gamad, Nanda; Kasudhan, Kripa Shanker; Kumar, Vivek; Rastogi, Ashu: Dose-dependent renoprotection efficacy of sglt2 inhibitors in type 2 diabetes: systematic review and network meta-analysis [248].

Published in: Acta Diabetologica (2023).

Link to original: https://doi.org/10.1007/s00592-023-02126-8

Copyright of the summarized publication:

If you want to cite the papers, please refer to the original.

For technical reasons we could not place the page where the original quote is coming from.

Abstract-Summary "The study searched different databases (PubMed, Embase, Scopus, and Web of Science) for studies comparing dose-dependent renoprotective efficacy defined as a decline in eGFR with the different "-flozins namely Empagliflozin, Canagliflozin, Dapagliflozin, Ertugliflozin, Ipragliflozin, Luseogliflozin, Remogliflozin and Sotagliflozin."

"The studies were compared with the Bayesian approach of network meta-analysis coupled with the random-effect model using the Cochrane risk of bias tool (RoB 2.0), and the surface under the cumulative ranking curve (SUCRA) score was allotted to each dosage of different SGLT-2i."

"A total of 43,434 citations were identified, out of which forty-five randomized trials with 48,067 patients, mentioning the flozin dose and eGFR as an endpoint, were found to be eligible for further analysis."

"Canagliflozin 100 mg demonstrated distinct eGFR benefit with an odds ratio of 2.3 (CI 0.72–3.9) compared to placebo."

"Canagliflozin 100 mg drug dose category showed the highest sucra rank probability score of 93%, followed by the Canagliflozin 300 mg and Dapagliflozin 5 mg with sucra rank probability scores of 69% and 65%, respectively."

"The Flozin-dose assessment against eGFR was similar to the albumin-creatinine ratios as the secondary endpoint in the SUCRA ranking."

Introduction

"SGLT2i have also shown a significant decrease in primary renal outcomes such as urine albumin-to-creatinine ratio, eGFR decline, risk of microalbuminuria, macroalbuminuria, and worsening nephropathy [249]."

"The antidiabetic efficacy of SGLT2i is dose-dependent, with an exponentially greater reduction in fasting plasma glucose and HbA1c at higher doses."

"It is observed that higher doses of SGLT2i are associated with more body weight and blood pressure reduction than the lower doses."

"Different RCTs have used varied parameters for assessing renal outcomes with SGLT2i, including a composite of doubling of creatinine, sustained decline in eGFR, and renal death or effect on albuminuria or end-stage kidney disease (ESKD) or others."

"No meta-analysis exists for the dose-dependent renal effects evaluation of various SGLT2i."

"We contemplated the present systematic review and network meta-analysis to synthesize evidence for a dose-related renal effect on the decline in eGFR and albuminuria with SGLTi, if any."

Methods

"Search efforts were made for the randomized controlled trials (RCTs) evaluating the presence or absence of the renal effect with the different dosages of the SGLT2i."

"The secondary study endpoints were the mean change in albumin creatinine ratio, measured similarly between pre- and post-flozin therapy."

"The study included only English language RCTs comparing different dosages of all flozins against placebo."

"We excluded studies reporting comparators as the standard of care other than placebo, e.g., sulfonylureas, single-arm studies, studies recruiting healthy volunteers or type 1 diabetes, studies reporting pooled analysis, unrelated studies, duplicate studies, studies either showing class effect or non-dose-dependent effect against placebo, observational studies, non-diabetic kidney disease, studies reporting eGFR in percent change format or qualitative data format using major adverse kidney event (MAKE) definition cut off for eGFR, narrative reviews, case reports/series, letter to the editor, and systematic reviews."

Results

"Search efforts for RCTs and eGFR outcome evaluation for Empagliflozin, Canagliflozin, Dapagliflozin, Sotagliflozin, Remogliflozin, Ipragliflozin, Ertugliflozin, Luseogliflozin showed 10,580, 10,208, 13,397, 1042, 433, 1794, 1583, and 1163 RCTs, respectively."

"Dapagliflozin was studied in the largest number of patients (n = 20,625), followed by Empagliflozin (n = 13,522), and only one study of sotagliflozin (n = 277) could be included."

"Sotagliflozin 200 mg, Sotagliflozin 400 mg, Dapagliflozin 2.5 mg, Ertugliflozin 5 mg, Ipragliflozin 50 mg, and Ertugliflozin 15 mg showed SUCRA scores of 44.1, 44, 34.5, 28.1, 22.6, and 18.6%, respectively, i.e., less than the placebo (46.8%)."

"Canagliflozin, Dapagliflozin, and empagliflozin showed similar renoprotection efficacy as compared to placebo, highest again for Canagliflozin 100 mg with a SUCRA score of 68.3%."

Discussion

"We report no dose-dependent difference in renal benefits in the present study, specifically looking at eGFR change from baseline with SGLT2i and similarly for albuminuria."

"There were no limits on specific doses of SGLT2i used in these studies, and the renal effects were presented as a combined effect of varied dosages [250–252]."

"No statistically significant renal benefit could be appreciated with higher doses of SGLT2i like 300 mg canagliflozin, 25 mg empagliflozin, or 10 mg dapagliflozin compared to the lower doses."

"The difference in renal benefits in our study could be due to the inclusion of RCTs that utilized various doses of SGLT2i, which are much less than clinically recommended dosages, like some studies with 2.5 mg of dapagliflozin."

"The renal benefits of SGLT2i are attributed as a class effect, the efficacy of certain gliflozins like remogliflozin and ertugliflozin has not been studied explicitly for renal outcomes."

Review of SGLT2i for the Treatment of Renal Complications: Experience in Patients with and Without T2D [253]

This is a machine-generated summary of:

González-Albarrán, Olga; Morales, Cristóbal; Pérez-Maraver, Manuel; Aparicio-Sánchez, José Juan; Simó, Rafael: Review of SGLT2i for the Treatment of Renal Complications: Experience in Patients with and Without T2D [253].

Published in: Diabetes Therapy (2022).

Link to original: https://doi.org/10.1007/s13300-022-01276-2

If you want to cite the papers, please refer to the original.

For technical reasons we could not place the page where the original quote is coming from.

Abstract-Summary "Diabetic kidney disease (DKD), defined as presence of albuminuria, impaired glomerular filtration, or both, is an insidious microvascular complication of diabetes that generates a substantial personal and clinical burden."

"Sodium–glucose cotransporter type 2 inhibitors (SGLT2i) reduce blood glucose concentrations by blocking the uptake of sodium and glucose in the proximal tubule and promoting glycosuria, and these agents now have an important role in the management of T2D. The results of several cardiovascular outcomes trials suggested that SGLT2i are associated with improvements in renal endpoints in addition to their reduction in cardiovascular events and mortality, which represents a major advance in the care of this population."

"The dedicated kidney outcomes trials have confirmed the renoprotective action of SGLT2i across different glomerular filtration and albuminuria values, even in patients with non-diabetic chronic kidney disease."

"This improvement in kidney function may indirectly benefit cardiac function through multifaceted interorgan cross talk, which can break the cardiorenal vicious circle linked to T2D. In this article, we briefly review the different mechanisms of action that may explain the renal beneficial effects of SGLT2i and disclose the results of the key renal outcome trials and the subsequent update of related clinical guidelines."

Introduction

"The management of type 2 diabetes (T2D) involves decreasing plasma glucose levels and reducing macrovascular and microvascular complications, including chronic kidney disease (CKD)."

"Sodium–glucose cotransporter type 2 inhibitors (SGLT2i) are the newest drug class for the management of hyperglycemia in T2D, as they lower blood glucose concentrations by blocking the uptake of sodium and glucose in the proximal tubule and promote glycosuria [254]."

"These agents were initially approved for use as glucose-lowering drugs for people with T2D and (nearly) preserved kidney function."

"On the basis of the findings of CVOTs, dedicated kidney outcomes trials (such as DAPA-CKD and CREDENCE) have been conducted, confirming the renoprotective benefit of SGLT2i across different glomerular filtration and albuminuria values [33, 34]."

CKD and T2D: Dance Partners in CV Disease

"Diabetic kidney disease (DKD), defined as presence of albuminuria, impaired glomerular filtration, or both, is an insidious microvascular complication of diabetes that develops in approximately 40% of patients with T2D and accounts for more than 50% of new patients beginning renal replacement therapy [255, 256]."

"As per chronic hyperglycemia, a classic study that followed patients with T2D during 11 years demonstrated a strong association between glycemic control and the incidence of CKD, regardless previous traditional risk factors for CKD and even in the absence of albuminuria and retinopathy [257]."

"Patients with DKD seem to concentrate most of the excess of all-cause and cardiovascular mortality risk among patients with T2D, with a sixfold higher risk for mortality associated with albuminuria and 15-fold higher risk with the combination of albuminuria and decreased GFR [153]."

"All this evidence indicates that patients with DKD require exhaustive control of the associated cardiovascular risk factors and that albuminuria may be considered as a relevant target for therapy."

Mechanisms of SGLT2i Effects on Renal Condition

"This stimulates SGLT2 expression and activity leading to an increase in proximal tubular glucose and sodium reabsorption and reduced sodium uptake at the juxtaglomerular macula densa, blunting the tubuloglomerular feedback (TGF), and dysregulating vasoactive substances."

"All these processes enhance preglomerular dilatation, postglomerular constriction, intraglomerular capillary pressure, and finally lead to hyperfiltration [258]."

"SGLT2i can correct TGF/intraglomerular hemodynamics by preventing sodium reabsorption, which partially explains the renoprotective effect of these agents."

Benefits of SGLT2i on Renal Function Beyond Their Glycemic Control

"In the whole patient sample, dapagliflozin treatment was associated with a significantly lower risk (− 47%) of the renal composite of decline in eGFR of ≥40% to less than 60 mL/min/1.73 m^2, ESKD or renal death, compared with placebo [259]."

"A total of 4304 patients with CKD were enrolled, 2906 (68%) of them with T2D. Dapagliflozin demonstrated a clear reduction (− 39% lower risk) in primary composite outcome events (sustained decline in the eGFR of ≥ 50%, ESKD, or death from renal or cardiovascular causes), regardless of the presence of diabetes."

"Regarding other renal outcomes trials with dapagliflozin, the DELIGHT study recruited patients with T2D and impaired renal function (UACR ≥ 30 mg/g and eGFR 25–75 mL/min/1.73 m^2) to assess the albuminuria-lowering effect of dapagliflozin with and without the dipeptidyl peptidase 4 inhibitor saxagliptin."

Current Recommendations for Treatment of Renal Complications with SGLT2i

"The American Diabetes Association (ADA) guidelines state: "For patients with type 2 diabetes and diabetic kidney disease, use of a SGLT2i in patients with an eGFR ≥ 25 mL/min/1.73 m^2 and urinary albumin ≥ 300 mg/g creatinine is recommended to reduce kidney disease progression and cardiovascular events."".

"The European Society of Cardiology, in collaboration with the European Association for the Study of Diabetes, have updated their guidelines to recommend SGLT2i as first-line therapy for the prevention and management of CKD (eGFR 30 to <90 mL/min/1.73 m^2) in patients with T2D and albuminuric kidney disease [260]."

"The Kidney Disease: Improving Global Outcomes (KDIGO) guidelines recommend the use of metformin in combination with SGLT2i (with GFR ≥ 30 mL/min/1.73 m^2) as first-line antihyperglycemic therapy for patients with T2D and CKD."

Changing Paradigm: The Cardiorenal and Metabolic Continuum

"These agents have demonstrated benefits in different clinical scenarios: patients with T2D with and without established cardiovascular disease [28], patients with T2D with CKD [261], patients with CKD with and without T2D [34], patients with heart failure with and without T2D [60], etc. Indeed, the populations included in the trials of dapagliflozin cover a wide range of diabetic patient profiles, going from those in the earlier stages of the cardiorenal continuum (DECLARE-TIMI 58) to those at more advanced stages (DAPA-CKD and DAPA-HF)."

"The diuretic effect facilitates a better management of volume status in patients with heart failure and may contribute to the long-term decrease of heart failure events reported with these agents [262]."

"Some authors have defined the cardiorenal disease in patients with T2D as the development of heart failure and CKD, and suggested a novel outcome, major adverse renal and cardiac events (MARCE), to be evaluated in future clinical trials [263, 264]."

"Patients with T2D suffer multiple comorbid conditions and usually receive several treatments such as antihypertensive agents, diuretics, insulin, or other glucose-lowering medications."

Conclusions

"The dedicated kidney outcomes trials of SGLT2i (such as DAPA-CKD and CREDECE) have confirmed the renoprotective benefit of these drugs across different glomerular filtration rates and albuminuria values."

"SGLT2i can correct TGF/intraglomerular hemodynamics by preventing sodium reabsorption, whereas other mechanisms such as ketone body production, lowering of serum uric acid concentrations, and increasing oxygen supply can contribute to their beneficial effects on cardiovascular outcomes."

"The multidisciplinary team should select the therapeutic strategy on the basis of the target organ of protection and patients' comorbidities and profile, going beyond glycemic control and ensuring that patients are able to benefit from the metabolic, cardiovascular, and kidney protection associated with SGLT2i."

Association of SGLT2 Inhibitors with Cardiovascular, Kidney, and Safety Outcomes Among Patients with Diabetic Kidney Disease: A Meta-Analysis [265]

This is a machine-generated summary of:

Kaze, Arnaud D.; Zhuo, Min; Kim, Seoyoung C.; Patorno, Elisabetta; Paik, Julie M.: Association of SGLT2 inhibitors with cardiovascular, kidney, and safety outcomes among patients with diabetic kidney disease: a meta-analysis [265].

Published in: Cardiovascular Diabetology (2022).

Link to original: https://doi.org/10.1186/s12933-022-01476-x

If you want to cite the papers, please refer to the original.

For technical reasons we could not place the page where the original quote is coming from.

Abstract-Summary "We conducted a systematic review and meta-analysis of the cardiovascular, kidney, and safety outcomes of sodium-glucose cotransporter 2 inhibitors (SGLT2i) among patients with diabetic kidney disease (DKD)."

"We searched electronic databases for major randomized placebo-controlled clinical trials published up to September 30, 2021 and reporting on cardiovascular and kidney outcomes of SGLT2i in patients with DKD."

"Random-effects meta-analysis models were used to estimate pooled hazard ratios (HR) and 95% confidence intervals (CI) for clinical outcomes including major adverse cardiovascular events (MACE: myocardial infarction [MI], stroke, and cardiovascular death), kidney composite outcomes (a combination of worsening kidney function, end-stage kidney disease, or death from renal or cardiovascular causes), hospitalizations for heart failure (HHF), deaths and safety events (mycotic infections, diabetic ketoacidosis [DKA], volume depletion, amputations, fractures, urinary tract infections [UTI], acute kidney injury [AKI], and hyperkalemia)."

"SGLT2i were associated with reduced risks of MACE (HR 0.83, 95% CI 0.75–0.93), kidney composite outcomes (HR 0.66, 95% CI 0.58–0.75), HHF (HR 0.62, 95% CI 0.55–0.71), cardiovascular death (HR 0.84, 95% CI 0.74–0.96), MI (HR 0.78, 95% CI 0.67–0.92), stroke (HR 0.76, 95% CI 0.59–0.97), and all-cause death (HR 0.86, 95% CI 0.77–0.96), with no significant heterogeneity detected."

"Among adults with DKD, SGLT2i were associated with reduced risks of MACE, kidney outcomes, HHF, and death."

"With a few exceptions of more clear safety signals, we found overall limited data on the associations between SGLT2i and safety outcomes."

Background

"Nearly 40% of patients with T2D develop DKD [63]."

"Sodium-glucose cotransporter 2 inhibitors (SGLT2i) have recently emerged as a new class of oral glucose-lowering agents with pleiotropic effects including reduction in cardiovascular and kidney outcomes among patients with T2D [27–30, 33, 34]."

"SGLT2i prescriptions have steadily increased among patients with DKD [266]."

"We performed a systematic review and meta-analysis of the major cardiovascular and kidney outcomes trials to summarize and update the currently available evidence on the effects of SGLT2i on cardiovascular, kidney and safety outcomes among patients with DKD."

Methods

"We conducted a comprehensive search of PubMed and Embase for major randomized, placebo-controlled clinical trials of SGLT2i published up to September 30, 2021 and reporting on cardiovascular and kidney outcomes as well as adverse events among adults with DKD."

"Studies were considered eligible if they met all of the following criteria: (1) the study design was a randomized controlled trial (RCT) of cardiovascular or kidney outcomes of SGLT2i; (2) the study reported on cardiovascular, kidney, or adverse events of SGLT2i among individuals with DKD; (3) the hazard ratio (HR) or relative risk (RR) and its corresponding 95% confidence interval (CI) or enough data to calculate them were reported."

"For each outcome, we sought to identify HRs and 95%CIs of the effects of SGLT2i in participants with DKD from individual studies."

Results

"Among participants with severely increased albuminuria, SGLT2i were associated with reduced risks of MACE (HR 0.73, 95% CI 0.65–0.83, $I^2 = 0.0\%$, P for heterogeneity = 0.444, n = 9,216), HHF (HR 0.62, 95% CI 0.51–0.75, $I^2 = 0.0\%$, P for heterogeneity = 0.915, n = 6,685), cardiovascular death (HR 0.72, 95% CI 0.59–0.87, $I^2 = 0.0\%$, P for heterogeneity = 0.408, n = 5,930), all-cause mortality (HR 0.77, 95% CI 0.65–0.90, $I^2 = 0.0\%$, P for heterogeneity = 0.415, n = 5,930), and kidney composite outcomes (HR 0.63, 95% CI 0.53–0.76, $I^2 = 0.8\%$, P for heterogeneity = 0.365, n = 8,447)."

Discussion

"We chose a random-effects meta-analysis approach as opposed to fixed-effects models used in prior meta-analyses [267, 268], due to the heterogeneity of patient populations included across the clinical trials of SGLT2i."

"Our observation of a beneficial effect of SGLT2i on HHF in patients with DKD is consistent with prior published meta-analyses of individuals with T2D [57, 268]."

"A recent meta-analysis of the effect of SGLT2i on the risk of stroke in patients with DKD observed a null association using the random-effects models, likely due to low statistical power [269]."

"The included SGLT2i trials did not always report the effect estimates for all the relevant outcomes specifically among participants with DKD (for example, the trials did not always report on individual kidney outcomes such as ESKD that would have been defined more consistently across trials); and we did not have access to individual participant data that could have been used to calculate the effect estimates for the unreported outcomes or perform meta-regression analyses."

Conclusions

"Our findings confirm the beneficial effects of the SGLT2i class on cardiovascular and kidney outcomes, as well as mortality in patients with T2D and DKD."

"Our data support the current recommendations to prioritize the prescriptions of SGLT2i in patients with DKD, independent of glycemic control [270]."

"Further research is warranted to explore the effects of SGLT2i in patients with advanced DKD and to better characterize the safety profile of SGLT2i in patients with DKD."

Sodium–Glucose Transporter-2 Inhibitors for Prevention and Treatment of Cardiorenal Complications of Type 2 Diabetes [271]

This is a machine-generated summary of:

Giugliano, Dario; Longo, Miriam; Scappaticcio, Lorenzo; Caruso, Paola; Esposito, Katherine: Sodium–glucose transporter-2 inhibitors for prevention and treatment of cardiorenal complications of type 2 diabetes [271].

Published in: Cardiovascular Diabetology (2021).

Link to original: https://doi.org/10.1186/s12933-021-01213-w

Abstract-Summary "Hospitalization for major diabetes complications, including myocardial infarction, stroke, lower-extremity amputation, and end-stage kidney disease, is on the rise and represents a great health burden for patients with type 2 diabetes (T2D), in particular for older people."

Introduction

"In the first half of the past decade, hospitalization for major diabetes complications, including myocardial infarction (MI), stroke, lower-extremity amputation, and end-stage kidney disease (ESKD), has increased substantially, subtracting much of the benefits obtained during the years between 1990 and 2010 [272]."

"The future of diabetes care may be darkened by this apparent resurgence of vascular complications, as well as by the evidence that heart failure (HF), once a neglected complication, may be as common as coronary heart disease in patients with T2D [273, 274]."

"These US data are consistent with both Swedish [275] and UK [276] data indicating that patients with T2D who obtained the control of five variables to optimal values (hemoglobin A1c [A1C], total cholesterol or LDL-cholesterol, blood pressure, absence of albuminuria or triglycerides, and abstinence from smoking) were at higher risk (31 to 45% higher risk) of hospitalization for HF."

"The natural history of HF in T2D seems to be unaffected by the optimal control of major metabolic and cardiovascular (CV) risk factors."

Glycemic Control Is Not Enough

"Only 9% of the risk of MACE (major adverse cardiovascular events) is eliminated after achievement of the best possible glycemic control in patients with T2D and the risk of HF is not influenced at all [273]."

"Among adults with T2D and pre-existing CVD, there is no difference in the risk of CV events in those allocated to intensive glucose control compared with those in the standard care arm (hazard ratio = 0.98, 95% confidence interval, 0.87–1.09) [277]."

"Paradoxically, tight glycemic control is ineffective on CV risk in those T2D patients who are at their maximum risk for future CV events."

"The contrast can only be apparent, as the CV risk in T2D can only be cleared off by the simultaneous control of the multiple factors at play, including glucose, lipids, blood pressure, albuminuria, and smoking."

SGLT-2 Inhibitors

"Sodium-glucose cotransporter 2 inhibitors (SGLT-2i) are a new class of orally active drugs approved for the management of T2D [254]."

"Inhibition of glucose reabsorption at the level of the proximal tubule results in enhanced glycosuria, osmotic diuresis and natriuresis, thereby improving glucose control, with a limited risk of hypoglycemia."

"Gordon and others [278] used the real-world data from 33,849 patients with T2D in UK and found that antihyperglycemic drugs associated with weight loss and lower incidence of hypoglycemia were generally associated with better medication adherence, which in turn was related to improved glycemic control."

"Medication non-adherence may also contribute for up to 75% to the gap between clinical efficacy from randomized controlled trials and real world results in lowering A1C levels [279, 280]."

Cardiorenal Effects

"We did a random effect meta-analysis including all the nine trials that evaluated the effect of the five SGLT-2i (empagliflozin, canagliflozin, dapagliflozin, ertugliflozin, sotagliflozin) in 67,190 patients with or without T2D, and with or without HF at baseline, on hospitalization for HF."

"An indirect support for this estimate comes from the results of the DAPA-CKD trial [34] evaluating 4304 patients with or without T2D, and with CKD randomized to dapagliflozin or placebo and followed for a median period of 2.4 years: the hazard ratio for the composite endpoint of CV death and hospitalization for HF was 0.71 (95% CI 0.55–0.92), but that for HF alone, although not presented in the results, should even be lower, as the HR for CV death alone was 0.81 (0.58–1.12)."

"Both SCORED [32] and SOLOIST-WHF [215] trials included a percentage of diabetic patients with HF and preserved ejection fraction (left ventricular ejection fraction of at least 50%); both trials found that sotagliflozin was effective in reducing hospitalization for HF, which may remove some hesitation to use SGLT-2i in T2D patients with HF and preserved ejection fraction."

The Effect of Age

"The post-hoc analysis of both EMPA-REG [281] and DECLARE [282] trials confirms that the efficacy/safety profile of these two SGLT-2i is unchanged by age, even with some signal of greater efficacy in patients older than 65 years of age."

"A significant interaction ($P = 0.01$) was reported in EMPA-REG trial [281] regarding the primary cardiovascular composite end point with better results in patients with T2D aged ≥ 65 years versus < 65 years."

"In the SCORED trial [32] with sotagliflozin, the primary efficacy endpoint of total occurrences of cardiovascular deaths, HF hospitalizations, and urgent visits for HF was not significantly different in the 3224 (30.5%) patients aged < 65 years (HR = 0.60, 95% CI 0.43–0.83) vs the 7360 (69.5%) patients aged ≥ 65 years (HR = 0.79, 0.66–0.95)."

Class Effect of SGLT-2i

"SGLT-2i are considered a class as they share a similar chemical structure derived from the ancestor phlorizin, a similar mechanism of action related to the inhibition of SGLT-2 located on the luminal membrane of proximal tubular cells (brush border), and similar pharmacological effects at the level of kidney, resulting in glycosuria and osmotic diuresis."

"For MACE, there seems to be no class effect, as both DECLARE and VERTIS-CV failed to reduce it significantly: on the other hand, a class effect is evident for hospitalization for HF, which at present remains the more striking therapeutic effect of SGLT-2i."

"Both VERTIS-CV and SCORED trials were unable to show any significant effect on DKD progression, a renal composite outcome of death from renal causes, kidney replacement therapy, or doubling of the serum creatinine level."

"Although comparison between trials should always be done with caution, the five trials are generally consistent with each other, showing reliable cardiorenal benefits (with the exception of VERTIS-CV and SCORED for DKD progression) and comparable expected adverse effects."

Primary vs Secondary Prevention

"The definition of secondary prevention usually refers to patients who suffered a previous acute ischemic event, whereas all other patients are categorized as requiring primary prevention."

"The CVOTs used to distinguish T2D patients with established CVD (secondary prevention), that is, those having experienced a previous event or with evidence of more than 50% stenosis in an epicardial coronary artery, and patients without established CVD (primary prevention), i.e. those with many risk factors for CVD."

"Definitions of established CVD varied across trials; although most patients had experienced a previous event at the level of coronary, cerebral or peripheral arteries, patients without events, but with clinical or instrumental evidence of the presence of CVD, were also included."

"Both EMPA-REG and VERTIS-CV trials included patients in secondary prevention only, and therefore an estimate of their effect in primary prevention of T2D is at present not possible."

What's the Road Ahead?

"The accumulated evidence suggests that SGLT-2i should be considered for control of hyperglycemia in patients with T2D, particularly in those with established CVD, given that they reduce the risk of MACE, hospitalization for HF and progression of DKD, regardless of whether patients are receiving or not metformin [283]."

"The results of post-hoc analyses [281, 282] or real-world databases [121] are reassuring about both the efficacy and safety of SGLT-2i in older patients with T2D, for whom the choice of the optimal drug is often limited by subjective (health state of patient) and objective (side effects of the antihyperglycemic drug) considerations."

"SGLT-2is can be used as an add-on therapy in selected and healthy older patients with T2D, especially those who are overweight and have uncontrolled hypertension."

"In a multinational observational study [284] including 1,006,577 new users of SGLT-2i or dipeptidyl peptidase-4 inhibitors (DPP-4i), the use of SGLT-2i was associated with a lower risk of HF and CKD versus DPP-4i in patients with T2D otherwise free from both cardiovascular and renal disease."

Balancing Benefits and Harms

"SGLT-2i have also been associated with a variety of adverse effects [285], inducing both the FDA and EMA to publish specific warnings regarding an increased risk of lower-limb amputation, diabetic ketoacidosis, bone fracture, acute renal injury and Fournier gangrene."

"A recent meta-analysis [286] of six trials (EMPA-REG, CANVAS, CREDENCE, DECLARE, DAPA-HF, VERTIS-CV) show that SGLT-2i were not significantly associated with an increased risk of amputation, including subgroups with or without established peripheral artery disease."

"The results of a large population-based cohort study [287] indicate that use of SGLT-2i is not associated with an overall increased risk of breast cancer compared with DPP-4 inhibitors, at least in the short term (median follow-up 2.6 years)."

Conclusions

"The cardiorenal benefits demonstrated by SGLT-2i are not only limited to patients with T2D, as a mounting evidence indicates that they can also be extended to patients without T2D who have CVD, HF, or CKD [27–30, 33, 34, 57, 59, 60, 63, 73, 139, 153, 216–222, 224–247, 249–252, 254–264, 266–270, 272–288]."

"The use of these agents will presumably be extended to other medical figures that cooperate in the management of T2D, including cardiologists and nephrologists, within the frame of a multidisciplinary approach, with the paramount aim to improve glycemic control and reduce the risk of cardiorenal events."

"It is sad to acknowledge that, despite the continuing accumulation of data regarding the benefits of SGLT-2i which are incorporated in newly updated guidelines, many eligible patients with T2D are still not receiving these agents, depriving them of protection against the progression of avoidable cardiorenal complications [289]."

Cardiorenal and Other Diabetes Related Outcomes with SGLT-2 Inhibitors Compared to GLP-1 Receptor Agonists in Type 2 Diabetes: Nationwide Observational Study [290]

This is a machine-generated summary of:

Lugner, Moa; Sattar, Naveed; Miftaraj, Mervete; Ekelund, Jan; Franzén, Stefan; Svensson, Ann-Marie; Eliasson, Björn: Cardiorenal and other diabetes related outcomes with SGLT-2 inhibitors compared to GLP-1 receptor agonists in type 2 diabetes: nationwide observational study [290].

Published in: Cardiovascular Diabetology (2021).

Link to original: https://doi.org/10.1186/s12933-021-01258-x

If you want to cite the papers, please refer to the original.

For technical reasons we could not place the page where the original quote is coming from.

Abstract-Summary "Major prospective randomized clinical safety trials have demonstrated beneficial effects of treatment with glucagon-like peptide-1 receptor agonists (GLP-1RA) and sodium–glucose co-transporter-2 inhibitors (SGLT-2i) in people with type 2 diabetes and elevated cardiovascular risk, and recent clinical treatment guidelines therefore promote early use of these classes of pharmacological agents."

"In this Swedish nationwide observational study, we compared cardiorenal outcomes and safety of new treatment with GLP-1RA and SGLT-2i in people with type 2 diabetes."

"The proportion of patients with a history of MACE were 15.8%, and 17.0% in patients treated with GLP-1RA and SGLT-2i, respectively."

"Mean HbA1c were 8.3% (67.6 mmol/mol) and 8.3% (67.2 mmol/mol), and mean BMI 33.3 and 32.5 kg/m^2 in patients treated with GLP-1RA or SGLT-2i, respectively."

"The risks of stroke and peripheral artery disease were higher in the SGLT-2i group relative to GLP-1RA, with HR 1.44 (95% CI 0.99–2.08) and 1.68 (95% CI 1.04–2.72), respectively."

"This observational study suggests that treatment with GLP-1RA and SGLT-2i result in very similar cardiorenal outcomes."

"In the short term, treatment with GLP-1RA seem to be associated with lower risks of stroke and peripheral artery disease, whereas SGLT-2i seem to be nominally associated with lower risk of heart failure and total mortality."

Background

"Major prospective randomized clinical safety trials have demonstrated beneficial effects of treatment with glucagon-like peptide-1 receptor agonists (GLP-1RA) and sodium–glucose co-transporter-2 inhibitors (SGLT-2i) in people with type 2 diabetes and elevated cardiovascular risk [120, 291]."

"The 2018 American Diabetes Association (ADA) and European Association for the Study of Diabetes (EASD) consensus report stated that patients with type 2 diabetes and established atherosclerotic cardiovascular disease (ASCVD) should use GLP-1RA or SGLT-2i as part of glycaemic management [292]."

"The updated version of the consensus report declares that in high-risk individuals with type 2 diabetes, the decision to treat with a GLP-1RA or SGLT-2i should be considered independently of baseline HbA1c, as the cardiovascular benefits of these drugs are independent of HbA1c."

"GLP-1RA is recommended in patients with type 2 diabetes and established ASCVD where major cardiovascular events (MACE) are considered the greatest threat, and in patients with indicators of high risk without established CVD, to reduce the risk of MACE."

Materials and Methods

"The clinical effects of the treatments as well as severe adverse events were captured using NDR, the national patient registry and the cause of death registry."

"The NDR is estimated to include almost 90% of all patients with type 2 diabetes aged $\geq$ 18 years in Sweden."

"Information on pre-existing comorbidities (hospitalizations from 1997 to index date), and conditions occurring during the study period, including severe hypoglycaemia and hyperglycaemia and carry data such as date of contact, diagnostic codes, and procedure codes, were obtained from the national patient register."

"To compare the effects in the two treatment groups, we used a propensity score adjusted analysis using inverse probability of treatment weighting (IPTW) to estimate the average treatment effect for everyone (ATE)."

Results

"The cumulative mortality risk was non-significantly lower in the group treated with SGLT-2i, HR 0.78 (95% CI 0.61–1.01)."

"The risks of HF and severe hypoglycemia were non-significantly lower in the group treated with SGLT-2i, HR 0.83 (95% CI 0.65–1.07) and 0.69 (95% CI 0.21–2.28), respectively."

"The risks of stroke and peripheral artery disease (PAD) were higher in the group treated with SGLT2-i relative to the group treated with GLP1-RA, HR 1.44 (95% CI 0.99–2.08) and 1.68 (95% CI 1.04–2.72), respectively."

"Patients treated with GLP-1RA had significantly lower risk of stroke in the group without established CVD compared to SGLT-2i, HR 1.73 (95% CI 1.11–2.68), as well as in the group without pre-existing cardiorenal disease, HR 2.08 (95% CI 1.21–3.58)."

Discussion

"Recent major cardiovascular outcome trials have shown quite comparable effects for these two classes of drugs in patients with type 2 diabetes with established cardiovascular disease or multiple risk factors, although hinting at better cardiorenal outcomes in the SGLT-2i class and more consistent atherothrombosis for the GLP-1RA class [29, 120, 291]."

"It did strongly hint at better potential and quite rapid effects of GLP-1RA on stroke and PAD, whereas total mortality and HF point estimates were lower for the SGLT-2i class, as they were for some renal outcomes."

"Although the differences were small between the groups in the present study, a recent meta-analysis has shown that GLP-1RA might be somewhat more effective reducing HbA1c than SGLT-2i [293]."

"This area needs to be examined in more detail, results suggest that co-treatment with SGLT-2i and GLP-1RA might attain beneficial effects on cardiovascular endpoints as well as on glycemic control and seems to be well tolerated by patients [294, 295]."

Conclusions

"The results of this observational pharmacoepidemiological study suggests that GLP-1RA and SGLT-2i are very similar with respect to risks of several major cardiovascular outcomes, such as MACE, acute myocardial infarction, and fatal CVD."

"Treatment with GLP-1RA seems to be associated with lower risks of PAD and stroke (including in those without prior ASCVD), whereas there is some hint of lower HF and total mortality in the short term in those prescribed SGLT-2i's."

"In the absence of dedicated head-to-head clinic trials, these results might provide further guidance for clinicians choosing between the two classes of drugs in patients with type 2 diabetes."

SGLT2 Inhibitors: Benefits for CKD and Cardiovascular Disease in Type 2 Diabetes [296]

This is a machine-generated summary of:

Singhal, Rohit; Hechanova, Lisa Aimee: SGLT2 Inhibitors: Benefits for CKD and Cardiovascular Disease in Type 2 Diabetes [296].

Published in: Current Cardiology Reports (2022).

Link to original: https://doi.org/10.1007/s11886-022-01637-0

If you want to cite the papers, please refer to the original.
For technical reasons we could not place the page where the original quote is coming from.

Abstract-Summary "The purpose of this review is to outline the key findings of the recent major outcome clinical trials on SGLT2 inhibitors, review the indications for their use, and improve adoption of these medications in patients with type 2 diabetes mellitus (T2DM)."

"Recent studies have shown a benefit for SGLT2 inhibitors in patients with heart failure (HF) and kidney disease both in the presence and absence of T2DM."

"Available data suggests that SGLT2 inhibitors should be used in all eligible patients with HFrEF and/or CKD with albuminuria to decrease progression of CKD, hospitalizations for heart failure, major atherosclerotic cardiovascular events, and cardiovascular death, with and without T2DM".

Introduction

"In patients with prevalent kidney disease at baseline, empagliflozin reduced the risk of cardiovascular death by 29% compared with placebo (HR, 0.71; 95% CI, 0.52–0.98), the risk of all-cause mortality by 24% (HR, 0.76; 95% CI, 0.59–0.99), the risk of hospitalization for heart failure by 39% (HR, 0.61; 95% CI, 0.42–0.87), and the risk of all-cause hospitalization by 19% (HR, 0.81; 95% CI, 0.72–0.92) [33] The reductions in risk of 3-point MACE, cardiovascular death, all-cause mortality, hospitalization for heart failure, and all-cause hospitalization with empagliflozin versus placebo were consistent between patients with eGFR < 60 and ≥ 60 ml per minute per 1.73 m^2 of body-surface area [33]."

"Empagliflozin also significantly reduced the risk for the composite renal end point which included progression to macroalbuminuria, doubling of serum creatinine, initiation of renal replacement therapy, or death resulting from renal disease, versus placebo in the subgroup of patients with prevalent kidney disease at baseline (HR, 0.58; 95% CI, 0.47–0.71) [33]."

"This trial showed that persons with chronic kidney disease who received dapagliflozin had a significantly lower risk of a composite of a sustained decline in the eGFR of at least 50%, end-stage kidney disease, or death from renal or cardiovascular causes than those who received placebo, independent of the presence or absence of T2DM."

Conclusion

"These trials established the superiority of an SGLT2 inhibitor added to the standard of care for CKD in T2DM for a primary outcome of kidney disease end points."

"Trials like DAPA-HF also showed cardiorenal endpoint benefits of SGLT2 inhibitors in patients without T2DM."

"It was concluded that SGLT2 inhibitors should be used when possible in patients with T2DM to reduce risks for CKD and CVD."

"The use of SGLT2 inhibitors should also be considered in all patients with HF and albuminuric kidney disease, even in the absence of T2DM."

Diabetes and Bone Fragility: SGLT2 Inhibitor Use in the Context of Renal and Cardiovascular Benefits [297]

This is a machine-generated summary of:

Jackson, Kristen; Moseley, Kendall F.: Diabetes and Bone Fragility: SGLT2 Inhibitor Use in the Context of Renal and Cardiovascular Benefits [297].

Published in: Current Osteoporosis Reports (2020).

Link to original: https://doi.org/10.1007/s11914-020-00609-z

If you want to cite the papers, please refer to the original.

For technical reasons we could not place the page where the original quote is coming from.

Abstract-Summary "Type 2 diabetes mellitus (T2DM) has been shown to negatively impact bone quality and increase fracture risk."

"To lowering blood glucose, there is evidence that these drugs offer cardiac and renal benefit to individuals with T2DM, leading to FDA-approved indications for use in at-risk individuals."

"There remain concerns that SGLT2 inhibitors, specifically canagliflozin, have adverse effects on bone metabolism and increase fracture risk in T2DM."

"The true long-term impact of SGLT2 inhibitors on the diabetic skeleton is still unclear; this review summarizes the results in studies investigating the impact of SGLT2 inhibitors on fracture risk in T2DM."

"Whereas studies performed with dapagliflozin and empagliflozin have not shown an increased risk of bone fractures compared with placebo, some studies have shown increased markers of bone turnover and reduced bone mineral density with canagliflozin treatment."

"There does not appear to be an increased fracture risk with the use of dapagliflozin or empagliflozin."

"Given the possible association between canagliflozin and adverse bone outcomes described in CANVAS, canagliflozin use should be pursued in individuals with T2DM only after careful consideration of the individual's skeletal risk."

Introduction

"It is well recognized that there are cardiac, renal, and ophthalmologic complications resulting from type 2 diabetes mellitus (T2DM)."

"Individuals with T2DM are at higher risk of hip, vertebral, and peripheral fracture compared with age and weight-matched non-diabetic controls [298]."

"T2DM affects over 30 million people in the USA, an improved understanding of the link between T2DM and fracture is imperative [299]."

T2DM and Fracture Risk

"In the Health Aging and Body Composition Study, which evaluated 2979 men and women ages 70–79, T2DM was associated with accelerated bone loss at the hip and an increased overall fracture risk (RR 1.64; 95% CI 1.07, 2.51) [300]."

"An increased risk of hip (RR 1.82; 95% CI:1.24, 2.69), proximal humerus (RR 1.94; 95% CI 1.24, 3.02), and foot fractures was observed in women with T2DM aged 65 years or older in the Study of Osteoporotic Fractures [301]."

"Even among younger women aged 24–59 in the Nurse's Health Study, the age-adjusted relative risk of hip fracture was 70% greater in individuals with T2DM compared with those without diabetes (RR 1.7; 95% CI 1.4, 2.0) [302]."

Pathophysiology of T2DM and Bone Fragility

"Paradoxically, individuals with T2DM fracture despite seemingly normal bone quantity, or BMD [303–308]."

"While bone mineral density (BMD) measured with dual-energy X-ray absorptiometry (DXA) should predict fracture risk, DXA and risk calculators underestimate the fracture risk among individuals with T2DM [309–312]."

"This discrepancy between normal bone quantity (BMD) and elevated fracture risk suggests there are additional factors contributing to increased bone fragility among persons with T2DM."

"AGEs have been shown to interfere with collagen cross-links in bone and lead to reduced osteoblast number and an increased fracture risk in diabetic individuals [313–317]."

Diabetes Medications and Bone Fragility

"In current practice, these agents have fallen out of favor due to concerns about cardiovascular safety as well as increased fracture risk."

"Most studies investigating other anti-hyperglycemic agents including metformin, sulfonylureas, dipeptidyl peptidase-4 (DPP-4) inhibitors, and glucagon-like peptide 1 (GLP-1) receptor agonists have shown neutral or beneficial effects on bone health [318]."

"While insulin has been shown to be anabolic to bone, the use of exogenous insulin also increases the frequency of hypoglycemic episodes, resulting in an increased rate of falls and fractures with insulin use [319]."

"The finding of increased fractures with insulin use is confounded by the fact that insulin is typically added when T2DM has advanced and glycemic control is poor, a state which independently contributes to bone fragility, as noted above."

SGLT2 Inhibitors for the Treatment of T2DM

"The study was concluded early at 2.6 years given significant renal benefit with canagliflozin; it showed that when compared with placebo, canagliflozin 100 mg/day resulted in a 30% reduction in the composite end point of end stage renal disease, doubling of serum creatinine from baseline, and death from renal or cardiovascular disease (HR 0.70; 95% CI 0.59–0.82; $p = 0.00001$) [320]."

"The cardiovascular benefits of dapagliflozin were evaluated in DECLARE-TIMI 58 trial, a phase 3 trial with 17,160 patients with T2DM and high risk for cardiovascular disease in which participants were randomized in a 1:1 ratio to dapagliflozin 10 mg daily or matching placebo [28]."

SGLT2 Inhibitors and Bone Fracture

"In this trial, secondary analysis of the data showed participants treated with canagliflozin 100 or 300 mg daily for a mean of 188 weeks demonstrated an increased risk of any fracture during the study period compared with placebo (15.4 vs. 11.9 participants with fracture per 1000 patient-years; HR 1.26; 95% CI 1.04, 1.52) [29]."

"The difference in fracture incidence in Watts' meta-analysis was driven by the large CANVAS trial data (where the adjudicated fracture adverse events were statistically higher in the canagliflozin group than placebo, 4.0% vs 2.6%); the pooled non-CANVAS studies did not show a significant difference in fracture incidence (1.7% vs 1.5%) [321]."

"Individual analysis of the meta-analyses by Cheng, Li, Ruanpeng, and Tang did not observe an increased risk in bone fractures with dapagliflozin treatment compared with placebo [322–325]."

Pathophysiology of SGLT2 Inhibitors and Bone Fracture

"The inconsistent results of these trials have prompted further evaluation of the potential mechanisms by which SGLT2 inhibitors could have negative effects on bone integrity."

"By inhibiting reabsorption of glucose at the proximal tubule, SGLT2 inhibitors lead to disruption of calcium, phosphate, and vitamin D homeostasis [326]."

"While elevations in PTH and FGF23 have opposing effects on the production of 1,25-dihydroxy vitamin D, data suggest that the net impact of SGLT2 inhibitors is to decrease 1,25-dihydroxyvitamin D levels [327, 328]."

"The resultant elevation in PTH and decrease in 1,25-dihydroxy vitamin D related to SGLT2 inhibitors would be expected to have negative implications for bone health [329]."

"Reduction in BMD with SGLT2 inhibitor use may be partially explained by modest weight loss caused by the agents, leading to increased bone turnover [330, 331]."

Discussion

"The 2020 American Diabetes Association Standards of Medical Care note that "for patients with type 2 diabetes and fracture risk factors … sodium-glucose cotransporter 2 inhibitors should be used with caution" [332]. In the data presented in this review, however, there was an increased fracture risk observed with canagliflozin in the CANVAS trial but no increase in fracture risk with dapagliflozin or empagliflozin in their respective cardiovascular safety trials; this discrepancy suggests that clinicians should consider the potential impact of SGLT2 inhibitors on bone fragility in the context of individual agents rather than as a class effect."

"Considering the findings of available studies on SGLT2 inhibitors' impact on bone, and until more long-term safety data are available to provide definitive answers on this subject, a patient's risk of fracture also merits pause prior to SGLT2 inhibitor use."

The Actions of SGLT2 Inhibitors on Metabolism, Renal Function and Blood Pressure [333]

This is a machine-generated summary of:

Thomas, Merlin C.; Cherney, David Z. I.: The actions of SGLT2 inhibitors on metabolism, renal function and blood pressure [333].

Published in: Diabetologia (2018).

Link to original: https://doi.org/10.1007/s00125-018-4669-0

If you want to cite the papers, please refer to the original.

For technical reasons we could not place the page where the original quote is coming from.

Abstract-Summary "Inhibition of the sodium–glucose cotransporter (SGLT) 2 in the proximal tubule of the kidney has a broad range of effects on renal function and plasma volume homeostasis, as well as on adiposity and energy metabolism across the entire body."

"Equally, the glucose-lowering effects of SGLT2 inhibitors are attenuated in individuals without diabetes and those with a reduced eGFR."

"Unlike the glucose-lowering effects of SGLT2 inhibitors, the spill-over of sodium and glucose beyond the proximal nephron following SGLT2 inhibition triggers dynamic and reversible realignment of energy metabolism, renal filtration and plasma volume without relying on losses into the urine."

"In the long term, the resetting of energy/salt/water physiology following SGLT2 inhibition has an impact, not only on adiposity, renal function and blood pressure control, but also on the health and survival of patients with type 2 diabetes."

Introduction

"Inhibitors of sodium–glucose cotransporter (SGLT) 2 have a wide range of clinically relevant actions in those with type 2 diabetes."

"We examine the effects of SGLT2 inhibitors on glucose metabolism and also explore their glucose-independent actions on adiposity, renal function and blood pressure."

"An intervention that reduces hyperglycaemia, aids weight loss and blood pressure control, and modulates kidney function has an important place in the management of type 2 diabetes."

SGLT2 Inhibitors and Glucose Control

"Smaller reductions in HbA_{1c} following SGLT2 inhibitor treatment are observed in participants with better control at baseline, especially at a low dose [334–336], and these reductions may be less than those with use of other agents for which the mechanism of action is not glucose-dependent."

"The glucose-lowering effect of SGLT2 inhibitors is dose-dependent, at least in patients with HbA_{1c} <64 mmol/mol (8%), in whom high-dose therapy produces superior glucose-lowering compared with low-dose formulations [252]."

"In those with poor glucose control, however, improvements in glycaemic control are statistically similar with both high- and low-dose SGLT2 inhibitors."

"As a corollary, the preferred strategy is to initiate patients with poor glucose control with low-dose formulations of SGLT2 inhibitors, escalating to higher doses as clinically indicated; although this approach remains to be formally studied."

"To maximise glucose-lowering effects in individuals with an eGFR < 60 ml min^{-1} $[1.73\ m]^{-2}$, initiating treatment with a high-dose formulation of an SGLT2 inhibitor may be preferred."

SGLT2 Inhibitors and Weight Control

"While SGLT2 inhibitors are not licensed for use in weight loss therapy, it is apparent that, by promoting glucosuria, they provide an opportunity to achieve a negative energy balance."

"Although clinical studies with SGLT2 inhibitors demonstrate an acute decline in body weight [252, 337], a nadir is reached after approximately 6 months and ongoing weight loss is not observed despite ongoing glucosuria and associated energy losses."

"A modest increase in energy intake may not balance initial heavy glucosuria, resulting in early weight loss with SGLT2 inhibitor use."

"As glucosuria declines with improving glucose control, (lesser) energy losses may become fully offset by increased food intake, achieving a new energy balance and plateau in weight."

"It is widely regarded that glucosuria, and its associated energy losses, is the primary driving factor for weight loss following SGLT2 inhibition."

SGLT2 Inhibitors and Renal Function

"~25 g of sodium (alongside ~180 g of glucose) is reabsorbed by SGLT-dependent pathways in the proximal tubule each day, amounting to 4–6% of the total filtered sodium load [338]."

"In diabetes, glucose-mediated renal hypertrophy, increased expression and activity of SGLT2 and full recruitment of SGLT1 mean that almost 50 g of sodium (over 10% of the filtered sodium load) may be reabsorbed via SGLT-dependent pathways [338]."

"In diabetes, energy-dependent sodium and glucose reabsorption in the proximal tubule increases hypoxia in the renal medulla, contributing to nephron dropout and functional decline."

"By transferring some of the energy burden of sodium reabsorption away from the proximal tubule, SGLT2 inhibitors may protect against AKI."

"The sodium and glucose not absorbed in the proximal tubule following SGLT2 inhibition also influences solute handling elsewhere in the nephron."

SGLT2 Inhibitors and Blood Pressure Control

"A reduction in blood pressure is also observed in individuals with reduced eGFR [339], even though the glucose-lowering efficacy of SGLT2 inhibitors is attenuated in this setting."

"SGLT2 inhibitors cause an acute contraction in plasma volume within hours of therapy initiation, manifested by a 3–7% increase in haemoglobin, albumin and urea concentrations."

"Unlike other causes of plasma volume loss, that induced by SGLT2 inhibitors continues, even over years of therapy [112]."

"Nor is it dependent on the osmotic diuretic effects of glucosuria, since similar changes in plasma volume are observed in SGLT2 inhibitor-treated individuals without diabetes, and those with a reduced eGFR, despite minimal glucosuria [339, 340]."

"It is likely that, following SGLT2 inhibition, the osmotic effect of glucose and increased sodium flow beyond the early proximal tubule, are interpreted by the nephron as signs of excessive filtration, such as may occur following inappropriate expansion of plasma volume or sodium loading."

Conclusions

"The spillover of sodium and glucose beyond the proximal nephron following SGLT2 inhibition triggers a dynamic and reversible realignment of energy metabolism, renal function and plasma volume."

"The much longer-term benefits of SGLT2 inhibitor use arising from improved glycaemic control, beta cell preservation, and reductions in adiposity, blood pressure and plasma volume, as well as better preservation of renal function may prove equally important and more broadly applicable."

"Unlike the glucose-lowering effects of SGLT2 inhibitors, effects on weight, renal function and plasma volume do not rely on ongoing losses into the urine, and occur in the absence of significant glucosuria [339] or ongoing natriuresis [341]."

"Subtle changes in the solute/water/energy balance in the proximal tubule following SGLT2 inhibition cause the kidney to take control of a perceived imbalance, modulating not only eGFR and plasma volume, but also metabolic processes across the entire body."

Bibliography

1. Salvatore T, Galiero R, Caturano A, Rinaldi L, Di Martino A, Albanese G, Di Salvo J, Epifani R, Marfella R, Docimo G, Lettieri M (2022) An overview of the cardiorenal protective mechanisms of SGLT2 inhibitors. Int J Mol Sci 23(7):3651
2. Nagahisa T, Saisho Y (2019) Cardiorenal protection: potential of SGLT2 inhibitors and GLP-1 receptor agonists in the treatment of type 2 diabetes. Diabetes Ther 10(5):1733–1752. https://doi.org/10.1007/s13300-019-00680-5
3. Hernandez AF, Green JB, Janmohamed S et al (2018) Albiglutide and cardiovascular outcomes in patients with type 2 diabetes and cardiovascular disease (Harmony Outcomes): a double-blind, randomised placebo-controlled trial. Lancet 392:1519–1529

4. Marso SP, Daniels GH, Brown-Frandsen K et al (2016) Liraglutide and cardiovascular outcomes in type 2 diabetes. N Engl J Med 375:311–322
5. Marso SP, Bain SC, Consoli A et al (2016) Semaglutide and cardiovascular outcomes in patients with type 2 diabetes. N Engl J Med 375:1834–1844
6. Gerstein HC, Colhoun HM, Dagenais GR et al (2019) Dulaglutide and cardiovascular outcomes in type 2 diabetes (REWIND): a double-blind, randomised placebo-controlled trial. Lancet 394:121–130
7. Davies MJ, D'Alessio DA, Fradkin J et al (2018) Management of hyperglycemia in type 2 diabetes, 2018. A consensus report by the American Diabetes Association (ADA) and the European Association for the Study of Diabetes (EASD). Diabetes Care 2018(41):2669–2701
8. UK Prospective Diabetes Study (UKPDS) Group (1998) Effect of intensive blood-glucose control with metformin on complications in overweight patients with type 2 diabetes (UKPDS 34). UK Prospective Diabetes Study (UKPDS) Group. Lancet 352:854–865
9. Gerstein HC, Miller ME, Byington RP et al (2008) Effects of intensive glucose lowering in type 2 diabetes. N Engl J Med 358:2545–2559
10. Patel A, MacMahon S, Chalmers J et al (2008) Intensive blood glucose control and vascular outcomes in patients with type 2 diabetes. N Engl J Med 24:2560–2572
11. Duckworth W, Abraira C, Moritz T et al (2009) Glucose control and vascular complications in veterans with type 2 diabetes. N Engl J Med 360:129–139
12. Kosiborod M, Lam CSP, Kohsaka S et al (2018) Cardiovascular events associated with SGLT-2 inhibitors versus other glucose-lowering drugs: the CVD-REAL 2 study. J Am Coll Cardiol 71:2628–2639
13. Tang H, Li D, Zhang J et al (2017) Sodium-glucose co-transporter-2 inhibitors and risk of adverse renal outcomes among patients with type 2 diabetes: a network and cumulative meta-analysis of randomized controlled trials. Diabetes Obes Metab 19:1106–1115
14. Margulies KB, Hernandez AF, Redfield MM et al (2016) Effects of liraglutide on clinical stability among patients with advanced heart failure and reduced ejection fraction: a randomized clinical trial. JAMA 316:500–508
15. Frias JP, Guja C, Hardy E et al (2016) Exenatide once weekly plus dapagliflozin once daily versus exenatide or dapagliflozin alone in patients with type 2 diabetes inadequately controlled with metformin monotherapy (DURATION-8): a 28 week, multicentre, double-blind, phase 3, randomised controlled trial. Lancet Diabetes Endocrinol 4:1004–1016
16. Ludvik B, Frias JP, Tinahones FJ et al (2018) Dulaglutide as add-on therapy to SGLT2 inhibitors in patients with inadequately controlled type 2 diabetes (AWARD-10): a 24-week, randomised, double-blind, placebo-controlled trial. Lancet Diabetes Endocrinol 6:370–381
17. DeFronzo RA (2017) Combination therapy with GLP-1 receptor agonist and SGLT2 inhibitor. Diabetes Obes Metab 19:1353–1362
18. Harashima SI, Inagaki N, Kondo K et al (2018) Efficacy and safety of canagliflozin as add-on therapy to a glucagon-like peptide-1 receptor agonist in Japanese patients with type 2 diabetes mellitus: a 52-week, open-label, phase IV study. Diabetes Obes Metab 20:1770–1775
19. Ishihara H, Yamaguchi S, Nakao I et al (2018) Ipragliflozin add-on therapy to a GLP-1 receptor agonist in Japanese patients with type 2 diabetes (AGATE): a 52-week open-label study. Diabetes Ther Res Treat Educ Diabetes Rel Disorders 9:1549–1567
20. Seino Y, Yabe D, Sasaki T et al (2018) Sodium-glucose cotransporter-2 inhibitor luseogliflozin added to glucagon-like peptide 1 receptor agonist liraglutide improves glycemic control with bodyweight and fat mass reductions in Japanese patients with type 2 diabetes: a 52-week, open-label, single-arm study. J Diab Investig 9:332–340
21. Liu H, Sridhar VS, Perkins BA, Rosenstock J, Cherney DZI (2022) SGLT2 inhibition in type 1 diabetes with diabetic kidney disease: potential cardiorenal benefits can outweigh preventable risk of diabetic ketoacidosis. Curr Diab Rep 22(7):317–332. https://doi.org/10.1007/s11892-022-01471-2

22. Helve J, Sund R, Arffman M, Harjutsalo V, Groop P-H, Grönhagen-Riska C et al (2018) Incidence of end-stage renal disease in patients with type 1 diabetes. Diabetes Care 41(3):434–439
23. Kristófi R, Bodegard J, Norhammar A, Thuresson M, Nathanson D, Nyström T et al (2021) Cardiovascular and renal disease burden in type 1 compared with type 2 diabetes: a two-country nationwide observational study. Diabetes Care 44(5):1211–1218
24. Rosenstock J, Ferrannini E (2015) Euglycemic diabetic ketoacidosis: a predictable, detectable, and preventable safety concern with SGLT2 inhibitors. Diabetes Care 38(9):1638–1642
25. Wolfsdorf JI, Ratner RE (2019) SGLT inhibitors for type 1 diabetes: proceed with extreme caution. Diabetes Care 42(6):991–993
26. Perkins BA, Rosenstock J, Skyler JS, Laffel LM, Cherney DZ, Mathieu C et al (2019) Exploring patient preferences for adjunct-to-insulin therapy in type 1 diabetes. Diabetes Care 42(9):1716–1723
27. Zinman B, Wanner C, Lachin JM, Fitchett D, Bluhmki E, Hantel S, Mattheus M, Devins T, Johansen OE, Woerle HJ, Broedl UC, Inzucchi SE (2015) Empagliflozin, cardiovascular outcomes, and mortality in type 2 diabetes. N Engl J Med 373:2117–2128
28. Wiviott SD, Raz I, Bonaca MP, Mosenzon O, Kato ET, Cahn A, Silverman MG, Zelniker TA, Kuder JF, Murphy SA, Bhatt DL, Leiter LA, McGuire DK, Wilding JPH, Ruff CT, Gause-Nilsson IAM, Fredriksson M, Johansson PA, Langkilde A-M, Sabatine MS (2018) Dapagliflozin and cardiovascular outcomes in type 2 diabetes. N Engl J Med 380:347–357
29. Neal B, Perkovic V, Mahaffey KW, de Zeeuw D, Fulcher G, Erondu N, Shaw W, Law G, Desai M, Matthews DR (2017) Canagliflozin and cardiovascular and renal events in type 2 diabetes. N Engl J Med 377:644–657
30. Cannon CP, Pratley R, Dagogo-Jack S, Mancuso J, Huyck S, Masiukiewicz U et al (2020) Cardiovascular outcomes with ertugliflozin in type 2 diabetes. N Engl J Med 383(15):1425–1435
31. Cherney DZI, Charbonnel B, Cosentino F, Dagogo-Jack S, McGuire DK, Pratley R et al (2021) Effects of ertugliflozin on kidney composite outcomes, renal function and albuminuria in patients with type 2 diabetes mellitus: an analysis from the randomised VERTIS CV trial. Diabetologia 64(6):1256–1267
32. Bhatt DL, Szarek M, Pitt B, Cannon CP, Leiter LA, McGuire DK et al (2021) Sotagliflozin in patients with diabetes and chronic kidney disease. N Engl J Med 384(2):129–139
33. Perkovic V, Jardine MJ, Neal B, Bompoint S, Heerspink HJL, Charytan DM, Edwards R, Agarwal R, Bakris G, Bull S, Cannon CP, Capuano G, Chu PL, de Zeeuw D, Greene T, Levin A, Pollock C, Wheeler DC, Yavin Y, Zhang H, Zinman B, Meininger G, Brenner BM, Mahaffey KW, CREDENCE Trial Investigators (2019) Canagliflozin and renal outcomes in type 2 diabetes and nephropathy. N Engl J Med 380(24):2295–2306
34. Heerspink HJL, Stefánsson BV, Correa-Rotter R, Chertow GM, Greene T, Hou F-F, Mann JFE, McMurray JJV, Lindberg M, Rossing P, Sjöström CD, Toto RD, Langkilde A-M, Wheeler DC (2020) Dapagliflozin in patients with chronic kidney disease. N Engl J Med 383(15):1436–1446. https://doi.org/10.1056/NEJMoa2024816
35. Cherney DZI, Zinman B, Inzucchi SE, Koitka-Weber A, Mattheus M, von Eynatten M et al (2017) Effects of empagliflozin on the urinary albumin-to-creatinine ratio in patients with type 2 diabetes and established cardiovascular disease: an exploratory analysis from the EMPA-REG OUTCOME randomised, placebo-controlled trial. Lancet Diabetes Endocrinol 5(8):610–621
36. Cherney DZI, Dekkers CCJ, Barbour SJ, Cattran D, Abdul Gafor AH, Greasley PJ et al (2020) Effects of the SGLT2 inhibitor dapagliflozin on proteinuria in non-diabetic patients with chronic kidney disease (DIAMOND): a randomised, double-blind, crossover trial. Lancet Diabetes Endocrinol 8(7):582–593
37. Cherney DZI, Heerspink HJL, Frederich R, Maldonado M, Liu J, Pong A et al (2020) Effects of ertugliflozin on renal function over 104 weeks of treatment: a post hoc analysis of two randomised controlled trials. Diabetologia 63(6):1128–1140

38. Van Raalte DH, Bjornstad P, Persson F, Powell DR, De Cassia CR, Wang PS et al (2019) The impact of sotagliflozin on renal function, albuminuria, blood pressure, and hematocrit in adults with type 1 diabetes. Diabetes Care 42(10):1921–1929
39. Tuttle KR, Brosius FC, Cavender MA, Fioretto P, Fowler KJ, Heerspink HJL et al (2021) SGLT2 inhibition for CKD and cardiovascular disease in type 2 diabetes: report of a scientific workshop sponsored by the national kidney foundation. Diabetes 70(1):1–16
40. Rosenstock J, Marquard J, Laffel LM, Neubacher D, Kaspers S, Cherney DZ et al (2018) Empagliflozin as adjunctive to insulin therapy in type 1 diabetes: The EASE trials. Diabetes Care 41(12):2560–2569. The EASE trials were one of the three large RCTs investigating the use of SGLT2 inhibitors (empagliflozin in the EASE trials) as an adjunctive to insulin therapy in patients with type 1 diabetes. This trial found that empagliflozin improved glycemic control and weight without increasing hypoglycemia, and provides concrete evidence of the benfits SGLT2 inhibitors provide in patients with type 1 diabetes.
41. Yamada T, Shojima N, Noma H, Yamauchi T, Kadowaki T (2018) Sodium-glucose co-transporter-2 inhibitors as add-on therapy to insulin for type 1 diabetes mellitus: Systematic review and meta-analysis of randomized controlled trials. Diabetes Obes Metab 20(7):1755–1761
42. Garg SK, Henry RR, Banks P, Buse JB, Davies MJ, Fulcher GR et al (2017) Effects of sotagliflozin added to insulin in patients with type 1 diabetes. N Engl J Med 377(24):2337–2348
43. Phillip M, Mathieu C, Lind M, Araki E, di Bartolo P, Bergenstal R et al (2021) Long-term efficacy and safety of dapagliflozin in patients with inadequately controlled type 1 diabetes: pooled 52-week outcomes from the DEPICT-1 and -2 studies. Diabetes Obes Metab 23(2):549–560
44. Fioretto P, Zambon A, Rossato M, Busetto L, Vettor R (2016) SGLT2 inhibitors and the diabetic kidney. Diabetes Care 39(Supplement 2):S165–S171
45. Danne T, Garg S, Peters AL, Buse JB, Mathieu C, Pettus JH et al (2019) International consensus on risk management of diabetic ketoacidosis in patients with type 1 diabetes treated with sodium-glucose cotransporter (SGLT) inhibitors. Diabetes Care 42(6):1147–1154. This Consensus Report written by an international team of physicians and researchers with expertise in using SGLT2 inhibitor therapy. The report summarizes and reviews the current research regarding SGLT2 inhibitor use in addition to providing recommendations and strategies to enhance the safety (mitigating risk of DKA in particular) of SGLT2 inhibitors in individuals with type 1 diabetes
46. Bailey CJ, Day C, Bellary S (2022) Renal protection with SGLT2 inhibitors: effects in acute and chronic kidney disease. Curr Diab Rep 22(1):39–52. https://doi.org/10.1007/s11892-021-01442-z
47. Wright EM, Loo DD, Hirayama BA (2011) Biology of human sodium glucose transporters. Physiol Rev 91:733–794
48. Ghezzi C, Loo DD, Wright EM (2018) Physiology of renal glucose handling via SGLT1, SGLT2 and GLUT2. Diabetologia 61:2087–2097. This clear, concise and highly informative review provides an ideal foundation for the study of SGLT2 inhibitor effects on the kidney
49. Bailey CJ (2011) Renal glucose reabsorption inhibitors to treat diabetes. Trends Pharmacol Sci 32:63–71
50. Zaccardi F, Webb DR, Htike ZZ, Youssef D, Khunti K, Davies MJ (2016) Efficacy and safety of sodium-glucose co-transporter-2 inhibitors in type 2 diabetes mellitus: systematic review and network meta-analysis. Diabetes Obes Metab 18:783–794
51. Scheen AJ (2020) Reduction in HbA1c with SGLT2 inhibitors vs. DPP-4 inhibitors as add-ons to metformin monotherapy according to baseline HbA1c: a systematic review of randomized controlled trials. Diabetes Metab 46:186–196
52. Yang L, Zhang L, He H, Zhang M, An Z (2019) Efficacy and safety of sodium-glucose cotransporter 2 inhibitors in east Asians with type 2 diabetes: a systematic review and meta-analysis. Diabetes Ther 10:1921–1934

53. Yang Y, Zhao C, Ye Y, Yu M, Qu X (2020) Prospect of sodium–glucose co-transporter 2 inhibitors combined with insulin for the treatment of type 2 diabetes. Front Endocrinol 10:3389. https://doi.org/10.3389/fendo.2020.00190
54. Chen J, Fan F, Wang JY, Long Y, Gao CL, Stanton RC, Xu Y (2017) The efficacy and safety of SGLT2 inhibitors for adjunctive treatment of type 1 diabetes: a systematic review and meta-analysis. Sci Rep 7:44128
55. Georgianos PI, Agarwal R (2019) Ambulatory blood pressure reduction with sglt-2 inhibitors: dose-response meta-analysis and comparative evaluation with low-dose hydrochlorothiazide. Diabetes Care 42:693–700
56. Bailey CJ, Day C (2019) The future of new drugs for diabetes management. Diabetes Res Clin Pract 155:107785
57. McGuire DK, Shih WJ, Cosentino F, Charbonnel B, Cherney DZ, Dagogo-Jack S et al (2021) Association of SGLT2 inhibitors with cardiovascular and kidney outcomes in patients with type 2 diabetes: a meta-analysis. JAMA Cardiol 6:148–158
58. Teo YH, Teo YN, Syn NL, Kow CS, Yoong CS, Tan BY et al (2021) Effects of sodium/glucose cotransporter 2 (SGLT2) inhibitors on cardiovascular and metabolic outcomes in patients without diabetes mellitus: a systematic review and meta-analysis of randomized-controlled trials. JAHA 10:e019463
59. Packer M, Anker SD, Butler J, Filippatos G, Pocock SJ, Carson P, Januzzi J, Verma S, Tsutsui H, Brueckmann M, Jamal W, Kimura K, Schnee J, Zeller C, Cotton D, Bocchi E, Böhm M, Choi D-J, Chopra V, Chuquiure E, Giannetti N, Janssens S, Zhang J, Gonzalez Juanatey JR, Kaul S, Brunner-La Rocca H-P, Merkely B, Nicholls SJ, Perrone S, Pina I, Ponikowski P, Sattar N, Senni M, Seronde M-F, Spinar J, Squire I, Taddei S, Wanner C, Zannad F (2020) Cardiovascular and renal outcomes with empagliflozin in heart failure. N Engl J Med 383:1413–1424
60. McMurray JJ, Solomon SD, Inzucchi SE, Køber L, Kosiborod MN, Martinez FA et al (2019) Dapagliflozin in patients with heart failure and reduced ejection fraction. N Engl J Med 381:1995–2008
61. Zannad F, Ferreira JP, Pocock SJ, Anker SD, Butler J, Filippatos G et al (2020) SGLT2 inhibitors in patients with heart failure with reduced ejection fraction: a meta-analysis of the EMPEROR-Reduced and DAPA-HF trials. Lancet 396:819–829
62. Bhatt DL, Szarek M, Steg PG, Cannon CP, Leiter LA, McGuire DK et al (2021) Sotagliflozin in patients with diabetes and recent worsening heart failure. N Engl J Med 384:117–128
63. Alicic RZ, Rooney MT, Tuttle KR (2017) Diabetic kidney disease: challenges, progress, and possibilities. Clin J Am Soc Nephrol 12:2032–2045
64. Vistisen D, Andersen GS, Hulman A, Persson F, Rossing P, Jørgensen ME (2019) Progressive decline in estimated glomerular filtration rate in patients with diabetes after moderate loss in kidney function—even without albuminuria. Diabetes Care 42:1886–1894
65. Canagliflozin prescribing information, USA (2016) https://www.accessdata.fda.gov/drugsatfda_docs/label/2016/204042s011lbl.pdf . Accessed 2 Jul 2021
66. Dapagliflozin prescribing information, USA (2020) https://www.accessdata.fda.gov/drugsatfda_docs/label/2020/202293s020lbl.pdf . Accessed 2 Jul 2021
67. Empagliflozin prescribing information, USA (2020) https://www.accessdata.fda.gov/drugsatfda_docs/label/2020/204629s023lbl.pdf. Accessed 2 Jul 2021
68. Ertugliflozin prescribing information, USA (2017) https://www.accessdata.fda.gov/drugsatfda_docs/label/2017/209803s000lbl.pdf . Accessed 2 Jul 2021
69. Wanner C, Inzucchi SE, Lachin JM, Fitchett D, von Eynatten M, Mattheus M et al (2016) Empagliflozin and progression of kidney disease in type 2 diabetes. N Engl J Med 375:323–334
70. Jhund PS, Solomon SD, Docherty KF, Heerspink HJ, Anand IS, Böhm M et al (2021) Efficacy of dapagliflozin on renal function and outcomes in patients with heart failure with reduced ejection fraction. Results of DAPA-HF Circulation 143:298–309

71. Zoungas S, Arima H, Gerstein HC, Holman RR, Woodward M, Reaven P et al (2017) Effects of intensive glucose control on microvascular outcomes in patients with type 2 diabetes: a meta-analysis of individual participant data from randomised controlled trials. Lancet Diabetes Endocrinol 5:431–437. An excellent analysis of studies detailing the effects of glycaemic control on the microvascular complications of type 2 diabetes
72. Kang HM, Ahn SH, Choi P, Ko YA, Han SH, Chinga F et al (2015) Defective fatty acid oxidation in renal tubular epithelial cells has a key role in kidney fibrosis development. Nat Med 21:37–46
73. Wilcox CS (2020) Antihypertensive and renal mechanisms of SGLT2 (sodium-glucose linked transporter 2) inhibitors. Hypertension 75:894–901
74. Onishi A, Fu Y, Darshi M, Crespo-Masip M (2019) Effect of renal tubule-specific knockdown of the Na+/H+ exchanger NHE3 in Akita diabetic mice. Am J Physiol Renal Physiol 317:F419–F434
75. Bailey CJ (2019) Uric acid and the cardio-renal effects of SGLT2 inhibitors. Diabetes Obes Metab 21:1291–1298
76. Donnan JR, Grandy CA, Chibrikov E, Marra CA, Aubrey-Bassler K, Johnston K et al (2019) Comparative safety of the sodium glucose co-transporter 2 (SGLT2) inhibitors: a systematic review and meta-analysis. BMJ Open 9:e022577
77. Gilbert RE, Thorpe KE (2019) Acute kidney injury with sodium-glucose co-transporter-2 inhibitors: a meta-analysis of cardiovascular outcome trials. Diabetes Obes Metab 21:1996–2000
78. Menne J, Dumann E, Haller H, Schmidt BMW (2019) Acute kidney injury and adverse renal events in patients receiving SGLT2-inhibitors: a systematic review and meta-analysis. PLoS Med 16:e1002983
79. Cherney DZ, Kanbay M, Lovshin JA (2020) Renal physiology of glucose handling and therapeutic implications. Nephrol Dial Transplant 35:i3–i12. This excellent review provides a clear and comprehensive account of the mechanisms that underlie the therapeutic effects of SGLT2 inhibitors on the kidney
80. Heerspink HJL, Kosiborod M, Inzucchi SE, Cherney DZI (2018) Renoprotective effects of sodium-glucose cotransporter-2 inhibitors. Kidney Int 94:26–39
81. Liu J, Tian J, Sodhi K, Shapiro JI (2021) The Na/K-ATPase signaling and SGLT2 inhibitor-mediated cardiorenal protection: a crossed road? J Membr Biol 254(5–6):513–529. https://doi.org/10.1007/s00232-021-00192-z
82. Margonato D, Galati G, Mazzetti S, Cannistraci R, Perseghin G, Margonato A, Mortara A (2020) Renal protection: a leading mechanism for cardiovascular benefit in patients treated with SGLT2 inhibitors. Heart Fail Rev 26(2):337–345. https://doi.org/10.1007/s10741-020-10024-2
83. Licic RZ, Rooney MT, Tuttle KR (2017) Diabetic kidney disease: challenges, progress and possibilities. Clin J Am Soc Nephrol 12:2032–2045
84. Arwar N, Gao P, Seshasai SR, Gobin R, Kaptoge S, Di Angelantonio E et al (2010) Diabetes mellitus, fasting blood glucose concentration, and risk of vascular disease: a collaborative meta-analysis of 102 prospective studies. Lancet 375:2215–2222
85. Cosentino F, Grant PJ, Aboyans V, Bailey CJ, Ceriello A, Delgado V, Federici M, Filippatos G, Grobbee DE, Hansen TB, Huikuri HV, Johansson I, Jüni P, Lettino M, Marx N, Mellbin LG, Östgren CJ, Rocca B, Roffi M, Sattar N, Seferović PM, Sousa-Uva M, Valensi P, Wheeler DC, ESC Scientific Document Group, Piepoli MF, Birkeland KI, Adamopoulos S, Ajjan R, Avogaro A, Baigent C, Brodmann M, Bueno H, Ceconi C, Chioncel O, Coats A, Collet JP, Collins P, Cosyns B, di Mario C, Fisher M, Fitzsimons D, Halvorsen S, Hansen D, Hoes A, RIG H, Home P, Katus HA, Khunti K, Komajda M, Lambrinou E, Landmesser U, Lewis BS, Linde C, Lorusso R, Mach F, Mueller C, Neumann FJ, Persson F, Petersen SE, Petronio AS, Richter DJ, GMC R, Rossing P, Rydén L, Shlyakhto E, Simpson IA, Touyz RM, Wijns W, Wilhelm M, Williams B, Aboyans V, Bailey CJ, Ceriello A, Delgado V, Federici M, Filippatos G, Grobbee DE, Hansen TB, Huikuri HV, Johansson I, Jüni P, Lettino M, Marx N,

Mellbin LG, Östgren CJ, Rocca B, Roffi M, Sattar N, Seferović PM, Sousa-Uva M, Valensi P, Wheeler DC, Windecker S, Aboyans V, Baigent C, Collet JP, Dean V, Delgado V, Fitzsimons D, Gale CP, Grobbee DE, Halvorsen S, Hindricks G, Iung B, Jüni P, Katus HA, Landmesser U, Leclercq C, Lettino M, Lewis BS, Merkely B, Mueller C, Petersen SE, Petronio AS, Richter DJ, Roffi M, Shlyakhto E, Simpson IA, Sousa-Uva M, Touyz RM, Zelveian PH, Scherr D, Jahangirov T, Lazareva I, Shivalkar B, Naser N, Gruev I, Milicic D, Petrou PM, Linhart A, Hildebrandt P, Hasan-Ali H, Marandi T, Lehto S, Mansourati J, Kurashvili R, Siasos G, Lengyel C, Thrainsdottir IS, Aronson D, di Lenarda A, Raissova A, Ibrahimi P, Abilova S, Trusinskis K, Saade G, Benlamin H, Petrulioniene Z, Banu C, Magri CJ, David L, Boskovic A, Alami M, Liem AH, Bosevski M, GFT S, Janion M, Gavina C, Vinereanu D, Nedogoda S, Mancini T, Ilic MD, Fabryova L, Fras Z, Jiménez-Navarro MF, Norhammar A, Lehmann R, Mourali MS, Ural D, Nesukay E, Chowdhury TA (2020) 2019 ESC guidelines on diabetes, pre-diabetes, and cardiovascular diseases developed in collaboration with the EASD. Eur Heart J 41:255–323

86. Tahrani AA, Barnett AH, Bailey CJ (2013) SGLT inhibitors in management of diabetes. Lancet Diabetes Endocrinol 1:140–151
87. Lee YJ, Lee YJ, Han HJ (2007) Regulatory mechanisms of Na+/glucose cotransporters in renal proximal tubule cells. Kidney Int 72:S27–S35
88. Griffin M, Rao VS, Ivey-Miranda J, Fleming J, Mahoney D, Maulion C, Suda N, Siwakoti K, Ahmad T, Jacoby D, Riello R, Bellumkonda L, Cox Z, Collins S, Jeon S, Turner JM, Wilson FP, Butler J, Inzucchi SE, Testani JM (2020) Empagliflozin in heart failure: diuretic and cardio-renal effects. Circulation 142(11):1028–1039. https://doi.org/10.1161/CIRCULATIONAHA.120.045691
89. Hallow KM, Helmlinger G, Greasley PJ, McMurray JJV, Boulton DW (2018) Why do SGLT2 inhibitors reduce heart failure hospitalization? A differential volume regulation hypothesis. Diabetes Obes Metab 20:479–487
90. Verma S, John JV (2018) McMurray SGLT2 inhibitors and mechanisms of cardiovascular benefit: a state-of-the-art review. Diabetologia 61:2108–2117
91. Wilcox CS, Shen W, Boulton DW, Leslie BR, Griffen SC (2018) Interaction between the sodium-glucose-linked transporter 2 inhibitor dapagliflozin and the loop diuretic bumetanide in normal human subjects. J Am Heart Assoc 7:e007046
92. Januzzi J, Ferreira JP, Böhm M, Kaul S, Wanner C, Brueckmann M, Petrie MC, Ofstad AP, Zeller C, George J, Fitchett D, Zannad F (2019) Empagliflozin reduces the risk of a broad spectrum of heart failure outcomes regardless of heart failure status at baseline. Eur J Heart Fail 21(3):386–388. https://doi.org/10.1002/ejhf.1419
93. Sabouret P, Galati G, Angoulvant D, Germanova O, Castelletti S, Pathak A et al (2020) The interplay between cardiology and diabetology: a renewed collaboration to optimize cardiovascular prevention and heart failure management. Eur Heart J Cardiovasc Pharmacother 13:pvaa051. https://doi.org/10.1093/ehjcvp/pvaa051
94. Hodrea J, Balogh DB, Hosszu A, Lenart L, Besztercei B, Koszegi S et al (2020) Reduced O-GlcNAcylation and tubular hypoxia contribute to the antifibrotic effect of SGLT2 inhibitor dapagliflozin in the diabetic kidney. Am J Physiol Renal Physiol 318(4):F1017–F1029
95. Woods TC, Satou R, Miyata K, Katsurada A, Dugas CM, Klingenberg NC, Fonseca VA, Navar LG (2019) Canagliflozin prevents intrarenal angiotensinogen augmentation and mitigates kidney injury and hypertension in mouse model of type 2 diabetes mellitus. Am J Nephrol 49:331–342
96. Yaribeygi H, Katsiki N, Butler AE, Sahebkar A (2019) Effects of antidiabetic drugs on NLRP3 inflammasome activity, with a focus on diabetic kidneys. Drug Discov Today 24:256–262
97. Castoldi G, Carletti R, Ippolito S, Colzani M, Barzaghi F, Stella A, Zerbini G, Perseghin G, di Gioia CRT (2020) Renal antifibrotic effect of sodium glucose cotransporter-2 inhibition in angiotensin II dependent hypertension. Am J Nephrol 51:119–129
98. Dekkers CCJ, Petrykiv S, Laverman GD, Cherney DZ, Gansevoort RT, Heerspink HJL (2018) Effects of the SGLT-2 inhibitor dapagliflozin on glomerular and tubular injury markers. Diabetes Obes Metab 20(8):1988–1993

99. Herat LY, Magno AL, Rudnicka C, Hricova J, Carnagarin R, Ward NC et al (2020) SGLT2 inhibitor–induced Sympathoinhibition a novel mechanism for cardiorenal protection. JACC Basic Transl Sci 5(2):169–179
100. Matthews V, Elliot R, Rudnicka C, Hricova J, Herat L, Schlaich M (2017) Role of the sympathetic nervous system in regulation of the sodium glucose co-transporter 2. J Hypertens 35:2059–2068
101. Scheen AJ, Delanaye P (2017) Effects of reducing blood pressure on renal outcomes in patients with type 2 diabetes: focus on SGLT2 inhibitors and EMPA-REG OUTCOME. Diabetes Metab 43(2):99–109
102. Coresh J, Heerspink HJL, Sang Y, Matsushita K, Arnlov J, Astor BC, Black C, Brunskill NJ, Carrero JJ, Feldman HI, Fox CS, Inker LA, Ishani A, Ito S, Jassal S, Konta T, Polkinghorne K, Romundstad S, Solbu MD, Stempniewicz N, Stengel B, Tonelli M, Umesawa M, Waikar SS, Wen CP, Wetzels JFM, Woodward M, Grams ME, Kovesdy CP, Levey AS, Gansevoort RT, Appel LJ, Greene T, Chen TK, Chalmers J, Arima H, Perkovic V, Levin A, Djurdjev O, Tang M, Nally J, Navaneethan SD, Schold JD, Weldegiorgis M, Herrington WG, Smith M, Hsu CY, Hwang SJ, Chang AR, Kirchner HL, Green JA, Ho K, Marks A, Prescott G, Clark LE, Fluck N, Shalev V, Chodick G, Blankestijn PJ, van Zuilen A, van den Brand JA, Sarnak MJ, Bottinger E, Nadkarni GN, Ellis SG, Nadukuru R, Metzger M, Flamant M, Houillier P, Haymann JP, Froissart M, Kenealy T, Elley RC, Collins JF, Drury PL, Cuddeback JK, Ciemins EL, Stempniewicz R, Nelson RG, Knowler WC, Bakker SJ, Major RW, Medcalf JF, Shepherd D, Barrett-Connor E, Bergstrom J, Ix JH, Molnar MZ, Sumida K, de Zeeuw D, Brenner B, Qureshi AR, Elinder CG, Runesson B, Evans M, Segelmark M, Stendahl M, Schön S, Naimark DM, Tangri N, Sud M, Hirayama A, Ichikawa K, Bilo HJG, Landman GWD, van Hateren KJJ, Kleefstra N, Hallan SI, Ballew SH, Chen J, Kwak L, Surapaneni A, Parving HH, Rodby RA, Rohde RD, Lewis JB, Lewis E, Perrone RD, Abebe KZ, Hou FF, Xie D, Hunsicker LG, Imai E, Kobayashi F, Makino H, Ito S, Remuzzi G, Ruggenenti P, Eckardt KU, Gudmundsdottir H, Maciulaitis R, Manley T, Smith K, Stockbridge N, Thompson A, Vetter T, Willis K, Zhang L (2019) Chronic kidney disease prognosis consortium and chronic kidney disease epidemiology collaboration. Change in albuminuria and subsequent risk of end-stage kidney disease: an individual participant-level consortium meta-analysis of observational studies. Lancet Diabetes Endocrinol 7:115–127
103. Heerspink HJL, Greene T, Tighiouart H, Gansevoort RT, Coresh J, Simon AL, Chan TM, Hou FF, Lewis JB, Locatelli F, Praga M, Schena FP, Levey AS, Inker LA, Sevillano A, Kamper AL, van Zuilen AD, Brenner BM, Maes B, Ihle BU, Barret B, Leung CB, Szeto CC, Fitzner C, Wanner C, Pozzi C, Montagnino CP, Xie D, de Zeeuw D, Lewis E, Verde E, Gutierrez E, Imai E, Hou FF, Caravaca F, Fervenza FC, Locatelli F, Schena FP, Kobayashi F, Moroni G, Becker GJ, Beck GJ, Appel GB, Frisch G, van Essen G, Maschio G, Remuzzi G, Montogrino G, Parving HH, Heerspink HJL, Makino H, Jehan I, Wetzels JFM, Donadio J, Dwyer J, van den Brand J, Kusek J, Lachin JM, Luño J, Lewis JB, Floege J, Abebe KZ, Chow KM, Hunsicker LG, del Vecchio L, Carlo M, Praga M, Goicoechea M, von Eynatten M, Poulter N, Chaturvedi N, Passerini P, de Jong PE, Blankestijn PJ, Li P, Ruggenenti P, Zucchelli P, Kincaid-Smith PS, Hilgers RD, Estacio RO, Rohde RD, Katafuchi R, Toto RD, Schrier RW, Rodby RA, Perrone RD, Ito S, Klahr S, Andrulli S, Strandgaard S, Chan TM, Hannedouche TP, Rauen T, Greene T, Verdalles U, Perkovic V, Keane W (2019) Chronic Kidney Disease Epidemiology Collaboration. Change in albuminuria as a surrogate endpoint for progression of kidney disease: a meta-analysis of treatment effects in randomised clinical trials. Lancet Diabetes Endocrinol 7:128–139
104. Cherney DZI, Heerspink HJL, Frederich R, Maldonado M, Liu J, Pong A, Xu ZJ, Patel S, Hickman A, Mancuso JP, Gantz I, Terra SG (2020) Effects of ertugliflozin on renal function over 104 weeks of treatment: a post hoc analysis of two randomised controlled trials. Diabetologia 63(6):1128–1140
105. Giorgino F, Vora J, Fenici P, Solini A (2020) Renoprotection with SGLT2 inhibitors in type 2 diabetes over a spectrum of cardiovascular and renal risk. Cardiovasc Diabetol 19(1):196. https://doi.org/10.1186/s12933-020-01163-9

106. Thomas MC, Cooper ME, Zimmet P (2016) Changing epidemiology of type 2 diabetes mellitus and associated chronic kidney disease. Nat Rev Nephrol 12(2):73–81
107. Arnold SV, Kosiborod M, Wang J, Fenici P, Gannedahl G, LoCasale RJ (2018) Burden of cardio-renal-metabolic conditions in adults with type 2 diabetes within the Diabetes Collaborative Registry. Diabetes Obes Metab 20(8):2000–2003
108. Brenner BM, Cooper ME, de Zeeuw D, Keane WF, Mitch WE, Parving HH et al (2001) Effects of losartan on renal and cardiovascular outcomes in patients with type 2 diabetes and nephropathy. N Engl J Med 345(12):861–869
109. Lewis EJ, Hunsicker LG, Clarke WR, Berl T, Pohl MA, Lewis JB et al (2001) Renoprotective effect of the angiotensin-receptor antagonist irbesartan in patients with nephropathy due to type 2 diabetes. N Engl J Med 345(12):851–860
110. Parving HH, Lehnert H, Brochner-Mortensen J, Gomis R, Andersen S, Arner P et al (2001) The effect of irbesartan on the development of diabetic nephropathy in patients with type 2 diabetes. N Engl J Med 345(12):870–878
111. Kohan DE, Fioretto P, Johnsson K, Parikh S, Ptaszynska A, Ying L (2016) The effect of dapagliflozin on renal function in patients with type 2 diabetes. J Nephrol 29(3):391–400
112. Wanner C, Inzucchi SE, Lachin JM, Fitchett D, von Eynatten M, Mattheus M, Johansen OE, Woerle HJ, Broedl UC, Zinman B (2016) EMPA-REG OUTCOME investigators. Empagliflozin and progression of kidney disease in type 2 diabetes. N Engl J Med 375(4):323–334. https://doi.org/10.1056/NEJMoa1515920
113. Kluger AY, Tecson KM, Lee AY, Lerma EV, Rangaswami J, Lepor NE et al (2019) Class effects of SGLT2 inhibitors on cardiorenal outcomes. Cardiovasc Diabetol 18(1):99
114. Cannon CP, Pratley R, Dagogo-Jack S, Mancuso J, Huyck S, Masiukiewicz U et al (2020) Cardiovascular outcomes with ertugliflozin in type 2 diabetes. New Engl J Med 28:96
115. Neuen BL, Young T, Heerspink HJL, Neal B, Perkovic V, Billot L et al (2019) SGLT2 inhibitors for the prevention of kidney failure in patients with type 2 diabetes: a systematic review and meta-analysis. Lancet Diabetes Endocrinol 7(11):845–854
116. Lo KB, Gul F, Ram P, Kluger AY, Tecson KM, McCullough PA et al (2020) The effects of SGLT2 inhibitors on cardiovascular and renal outcomes in diabetic patients: a systematic review and meta-analysis. Cardiorenal Med 10(1):1–10
117. Toyama T, Neuen BL, Jun M, Ohkuma T, Neal B, Jardine MJ et al (2019) Effect of SGLT2 inhibitors on cardiovascular, renal and safety outcomes in patients with type 2 diabetes mellitus and chronic kidney disease: a systematic review and meta-analysis. Diabetes Obes Metab 21(5):1237–1250
118. Packer M, Anker SD, Butler J, Filippatos G, Pocock SJ, Carson P et al (2020) Cardiovascular and renal outcomes with empagliflozin in heart failure. N Engl J Med 26:87
119. Mosenzon O, Wiviott SD, Cahn A, Rozenberg A, Yanuv I, Goodrich EL et al (2019) Effects of dapagliflozin on development and progression of kidney disease in patients with type 2 diabetes: an analysis from the DECLARE-TIMI 58 randomised trial. Lancet Diabetes Endocrinol 7(8):606–617. https://doi.org/10.1016/S2213-8587(19)30180-9. Erratum in: Lancet Diabetes Endocrinol 2019 Aug;7(8):e20
120. Zelniker TA, Wiviott SD, Raz I, Im K, Goodrich EL, Bonaca MP et al (2019) SGLT2 inhibitors for primary and secondary prevention of cardiovascular and renal outcomes in type 2 diabetes: a systematic review and meta-analysis of cardiovascular outcome trials. Lancet 393(10166):31–39. https://doi.org/10.1016/S0140-6736(18)32590-X. Erratum in: Lancet 2019 Jan 5;393(10166):30
121. Ryan PB, Buse JB, Schuemie MJ, DeFalco F, Yuan Z, Stang PE et al (2018) Comparative effectiveness of canagliflozin, SGLT2 inhibitors and non-SGLT2 inhibitors on the risk of hospitalization for heart failure and amputation in patients with type 2 diabetes mellitus: A real-world meta-analysis of 4 observational databases (OBSERVE-4D). Diabetes Obes Metab 20(11):2585–2597

122. Li D, Yang JY, Wang T, Shen S, Tang H (2018) Risks of diabetic foot syndrome and amputation associated with sodium glucose co-transporter 2 inhibitors: a meta-analysis of randomized controlled trials. Diabetes Metab 44(5):410–414
123. Leiter LA, Cefalu WT, de Bruin TW, Gause-Nilsson I, Sugg J, Parikh SJ (2014) Dapagliflozin added to usual care in individuals with type 2 diabetes mellitus with preexisting cardiovascular disease: a 24-week, multicenter, randomized, double-blind, placebo-controlled study with a 28-week extension. J Am Geriatr Soc 62(7):1252–1262
124. Kambara T, Shibata R, Osanai H, Nakashima Y, Asano H, Sakai K et al (2018) Use of sodium-glucose cotransporter 2 inhibitors in older patients with type 2 diabetes mellitus. Geriatr Gerontol Int 18(1):108–114
125. Lahnwong S, Chattipakorn SC, Chattipakorn N (2018) Potential mechanisms responsible for cardioprotective effects of sodium–glucose co-transporter 2 inhibitors. Cardiovasc Diabetol 17(1):101. https://doi.org/10.1186/s12933-018-0745-5
126. Kosiborod M, Cavender MA, Fu AZ, Wilding JP, Khunti K, Holl RW et al (2017) Lower risk of heart failure and death in patients initiated on sodium–glucose cotransporter-2 inhibitors versus other glucose-lowering drugs: the CVD-REAL Study (comparative effectiveness of cardiovascular outcomes in new users of sodium–glucose cotransporter-2 inhibitors). Circulation 136:249–259
127. Lin B, Koibuchi N, Hasegawa Y, Sueta D, Toyama K, Uekawa K et al (2014) Glycemic control with empagliflozin, a novel selective SGLT2 inhibitor, ameliorates cardiovascular injury and cognitive dysfunction in obese and type 2 diabetic mice. Cardiovasc Diabetol 13:148
128. Habibi J, Aroor AR, Sowers JR, Jia G, Hayden MR, Garro M et al (2017) Sodium glucose transporter 2 (SGLT2) inhibition with empagliflozin improves cardiac diastolic function in a female rodent model of diabetes. Cardiovasc Diabetol 16:9
129. Ye Y, Bajaj M, Yang H-C, Perez-Polo JR, Birnbaum Y (2017) SGLT-2 inhibition with dapagliflozin reduces the activation of the Nlrp3/ASC inflammasome and attenuates the development of diabetic cardiomyopathy in mice with type 2 diabetes. Further augmentation of the effects with saxagliptin, a DPP4 inhibitor. Cardiovasc Drugs Ther 31:119–132
130. Zhou Y, Wu W (2017) The sodium–glucose co-transporter 2 inhibitor, empagliflozin, protects against diabetic cardiomyopathy by inhibition of the endoplasmic reticulum stress pathway. Cell Physiol Biochem Int J Exp Cell Physiol Biochem Pharmacol 41:2503–2512
131. Lee T-M, Chang N-C, Lin S-Z (2017) Dapagliflozin, a selective SGLT2 Inhibitor, attenuated cardiac fibrosis by regulating the macrophage polarization via STAT3 signaling in infarcted rat hearts. Free Radic Biol Med 104:298–310
132. Tanajak P, Sa-Nguanmoo P, Sivasinprasasn S, Thummasorn S, Siri-Angkul N, Chattipakorn SC et al (2018) Cardioprotection of dapagliflozin and vildagliptin in rats with cardiac ischemia-reperfusion injury. J Endocrinol 236:69–84
133. Vrhovac I, Balen Eror D, Klessen D, Burger C, Breljak D, Kraus O et al (2015) Localizations of Na(+)-d-glucose cotransporters SGLT1 and SGLT2 in human kidney and of SGLT1 in human small intestine, liver, lung, and heart. Pflugers Arch 467:1881–1898
134. Zhou L, Cryan EV, D'Andrea MR, Belkowski S, Conway BR, Demarest KT (2003) Human cardiomyocytes express high level of Na+/glucose cotransporter 1 (SGLT1). J Cell Biochem 90:339–346
135. Chen J, Williams S, Ho S, Loraine H, Hagan D, Whaley JM et al (2010) Quantitative PCR tissue expression profiling of the human SGLT2 gene and related family members. Diab Ther 1:57–92
136. Baker WL, Smyth LR, Riche DM, Bourret EM, Chamberlin KW, White WB (2014) Effects of sodium–glucose co-transporter 2 inhibitors on blood pressure: a systematic review and meta-analysis. J Am Soc Hypertens JASH 8(262–275):e9
137. Mazidi M, Rezaie P, Gao H-K, Kengne AP (2017) Effect of sodium–glucose cotransport-2 inhibitors on blood pressure in people with type 2 diabetes mellitus: a systematic review and meta-analysis of 43 randomized control trials with 22 528 patients. J Am Heart Assoc 6:e004007

138. Baker WL, Buckley LF, Kelly MS, Bucheit JD, Parod ED, Brown R et al (2017) Effects of sodium–glucose cotransporter 2 inhibitors on 24-hour ambulatory blood pressure: a systematic review and meta-analysis. J Am Heart Assoc 6:e005686
139. Baartscheer A, Schumacher CA, Wüst RCI, Fiolet JWT, Stienen GJM, Coronel R et al (2017) Empagliflozin decreases myocardial cytoplasmic Na(+) through inhibition of the cardiac Na(+)/H(+) exchanger in rats and rabbits. Diabetologia 60:568–573
140. Anson M, Zhao SS, Austin P, Ibarburu GH, Malik RA, Alam U (2023) SGLT2i and GLP-1 RA therapy in type 1 diabetes and reno-vascular outcomes: a real-world study. Diabetologia 66(10):1869–1881. https://doi.org/10.1007/s00125-023-05975-8
141. Holt RIG, DeVries JH, Hess-Fischl A et al (2021) The management of type 1 diabetes in adults. A consensus report by the American Diabetes Association (ADA) and the European Association for the Study of Diabetes (EASD). Diabetes Care 44(11):2589–2625. https://doi.org/10.2337/dci21-0043
142. Fang M, Jeon Y, Echouffo-Tcheugui JB, Selvin E (2023) Prevalence and management of obesity in U.S. adults with type 1 diabetes. Ann Intern Med 176(3):427–429. https://doi.org/10.7326/M22-3078
143. Edwards K, Li X, Lingvay I (2022) Clinical and safety outcomes with GLP-1 receptor agonists and SGLT2 inhibitors in type 1 diabetes: a real-world study. J Clin Endocrinol Metab 108(4):920–930. https://doi.org/10.1210/clinem/dgac618
144. FDA (2022) FDA revises labels of SGLT2 inhibitors for diabetes to include warnings about too much acid in the blood and serious urinary tract infections. https://www.fda.gov/drugs/drug-safety-and-availability/fda-revises-labels-sglt2-inhibitors-diabetes-include-warnings-about-too-much-acid-blood-and-serious#:~:text=Safety%20and%20Availability-,FDA%20revises%20labels%20of%20SGLT2%20inhibitors%20for%20diabetes%20to%20include,and%20serious%20urinary%20tract%20infections&text=To%20lessen%20the%20risk%20of,information%20for%20SGLT2%20inhibitor%20medicines. Accessed 1 Mar 2023
145. Brown E, Heerspink HJL, Cuthbertson DJ, Wilding JPH (2021) SGLT2 inhibitors and GLP-1 receptor agonists: established and emerging indications. Lancet 398(10296):262–276. https://doi.org/10.1016/S0140-6736(21)00536-5
146. Wheeler DC, James J, Patel D, Viljoen A, Ali A, Evans M, Fernando K, Hicks D, Milne N, Newland-Jones P, Wilding J (2020) SGLT2 inhibitors: slowing of chronic kidney disease progression in type 2 diabetes. Diabetes Ther 11(12):2757–2774. https://doi.org/10.1007/s13300-020-00930-x
147. Wilding J, Fernando K, Milne N et al (2018) SGLT2 inhibitors in type 2 diabetes management: key evidence and implications for clinical practice. Diabetes Ther 9:1757–1773
148. Ali A, Bain S, Hicks D et al (2019) SGLT2 inhibitors: cardiovascular benefits beyond HbA1c-translating evidence into practice. Diabetes Ther 10:1595–1622
149. Ito M, Tanaka T (2018) The anticipated renoprotective effects of sodium-glucose cotransporter 2 inhibitors. Intern Med 57:2105–2114
150. Wu B, Bell K, Stanford A et al (2016) Understanding CKD among patients with T2DM: prevalence, temporal trends, and treatment patterns-NHANES 2007–2012. BMJ Open Diabetes Res Care 4(1):e000154
151. Kainz A, Hronsky M, Stel VS et al (2015) Prediction of prevalence of chronic kidney disease in diabetic patients in countries of the European Union up to 2025. Nephrol Dial Transplant 30(Suppl 4):113–118
152. Assogba FG, Couchoud C, Hannedouche T et al (2014) Trends in the epidemiology and care of diabetes mellitus-related end-stage renal disease in France, 2007–2011. Diabetologia 57:718–728
153. Afkarian M, Sachs MC, Kestenbaum B et al (2013) Kidney disease and increased mortality risk in type 2 diabetes. J Am Soc Nephrol 24:302–308
154. MacIsaac RJ, Ekinci EI, Jerums G (2014) Markers of and risk factors for the development and progression of diabetic kidney disease. Am J Kidney Dis 63:S39–S62

155. National Institute for Health and are Excellence (2015) Clinical guideline (CG182). Chronic kidney disease in adults: assessment and management. https://www.nice.org.uk/guidance/cg182/resources/chronic-kidney-disease-in-adults-assessment-and-management-pdf-35109809343205. Accessed Jul 2020
156. National Institute for Health and are Excellence (2015) Clinical guideline type 2 diabetes in adults: management (NG28). https://www.nice.org.uk/guidance/ng28. Accessed Jul 2020
157. Muskiet MHA, Tonneijck L, Smits MM et al (2015) Pleiotropic effects of type 2 diabetes management strategies on renal risk factors. Lancet Diabetes Endocrinol 3:367–381
158. Heerspink HJL, Karasik A, Thuresson M, Melzer-Cohen C, Chodick G, Khunti K et al (2020) Kidney outcomes associated with use of SGLT2 inhibitors in real-world clinical practice (CVD-REAL 3): a multinational observational cohort study. Lancet Diabetes Endocrinol 8(1):27–35
159. Cannon CP, McGuire DK, Pratley R et al (2020) The VERTIS CV trial. Cardiovascular outcomes following ertugliflozin treatment in patients with type 2 diabetes mellitus and atherosclerotic cardiovascular disease. Presented during American Diabetes Association (ADA) Virtual 88th Scientific Sessions. https://www.acc.org/education-and-meetings/image-and-slide-gallery/media-detail?id=307A7E103BC04A588A3370709253FC35 . Accessed Jul 2020
160. Heerspink HJ, Perkins BA, Fitchett DH, Husain M, Cherney DZ (2016) Sodium glucose cotransporter 2 inhibitors in the treatment of diabetes mellitus: cardiovascular and kidney effects, potential mechanisms, and clinical applications. Circulation 134(10):752–772
161. Cherney DZ, Perkins BA, Soleymanlou N, Maione M, Lai V, Lee A et al (2014) Renal hemodynamic effect of sodium-glucose cotransporter 2 inhibition in patients with type 1 diabetes mellitus. Circulation 129(5):587–597
162. 2019/20 General Medical Services (GMS) contract Quality and Outcomes Framework (QOF) (2019) Guidance for GMS contract 2019/20 in England. https://www.england.nhs.uk/wp-content/uploads/2019/05/gms-contract-qof-guidance-april-2019.pdf. Accessed Jul 2020
163. KDIGO clinical practice guideline on diabetes management in chronic kidney disease (2019) [Public review draft] and Wedbinar. https://www.kdigo.org/guidelines/diabetes-ckd/. Accessed Jul 2020
164. National Institute for Health and are Excellence (2014) NICE guideline (CG181). Cardiovascular disease: risk assessment and reduction, including lipid modification. https://www.nice.org.uk/guidance/cg181. Accessed Jul 2020
165. Davies MJ, D'Alessio DA, Fradkin JM et al (2018) Management of hyperglycemia in type 2 diabetes, 2018. Consensus report by the American Diabetes Association (ADA) and the European Association for the Study of Diabetes (EASD). Diabetes Care 2018(41):2669–2701
166. Schernthaner G, Groop PH, Kalra PA, Ronco C, Taal MW (2020) Sodium-glucose linked transporter-2 inhibitor renal outcome modification in type 2 diabetes: evidence from studies in patients with high or low renal risk. Diabetes Obes Metab 22:1024
167. Lin F-J, Wang C-C, Hsu C-N, Yang C-Y, Wang C-Y, Ou H-T (2021) Renoprotective effect of SGLT-2 inhibitors among type 2 diabetes patients with different baseline kidney function: a multi-center study. Cardiovasc Diabetol 20(1):203. https://doi.org/10.1186/s12933-021-01396-2
168. Roy A, Maiti A, Sinha A, Baidya A, Basu AK, Sarkar D, Sanyal D, Biswas D, Maisnam I, Pandit K, Raychaudhuri M, Sengupta N, Chakraborty PP, Mukhopadhyay P, Raychaudhuri P, Sahana PK, Chatterjee P, Bhattacharjee R, Dasgupta R, Saraogi RK, Pal SK, Mukhopadhyay S, Mukhopadhyay S, Goswami S, Chowdhury S, Ghosh S (2020) Kidney disease in type 2 diabetes mellitus and benefits of sodium-glucose cotransporter 2 inhibitors: a consensus statement. Diabetes Ther 11(12):2791–2827. https://doi.org/10.1007/s13300-020-00921-y
169. Arnold SV, Hunt PR, Chen H et al (2018) Cardiovascular outcomes and mortality in type 2 diabetes with associated cardio-renal-metabolic comorbidities. Diabetes 67(Suppl 1):1582
170. Webster AC, Nagler EV, Morton RL, Masson P (2017) Chronic kidney disease. Lancet 389:1238–1252

171. KDIGO Working Group (2011) Chapter 1: definition and classification of CKD. Kidney Int Suppl 2013(3):19–62
172. Inker LA, Astor BC, Fox CH et al (2014) KDOQI US commentary on the 2012 KDIGO clinical practice guideline for the evaluation and management of CKD. Am J Kidney Dis 63:713–735
173. The Diabetes Control and Complications Trial Research Group (1993) The effect of intensive treatment of diabetes on the development and progression of long-term complications in insulin-dependent diabetes mellitus. N Engl J Med 329:977–986
174. Perkovic V, Heerspink HL, Chalmers J et al (2013) Intensive glucose control improves kidney outcomes in patients with type 2 diabetes. Kidney Int 83:517–523
175. Parving HH, Brenner BM, McMurray JJ et al (2012) Cardiorenal end points in a trial of aliskiren for type 2 diabetes. N Engl J Med 367(23):2204–2213
176. Liakos A, Karagiannis T, Athanasiadou E et al (2014) Efficacy and safety of empagliflozin for type 2 diabetes: a systematic review and meta-analysis. Diabetes Obes Metab 16:984–993
177. Devi R, Mali G, Chakraborty I, Unnikrishnan MK, Abdulsalim S (2017) Efficacy and safety of empagliflozin in type 2 diabetes mellitus: a meta-analysis of randomized controlled trials. Postgrad Med 129:382–392
178. Cefalu WT, Stenlöf K, Leiter LA et al (2015) Effects of canagliflozin on body weight and relationship to HbA1c and blood pressure changes in patients with type 2 diabetes. Diabetologia 58:1183–1187
179. Wilding JP, Blonde L, Leiter LA et al (2015) Efficacy and safety of canagliflozin by baseline HbA1c and known duration of type 2 diabetes mellitus. J Diabetes Complications 29:438–444
180. Fioretto P, Del Prato S, Buse JB et al (2018) Efficacy and safety of dapagliflozin in patients with type 2 diabetes and moderate renal impairment (chronic kidney disease stage 3A): the DERIVE Study. Diabetes Obes Metab 20:2532–2540
181. Qiu M, Ding L-L, Zhou H-R (2021) Comparative efficacy of five SGLT2i on cardiorenal events: a network meta-analysis based on ten CVOTs. Am J Cardiovasc Drugs 22(1):69–81. https://doi.org/10.1007/s40256-021-00484-8
182. Dostanic-Larson I, Van Huysse JW, Lorenz JN, Lingrel JB (2005) The highly conserved cardiac glycoside binding site of Na, K-ATPase plays a role in blood pressure regulation. Proc Natl Acad Sci U S A 102(15845–15):850
183. Dostanic I, Paul RJ, Lorenz JN, Theriault S, Van Huysse JW, Lingrel JB (2005) The alpha2-isoform of Na-K-ATPase mediates ouabain-induced hypertension in mice and increased vascular contractility in vitro. Am J Physiol Heart Circ Physiol 288:H477–H485
184. Hamlyn JM, Blaustein MP, Bova S, DuCharme DW, Harris DW, Mandel F, Mathews WR, Ludens JH (1991) Identification and characterization of a ouabain-like compound from human plasma. Proc Natl Acad Sci U S A 88:6259–6263
185. Loreaux EL, Kaul B, Lorenz JN, Lingrel JB (2008) Ouabain-Sensitive alpha1 Na, K-ATPase enhances natriuretic response to saline load. J Am Soc Nephrol 19:1947–1954
186. Aperia A (2007) New roles for an old enzyme: Na, K-ATPase emerges as an interesting drug target. J Intern Med 261:44–52
187. Bagrov AY, Shapiro JI (2008) Endogenous digitalis: pathophysiologic roles and therapeutic applications. Nat Clin Pract Nephrol 4:378–392
188. Bagrov AY, Shapiro JI, Fedorova OV (2009) Endogenous cardiotonic steroids: physiology, pharmacology, and novel therapeutic targets. Pharmacol Rev 61:9–38
189. Schoner W (2002) Endogenous cardiac glycosides, a new class of steroid hormones. Eur J Biochem 269:2440–2448
190. Yatime L, Buch-Pedersen MJ, Musgaard M, Morth JP, Lund Winther AM, Pedersen BP, Olesen C, Andersen JP, Vilsen B, Schiott B, Palmgren MG, Moller JV, Nissen P, Fedosova N (2009) P-type ATPases as drug targets: tools for medicine and science. Biochim Biophys Acta 1787:207–220
191. Brown GK (2000) Glucose transporters: structure, function and consequences of deficiency. J Inherit Metab Dis 23:237–246
192. Hediger MA, Rhoads DB (1994) Molecular physiology of sodium-glucose cotransporters. Physiol Rev 74:993–1026

193. Lee YJ, Lee YJ, Han HJ (2007) Regulatory mechanisms of Na(+)/glucose cotransporters in renal proximal tubule cells. Kidney Int 72:S27–S35
194. Wright EM, Hirayama BA, Loo DF (2007) Active sugar transport in health and disease. J Intern Med 261:32–43
195. Vestri S, Okamoto MM, de Freitas HS, Aparecida Dos Santos R, Nunes MT, Morimatsu M, Heimann JC, Machado UF (2001) Changes in sodium or glucose filtration rate modulate expression of glucose transporters in renal proximal tubular cells of rat. J Membr Biol 182:105–112
196. Mosenzon O, Wiviott SD, Cahn A, Rozenberg A, Yanuv I, Goodrich EL, Murphy SA, Heerspink HJL, Zelniker TA, Dwyer JP, Bhatt DL, Leiter LA, McGuire DK, Wilding JPH, Kato ET, Gause-Nilsson IAM, Fredriksson M, Johansson PA, Langkilde AM, Sabatine MS, Raz I (2019) Effects of dapagliflozin on development and progression of kidney disease in patients with type 2 diabetes: an analysis from the DECLARE-TIMI 58 randomised trial. Lancet Diabetes Endocrinol 7:606–617
197. Wheeler DC, Stefánsson BV, Jongs N, Chertow GM, Greene T, Hou FF, McMurray JJV, Correa-Rotter R, Rossing P, Toto RD, Sjöström CD, Langkilde AM, Heerspink HJL (2021) Effects of dapagliflozin on major adverse kidney and cardiovascular events in patients with diabetic and non-diabetic chronic kidney disease: a prespecified analysis from the DAPA-CKD trial. Lancet Diabetes Endocrinol 9:22–31
198. Jhund PS, Solomon SD, Docherty KF, Heerspink HJL, Anand IS, Böhm M, Chopra V, Boer RA, Desai AS, Ge J, Kitakaze M, Merkley B, O'Meara E, Shou M, Tereshchenko S, Verma S, Vinh PN, Inzucchi SE, Køber L, Kosiborod MN, Martinez FA, Ponikowski P, Sabatine MS, Bengtsson O, Langkilde AM, Sjöstrand M, McMurray JJV (2021) Efficacy of dapagliflozin on renal function and outcomes in patients with heart failure with reduced ejection fraction. Circulation 143:298–309
199. Ye N, Jardine MJ, Oshima M, Hockham C, Heerspink HJL, Agarwal R, Bakris G, Schutte AE, Arnott C, Chang TI, Górriz JL, Cannon CP, Charytan DM, Zeeuw D, Levin A, Mahaffey KW, Neal B, Pollock C, Wheeler DC, Tanna GLD, Cheng H, Perkovic V, Neuen BL (2021) Blood pressure effects of canagliflozin and clinical outcomes in type 2 diabetes and chronic kidney disease: insights from the CREDENCE trial. Circulation 143:1735
200. Cai H, Wu L, Qu W, Malhotra D, Xie Z, Shapiro JI, Liu J (2008) Regulation of apical NHE3 trafficking by ouabain-induced activation of the basolateral Na+-K+-ATPase receptor complex. Am J Physiol Cell Physiol 294:C555–C563
201. Liu J, Kesiry R, Periyasamy SM, Malhotra D, Xie Z, Shapiro JI (2004) Ouabain induces endocytosis of plasmalemmal Na/K-ATPase in LLC-PK1 cells by a clathrin-dependent mechanism. Kidney Int 66:227–241
202. Liu J, Liang M, Liu L, Malhotra D, Xie Z, Shapiro JI (2005) Ouabain-induced endocytosis of the plasmalemmal Na/K-ATPase in LLC-PK1 cells requires caveolin-1. Kidney Int 67:1844–1854
203. Liu J, Yan Y, Liu L, Xie Z, Malhotra D, Joe B, Shapiro JI (2011) Impairment of Na/K-ATPase signaling in renal proximal tubule contributes to Dahl salt-sensitive hypertension. J Biol Chem 286(22806–22):813
204. Liu J, Shapiro JI (2007) Regulation of sodium pump endocytosis by cardiotonic steroids: molecular mechanisms and physiological implications. Pathophysiology 14:171–181
205. Periyasamy SM, Liu J, Tanta F, Kabak B, Wakefield B, Malhotra D, Kennedy DJ, Nadoor A, Fedorova OV, Gunning W, Xie Z, Bagrov AY, Shapiro JI (2005) Salt loading induces redistribution of the plasmalemmal Na/K-ATPase in proximal tubule cells. Kidney Int 67:1868–1877
206. Liu J, Nie Y, Chaudhry M, Bai F, Chuang J, Sodhi K, Shapiro JI (2020) The redox-sensitive Na/K-ATPase signaling in uremic cardiomyopathy. Int J Mol Sci 21:1256
207. Liu J, Tian J, Chaudhry M, Maxwell K, Yan Y, Wang X, Shah PT, Khawaja AA, Martin R, Robinette TJ, El-Hamdani A, Dodrill MW, Sodhi K, Drummond CA, Haller ST, Kennedy DJ, Abraham NG, Xie Z, Shapiro JI (2016a) Attenuation of Na/K-ATPase mediated oxidant AMPLIFICATION with pNaKtide ameliorates experimental uremic cardiomyopathy. Sci Rep 6:34592

208. Liu L, Wu J, Kennedy DJ (2016b) Regulation of cardiac remodeling by cardiac Na(+)/K(+)-ATPase Isoforms. Front Physiol 7:382
209. Pratt RD, Brickman CR, Cottrill CL, Shapiro JI, Liu J (2018) The Na/K-ATPase signaling: from specific ligands to general reactive oxygen species. Int J Mol Sci 19:2600
210. Sodhi K, Wang X, Chaudhry MA, Lakhani HV, Zehra M, Pratt R, Nawab A, Cottrill CL, Snoad B, Bai F, Denvir J, Liu J, Sanabria JR, Xie Z, Abraham NG, Shapiro JI (2020) Central role for adipocyte Na, K-ATPase oxidant amplification loop in the pathogenesis of experimental uremic cardiomyopathy. J Am Soc Nephrol 31:1746–1760
211. Wang X, Shapiro JI (2019) Evolving concepts in the pathogenesis of uraemic cardiomyopathy. Nat Rev Nephrol 15:159–175
212. Yan Y, Wang J, Chaudhry MA, Nie Y, Sun S, Carmon J, Shah PT, Bai F, Pratt R, Brickman C, Sodhi K, Kim JH, Pierre S, Malhotra D, Rankin GO, Xie ZJ, Shapiro JI, Liu J (2019) Metabolic syndrome and salt-sensitive hypertension in polygenic obese TALLYHO/JngJ mice: role of Na/K-ATPase signaling. Int J Mol Sci 20(14):3495. https://doi.org/10.3390/ijms20143495
213. Drummond CA, Fan X, Haller ST, Kennedy DJ, Liu J, Tian J (2018) Na/K-ATPase signaling mediates miR-29b-3p regulation and cardiac fibrosis formation in mice with chronic kidney disease. PLoS One 13:e0197688
214. de Zeeuw D, Heerspink HJL (2016) Unmet need in diabetic nephropathy: failed drugs or trials? Lancet Diabetes Endocrinol 4:638–640
215. Bhatt DL, Szarek M, Steg PG et al (2021) Sotagliflozin in patients with diabetes and recent worsening heart failure. N Engl J Med 384:117–128
216. Hutton B, Salanti G, Caldwell DM et al (2015) The PRISMA extension statement for reporting of systematic reviews incorporating network meta-analyses of health care interventions: checklist and explanations. Ann Intern Med 162:777–784
217. Täger T, Atar D, Agewall S et al (2020) Comparative efficacy of sodium-glucose cotransporter-2 inhibitors (SGLT2i) for cardiovascular outcomes in type 2 diabetes: a systematic review and network meta-analysis of randomised controlled trials. Heart Fail Rev 26(6):1421–1435. https://doi.org/10.1007/s10741-020-09954-8
218. Wei XB, Wei W, Ding LL et al (2021) Comparison of the effects of 10 GLP-1 RA and SGLT2 inhibitor interventions on cardiovascular, mortality, and kidney outcomes in type 2 diabetes: a network meta-analysis of large randomized trials. Prim Care Diabetes 15:208–211
219. Qiu M, Ding LL, Wei XB et al (2021) Comparative efficacy of glucagon-like peptide 1 receptor agonists and sodium glucose cotransporter 2 inhibitors for prevention of major adverse cardiovascular events in Type 2 diabetes: a network meta-analysis. J Cardiovasc Pharmacol 77:34–37
220. Fei Y, Tsoi MF, Cheung B (2019) Cardiovascular outcomes in trials of new antidiabetic drug classes: a network meta-analysis. Cardiovasc Diabetol 18:112
221. Hussein H, Zaccardi F, Khunti K et al (2019) Cardiovascular efficacy and safety of sodium-glucose co-transporter-2 inhibitors and glucagon-like peptide-1 receptor agonists: a systematic review and network meta-analysis. Diabet Med 36:444–452
222. Alfayez OM, Al YM, Alshibani M et al (2019) Network meta-analysis of nine large cardiovascular outcome trials of new antidiabetic drugs. Prim Care Diabetes 13:204–211
223. Hoehlschen J, Hofreither D, Tomin T, Birner-Gruenberger R (2023) Redox-driven cardioprotective effects of sodium-glucose co-transporter-2 inhibitors: comparative review. Cardiovasc Diabetol 22:101. https://doi.org/10.1186/s12933-023-01822-7
224. Chatterjee S, Khunti K, Davies MJ (2017) Type 2 diabetes. The Lancet 389(10085):2239–2251
225. Rieg T, Vallon V (2018) Development of SGLT1 and SGLT2 inhibitors. Diabetologia 61(10):2079–2086
226. Aguillón AR, Mascarello A, Segretti ND, de Azevedo HFZ, Guimaraes CRW, Miranda LSM et al (2018) Synthetic strategies toward SGLT2 inhibitors. Org Process Res Dev 22(4):467–488

227. Hallow KM, Gebremichael Y, Helmlinger G, Vallon V (2017) Primary proximal tubule hyperreabsorption and impaired tubular transport counterregulation determine glomerular hyperfiltration in diabetes: a modeling analysis. Am J Physiol Renal Physiol 312(5):F819–F835
228. Jo HA, Seo JH, Lee S, Yu MY, Bae E, Kim DK et al (2023) Metabolomic profiling in kidney cells treated with a sodium glucose-cotransporter 2 inhibitor. Sci Rep 4(1):2026
229. Lu YP, Zhang ZY, Wu HW, Fang LJ, Hu B, Tang C et al (2022) SGLT2 inhibitors improve kidney function and morphology by regulating renal metabolic reprogramming in mice with diabetic kidney disease. J Transl Med 14(1):420
230. Nakamura M, Sadoshima J (2018) Mechanisms of physiological and pathological cardiac hypertrophy. Nat Rev Cardiol 15(7):387–407
231. Tran DH, Wang Z, v. (2019) Glucose metabolism in cardiac hypertrophy and heart failure. J Am Heart Assoc 8(12):e012673
232. Pereira RO, Wende AR, Olsen C, Soto J, Rawlings T, Zhu Y et al (2013) Inducible overexpression of GLUT1 prevents mitochondrial dysfunction and attenuates structural remodeling in pressure overload but does not prevent left ventricular dysfunction. J Am Heart Assoc 2(5):e000301
233. Zhang L, Jaswal JS, Ussher JR, Sankaralingam S, Wagg C, Zaugg M et al (2013 Sep) Cardiac insulin-resistance and decreased mitochondrial Energy production precede the development of systolic heart failure after pressure-overload hypertrophy. Circ Heart Fail 6(5):1039–1048
234. Makarewich CA, Zhang H, Davis J, Correll RN, Trappanese DM, Hoffman NE et al (2014) Transient receptor potential channels contribute to pathological structural and functional remodeling after myocardial infarction. Circ Res 115(6):567–580
235. Ritterhoff J, Tian R (2017) Metabolism in cardiomyopathy: every substrate matters. Cardiovasc Res 113(4):411–421
236. Makrecka-Kuka M, Liepinsh E, Murray AJ, Lemieux H, Dambrova M, Tepp K et al (2020) Altered mitochondrial metabolism in the insulin-resistant heart. Acta Physiologica 228(3):e13430
237. Giordano FJ (2005) Oxygen, oxidative stress, hypoxia, and heart failure. J Clin Invest 115(3):500–508
238. Izzo C, Vitillo P, di Pietro P, Visco V, Strianese A, Virtuoso N et al (2021) The role of oxidative stress in cardiovascular aging and cardiovascular diseases. Life 11(1):60
239. Kiyuna LA, Albuquerque RPE, Chen CH, Mochly-Rosen D, Ferreira JCB (2018) Targeting mitochondrial dysfunction and oxidative stress in heart failure: challenges and opportunities. Free Radic Biol Med 129:155–168
240. Noordali H, Loudon BL, Frenneaux MP, Madhani M (2018) Cardiac metabolism—a promising therapeutic target for heart failure. Pharmacol Ther 182:95–114
241. Zinman B, Inzucchi SE, Lachin JM, Wanner C, Ferrari R, Fitchett D et al (2014) Rationale, design, and baseline characteristics of a randomized, placebo-controlled cardiovascular outcome trial of empagliflozin (EMPA-REG OUTCOME™). Cardiovasc Diabetol 13(1):102
242. Uthman L, Baartscheer A, Bleijlevens B, Schumacher CA, Fiolet JWT, Koeman A et al (2018) Class effects of SGLT2 inhibitors in mouse cardiomyocytes and hearts: inhibition of Na+/H + exchanger, lowering of cytosolic Na + and vasodilation. Diabetologia 61(3):722–726
243. Hawley SA, Ford RJ, Smith BK, Gowans GJ, Mancini SJ, Pitt RD et al (2016) The Na+/glucose cotransporter inhibitor canagliflozin activates AMPK by inhibiting mitochondrial function and increasing cellular AMP levels. Diabetes 65(9):2784–2794
244. Li C, Zhang J, Xue M, Li X, Han F, Liu X et al (2019) SGLT2 inhibition with empagliflozin attenuates myocardial oxidative stress and fibrosis in diabetic mice heart. Cardiovasc Diabetol 2(1):15
245. Zhou H, Wang S, Zhu P, Hu S, Chen Y, Ren J (2018) Empagliflozin rescues diabetic myocardial microvascular injury via AMPK-mediated inhibition of mitochondrial fission. Redox Biol 15:335–346
246. Zelniker TA, Braunwald E (2020) Mechanisms of cardiorenal effects of sodium-glucose cotransporter 2 inhibitors. J Am Coll Cardiol 75(4):422–434

247. Zannad F, Ferreira JP, Butler J, Filippatos G, Januzzi JL, Sumin M et al (2022) Effect of empagliflozin on circulating proteomics in heart failure: mechanistic insights into the EMPEROR programme. Eur Heart J 43(48):4991–5002
248. Hegde NC, Kumar A, Patil AN, Bhattacharjee S, Gamad N, Kasudhan KS, Kumar V, Rastogi A (2023) Dose-dependent renoprotection efficacy of sglt2 inhibitors in type 2 diabetes: systematic review and network meta-analysis. Acta Diabetol 60(10):1311–1331. https://doi.org/10.1007/s00592-023-02126-8
249. Xiang B, Zhao X, Zhou X (2021) Cardiovascular benefits of sodium-glucose cotransporter 2 inhibitors in diabetic and nondiabetic patients. Cardiovasc Diabetol 20:78
250. Bae JH, Park E-G, Kim S, Kim SG, Hahn S, Kim NH (2019) Effects of Sodium-glucose cotransporter 2 inhibitors on renal outcomes in patients with type 2 diabetes: a systematic review and meta-analysis of randomized controlled trials. Sci Rep 9(1):13009
251. Mearns ES, Sobieraj DM, White CM et al (2015) Comparative efficacy and safety of antidiabetic drug regimens added to metformin monotherapy in patients with type 2 diabetes: a network meta-analysis. PLoS One 10(4):e0125879
252. Zaccardi F, Webb DR, Htike ZZ, Youssef D, Khunti K, Davies MJ (2016) Efficacy and safety of sodium-glucose co-transporter-2 inhibitors in type 2 diabetes mellitus: systematic review and network meta-analysis. Diabetes Obes Metab 18(8):783–794
253. González-Albarrán O, Morales C, Pérez-Maraver M, Aparicio-Sánchez JJ, Simó R (2022) Review of SGLT2i for the treatment of renal complications: experience in patients with and without T2D. Diabetes Ther 13(Suppl 1):35–49. https://doi.org/10.1007/s13300-022-01276-2
254. Kramer CK, Zinman B (2019) Sodium–glucose cotransporter-2 (SGLT-2) inhibitors and the treatment of type 2 diabetes. Annu Rev Med 70:323–334
255. Xie Y, Bowe B, Mokdad AH et al (2018) Analysis of the global burden of disease study highlights the global, regional, and national trends of chronic kidney disease epidemiology from 1990 to 2016. Kidney Int 94:567–581
256. Saran R, Robinson B, Abbott KC et al (2019) Annual data report: epidemiology of kidney disease in the United States. Am J Kidney Dis 2020:A6–A7
257. Bash LD, Selvin E, Steffes M, Coresh J, Astor BC (2008) Poor glycemic control in diabetes and the risk of incident chronic kidney disease even in the absence of albuminuria and retinopathy: Atherosclerosis Risk in Communities (ARIC) Study. Arch Intern Med 168:2440–2447
258. De Pascalis A, Cianciolo G, Capelli I, Brunori G, La Manna G (2021) SGLT2 inhibitors, sodium and off-target effects: an overview. J Nephrol 34:673–680
259. Mosenzon O, Wiviott SD, Cahn A et al (2019) Effects of dapagliflozin on development and progression of kidney disease in patients with type 2 diabetes: an analysis from the DECLARE-TIMI 58 randomised trial. Lancet Diabetes Endocrinol 7:606–617
260. Cosentino F, Grant PJ, Aboyans V et al (2020) 2019 ESC guidelines on diabetes, pre-diabetes, and cardiovascular diseases developed in collaboration with the EASD. Eur Heart J Engl 41:255–323
261. Perkovic V, de Zeeuw D, Mahaffey KW et al (2018) Canagliflozin and renal outcomes in type 2 diabetes: results from the CANVAS Program randomised clinical trials. Lancet Diabetes Endocrinol 6:691–704
262. Vaduganathan M, Claggett BL, Jhund PS et al (2020) Estimating lifetime benefits of comprehensive disease-modifying pharmacological therapies in patients with heart failure with reduced ejection fraction: a comparative analysis of three randomised controlled trials. Lancet 396:121–128
263. Birkeland KI, Bodegard J, Eriksson JW et al (2020) Heart failure and chronic kidney disease manifestation and mortality risk associations in type 2 diabetes: a large multinational cohort study. Diabetes Obes Metab 22:1607–1618
264. Ronco C, Ronco F, McCullough PA (2017) A call to action to develop integrated curricula in cardiorenal medicine. Blood Purif 44:251–259
265. Kaze AD, Zhuo M, Kim SC, Patorno E, Paik JM (2022) Association of SGLT2 inhibitors with cardiovascular, kidney, and safety outcomes among patients with diabetic kidney disease: a meta-analysis. Cardiovasc Diabetol 21(1):47. https://doi.org/10.1186/s12933-022-01476-x

266. Harris ST, Patorno E, Zhuo M, Kim SC, Paik JM (2021) Prescribing trends of antidiabetes medications in patients with type 2 diabetes and diabetic kidney disease, a cohort study. Diabetes Care 44(10):2293–2301. https://doi.org/10.2337/dc21-0529
267. Zhao L-M, Huang J-N, Qiu M, Ding L-L, Zhan Z-L, Ning J (2021) Gliflozins for the prevention of stroke in diabetes and cardiorenal diseases: a meta-analysis of cardiovascular outcome trials. Medicine (Baltimore) 100:e27362
268. Arnott C, Li Q, Kang A, Neuen BL, Bompoint S, Lam CSP et al (2020) Sodium-glucose cotransporter 2 inhibition for the prevention of cardiovascular events in patients with type 2 diabetes mellitus: a systematic review and meta-analysis. J Am Heart Assoc 9:e014908
269. Zhou Z, Jardine MJ, Li Q, Neuen BL, Cannon CP, de Zeeuw D et al (2021) Effect of SGLT2 inhibitors on stroke and atrial fibrillation in diabetic kidney disease: results from the CREDENCE trial and meta-analysis. Stroke 52:1545–1556
270. Li J, Albajrami O, Zhuo M, Hawley CE, Paik JM (2020) Decision algorithm for prescribing SGLT2 inhibitors and GLP-1 receptor agonists for diabetic kidney disease. Clin J Am Soc Nephrol 15:1678–1688
271. Giugliano D, Longo M, Scappaticcio L, Caruso P, Esposito K (2021) Sodium–glucose transporter-2 inhibitors for prevention and treatment of cardiorenal complications of type 2 diabetes. Cardiovasc Diabetol 20(1):17. https://doi.org/10.1186/s12933-021-01213-w
272. Gregg EW, Hora I, Benoit SR (2019) Resurgence in diabetes-related complications. JAMA 321:1867–1868
273. Giugliano D, Meier JJ, Esposito K (2019) Heart failure and type 2 diabetes: from cardiovascular outcome trials, with hope. Diabetes Obes Metab 21:1081–1087
274. Sacre JW, Magliano DJ, Shaw JE (2020) Incidence of hospitalization for heart failure relative to major atherosclerotic events in type 2 diabetes: a meta-analysis of cardiovascular outcomes trials. Diabetes Care 43:2614–2623
275. Rawshani A, Rawshani A, Franzén S et al (2018) Risk factors, mortality, and cardiovascular outcomes in patients with type 2 diabetes. N Engl J Med 379:633–644
276. Wright AK, Suarez-Ortegon MF, Read SH et al (2020) Risk factor control and cardiovascular event risk in people with type 2 diabetes in primary and secondary prevention settings. Circulation 142:1925–1936
277. Barer Y, Cohen O, Cukierman-Yaffe T (2019) Effect of glycaemic control on cardiovascular disease in individuals with type 2 diabetes with pre-existing cardiovascular disease: a systematic review and meta-analysis. Diabetes Obes Metab 21:732–735
278. Gordon J, McEwan P, Idris I, Evans M, Puelles J (2018) Treatment choice, medication adherence and glycemic efficacy in people with type 2 diabetes: a UK clinical practice database study. BMJ Open Diabetes Res Care 6:e000512
279. Edelman SV, Polonsky WH (2017) Type 2 diabetes in the real world: the elusive nature of glycemic control. Diabetes Care 40:1469–1478
280. Giugliano D, Maiorino MI, Bellastella G, Esposito K (2017) Comment on Edelman and Polonsky. Type 2 diabetes in the real world: the elusive nature of glycemic control. Diabetes Care 40:1425–1432. Diabetes Care (2018) 41:e17
281. Monteiro P, Bergenstal RM, Toural E et al (2019) Efficacy and safety of empagliflozin in older patients inthe EMPA-REG OUTCOME® trial. Age Ageing 48:859–866
282. Cahn A, Mosenzon O, Wiviott SD et al (2020) Efficacy and safety of dapagliflozin in the elderly: analysis from the DECLARE-TIMI 58 Study. Diabetes Care 43:468–475
283. Neuen BL, Arnott C, Perkovic V et al (2020) Sodium-glucose co-transporter-2 inhibitors with and without metformin: a meta-analysis of cardiovascular, kidney and mortality outcomes. Diabetes Obes Metab 23(2):382–390. https://doi.org/10.1111/dom.14226
284. Birkeland KI, Bodegard J, Banerjee A et al (2020) Lower cardiorenal risk with sodium-glucose cotransporter-2 inhibitors versus dipeptidyl peptidase-4 inhibitors in patients with type 2 diabetes without cardiovascular and renal diseases: a large multinational observational study. Diabetes Obes Metab 23(1):75–85. https://doi.org/10.1111/dom.14189
285. Fitchett D (2019) A safety update on sodium glucose co-transporter 2 inhibitors. Diabetes Obes Metab 21:34–42

286. Huang CY, Lee JK (2020) Sodium-glucose co-transporter-2 inhibitors and major adverse limb events: a trial-level meta-analysis including 51,713 individuals. Diabetes Obes Metab 22(12):2348–2355. https://doi.org/10.1111/dom.14159
287. Suissa M, Yin H, Yu OHY, Wong SM, Azoulay L (2020) Sodium–glucose cotransporter 2 inhibitors and the short-term risk of breast cancer among women with type 2 diabetes. Diabetes Care 44(1):e9–e11. https://doi.org/10.2337/dc20-1073
288. Docherty KF, Jhund PS, Anand I et al (2020) Effect of dapagliflozin on outpatient worsening of patients with heart failure and reduced ejection fraction: a prespecified analysis of DAPA-HF. Circulation 142:1623–1632
289. Schernthaner G, Shehadeh N, Ametov AS et al (2020) Worldwide inertia to the use of cardiorenal protective glucose-lowering drugs (SGLT2i and GLP-1 RA) in high-risk patients with type 2 diabetes. Cardiovasc Diabetol 19:185
290. Lugner M, Sattar N, Miftaraj M, Ekelund J, Franzén S, Svensson A-M, Eliasson B (2021) Cardiorenal and other diabetes related outcomes with SGLT-2 inhibitors compared to GLP-1 receptor agonists in type 2 diabetes: nationwide observational study. Cardiovasc Diabetol 20(1):67. https://doi.org/10.1186/s12933-021-01258-x
291. Kristensen SL, Rorth R, Jhund PS, Docherty KF, Sattar N, Preiss D et al (2019) Cardiovascular, mortality, and kidney outcomes with GLP-1 receptor agonists in patients with type 2 diabetes: a systematic review and meta-analysis of cardiovascular outcome trials. Lancet Diabetes Endocrinol 7(10):776–785
292. Dietlein M (2019) Management of hyperglycaemia in type 2 diabetes. Consensus Report 2018 by the ADA and EASD. MMW Fortschr Med 161(16):55–56
293. Patoulias D, Katsimardou A, Kalogirou MS, Zografou I, Toumpourleka M, Imprialos K et al (2020) Glucagon-like peptide-1 receptor agonists or sodium–glucose cotransporter-2 inhibitors as add-on therapy for patients with type 2 diabetes? A systematic review and meta-analysis of surrogate metabolic endpoints. Diabetes Metab 46(4):272–279
294. Frías J, Guja C, Hardy E, Ahmed A, Dong F, Öhman P, Jabbour SA (2016) Exenatide once weekly plus dapagliflozin once daily versus exenatide or dapagliflozin alone in patients with type 2 diabetes inadequately controlled with metformin monotherapy (DURATION-8): a 28 week, multicentre, double-blind, phase 3, randomised controlled trial. Lancet Diabetes Endocrinol 4(12):1004–1016
295. Dave CV, Kim SC, Goldfine AB, Glynn RJ, Tong A, Patorno E (2021) Risk of cardiovascular outcomes in patients with type 2 diabetes after addition of SGLT2 inhibitors versus sulfonylureas to baseline GLP-1RA therapy. Circulation 143(8):770–779
296. Singhal R, Hechanova LA (2022) SGLT2 inhibitors: benefits for CKD and cardiovascular disease in type 2 diabetes. Curr Cardiol Rep 24(3):183–189. https://doi.org/10.1007/s11886-022-01637-0
297. Jackson K, Moseley KF (2020) Diabetes and bone fragility: SGLT2 inhibitor use in the context of renal and cardiovascular benefits. Curr Osteoporos Rep 18(5):439–448. https://doi.org/10.1007/s11914-020-00609-z
298. Moayeri A, Mohamadpour M, Mousavi SF, Shirzadpour E, Mohamadpour S, Amraei M (2017) Fracture risk in patients with type 2 diabetes mellitus and possible risk factors: a systematic review and meta-analysis. Ther Clin Risk Manag 13:455–468
299. National diabetes Statistics Report. PDF file (2017) https://dev.diabetes.org/sites/default/files/2019-06/cdc-statistics-report-2017.pdf. Accessed 5 May 2020
300. Strotmeyer ES, Cauley JA, Schwartz AV, Nevitt MC, Resnick HE, Bauer DC et al (2005) Nontraumatic fracture risk with diabetes mellitus and impaired fasting glucose in older white and black adults: the health, aging, and body composition study. Arch Intern Med 165:1612–1617
301. Schwartz AV, Sellmeyer DE, Ensrud KE, Cauley JA, Tabor HK, Schreiner PJ et al (2001) Older women with diabetes have an increased risk of fracture: a prospective study. J Clin Endocrinol Metab 86:32–38
302. Janghorbani M, Feskanich D, Willett WC, Hu F (2006) Prospective study of diabetes and risk of hip fracture: the Nurses' Health Study. Diabetes Care 29:1573–1578

303. Duan Y, Beck TJ, Wang XF, Seeman E (2003) Structural and biomechanical basis of sexual dimorphism in femoral neck fragility has its origins in growth and aging. J Bone Miner Res 18:1766–1774
304. Beck TJ, Oreskovic TL, Stone KL, Ruff CB, Ensrud K, Nevitt MC et al (2001) Structural adaptation to changing skeletal load in the progression toward hip fragility: the study of osteoporotic fractures. J Bone Miner Res 16:1108–1119
305. Barrett-Connor E, Kritz-Silverstein D (1996) Does hyperinsulinemia preserve bone? Diabetes Care 19:1388–1392
306. Thrailkill KM, Lumpkin CK Jr, Bunn RC, Kemp SF, Fowlkes JL (2005) Is insulin an anabolic agent in bone? Dissecting the diabetic bone for clues. Am J Physiol Endocrinol Metab 289:E735–E745
307. van Daele PL, Stolk RP, Burger H, Algra D, Grobbee DE, Hofman A et al (1995) Bone density in noninsulin-dependent diabetes mellitus. The Rotterdam Study. Ann Intern Med 122:409–414
308. Rakic V, Davis WA, Chubb SA et al (2006) Bone mineral density and its determinants in diabetes: the Fremantle Diabetes Study. Diabetologia 49:863–871
309. Schwartz AV, Vittinghoff E, Bauer DC, Hillier TA, Strotmeyer ES, Ensrud KE et al (2011) Association of BMD and FRAX score with risk of fracture in older adults with type 2 diabetes. JAMA 305:2184–2192
310. Montagnani A, Gonnelli S, Alessandri M, Nuti R (2011) Osteoporosis and risk of fracture in patients with diabetes: an update. Aging Clin Exp Res 23:84–90
311. Isidro ML, Ruano B (2010) Bone disease in diabetes. Curr Diabetes Rev 6:144–155
312. Schwartz AV, Sellmeyer DE (2007) Diabetes, fracture, and bone fragility. Curr Osteoporos Rep 5:105–111
313. Wang X, Shen X, Li X, Agrawal CM (2002) Age-related changes in the collagen network and toughness of bone. Bone 31:1–7
314. Viguet-Carrin S, Roux JP, Arlot ME, Merabet Z, Leeming DJ, Byrjalsen I et al (2006) Contribution of the advanced glycation end product pentosidine and of maturation of type I collagen to compressive biomechanical properties of human lumbar vertebrae. Bone 39:1073–1079
315. Saito M, Marumo K (2010) Collagen cross-links as a determinant of bone quality: a possible explanation for bone fragility in aging, osteoporosis, and diabetes mellitus. Osteoporos Int 21:195–214
316. Schwartz AV, Garnero P, Hillier TA, Sellmeyer DE, Strotmeyer ES, Feingold KR et al (2009) Pentosidine and increased fracture risk in older adults with type 2 diabetes. J Clin Endocrinol Metab 94:2380–2386
317. Yamamoto M, Yamaguchi T, Yamauchi M, Yano S, Sugimoto T (2008) Serum pentosidine levels are positively associated with the presence of vertebral fractures in postmenopausal women with type 2 diabetes. J Clin Endocrinol Metab 93:1013–1019
318. Paschou SA, Dede AD, Anagnostis PG, Vryonidou A, Morganstein D, Goulis DG (2017) Type 2 diabetes and osteoporosis: a guide to optimal management. J Clin Endocrinol Metab 102(10):3621–3634
319. Kheniser KG, Polanco Santos CM, Kashyap SR (2018) The effects of diabetes therapy on bone: a clinical perspective. J Diabetes Complications 32(7):713–719
320. Perkovic V, Jardine MJ, Neal B, Bompoint S, Heerspink HJL, Charytan DM et al (2019) CREDENCE Trial Investigators. Canagliflozin and renal outcomes in diabetic nephropathy. N Engl J Med 380(24):2295–2306
321. Watts NB, Bilezikian JP, Usiskin K et al (2016) Effects of canagliflozin on fracture risk in patients with type 2 diabetes mellitus. J Clin Endocrinol Metab 101(1):157–166. Randomized phase 3 study of fracture risk with canagliflozin compared with placebo. Fracture risk was found to be increased with canagliflozin treatment, driven by the CANVAS data; the incidence of fractures was similar in canagliflozin and noncanagliflozin groups in the pooled non-CANVAS studies

322. Li X, Li T, Cheng Y, Lu Y, Xue M, Xu L et al (2019) Effects of SGLT2 inhibitors on fractures and bone mineral density in type 2 diabetes: an updated meta-analysis. Diabetes Metab Res Rev 35(7):e3170. https://doi.org/10.1002/dmrr.3170
323. Tang HL, Li DD, Zhang JJ, Hsu YH, Want TS, Zhai SD et al (2016) Lack of evidence for a harmful effect of sodium-glucose co-transporter 2 (SGLT2) inhibitors on fracture risk among type 2 diabetes patients: a network and cumulative meta-analysis of randomized controlled trials. Diabetes Obes Metab 18(12):1199–1206
324. Ruanpeng D, Ungprasert P, Sangtian J, Harindhanavudhi T (2017) Sodium-glucose cotransporter 2 (SGLT2) inhibitors and fracture risk in patients with type 2 diabetes mellitus: a meta-analysis. Diabetes Metab Res Rev 33(6). https://doi.org/10.1002/dmrr.2903
325. Cheng L, Li YY, Hu W, Bai F, Hao HR, Yu WN et al (2019) Risk of bone fracture associated with sodium-glucose cotransporter-2 inhibitor treatment: a meta-analysis of randomized controlled trials. Diabetes Metab 45(5):436–445. This large meta-analysis of over 20,000 patients across 30 studies did not find evidence that individual SGLT2 inhibitors were associated with increased risk of bone fracture compared with placebo
326. Ye Y, Zhao C, Liang J, Yang Y, Yu M, Qu X (2018) Effect of sodium-glucose co-transporter 2 inhibitors on bone metabolism and fracture risk. Front Pharmacol 9:1517
327. Taylor SI, Blau JE, Rother KI (2015) Possible adverse effects of SGLT2 inhibitors on bone. Lancet Diabetes Endocrinol 3:8–10
328. Kwon H. Canagliflozin: clinical efficacy and safety. Endocrinology and Metabolic Drugs Advisory Committee Meeting 2013. www.fda.gov/downloads/AdvisoryCommittees/CommitteesMeetingMaterials/Drugs/EndocrinologicandMetabolicDrugsAdvisoryCommittee/UCM336234.pdf . Accessed 5 May 2020
329. Blau JE, Taylor SI (2018) Adverse effects of SGLT2 inhibitors on bone. Nat Rev Nephrol 14(8):473–474
330. Bilezikian JP, Watts NB, Usiskin K, Polidori D, Fung A, Sullivan D et al (2016) Evaluation of bone mineral density and bone biomarkers in patients with type 2 diabetes treated with canagliflozin. J Clin Endocrinol Metab 101:44–51
331. Zibellini J, Seimon RV, Lee CM, Gibson AA, Hsu MS, Shapses SA et al (2015) Does diet-induced weight loss lead to bone loss in overweight or obese adults? A systematic review and meta-analysis of clinical trials. J Bone Miner Res 30:2168–2178
332. American Diabetes Association (2020) 4. Comprehensive medical evaluation and assessment of comorbidities: standards of medical care in diabetes-2020. Diabetes Care 43(Suppl 1):S37–S47
333. Thomas MC, Cherney DZI (2018) The actions of SGLT2 inhibitors on metabolism, renal function and blood pressure. Diabetologia 61:2098–2107. https://doi.org/10.1007/s00125-018-4669-0
334. Roden M, Weng J, Eilbracht J, Delafont B, Kim G, Woerle HJ et al (2013) Empagliflozin monotherapy with sitagliptin as an active comparator in patients with type 2 diabetes: a randomised, double-blind, placebo-controlled, phase 3 trial. Lancet Diabetes Endocrinol 1(3):208–219
335. Bujac S, Del Parigi A, Sugg J et al (2014) Patient characteristics are not associated with clinically important differential response to dapagliflozin: a staged analysis of phase 3 data. Diab Ther 5:471–482
336. Abe T, Matsubayashi Y, Yoshida A et al (2018) Predictors of the response of HbA1c and body weight after SGLT2 inhibition. Diabete Metab 44:172–174
337. Cai X, Yang W, Gao X, Chen Y, Zhou L, Zhang S et al (2018) The Association between the dosage of SGLT2 inhibitor and weight reduction in type 2 diabetes patients: a meta-analysis. Obesity (Silver Spring, Md) 26(1):70–80
338. Brady JA, Hallow KM (2017) Model-based evaluation of proximal sodium reabsorption through SGLT2 in health and diabetes and the effect of inhibition with canagliflozin. J Clin Pharmacol 58(3):377–385. https://doi.org/10.1002/jcph.1030

339. Cherney DZI, Cooper ME, Tikkanen I, Pfarr E, Johansen OE, Woerle HJ et al (2018) Pooled analysis of Phase III trials indicate contrasting influences of renal function on blood pressure, body weight, and HbA1c reductions with empagliflozin. Kidney Int 93(1):231–244
340. Ferrannini E, Baldi S, Frascerra S et al (2017) Renal handling of ketones in response to sodium-glucose cotransporter 2 inhibition in patients with type 2 diabetes. Diabetes Care 40:771–776
341. Tanaka H, Takano K, Iijima H, Kubo H, Maruyama N, Hashimoto T et al (2017) Factors affecting canagliflozin-induced transient urine volume increase in patients with type 2 diabetes mellitus. Adv Ther 34(2):436–451

Chapter 4
SGLT2 Inhibitors: Emerging Opportunities for the Treatment of Myocardial Infarction

Mukesh Nandave

Introduction by the Editor

The relationship between SGLT2i and myocardial infarction has the most research out of all the anti-diabetic drugs. According to several investigations, SGLT2i has been proven to provide cardiorenal advantages in diabetic individuals with severe kidney disease and heart failure, as shown in Fig. 4.1. SGLT2i aids in lowering the risk of cardiorenal disease mortality in diabetes individuals with a history of myocardial infarction.

SGLT2i, corresponding empagliflozin, canagliflozin, and the newly developed dapagliflozin have produced positive outcomes in diabetic individuals with chronic heart failure and a condensed ejection fraction. This has sparked an impressive interest in researching brief cardiac mechanisms associated with clinical aids and drawn more consideration of SGLT2i in several cardiovascular events. There are few experimental studies on SGLT2i therapy for myocardial infarction. The clinical and preclinical effects of SGLT2i are the subject of this chapter, which also provides a brief description of ongoing trials. It concentrates on the information that is currently known about the effects of SGLT2i in myocardial infarction patients.

Approximately 29 clinical investigations, consisting of 4 trials in Phase IV, 13 trials in Phase III trials, and 4 in Phase II, have been published regarding the regular use of SGLT2i to treat myocardial infarction. The most recent status of all trials involving SGLT2i used to treat myocardial infarction is displayed in clinical trials Table 4.1. These trials were chosen from the clinical trials database based on how SGLT2i interacted with patients at risk of heart failure to prevent myocardial infarction.

M. Nandave (✉)
Department of Pharmacology and Pharmaceutical Biotechnology, Delhi Pharmaceutical Sciences and Research University (DPSRU), New Delhi, Delhi, India

M. Nandave (ed.), *Sodium-glucose Cotransporter-2 (SGLT2) Inhibitors in Heart Failure*, https://doi.org/10.1007/978-981-97-7568-2_4

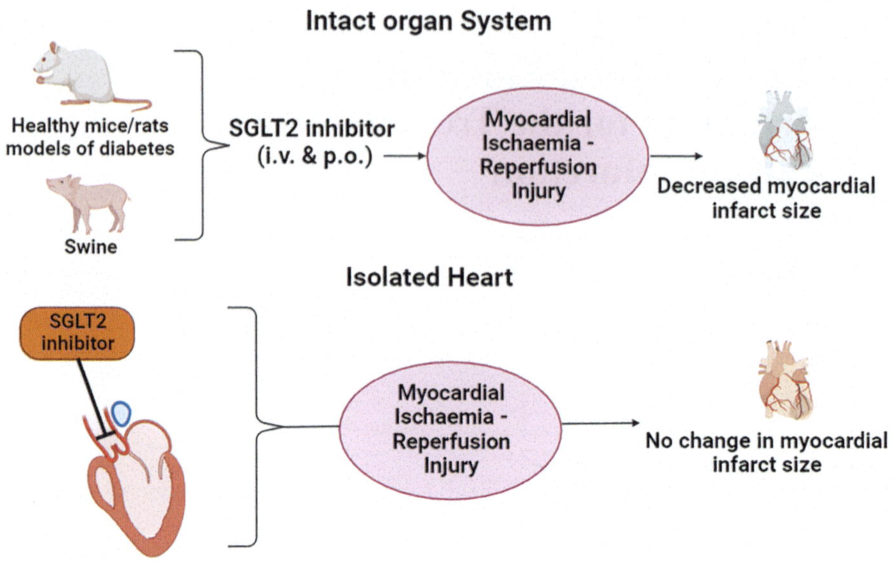

Fig. 4.1 SGLT2i reduces myocardial infarct size in preclinical animal models of myocardial ischemia-reperfusion injury

Regarding T2D, nephropathy, and chronic HF, the suggestion for SGLT2i as the most recent cohort of cardiorenal protective medicines is growing and comparable to (renin-angiotensin-aldosterone system) RAAS inhibitor treatment. A cohort at high risk for primary and advanced HF or cardiac mortality includes those with complex acute myocardial infarction (MI).

These individuals have a clear unmet need for additional risk reduction while receiving current medical treatment, especially in the important early stages after an acute MI to stop unfavorable cardiac remodeling, chronic HF, and cardiac mortality. Patients with acute MI may benefit especially from the possible molecular benefits of SGLT2i medication. Contrary to popular belief, acute MI patients have, up to this point, received very little attention in SGLT2i outcome studies. As a result, research is still being done to determine the effectiveness and safety of starting SGLT2i early, within days after an acute MI. The ordinary therapy for this frequent cardiovascular illness that entails significant morbidity and mortality will undergo another paradigm change if SGLT2 inhibition for acute MI is successful [1].

Machine Generated Summaries

Disclaimer: The summaries in this chapter were generated from Springer Nature publications using extractive AI auto-summarization: An extraction-based summarizer aims to identify the most important sentences of a text using an algorithm and

Table 4.1 Summary of current status of phase 4 clinical trials of SGLT2i-associated myocardial infarction

	Objective	Sponsor ID	Intervention	Phase	Descriptions
Based on cardiac infarction and remodelling in individuals susceptible for heart failure	To determine the efficacy of SGLT-2i via lowering the myocardial remodeling and infarction size in patients having chances of heart failure and mild myocardial infarction	NCT04899479	SGLT2i + Control	IV	The safety and effectiveness of SGLT-2i may be ascertained by CMR measures, which also show that it reduces the causes and severity of myocardial remodelling and infarction
	Dapagliflozin is expected to lessen left ventricular remodeling in individuals who have experienced a myocardial infarction, according to the main hypothesis of the research	NCT04783870	Dapagliflozin + Placebo	Phase IV	SGLT2i has been demonstrated to reduce remodeling in individuals with heart failure. The current trial will investigate the idea that in individuals who have experienced a myocardial infarction (<7 days), dapagliflozin will lessen left ventricular remodeling
	To compare dapagliflozin to a placebo in terms of how patients with acute myocardial infarction fare in the short term	NCT05050500	Dapagliflozin + Placebo	IV	These studies suggest that dapagliflozin may be beneficial for individuals experiencing an acute myocardial infarction
	To assess the clinical effect of cardiovascular mortality or deteriorating heart failure by comparing the effects of dapagliflozin against placebo when started in the hospital	NCT04363697	Dapagliflozin + Placebo	IV	Dapagliflozin may reduce the mortality of CV patients who have been stabilized during hospitalization

uses those original sentences to create the auto-summary (unlike generative AI). As the constituted sentences are machine selected, they may not fully reflect the body of the work, so we strongly advise that the original content is read and cited. The auto generated summaries were curated by the editor to meet Springer Nature publication standards. To cite this content, please refer to the original papers.

Machine generated keywords: sglti, ami, hospitalisation, tdm, hfref, antidiabetic drug, acute myocardial, ketone, sgltis, fatty, ischemia, fatty acid, acute, dcm, without diabetes.

SGLT2 Inhibitors: New Hope for the Treatment of Acute Myocardial Infarction? [2]

This is a machine-generated summary of:

Wu, Yu-Jie; Wang, Si-Bo; Wang, Lian-Sheng: SGLT2 Inhibitors: New Hope for the Treatment of Acute Myocardial Infarction? [2].

Published in: American Journal of Cardiovascular Drugs (2022).

Link to original: https://doi.org/10.1007/s40256-022-00545-6

If you want to cite the papers, please refer to the original.

For technical reasons we could not place the page where the original quote is coming from.

Abstract-Summary "Experimental and clinical data on SGLT2i treatment after AMI is limited."

"This is a review of the clinical and preclinical effects of SGLT2i, focusing on available data on the effects of SGLT2i in AMI patients with a brief overview of ongoing trials."

Introduction

"The role of SGLT2i on patients with heart failure (HF) is confirmed, especially for those with reduced ejection fraction (HFrEF), while an increasing number of studies try to fill the gap in the field of acute myocardial infarction (AMI)."

"Complications are one of the major risk factors after AMI, including DM, renal failure, and so on [3]."

"Although the current treatment of AMI can improve survival, the existence of DM may increase mortality (the fatality rate) during the whole phase of AMI."

"Within the infarcted area, acute ischemia can lead to energy depletion and risk of irreversible necrotic cell damage and neurohumoral response triggered by AMI, mainly driven by an upregulation of the renin-angiotensin-aldosterone system and activation of the sympathetic nervous system."

"Among the new antidiabetic drugs, we will review all experimental and the latest clinical studies related to SGLT2i to explore whether SGLT2i has an effect on AMI and, if so, how it may be achieved."

Mechanism of Sodium-Glucose Cotransporter 2 Inhibitors

"Despite the lack of direct evidence on AMI models, these results obtained in studies on HF and DM models could help explain the beneficial effects of SGLT2i in AMI patients that we observed in clinical studies."

"The EMBODY trial [4], which evaluated the effect of empagliflozin on cardiac sympathetic and parasympathetic activity in patients with T2DM combined with AMI, showed that SGLT2i was effective in improving cardiac neural activity as assessed by surrogate markers of sudden cardiac death (SCD), HRV, and heart rate turbulence (HRT)."

"A meta-analysis of randomized controlled trials [5] which included a total of 62 studies and comprised 34,941 patients found that the SGLT2 inhibitors (empagliflozin, canagliflozin, dapagliflozin, tofogliflozin, luseogliflozin or ipragliflozin) significantly decreased SUA levels compared with control and the effect persisted during long-term treatment."

Clinical Trials from 2017 to 2024

"The EMBODY trial is a prospective, multicenter, randomized, placebo-controlled, double-blind trial designed to investigate the effects of empagliflozin versus placebo on cardiac sympathetic activity in AMI patients with T2DM."

"As the first clinical randomized trial to provide data on the effect of empagliflozin on cardiac sympathetic and parasympathetic activity in patients with T2DM and AMI, the EMBODY trial showed that early SGLT2i administration might be effective in improving cardiac nerve activity without any adverse events."

"In patients with AMI and T2DM, whether the combination of empagliflozin with standard AMI therapy was related to a reduction in LV mass and favorable changes in diastolic function parameters compared with patients without SGLT2i initiation therapy still needed further investigation with a large sample size."

"These trials focus mainly on the effectiveness of empagliflozin on cardiac-renal injury, hospitalization for HF, and mortality in patients with AMI."

Adverse Effect of SGLT2i

"SGLT2i are a class of novel antidiabetic drugs with positive effects on the cardiovascular and kidney systems; however, traces of SGLT2i side effects have been found in several clinical studies of SGLT2i in patients with cardiovascular disease with or without DM."

"An adverse effect reported by major trial CANVAS is that canagliflozin seems to raise the risk of amputations of toes, feet, and legs [6]."

"The occurrence of toe amputations shows the same trend."

"Although the current evidence does not suggest a class effect, the increased risk of amputation is confined only to canagliflozin."

"Another common adverse effect is mycotic genitourinary infections, and all agents (canagliflozin, empagliflozin, and dapagliflozin) increase the risk [7–9]."

Conclusion

"Despite numerous studies showing that downregulation of SGLT1 reduces myocardial nitrogen oxidative stress and inflammatory responses [10, 11] and improves cardiac function, it remains to be determined whether SGLT1 inhibitors provide more cardiovascular benefit than SGLT2i."

"Although most studies have shown a clear ameliorative effect of SGLT2i on AMI, some studies [12] claimed that the addition of SGLT2i to myocardial perfusion fluid didn't directly reduce the size of MI, but the oral administration of canagliflozin for 4 weeks could effectively reduce the size of myocardial infarcts, which made us think deeply about what mode of administration could maximize the protective effect of SGLT2i on the heart."

"Regardless of the mode of administration, most of the investigators concluded that the cardiovascular protection of SGLT2i didn't reduce the occurrence of AMI, but rather improved the immediate and long-term survival after AMI by ameliorating the myocardial damage caused by these events through direct cytoprotective effects, thereby reducing the progression of ischemic cardiomyopathy and heart failure."

SGLT-2 Inhibitors and In-Stent Restenosis-Related Events After Acute Myocardial Infarction: An Observational Study in Patients with Type 2 Diabetes [13]

This is a machine-generated summary of:

Marfella, Raffaele; Sardu, Celestino; D'Onofrio, Nunzia; Fumagalli, Carlo; Scisciola, Lucia; Sasso, Ferdinando Carlo; Siniscalchi, Mario; Marfella, Ludovica Vittoria; D'Andrea, Davide; Minicucci, Fabio; Signoriello, Giuseppe; Cesaro,

Arturo; Trotta, Maria Consiglia; Frigé, Chiara; Prattichizzo, Francesco; Balestrieri, Maria Luisa; Ceriello, Antonio; Calabrò, Paolo; Mauro, Ciro; del Viscovo, Luca; Paolisso, Giuseppe: SGLT-2 inhibitors and in-stent restenosis-related events after acute myocardial infarction: an observational study in patients with type 2 diabetes [13].

Published in: BMC Medicine (2023).

Link to original: https://doi.org/10.1186/s12916-023-02781-2

If you want to cite the papers, please refer to the original.

For technical reasons we could not place the page where the original quote is coming from.

Abstract-Summary "No study evaluated the incidence of intra-stent restenosis (ISR)-related events in patients with type 2 diabetes (T2DM) and acute myocardial infarction (AMI) treated or not with sodium/glucose cotransporter 2 inhibitors (SGLT2i)."

"Glycemic control was similar in SGLT2i-treated patients and never SGLT2i-users."

"The incidence of ISR-related MACE was higher in never SGLT2i-users compared with SGLT2i-treated patients, an effect independent of glycemic status (HR = 0.418, 95% CI = 0.241–0.725, P = 0.002) and observed also in the subgroup of patients with HbA1c < 7% (HR = 0.393, 95% CI = 0.157–0.984, P = 0.027)."

"In patients without the event, the stent patency was greater in SGLT2i-treated patients compared with never SGLT2i-users at 1-year follow-up."

"SGLT2i treatment in T2DM is associated with a reduced incidence of ISR-related events, independently of glycemic control."

Background

“Patients with type 2 diabetes (T2DM) have an accelerated rate of late loss of lumen diameter and an increased incidence of intra-stent restenosis (ISR) [14, 15], with T2DM being an independent predictor of recurrent restenosis [16, 17].”

“Although several large clinical trials have convincingly demonstrated that sodium-glucose co-transporter2 inhibitors (SGLT2i) improve cardiovascular outcomes in both T2DM and non-DM patients [18] and atherosclerosis progression [19], no data are available investigating the effects of SGLT2i on intra-stent restenosis in patients with AMI treated with revascularization and the possible relationships with glycemic status.”

“We evaluated whether SGLT2i therapy is associated with lower rates of ISR-related events independently of glycemic control in T2DM patients with acute myocardial infarction (AMI).”

Methods

“The current SGLT2i-users were patients with ongoing SGLT2i therapy without discontinuation for at least 6 months before AMI and continued SGLT2i therapy without discontinuation during the follow-up.”

“PCI was performed via the femoral or radial approach after an intravenous bolus dose of heparin (50–100 U/kg) to achieve an activated clotting time of > 250 s. DAPT (a combination of aspirin 100 mg/day with clopidogrel 75 mg/day or ticagrelor 90 mg twice daily or prasugrel 5–10 mg/day) was recommended for > 12 months for patients who underwent PCI.”

“Coronary CT angiography (CCTA) was performed in all patients at 1-year follow-up.”

“Datasets of each coronary CCTA examination were transferred to an image-processing workstation (VitreaTM Advanced Visualization, Canon Medical Europe) and analyzed by 2 readers, both with > 10 years of clinical experience in coronary CTA performance and analysis, blinded to the clinical findings.”

Results

“There were no differences in the mean age, BMI, sex distribution, smoking habits, HbA1c, admission glucose level, plasma cholesterol, and triglyceride levels among the groups.”

“Multiple logistic regression was then performed to evaluate the relationship between the use of SGLT-2i and ISR-related MACE, adjusted for glycemic control (admission HbA1c and 1-year HbA1c mean), age, BMI, and sex.”

“The probability of ISR-related MACE in patients treated with SGLT2i was reduced by 58 % regardless of glycemic control, age, BMI, and sex (OR, 0.42; 95% CI, 0.23–0.76).”

"To evaluate whether SGLT2i therapy was effective in patients with good glycemic control (1-year HbA1c mean < 7%), we performed a Cox regression analysis in this subgroup of patients, adjusted for admission age, hypertension, cigarette smoking, BMI, HDL, LDL-cholesterol levels, triglycerides, antithrombotic, and lipid-lowering and glucose-lowering therapies."

Discussion

"The effect of SGLT2i treatment on ISR outcomes was independent of the glycated hemoglobin levels at admission and during 1-year follow-up, thus suggesting that the benefit observed with SGLT2 inhibition on coronary reperfusion might be independent of their glucose-lowering properties."

"For the first time, our data evidenced a reduction in ISR-related events in patients with T2DM and acute coronary syndrome treated with SGLT2i."

"The SGLT2i results on ISR were independent of glycemic control suggesting that SGLT2 inhibitors might favorably affect the coronary remodeling after stent implantation, possibly through the regulation of a large range of metabolic, molecular, and hemodynamic mechanisms irrespectively of their glucose-lowering effects [19–21]."

"These data might suggest that the anti-inflammatory effect of SGLT2i eventually contribute to their putative protective effect against restenosis."

"Consistently, our data suggest also that the protective effect of SGLT2i on ISR-related MACE is maintained in the subgroup of patients with good glycemic control."

Conclusions

"The use of SGLT2i is associated with a reduced incidence of cardiovascular events related to ISR in patients with diabetes."

"The SGLT2i protective effects extend beyond glycemic control, suggesting their potential use in a larger range of patients."

"Clinical trials are clearly needed to substantiate the findings of this study while future studies characterizing the functional, metabolic, and molecular actions of SGLT2i in the vasculature might furnish insights into how these drugs eventually prevent the development of ISR-related events, overall providing the foundation and the rationale for a potential use of SGLT2i to prevent ISR in AMI patients with and, eventually, without diabetes."

The Role of Combined SGLT1/SGLT2 Inhibition in Reducing the Incidence of Stroke and Myocardial Infarction in Patients with Type 2 Diabetes Mellitus [22]

This is a machine-generated summary of:

Pitt, Bertram; Steg, Gabriel; Leiter, Lawrence A.; Bhatt, Deepak L.: The Role of Combined SGLT1/SGLT2 Inhibition in Reducing the Incidence of Stroke and Myocardial Infarction in Patients with Type 2 Diabetes Mellitus [22].

Published in: Cardiovascular Drugs and Therapy (2021).

Link to original: https://doi.org/10.1007/s10557-021-07291-y

If you want to cite the papers, please refer to the original.

For technical reasons we could not place the page where the original quote is coming from.

Abstract-Summary "This paper will briefly compare the effect of SGLT2is and GLP-1 RAs to that of the SGLT1/2 inhibitor sotagliflozin on the incidence of myocardial infarction (MI) and stroke in patients with T2DM and further postulate mechanisms to account for these findings."

"The results from SCORED and SOLOIST (trials studying the SGLT1/2 inhibitor sotagliflozin) suggest that an increase in SGLT1 inhibition when added to SGLT2 inhibition may contribute to reductions in MI and stroke in patients with T2DM."

"Larger and longer studies are required to confirm the effectiveness of SGLT1/SGLT2 inhibition in reducing MI and stroke in patients with T2DM and elucidate the mechanisms associated with this finding."

"The role of SGLT1/2 inhibition as an addition to GLP-1 RAs in patients with and without T2DM at increased risk for MI and stroke requires further study."

[Section 1]

"The recent findings from the SCORED (10,584 patients with type 2 diabetes and CKD randomized to sotagliflozin or placebo) and SOLOIST (1222 patients with type 2 diabetes admitted with worsening heart failure randomized to sotagliflozin or placebo) trials suggest that like SGLT2is, SGLT1/2 s reduce the composite of deaths from cardiovascular causes, hospitalization for heart failure, and urgent visits for heart failure but may provide greater reduction in MI and stroke [23, 24]."

"This paper will briefly compare the effect of SGLT2is and GLP-1 RAs to that of the SGLT1/2 inhibitor sotagliflozin on the incidence of MI and stroke in patients with type 2 diabetes and further postulate mechanisms associated with SGLT1 inhibition that could account for these findings."

"The role of SGLT1/2 inhibition with sotagliflozin as an addition to GLP-1 RA in patients with and without type 2 diabetes at increased risk for stroke and MI remains to be studied."

Impact of the SGLT2-Inhibitor Empagliflozin on Inflammatory Biomarkers After Acute Myocardial Infarction—A Post-hoc Analysis of the EMMY Trial [25]

This is a machine-generated summary of:

Benedikt, Martin; Mangge, Harald; Aziz, Faisal; Curcic, Pero; Pailer, Sabine; Herrmann, Markus; Kolesnik, Ewald; Tripolt, Norbert J.; Pferschy, Peter N.; Wallner, Markus; Zirlik, Andreas; Sourij, Harald; von Lewinski, Dirk: Impact of the SGLT2-inhibitor empagliflozin on inflammatory biomarkers after acute myocardial infarction—a post-hoc analysis of the EMMY trial [25].

Published in: Cardiovascular Diabetology (2023).

Link to original: https://doi.org/10.1186/s12933-023-01904-6

If you want to cite the papers, please refer to the original.

For technical reasons we could not place the page where the original quote is coming from.

Abstract-Summary "The EMMY trial was the first to show a significant reduction in NTproBNP levels as well as improved cardiac structure and function in post-AMI patients treated with Empagliflozin compared to placebo."

"The EMMY trial is an investigator-initiated, multicentre, double-blind, placebo-controlled trial, which enrolled patients after AMI, receiving either 10 mg Empagliflozin once daily or placebo over a period of 26 weeks on top of standard guideline-recommended therapy starting within 72 h after percutaneous coronary intervention."

"In this post-hoc subgroup analysis of the EMMY trial, we investigated inflammatory biomarkers of 374 patients."

"The endpoints investigated were the mean change in inflammatory biomarkers such as high-sensitive c-reactive protein (hsCRP), interleukin-6 (IL-6), neutrophils, leukocytes, neutrophile/lymphocyte ratio (NLR) and platelet to lymphocyte ratio (PLR) from baseline to 26 weeks."

"At week 26, a significant mean reduction in inflammatory biomarkers was observed, being 35.1 ± 3.2% ($p < 0.001$) for IL-6, 57.4 ± 0.7% ($p < 0.001$) for hsCRP, 26.1 ± 0.7% ($p <0.001$) for neutrophils, 20.5 ± 0.6% ($p < 0.001$) for leukocytes, 10.22 ± 0.50% ($p < 0.001$) for NLR, and − 2.53 ± 0.92% for PLR ($p = 0.006$) with no significant difference between Empagliflozin and placebo treatment."

Introduction

"Apart from the molecular associations, specific blood cells, like neutrophils and leukocytes, were also identified to be an independent predictor for cardiovascular outcome showing positive correlations to infarct size and Troponin T levels, negative correlations were observed for the left ventricular ejection fraction (LVEF) [26–28]."

"The SGLT2-I AMI Protect registry showed that chronic application of sodium glucose linked transporter 2 inhibitors (SGLT2-I) significantly lowered inflammatory parameters at the time of admission and 24 h after AMI in patients with diabetes as compared to other oral anti-hyperglycaemic agents as a significant predictor of reduced inflammatory response (OR 0.457, 95% CI 0.275–0.758, $p = 0.002$) levels."

"The EMMY trial showed a significant reduction in NTproBNP levels in patients with acute coronary syndrome for Empagliflozin compared to placebo, independent of diabetes status [29]."

Materials and Methods

"In this post-hoc analysis, the outcome variables were inflammatory biomarkers (leukocytes, interleukin-6, hsCRP, neutrophil granulocytes, neutrophil-to-lymphocyte ratio) defined as mean changes from baseline to 26 weeks."

"Explanatory variables in this post-hoc analysis include age, sex, treatment groups (Empagliflozin vs. placebo), hypertension, T2DM, smoking behaviour, NTproBNP, systolic function (LVEF), and diastolic function (E/E'), smoking status, body mass index (BMI), estimated glomerular filtration rate (eGFR), and lipid status."

"A complete case analysis of the inflammatory biomarkers in all patients participating in the EMMY trial with available frozen biomarker samples for all visits was performed."

"A linear mixed effect model (LMEM) was established to analyse mean and percentage changes in inflammatory biomarker levels over visits including correlations with explanatory clinical variables (age, sex, T2DM, hyperlipidemia, smoking behavior, BMI, and hypertension) and biomarkers (functional cardiac parameters, eGFR, and NTproBNP)."

Results

"Inflammatory biomarkers decreased in both groups from baseline up to 26 weeks showing significant mean reduction of $35.1 \pm 3.2\%$ ($p < 0.001$) for IL-6, $57.4 \pm 0.7\%$ ($p < 0.001$) for hsCRP, $26.1 \pm 0.7\%$ (0.001) for neutrophils, $20.5 \pm 0.6\%$ ($p < 0.001$) for leukocytes, $10.2 \pm 0.5\%$ ($p < 0.001$) for NLR, and $-2.53 \pm 0.92\%$ for PLR ($p = 0.006$), but no significant difference between the Empagliflozin group and placebo was noted after 26 weeks."

"Univariable linear mixed effect analysis of inflammatory biomarkers showed significant correlations of IL-6, hsCRP, and NLR with NTproBNP levels ($p < 0.001$) and high-sensitive troponin T ($p < 0.001$), LVEF was only observed to be significantly correlated with hsCRP ($p < 0.001$) and IL-6 ($p < 0.001$)."

Discussion

"The post-hoc analysis showed elevated inflammatory biomarkers when initially presenting with AMI and showed a significant decrease up to 26 weeks, however, this effect was already evident at week 6."

"The only available data regarding the effects of SGLT2-inhibitors on inflammatory biomarkers in acute myocardial infarction derive from the SGLT2-I AMI Protect international registry, which investigated the impact of chronic SGLT2-I treatment on inflammatory biomarkers in patients with diabetes presenting with AMI."

"Patients with diabetes, receiving SGLT2-I, were identified to have lower initial NLR in AMI as well as smaller infarct size [30]; however, the EMMY sub-analysis did not exhibit such differences in NLR between Empagliflozin and placebo group post-MI."

"Inflammation plays a crucial role in ventricular cardiac remodeling [31] and numerous reactants as well as immune cells are involved in this complex process [31–35], but no difference in trajectories of inflammatory biomarkers between the SGLT2-inhibitor Empagliflozin and placebo was observed in the EMMY subgroup-analysis."

Conclusion

"The results of the recently published EMMY trial presented first evidence for the administration of SGLT2-I after AMI in addition to guideline-recommended post-MI therapy showing significant reduction in NTproBNP levels at weeks 26 compared to placebo independent of diabetic status."

"In this post-hoc analysis, a great extend in inflammatory biomarkers was identified at initial presentation with AMI with a significant decline up to week 26 that was already evident at week 6."

"No difference between SGLT2-I and placebo was observed with regards to inflammatory biomarkers suggesting that inflammatory response post-MI is not significantly altered by Empagliflozin."

Characterization of Left Ventricular Myocardial Sodium-Glucose Cotransporter 1 Expression in Patients with End-Stage Heart Failure [36]

This is a machine-generated summary of:

Sayour, Alex Ali; Oláh, Attila; Ruppert, Mihály; Barta, Bálint András; Horváth, Eszter Mária; Benke, Kálmán; Pólos, Miklós; Hartyánszky, István; Merkely, Béla; Radovits, Tamás: Characterization of left ventricular myocardial sodium-glucose cotransporter 1 expression in patients with end-stage heart failure [36].

Published in: Cardiovascular Diabetology (2020).

Link to original: https://doi.org/10.1186/s12933-020-01141-1

If you want to cite the papers, please refer to the original.

For technical reasons we could not place the page where the original quote is coming from.

Abstract-Summary "Despite its clinical relevance, data are scarce regarding left ventricular (LV) SGLT1 expression in distinct heart failure (HF) pathologies."

"We aimed to characterize LV SGLT1 expression in human patients with end-stage HF, in context of the other two major glucose transporters: GLUT1 and GLUT4."

"We measured LV SGLT1, GLUT1 and GLUT4 gene expressions with qRT-PCR."

"Compared with controls, LV SGLT1 mRNA and protein expressions were significantly and comparably upregulated in HF patients with DCM, IHD and IHD + T2DM (all $P < 0.05$), but not in HCM."

"LV SGLT1 mRNA and protein expressions positively correlated with LVEDD and negatively correlated with EF (all $P < 0.01$)."

"Whereas AMPKα phosphorylation was positively associated with SGLT1 protein expression, ERK1/2 phosphorylation showed a negative correlation (both $P < 0.01$)."

"CRT was associated with reduction of LV SGLT1 expression, especially in patients with DCM."

"Myocardial LV SGLT1 is upregulated in patients with HF (except in those with HCM), correlates significantly with parameters of cardiac remodeling (LVEDD) and systolic function (EF), and is downregulated in DCM patients with CRT."

"The possible role of SGLT1 in LV remodeling needs to be elucidated."

Introduction

"Recent cardiovascular outcome trials in patients with type 2 diabetes mellitus (T2DM) [6–12, 14–21, 23, 24, 26–35, 37–39], and dedicated heart failure (HF) trials in patients with HF and reduced ejection fraction (HFrEF) with or without T2DM [40–42] have demonstrated a consistently significant reduction in hospitalization for HF with SGLT2 inhibitor treatment versus placebo."

"The currently marketed SGLT2 inhibitors are selective for SGLT2 over SGLT1 to different extent, of which canagliflozin is capable of slightly inhibiting SGLT1 in the small intestine at clinically relevant doses [43, 44]."

"Dual SGLT1/2 inhibitors have been developed to reduce postprandial glucose absorption via blockade of SGLT1 in the small intestine, while at the same time preserving the beneficial renal glucosuric effect by SGLT2 inhibition [45]."

"The dual SGLT1/2 inhibitor sotagliflozin is currently being tested in cardiovascular outcome trial in patients with T2DM [45, 46]."

"Its expression needs to be further characterized in patients with end-stage HF of distinct etiologies in order to better predict and understand the putative direct cardiac effects of SGLT1 inhibition in these patient groups."

Materials and Methods

"Myocardial LV samples from end-stage HF patients (n = 71) were collected during heart transplantation (HTx) from the diseased hearts of the recipients immediately after explantation."

"End-stage HF patients not receiving CRT (n = 44): a. Hypertrophic cardiomyopathy (HCM, n = 7): severe LV hypertrophy; absence of relevant comorbidities (hypertension, T2DM); no relevant coronary atherosclerosis b. Dilated cardiomyopathy (DCM, n = 12): severe LV dilation not explained by valvular disease; no history of myocarditis; no relevant comorbidities (hypertension, T2DM); no relevant coronary atherosclerosis c. Ischemic heart disease (IHD, n = 14): severe diffuse coronary atherosclerosis at multiple sites, with or without prior revascularization therapy; no T2DM as comorbidity d. Ischemic heart disease and T2DM (IHD-T2DM, n = 11): severe diffuse coronary atherosclerosis at multiple sites, with or without prior revascularization therapy; T2DM as comorbidity 3."

"Myocardial LV tissue samples were homogenized in RIPA buffer (Bio-Rad Laboratories, Hercules, CA, USA) containing protease and phosphatase inhibitor cocktail (Roche, Basel, Switzerland), using Bertin Precellys 24 Tissue Homogenizer with Bertin Cryolys cooling system (Bertin Technologies)."

Results

"We found no detectable LV SGLT2 mRNA expression in any of the studied groups (data not depicted)."

"We investigated the effect of CRT on mRNA expression of SGLT1, GLUT1 and GLUT4 in LV samples from patients with DCM, IHD and IHD-T2DM."

"According to ANCOVA, this difference remained significant even after adjusting for age, sex, and BMI (estimated marginal means: 1.515 ± 0.205 vs. 0.774 ± 0.219, P = 0.048)."

Discussion

"This is the first study to provide a comprehensive evaluation of myocardial LV SGLT1 expression in context of the other two major myocardial glucose transporters, GLUT1 and GLUT4, in a relatively large number of myocardial LV human samples representing patients with end-stage HF."

"We observed that non-diabetic and diabetic IHD patients showed comparable upregulation of LV SGLT1 expressions, indicating that T2DM itself might not further increase the already elevated SGLT1 expression in HF."

"This reduced ERK1/2 phosphorylation in patients with HF was accompanied by the counter-upregulation of SGLT1 expression, showing significant negative correlation."

"We found that despite a ~ twofold upregulation of SGLT1, the mRNA expression of GLUT1 was only slightly increased compared with controls (after adjusting for baseline characteristics) and we found no correlation between SGLT1 and GLUT1 expressions in end-stage HF patients."

Conclusions

"LV SGLT1 expression shows etiology-dependent alterations in human patients with end-stage HF, and correlates significantly with LV dilation and with the deterioration of LV systolic function."

"AMPK and ERK1/2 might play antagonistic role in the regulation of SGLT1 expression."

"The potential causal role of SGLT1 in HF development and whether its pharmacological blockade exerts cardioprotection need to be further elucidated."

Inhibition of Sodium–Glucose Cotransporter-2 Preserves Cardiac Function During Regional Myocardial Ischemia Independent of Alterations in Myocardial Substrate Utilization [47]

This is a machine-generated summary of:

Baker, Hana E.; Kiel, Alexander M.; Luebbe, Samuel T.; Simon, Blake R.; Earl, Conner C.; Regmi, Ajit; Roell, William C.; Mather, Kieren J.; Tune, Johnathan D.; Goodwill, Adam G.: Inhibition of sodium–glucose cotransporter-2 preserves cardiac function during regional myocardial ischemia independent of alterations in myocardial substrate utilization [47].

Published in: Basic Research in Cardiology (2019).

Link to original: https://doi.org/10.1007/s00395-019-0733-2

Copyright of the summarized publication:

If you want to cite the papers, please refer to the original.

For technical reasons we could not place the page where the original quote is coming from.

Abstract-Summary "The goal of the present study was to evaluate the effects of SGLT2i on cardiac contractile function, substrate utilization, and efficiency before and during regional myocardial ischemia/reperfusion injury in normal, metabolically healthy swine."

"At the onset of ischemia, canagliflozin produced acute large increases in left ventricular end-diastolic and systolic volumes which returned to baseline with reperfusion."

"Canagliflozin-mediated increases in end-diastolic volume were directly associated with increases in stroke volume and stroke work relative to controls during ischemia."

"Canagliflozin also increased cardiac work efficiency during ischemia relative to control swine."

"In separate experiments using a longer 60 min coronary occlusion followed by 2 h of reperfusion, canagliflozin increased end-diastolic volume and stroke volume and significantly diminished myocardial infarct size relative to control swine."

"These data demonstrate that SGLT2i with canagliflozin preserves cardiac contractile function and efficiency during regional myocardial ischemia and provides ischemia protection independent of alterations in myocardial substrate utilization."

Introduction

"SGLT2i have been shown to improve cardiac function and mitigate myocardial infarct size in metabolically normal animal models [12, 48]."

"Improved arterial stiffness [49] and reduced blood pressure [50] have been reported with chronic SGLT2i treatment; however, it is unclear whether these effects are sufficient to explain the observed cardiovascular benefits."

"Some support for the plausibility of this ketone hypothesis in improving cardiac function and efficiency in response to pathologic stimuli such as ischemia has been presented [51]."

"Studies to directly assess the effects of SGLT2i on myocardial substrate utilization during ischemia are presently lacking."

"The goal of the present study was to evaluate the effects of SGLT2i on cardiac contractile function, substrate utilization, and efficiency before and during regional myocardial ischemia/reperfusion injury in normal, metabolically healthy swine."

"We tested the hypothesis that SGLT2i improves cardiac function and efficiency during ischemia/reperfusion injury via shifts in myocardial substrate selection toward ketone utilization."

Methods

"Depth of anesthesia was monitored by observing continuous measurements of arterial blood pressure and heart rate as well as regular (15-min intervals) reflex tests (corneal, jaw, and limb withdrawal), beginning after induction of anesthesia and continuing throughout the experimental protocol."

"These samples were collected every 15 min during baseline and the coronary occlusion, and every 30 min during reperfusion; total blood samples across the 2–3 h experimental protocol summed to < 100 mL from an estimated ~ 4 to 5 L total circulating blood volume."

"Four swine fibrillated during the LAD coronary occlusion portion of this protocol (n = 2 in each group) and thus were not included in infarct analyses."

"No measurable infarct was detected in animals subjected to LCX occlusion regardless of treatment (control n = 3; SGLT2i n = 4) and those animals are, accordingly, not included in infarct analyses."

Results

"No evidence of myocardial infarction was detected in either control (n = 3) or SGLT2i (n = 4)-treated hearts following the 30 min LCX occlusion protocol."

"To better assess potential effects on magnitude of myocardial infarction, a 60 min occlusion with 2 h reperfusion was performed in a separate cohort of animals in the distal LAD region."

"Our additional cohort of animals was modeled after established protocols demonstrating reliable induction of myocardial infarction with higher survival rates following 60 min occlusion of the distal LAD in swine [52, 53]."

"Canagliflozin treatment produced similar effects following the onset (15 and 30 min) of the distal LAD occlusion, including a significant increase in left ventricular end-diastolic volume and stroke volume (Supplemental Figure; P = 0.01) compared to control swine."

Discussion

"We set out to evaluate the effects of the SGLT2i canagliflozin on cardiac contractile function, substrate utilization, and efficiency before and during regional myocardial ischemia/reperfusion injury in normal, metabolically healthy swine."

"We observed effects of canagliflozin to augment cardiac function during regional myocardial ischemia and reduce myocardial infarct size, but these effects were independent of alterations myocardial substrate utilization."

"It is unclear whether the SGLT2i-mediated effects in this study are the result of direct and/or indirect actions on the heart."

"The current observations are not consistent with beneficial effects of diuresis, as any reduction in plasma volume would be expected to reduce overall ventricular filling volumes, in contrast to our observed ~ 50% increase in end-diastolic volume during ischemia."

"These data are directionally consistent with our present observations, and suggest a direction for further systematic in vivo and in vitro studies to explore the potential mechanisms of SGLT2i-mediated cardioprotection."

Conclusion

"Data from these studies demonstrate that canagliflozin preserves cardiac contractile function and efficiency during acute regional myocardial ischemia through acute effects on cardiac volume regulation that cannot be explained by myocardial fuel switching."

"SGLT2i reduces infarct size following 60 min ischemia."

"Findings from this study highlight the therapeutic potential for SGLT2i in metabolically normal subjects [48] and demonstrate the need for further investigations to both elucidate the mechanisms responsible for improvements in cardiac function during ischemia and to extend these studies into metabolically deranged cohorts as well as cohorts with normal glucose metabolism but abnormal cardiac function."

SGLT2 Inhibition and Heart Failure—Current Concepts [54]

This is a machine-generated summary of:

Custodio, Joaquim Silva; Duraes, Andre Rodrigues; Abreu, Marconi; Albuquerque Rocha, Natalia; Roever, Leonardo: SGLT2 inhibition and heart failure—current concepts [54].

Published in: Heart Failure Reviews (2018).

Link to original: https://doi.org/10.1007/s10741-018-9703-2

If you want to cite the papers, please refer to the original.

For technical reasons we could not place the page where the original quote is coming from.

Abstract-Summary "Type 2 diabetes mellitus (T2DM) is a major risk factor for several cardiovascular (CV) conditions, including heart failure (HF)."

"Until recently, no therapy to treat patients with diabetes could also reduce CV risks related to HF."

"Its impressive 35% reduction in hospitalizations for HF drew the attention of the scientific community to the possibility that pharmacologic sodium-glucose cotransporter 2 (SGLT2) inhibition could be part of the armamentarium for treating patients with HF, with and without diabetes."

Introduction

"The CHARM (Candesartan in Heart failure—Assessment of moRtality and Morbidity) study found that T2DM is an independent predictor of mortality in HF patients, and that each 1% increase in glycosylated hemoglobin A1c (HbA1c) is associated with a 25% increase in the risk for cardiovascular events or death [55]."

"In the EMPA-REG OUTCOME trial, empagliflozin resulted in a significantly lower risk of death from cardiovascular causes when compared to placebo (hazard ratio, 0.62; 95% CI, 0.49 to 0.77; $p < 0.001$) and a lower rate of hospitalization for HF (hazard ratio, 0.65 (95% CI, 0.50–0.85) $p = 0.002$), with no statistically significant between-group difference in the risk of myocardial infarction or stroke [38]."

"Researchers hypothesized a direct effect of SGLT2 inhibitor on myocyte intracellular sodium concentration, previously recognized as an early pathophysiological alteration in patients with HF [56–58]."

Conclusions

"Pharmacologic SGLT2 inhibition has many effects beyond glycemic control."

"It reduces body weight and blood pressure and reduces CV risk, HF hospitalization, and progression of kidney disease."

"Present evidence suggests that, if not contraindicated, SGLT2 inhibitors should be the preferred therapy for treating patients who have both T2DM and HF, adding substantial improvement in clinical parameters and longevity."

"Trials in progress including HF subjects could produce new data regarding the possibility of expanding use of SGLT2 inhibitors to all patients with HF, irrespective of glycemic status."

Mechanisms and Evidence for Heart Failure Benefits from SGLT2 Inhibitors [59]

This is a machine-generated summary of:

Wojcik, Cezary; Warden, Bruce A.: Mechanisms and Evidence for Heart Failure Benefits from SGLT2 Inhibitors [59].

Published in: Current Cardiology Reports (2019).

Link to original: https://doi.org/10.1007/s11886-019-1219-4

If you want to cite the papers, please refer to the original.

For technical reasons we could not place the page where the original quote is coming from.

Abstract-Summary "To review the clinical trial data and underlying mechanistic principles in support of the robust cardiovascular (CV) benefits, in particular, heart failure (HF) outcomes association with sodium-glucose co-transporter-2 (SGLT2) inhibitors."

"Several large CV outcome trials in patients with type 2 diabetes mellitus (T2DM) and with either established atherosclerotic CV disease (ASCVD) or at high risk for ASCVD reveal that SGLT2 inhibitors cause reductions in CV and HF endpoints."

"Recent evidence has unveiled the irrefutable data that SGLT2 inhibitors reduce CV events in patients with T2DM, with a profound effect on reductions in hospitalization for HF."

"The arrival of SGLT2 inhibitors has ushered in a new era of CV risk reductions therapies."

Introduction

"A recent meta-analysis of the three CVOT which included almost 35,000 patients (60.2% with established ASCVD) did show that SGLT2 inhibitors reduced major adverse cardiovascular events (MACE) by 11% (95% confidence interval [CI], 0.83–0.96, $p = 0.0014$), with statistically significant benefit seen only in patients with ASCVD (14% relative risk reduction [RRR], 95% CI, 0.80–0.93, $p < 0.001$)."

"SGLT2 inhibitors reduced the risk of CV death or HF hospitalization by 23% (95% CI, 0.71–0.84, $p < 0.0001$) regardless of pre-existing ASCVD or HF."

"The results of this meta-analysis contrast with data from a large observational study CVD-REAL (Comparative Effectiveness of Cardiovascular Outcomes in New Users of SGLT2 Inhibitors), which demonstrated benefit in reduction of CV events also in patients without pre-existing ASCVD."

Clinical Trial Evidence

"In this high-risk, secondary prevention population, empagliflozin lowered the primary composite outcome of myocardial infarction (MI), stroke, and CV death by 14% (95% CI, 0.74–0.99; $p < 0.001$), CV death by 38% (95% CI, 0.49–0.77; $p < 0.001$), death from any cause by 32% (95% CI, 0.57–0.82, $p < 0.001$), and reduced HF hospitalizations by 35% (95% CI, 0.50 – 0.85; $p = 0.002$) [60]."

"To empagliflozin, canagliflozin lowered the primary composite outcome of MI, stroke, and CV death by 14% (95% CI, 0.75–0.97; $P < 0.001$) and reduced HF hospitalizations by 33% (95% CI, 0.52–0.87, $p < 0.001$)."

"Compared to GLP-1 RA, the hazard ratio (HR) for the composite CV outcome (MI, stroke, mortality, and hospitalization for HF) was 1.10 (95% CI 0.95–1.26) for patients with ASCVD, and 1.23 (95% CI, 1.08–1.41) for patients without ASCVD."

Mechanism of Action: Glucose Reduction

"In the absence of diabetes, glucosuria appears when blood glucose levels exceed 180 mg/dL. However, in those with diabetes, SLGT2 is paradoxically upregulated, leading to increased glucose reabsorption in the PCT and therefore shifting the threshold of glycosuria up to ≈ 220 mg/dL. SGLT2 activity requires energy provided by the sodium gradient created by the Na^+/K^+ ATPase located in the basolateral surface of PCT epithelial cells, in contrast to the passive transport of glucose from cytoplasm towards plasma via GLUT2 [61, 62]."

"Inhibition of SGLT2 causes glucosuria with glucose levels much lower than ≈ 220 mg/dL as long as they are above 40–80 mg/dL (depending on the SGLT2 inhibitor studied)."

"As blood glucose levels drop, glucosuria caused by SGLT2 inhibitors decreases, preventing the occurrence of hypoglycemia."

"SGLT2 inhibitors display a modest efficacy in lowering plasma glucose levels, reducing HbA1C by ≈ 0.5–1%."

Mechanism of Action: Cardiovascular Protection

"SGLT2 inhibitors have a more robust and consistent effect on the prevention of HF and renal outcomes than on ASCVD."

"Although treatment with SGLT2 inhibitors appears to result in a moderate reduction in the risk of MACE solely in patients with established ASCVD, reductions in the risk of HF and renal outcomes occur regardless of patient characteristics [63]."

"SGLT2 inhibitors reduce renal afferent nervous activity and suppress associated central reflex mechanisms that contribute to generalized sympathetic activation."

"Published studies of SGLT2 inhibitors demonstrated their ability to induce a reduction in epicardial fat and thus providing another possible mechanism for the beneficial CV and HF outcomes [64–66]."

"SGLT2 inhibitors, by way of inducing glycosuria, reduce the workload of the renal PCT and reverse the downstream consequences, resulting in erythropoiesis and improved oxygen delivery to tissues [67]."

Conclusion

"The T2DM epidemic is on the rise with associated increases in morbidity and mortality, predominantly associated with CV complications, such as ASCVD events and HF."

"Through their unique mechanism of action, SGLT2 inhibitors significantly improve HF-related outcomes, decreasing the frequency of HF-related hospitalizations as well as CV-related death."

"The theorized protective CV mechanisms induced by SGLT2 inhibitors are several fold and include optimization of ASCVD risk factors, improvement in hemodynamics, prevention of cardiac and renal remodeling, inhibiting hormone dysregulation, use of a more efficient metabolic substrate, NHE inhibition, anti-inflammatory effects, and anti-oxidant effects."

"The future of SGLT2 inhibitors and its role in preventing catastrophic CV events is bright."

"Dual SGLT1/SGLT2 inhibitors are theorized to be even more beneficial through additional effects."

Addendum

"A recent subanalysis of DECLARE-TIMI 58 has shown that dapagliflozin reduced HF hospitalizations both in those with HFrEF (HR, 0.64 [95% CI, 0.43–0.95]) and in those without HFrEF (HR, 0.76 [95% CI, 0.62–0.92]); however, it reduced CV death (HR, 0.55 [95% CI, 0.34–0.90]) and all-cause mortality (HR, 0.59 [95% CI, 0.40–0.88]) only in patients with HFrEF [68]."

"Dapagliflozin reduced the relative risk of MACE by 16% (15.2% versus 17.8%; hazard ratio [HR], 0.84; 95% CI, 0.72–0.99; P = 0.039) in patients with previous MI, whereas there was no effect in patients without previous MI including in patients with established ASCVD but no history of MI [69]."

Promising Roles of Sodium–Glucose Cotransporter 2 Inhibitors in Heart Failure Prevention and Treatment [70]

This is a machine-generated summary of:

Tanaka, Atsushi; Node, Koichi: Promising roles of sodium–glucose cotransporter 2 inhibitors in heart failure prevention and treatment [70].

Published in: Diabetology International (2020).

Link to original: https://doi.org/10.1007/s13340-020-00445-7

If you want to cite the papers, please refer to the original.

For technical reasons we could not place the page where the original quote is coming from.

Abstract-Summary "Their results have shown that sodium–glucose cotransporter 2 (SGLT2) inhibitors are hypoglycemic drugs that could potentially greatly improve the heart failure-related outcomes in type 2 diabetes patients with a high cardiovascular risk."

"A clear concept has globally emerged with SGLT2 inhibitors as drugs of choice in clinical practice to prevent heart failure in type 2 diabetes patients."

"This paper outlines (1) the current evidence of heart failure prevention by SGLT2 inhibitors based on the results of recent large-scale cardiovascular outcome trials and (2) future research topics on their further applications in clinical practice."

Introduction

"One reason behind this attention is that HF-related outcomes are becoming evaluated in large-scale clinical trials of antidiabetic drugs in addition to macroangiopathy from conventional arteriosclerosis."

"Large-scale clinical trials using SGLT2 inhibitors have indicated the potential in their strong preventive effect against HF, thereby building an expectation of a major breakthrough in the HF prevention strategy for diabetic patients."

"This paper outlines (1) the current state of HF prevention in diabetic patients based on evidence of such prevention, focusing on SGLT2 inhibitors used in large-scale clinical trials, and (2) future topics of research."

Clinical Relevance of Diabetes and HF

"Another study examined type 2 diabetes patients without a past diagnosis of HF and found that 28% of these patients were diagnosed with HF after detailed examination, the majority of whom had HFpEF [71]."

"Another study has reported that the mortality rate was ten times higher in diabetic patients with comorbid HF than those without, and the former had a 5-year survival rate of only 12.5% [72]."

"HF itself is closely associated with the onset of diabetes, and approximately 20–40% of HF patients have been reported to have comorbid diabetes based on Japanese studies, including the Chronic Heart Failure Analysis and Registry in the Tohoku District (CHART)-2 Study and the Japanese Cardiac Registry of Heart Failure in Cardiology (JCARE-CARD)."

"When the background was examined for registered patients in past multiple large-scale clinical trials, the diabetes comorbidity rate increased with the severity of HF (New York Heart Association functional classification)."

Existing HF Prevention Strategies in Diabetes

"In diabetic patients, HF prevention strategies (including primary and secondary prevention) can be thought to have two aspects, diabetes treatment and HF treatment."

"There is presently no clear difference in HF treatment between diabetic patients and non-diabetic patients."

"They are contraindicated in HF patients."

"However, European and US studies have examined diabetic patients with HF and have shown that biguanides improved their HHF rate and mortality rate [73, 74]."

"In Japan, they continue to be relatively contraindicated, because clear evidence on their effectiveness is limited in patients with chronic HF."

"Based on such a background, the Japanese Circulation Society has stated in its Guidelines for Treatment of Chronic Heart Failure (2010 revised version) that there is no firm evidence to recommend a particular diabetes treatment in patients with chronic HF with comorbid diabetes."

Incretin-Based Drugs and HF Outcomes in Large-Scale Clinical Trials

"In the Examination of Cardiovascular Outcomes with Alogliptin versus Standard of Care in Patients with Type 2 Diabetes Mellitus and Acute Coronary Syndrome (EXAMINE) trial, HHF tended to increase, although not significantly, in diabetic patients with recent acute coronary syndrome and taking alogliptin [75]."

"An increase in HF risk was not seen in large-scale outcome trials using other DPP-4 inhibitors and glucagon-like peptide-1 (GLP-1) receptor agonists, and these drugs showed neutral results compared with the placebo."

"In the Cardiovascular and Renal Microvascular Outcome Study With Linaglipin (CARMELINA) trail, linagliptin at least did not increase the risk of HHF in patients with type 2 diabetes and established cardiovascular disease with albuminuria and/or kidney disease (HR 0.90; 95% CI 0.74–1.08) [76], suggesting its safety for HF."

Basic Pharmacological Effects of SGLT2 Inhibitors

"These inhibitors are antidiabetic drugs with the plain and simple effect of increasing urinary glucose excretion, thereby decreasing glucose reabsorption into the blood."

"When SGLT2 inhibitors are compared with conventional antidiabetic drugs, the most characteristic feature of SGLT2 inhibitors is their unique and efficient pharmacological effect which enables glucose (+ sodium) excretion in the urine in an insulin-independent manner."

"Although SGLT2 inhibitors have this seemingly simple effect, they are also considered to have a complex effect on the pathology of diabetes."

"This point indicates the characteristic pharmacological effect of SGLT2 inhibitors, that is not seen in other hypoglycemic drugs."

Summaries of Large-Scale Cardiovascular Outcome Trials

"Empagliflozin Cardiovascular Outcome Event Trial in Type 2 Diabetes Mellitus Patients (EMPA-REG OUTCOME) trial [77] The subjects were 7020 high-risk type 2 diabetes patients with a history of cardiovascular disease (all patients were secondary prevention cases)."

"When a stratified analysis was performed on the presence/absence of history of cardiovascular disease [78], no statistical evidence of heterogeneity was observed for the effects of canagliflozin on either outcome of MACE or HHF in the primary and secondary prevention groups."

"When a stratified analysis was performed on the presence/absence of HF history (14% of the total patients had an HF history), more remarkable reductions of HHF risk and cardiovascular mortality risk were seen in patients with HF history than patients without [79]."

"When a stratified analysis was performed by the presence/absence of history of myocardial infarction [69], dapagliflozin tended to show a strong risk-reduction effect for cardiovascular death or HHF in patients with a history of myocardial infarction."

Inhibition of Cardiovascular Event and HF Prevention Using SGLT2 Inhibitors

"These inhibitors not only are effective in patients at high risk for cardiovascular events, but also have a high potential to be similarly effective in type 2 diabetes patients with a history of CKD (details are not presented in our paper)."

"The dramatic effects of SGLT2 inhibitors have clearly been demonstrated for the prevention of HF, which is the theme of our paper, and for renal events."

"The above results have led to a high level of global attention on SGLT2 inhibitors' positioning in diabetes treatment strategy, which aims to improve outcomes, such as renal prognosis, and to prevent HF in diabetic patients."

"In Japan, the Guidelines for Diagnosis and Treatment of Acute and Chronic Heart Failure (revised 2017) indicate SGLT2 inhibitors, with a high level of evidence and class of recommendation, as a treatment for diabetic patients with HF and HF prevention in obese and diabetic patients [80]."

What Is the Mechanism of HF Prevention?

"SGLT2 inhibitors have a very characteristic preventive effect on HF."

"In clinical practice, the diuretic effect of SGLT2 inhibitors is temporary, occurring only in the initial stage of their administration."

"We clinicians may think that the main mechanism of SGLT2 inhibitors in HF prevention involves their effect on macro-hemodynamic parameters, such as those causing body weight and blood pressure reduction due to their diuretic effect."

"The greatest potential of SGLT2 inhibitors is not limited to such macro-effects, but also extends to the improvement of glucose and lipid metabolism and triggering of various micro-effects on metabolic and biological remodeling in many organs and tissues."

"In the DAPA-HF trial, an SGLT2 inhibitor also showed effectiveness against HF in non-diabetic patients, and the mechanism is predicted to be at the least independent of glucose metabolism improvement and elimination of glucotoxicity."

Future Research Topic and Outlook

"The effects of SGLT2 inhibitors on HF itself have not yet been fully elucidated."

"Specific effects have not yet been fully examined on clinical indicators related to HF, such as biomarkers and cardiac function, and there are only limited reports on patients irrespective of HF at baseline [81–83]."

"Effective treatment strategy and drugs have not yet been established for HFpEF, resulting in unmet clinical needs in HF treatment."

"A multinational clinical trial is also presently being conducted to examine the effects of SGLT2 inhibitors on HFpEF [84], resulting in great anticipation among cardiologists for the potential of these inhibitors in HFpEF treatment."

"We anticipate further accumulation of evidence for the scope of indications, examination of effectiveness in clinical practice, and the elucidation of mechanism of action against a specific type of HF."

Conclusions

"The recent results of large-scale clinical trials have attracted major attention in the treatment of HF as a cardiovascular complication in diabetic patients."

"Under such a circumstance, there has been great anticipation for SGLT2 inhibitors in a strategy for HF prevention in diabetic patients."

"The concept of such SGLT2-inhibitor use has just begun to be advanced in the light of major evidence being accumulated."

"It will be necessary to elucidate the effectiveness and mechanism of action against more specific types of HF such as HFpEF, to examine clinical long-term safety, and to carefully examine the scope of clinical indications."

SGLT-2 Inhibitors in Heart Failure: Guide for Prescribing and Future Perspectives [85]

This is a machine-generated summary of:

Garla, Vishnu Vardhan; Butler, Javed; Lien, Lillian F.: SGLT-2 Inhibitors in Heart Failure: Guide for Prescribing and Future Perspectives [85].

Published in: Current Cardiology Reports (2021).

Link to original: https://doi.org/10.1007/s11886-021-01486-3

Copyright of the summarized publication:

If you want to cite the papers, please refer to the original.

For technical reasons we could not place the page where the original quote is coming from.

Abstract-Summary "Sodium-glucose cotransporter-2 (SGLT-2) inhibitors are novel agents approved for the treatment of diabetes mellitus; in recent clinical trials, these agents have shown a significant reduction in cardiovascular death and hospitalization secondary to heart failure."

"Clinical trials with specific heart failure outcomes have shown the benefit of SGLT-2 inhibitors in reducing the mortality and morbidity associated with heart failure."

"SGLT-2 inhibitors are potential game changers in the treatment of heart failure."

Introduction

"Heart failure (HF) affects 5.7 million people in the USA [86]."

"DM and HF are intricately intertwined, with either one increasing the likelihood of developing the other."

"In the Framingham Heart Study, men (fivefold) and women (twofold) were more likely to develop HF in the presence of DM [87]."

"HF can also increase the rate of incident DM, as evidenced in the Candesartan in Heart Failure Assessment of Reduction in Mortality and Morbidity (CHARM) trial [88]."

"This article will review the pharmacological action, safety issues, clinical trials, and recommendations for using SGLT-2 inhibitors in HF."

Mechanism of Action

"SGLT-2 inhibitors lower glucose by inhibiting the SGLT-2 channels located in the proximal tubule of the kidney and inducing glycosuria [89]."

"There are several hypothesized mechanisms proposed to explain the efficacy of SGLT-2 inhibitors in reducing the mortality and morbidity associated with HF."

"SGLT-2 inhibitors by inducing diuresis reduce preload and improve cardiac contractility."

"SGLT-2 inhibitors also decrease intraglomerular hypertension, and tubuloglomerular feedback, helping improve renal hemodynamics."

"SGLT-2 inhibitors also directly inhibit the sodium hydrogen exchange pump 3 (NH3) in the kidneys resulting in natriuresis."

"SGLT-2 inhibitors induce ketogenesis due to an increased glucagon/insulin ratio which can improve myocardial contractility [51, 90]."

"SGLT-2 inhibitors have both direct and indirect actions to prevent cardiac fibrosis and reduce inflammation."

"Indirectly, SGLT-2 inhibitors by decreasing epicardial fat mass and by inhibiting NLRP3 inflammasome decrease production of inflammatory mediators like interleukin-1 (IL-1), interleukin-6 (IL-6), and tumor necrosis factor-α (TNF-α) [91–93]."

Safety of SGLT-2 Inhibitors

"SGLT-2 inhibitors in the EMPAREG-OUTCOME, DECLARE-TIMI58, and CANVAS clinical trials were not associated with increased hypoglycemic events when compared to the control groups."

"SGLT-2 inhibitors are associated with an increase in the occurrence of mycotic genital infections."

"All the major cardiovascular outcome trials (CVOT) with SGLT-2 inhibitors have shown a significantly higher infection rate in the treatment group than the control group."

"OBSERVE 4D, a meta-analysis of four observational studies evaluating canagliflozin, did not show any increase in LLA incidence with canagliflozin compared to other SGLT-2 inhibitors non-SGLT-2 glucose-lowering agents [94]."

"Among all the glucose-lowering agents, the proportionality reporting ratio was increased only for SGLT-2 inhibitors [95]."

"Between 2013 and 2019, the FDA identified fifty-five cases of FG in patients on SGLT-2 inhibitors, while only nineteen cases of FG were identified in patients using other antihyperglycemic agents [96]."

"None of the four major CVOT trials with SGLT-2 inhibitors identified any cases of FG."

Evidence from Clinical Trials

"A statistically significant reduction in CVHF was observed only in the EMPAREG-OUTCOME and DECLARE-TIMI 58 trials."

"In secondary analyses of the EMPAREG-OUTCOME trial based on the presence or absence of preexisting HF empagliflozin reduced CVHF (28%) and HHF (25%); however, these results were not statistically significant."

"In the CANVAS trial, canagliflozin failed to show a significant reduction in CVHF and HHF in the overall trial population but did decrease CVHF (39%) and HHF (49%) significantly in those with preexisting HF."

"In the DECLARE-TIMI 58 trial, dapagliflozin reduced CVHF (38%) significantly in those with HF and reduced left ventricular ejection fraction but not in the HF without known reduced left ventricular ejection fraction or no HF groups."

"As in the DAPA-HF study, the primary outcome reduction was significant in NYHA class II (29%) but not III or IV [42]."

Guidelines and Approach to SGLT-2 Inhibitors Therapy

"SGLT-2 inhibitors are recommended as an add-on therapy to metformin in patients with established atherosclerotic cardiovascular disease (ASCVD) or chronic kidney disease (eGFR 30–60 ml/min) [97]."

"The European Society of Cardiology (ESC) and the European Association for the Study of Diabetes (EASD) in their guidelines on DM in 2019 recommended that: Metformin should be considered in T2DM patients who are overweight with no established cardiovascular disease but at moderate risk for cardiovascular disease."

"SGLT-2 inhibitors are recommended as initial therapy for DM in patients with T2DM with established cardiovascular disease or those with high/very high risk for cardiovascular disease to reduce cardiovascular events."

"Above, the significant difference between the ADA and ESC/EASD guidelines is the use of SGLT-2 inhibitors as the initial choice of therapy in T2DM as well as expanding the use of SGLT-2 inhibitors for not only for established cardiovascular disease but also those at high/very high risk."

Future Directions

"SGLT-2 inhibitors are being studied for the treatment of HF with preserved left ventricular ejection fraction in the EMPEROR-PRESERVED (empagliflozin) and DELIVER (dapagliflozin) trials."

"The DICTATE clinical trial evaluates the role of dapagliflozin in patients admitted with acute HF."

"The EMPA-tropism trial studies the efficacy of empagliflozin in HF patients without DM in improving cardiac function and HF parameters."

"Studies are also needed to evaluate the role of SGLT-2 inhibitors in advanced HF."

Conclusion

"SGLT-2 inhibitors are potential game changers in the treatment of HF."

"Most of the safety issues identified have been relatively rare and can be addressed effectively with provider and patient education or not consistently associated with SGLT-2 inhibitors."

"Several new trials are underway, which will help us better elucidate the role of SGLT-2 inhibitors in the management of HF."

Sodium-Glucose Co-transporter 2 Inhibitors in the Failing Heart: A Growing Potential [98]

This is a machine-generated summary of:

Brito, Dulce; Bettencourt, Paulo; Carvalho, Davide; Ferreira, Jorge; Fontes-Carvalho, Ricardo; Franco, Fátima; Moura, Brenda; Silva-Cardoso, José Carlos; de Melo, Rachel Tavares; Fonseca, Cândida: Sodium-Glucose Co-transporter 2 Inhibitors in the Failing Heart: a Growing Potential [98].

Published in: Cardiovascular Drugs and Therapy (2020).

Link to original: https://doi.org/10.1007/s10557-020-06973-3

If you want to cite the papers, please refer to the original.

For technical reasons we could not place the page where the original quote is coming from.

Abstract-Summary "These benefits appear to be independent of glycaemic control and have recently been demonstrated in the HF population with reduced ejection fraction (HFrEF), with or without T2D. This comprehensive, evidence-based review focuses on the published studies concerning HF outcomes with SGLT2i, discussing issues that may underlie the different results, along with the impact of these new drugs in clinical practice."

"We focus on practical management issues regarding SGLT2i use in association with other T2D and HFrEF common pharmacological therapies."

"Considering the paradigm shift in T2D management, from a focus on glycaemic control to a broader approach on cardiovascular protection and event reduction, including the potential for wide SGLT2i implementation in HF patients, with or without T2D, we are facing a promising time for major changes in the global management of cardiovascular disease."

Diabetes and Heart Failure

"The relationship between T2D and HF has been well established since the Framingham study, which reported a 2- and 5-fold higher risk of HF in men and women with T2D, respectively, compared with individuals without T2D [99]."

"T2D adversely affects outcomes amongst patients with HF, has a substantial influence on the costs of managing HF patients, extends hospital stay and worsens prognosis [100, 101]."

"HF increases the risk of fatal and non-fatal cardiovascular (CV) events in T2D patients [102]."

"Sodium-glucose co-transporter 2 inhibitors (SGLT2i) have emerged as a new class of drugs designed to treat patients with T2D, but have also been shown to be protective against HF-related events and CV mortality."

"We present a comprehensive, evidence-based overview concerning the use of SGLT2i in patients with or without T2D at risk for CV events, focusing on HF outcomes."

Improving Prognosis: The Clinical Research Arena

"The EMPA-REG OUTCOME trial analysed the outcomes of the SGLT2i empagliflozin vs. placebo in patients with T2D and established CVD at baseline, and demonstrated the superiority of empagliflozin in reducing the risk of 3-point MACE, with significant reductions in CV death, all-cause death and in hospitalization for HF (HHF)."

"Post hoc analyses of the EMPA-REG OUTCOME trial revealed that besides the higher incident rates of HHF, CV death and all-cause mortality in patients with HF at baseline compared with patients without HF, the risk reductions of these outcomes with empagliflozin were consistent in both subgroups (hazard ratio (HR): 0.67, 95% confidence interval (CI) 0.47–0.97 in patients with HF burden (defined as HF at baseline, HHF or incident HF without hospitalization during the trial); HR 0.63, 95% CI 0.48–0.84 in patients without HF burden) [103]."

"These trials showed that both SGLT2i also reduced the composite endpoint of CV death and HHF in T2D patients, with similar results observed with dapagliflozin for patients with and without HF at baseline [39]."

From Clinical Trials to the Real World

"The SGLT2i positive impact on CV outcomes observed in CVOTs, specifically regarding HHF, was also observed in the real-world evidence (RWE) studies CVD-REAL and EMPRISE [69, 104]."

"CVD-REAL study included 309,056 T2D patients with or without CVD at baseline, newly treated with SGLT2i or other glucose-lowering drugs, from registries within six countries."

"The available data on SGLT2i, both from CVOTs and from RWE, has undoubtedly shifted the paradigm of T2D management in clinical practice from a focus on glycaemic control to a broader approach on CV event reduction, and also as a potential new class of drugs for HF treatment even in people without T2D. Given the impressive cardioprotective effects of SGLT2i, the results of the DAPA-HF trial were enthusiastically received."

Potential Mechanisms Behind the Cardio-renal Benefits Observed with SGLT2i

"Their effects consequently include reductions in HbA1c, blood glucose levels and blood pressure (BP), but also reductions in body weight and adiposity, all mechanisms that may contribute to reducing cardiovascular risk and HF [105, 106]."

"The glucose and BP-lowering effects of SGLT2i compared with placebo are not sufficient to explain the outcomes observed in randomized clinical trials (RCT)."

"This differs from the drastic reduction in intravascular volume observed with loop diuretics, which may lead to compensatory mechanisms and neurohormonal activation, associated with deleterious effects [107]."

"Multiple other mechanisms have been proposed to explain the early cardiorenal benefits of SGLT2i, including hypotheses that rely on leptin, calcium-calmodulin inhibition, visceral adipose tissue loss and direct vascular (arterial rigidity and central pressure) effects."

"EMPA-HEART aimed to determine whether the CV benefits of SGLT2i could be secondary to a reduction in LV mass, an important and independent predictor of MI, HF and mortality."

Practical Considerations for SGLT2i Management in T2D Patients with HF

"Although in the HFA expert consensus, no specific recommendations for the use of SGLT2i could be made for patients with established HF, some practical considerations were highlighted."

"This remains to be confirmed specifically in HF patients with or without T2D. The observed effects of SGLT2i in eGFR may be similar to the effect noted upon initiation of angiotensin-converting enzyme inhibitors (ACEi) or angiotensin receptor blockers (ARB) therapy, and therefore caution may be recommended upon concomitant initiation of SGLT2i and renin-angiotensin-aldosterone system (RAAS) modulating therapies."

"As most HF patients are managed with loop diuretics for congestion, adjustments to baseline diuretic therapy may be necessary upon SGLT2i initiation, based on adequate volume assessment and definition of volume status."

"No specific recommendations are considered for the concomitant use of SGLT2i and other diuretics in the ambulatory chronic HF setting, where SGLT2i therapy will most often be implemented [108]."

Unmet Medical Needs and Conclusions

"Despite the close pathophysiological relation between T2D and HF, cardiovascular outcome trials with SGLT2i were not designed to test their efficacy and safety, specifically in HF patients."

"The results from ongoing SGLT2i HF-dedicated outcomes trials are expected to lead to a growing potential for SGLT2i use in HF clinical practice (in the same way that the EMPA-REG OUTCOME trial drove a major shift in T2D management) and will answer the remaining questions of whether the results observed in DAPA-HF extend to other SGLT2i, and if the beneficial effects also include the HFpEF population."

"The EMPA Acute Heart Failure, EMPAG-HF and EMPULSE trials are underway to study the effects of SGLT2i on clinical outcomes in the AHF population (ClinicalTrials.gov Identifiers: NCT03554200, NCT04049045 and NCT04157751, respectively), while the EMPA-RESPONSE study has been published recently [109]."

Optimising the Heart Failure Treatment Pathway: The Role of SGLT2 Inhibitors [110]

This is a machine-generated summary of:

Evans, Marc; Morgan, Angharad R.; Yousef, Zaheer; Ellis, Gethin; Dashora, Umesh; Patel, Dipesh C.; Brown, Pam; Hanif, Wasim; Townend, Johnathan N.; Kanumilli, Naresh; Moore, Jim; Wilding, John P. H.; Bain, Stephen C.: Optimising the Heart Failure Treatment Pathway: The Role of SGLT2 Inhibitors [110].

Published in: Drugs (2021).

Link to original: https://doi.org/10.1007/s40265-021-01538-6

If you want to cite the papers, please refer to the original.

For technical reasons we could not place the page where the original quote is coming from.

Abstract-Summary "Sodium-glucose cotransporter 2 (SGLT2) inhibitors were first developed as glucose-lowering therapies for the treatment of diabetes."

"Despite robust clinical trial data demonstrating favourable outcomes with SGLT2 inhibitors for patients with HFrEF, there is a lack of familiarity with the HF indication for these drugs, which have been the remit of diabetologists to date."

"We use consensus expert opinion alongside the available evidence and label indication to provide support for the healthcare community treating people with HF regarding positioning of SGLT2 inhibitors within the treatment pathway."

Introduction

"To the glucose-lowering effect of SGLT2 inhibitors, several clinical trials have also demonstrated a cardioprotective benefit, including a reduced incidence of cardiovascular (CV) events and hospitalisation for heart failure (HF) in individuals with and without diabetes, including those with and without chronic HF [111]."

"It is notable that prior to the SGLT2 inhibitor trials, the last drug shown to improve mortality in chronic HF was sacubitril-valsartan in 2014; advances in HF management have stalled for over 7 years."

"With the emergence of new clinical evidence supporting the use of SGLT2 inhibitors in the management of HFrEF in people with and without diabetes, and as licensing and guidelines for SGLT2 inhibitors are updated, there is an immediate requirement to adapt HF treatment pathways and to encourage clinicians to start using this class of drugs as part of standard care for the treatment of HF."

Efficacy of Sodium-Glucose Cotransporter 2 (SGLT2) Inhibitors in People with Heart Failure (HF)

"Whilst these previous clinical trials have shown that SGLT2 inhibitors reduce the risk of new-onset HF in people with T2D, data from the DAPA-HF (Dapagliflozin and Prevention of Adverse Outcomes in Heart Failure) trial [41], which included patients with New York Heart Association (NYHA) class II-IV HFrEF (EF $\leq$ 40%) and N-terminal prohormone B-type natriuretic peptide (NT-proBNP) $\geq$ 600 pg/ml, 55% of whom did not have T2D, demonstrated that dapagliflozin improved outcomes among individuals with established HFrEF."

"This reduction in the primary outcome was similar in patients irrespective of the presence of T2D. Post hoc analysis of the DAPA-HF trial data has suggested an early benefit with dapagliflozin, with a sustained statistically significant benefit of a reduction in the primary outcome observed 28 days after randomisation (HR 0.51; 95% CI 0.28–0.94) [112]."

Safety Profile of SGLT2 Inhibitors

"Most of the adverse events associated with SGLT2 inhibitors in the HF population are consistent with the glycosuria mechanism of action of this drug class and include minor complications such as genital mycotic infections and volume depletion."

"A systematic review of population-based studies investigating SGLT2 inhibitor effectiveness and safety, that included 37 studies, reported that SGLT2 inhibitors were not associated with an increased risk of acute kidney injury, fractures, hypoglycaemia, or urinary tract infection."

"Other adverse effects such as urinary tract infections or genital infections were not routinely collected in DAPA-HF as extensive safety information was obtained from the DECLARE–TIMI 58 trial."

"The frequency of urinary tract infections was no different between SGLT2 inhibitor and placebo; however, the frequency of genital mycotic infections was increased with SGLT2 inhibitor use [39]."

The Positioning of SGLT2 Inhibitors Within the HF Treatment Pathway

"Support for such a strategy has recently been provided by a cross-trial analysis that included patient-level data from three randomized, controlled trials (EMPHASIS-HF, PARADIGM-HF and DAPA-HF) to estimate the treatment effects of comprehensive therapy (ARNI, beta-blocker, MRA and SGLT2 inhibitor) versus conventional therapy (ACE inhibitor or ARB and beta-blocker) in people with chronic HFrEF."

"For HF patients without T2D with a history of myocardial infarction or arrhythmia/rapid ventricular rates in atrial fibrillation we recommend a beta-blocker-first strategy followed by an ACE inhibitor, then an SGLT2 inhibitor, and then an MRA, as trial data for this population has demonstrated beta-blocker therapy to be more effective than ACE inhibitors as initiation therapy [113, 114]."

"For HF patients with a history of hypotension treatment we suggest the order of therapy to be ACE inhibitor or ARNI first followed by a beta-blocker, then an SGLT2 inhibitor and then an MRA."

Appropriate Prescribing of an SGLT2 Inhibitor in HF Patients

"The checklist follows a traffic light system that recommends that clinicians should consider prescribing an SGLT2 inhibitor for people in the green section, in accord with patients included in the DAPA-HF and EMPEROR-Reduced trials, and in alignment with the licence, that is, symptomatic stable chronic HF patients with an EF $\leq$ 40% (HFrEF) and eGFR > 30 mL/min/1.73 m^2."

"SGLT2 inhibitors should be considered for patients with or without T2D. As there is limited experience with SGLT2 inhibitors for the treatment of HF in patients with eGFR < 30 mL/min/1.73 m^2, prescription of SGLT2 inhibitors in those with eGFR 20–30 mL/min/1.73 m^2 should be with caution (amber section of the checklist)."

Practical Considerations

"Although SGLT2 inhibitors are unlikely to cause hypoglycaemia independently, when combined with other therapies especially insulin, sulphonylureas or glinides in patients with concomitant diabetes, hypoglycaemia may occur."

"When initiating SGLT2 inhibitors in HF patients who also have diabetes, reducing the dose of these background anti-diabetes therapies should be considered."

"Based on post-marketing surveillance, concerns were initially raised that SGLT2 inhibitors may increase the risk of Fournier's gangrene for patients with diabetes."

"If Fournier's gangrene is suspected (a combination of pain, tenderness, erythema, or swelling in the genital or perineal area, with fever or malaise), patients are advised to stop SGLT2 inhibitor treatment and immediately seek medical assessment."

"Regardless of the SGLT2 inhibitor used, annual foot review and regular self-examination should be encouraged particularly for HF patients with diabetes who are at higher risk than those without diabetes."

Future HF Indications for SGLT2 Inhibitors

"For patients with acute HF data, although clinical guidelines currently recommend intravenous diuretic therapy via either a bolus or infusion strategy as initial pharmacological treatment [115], data are emerging regarding the potential role of SGLT2 inhibitors; the EMPULSE trial (NCT04157751) is a superiority study that is currently in progress and that aims to determine whether in-hospital administration of empagliflozin results in improvements in HF-related clinical events and patient-reported outcomes in patients hospitalised for acute HF (de novo or decompensated chronic HF)."

"Recent results from SOLOIST-WHF [116] and SCORED [117] have demonstrated for the first time, in a prospective trial, improved outcomes for patients with HFpEF with sotagliflozin (a dual SGLT2/1 inhibitor)."

"Demonstration of a benefit of SGLT2 inhibitors on HF events in these studies would dramatically broaden the clinical impact of SGLT2 inhibitors."

Summary

"SGLT2 inhibitors are generally well tolerated with a low risk of serious adverse effects and these should not overshadow the significant cardioprotective benefits."

"Considering the benefits observed with SGLT2 inhibitors in patients with HF, both with and without T2D, SGLT2 inhibitors should no longer be considered only as glucose-lowering therapy, and cardiologists and HF specialists should familiarise themselves with their use and begin to prescribe an appropriate SGLT2 inhibitor as a new pillar of therapy for HFrEF, alongside an ACE inhibitor/ARB/ARNI, a beta-blocker and MRA."

"There are a number of practical considerations to bear in mind to support the optimal use of these drugs in routine clinical practice regarding appropriate prescribing and counselling of patients regarding potential side effects and sick-day guidance, particularly in those with concomitant T2D. However, adding an SGLT2 inhibitor to standard of care in HF represents an opportunity to significantly modify the clinical course and improve symptoms and outcomes for patients."

Practical Considerations and Opportunities for SGLT2 Inhibitor Prescription in Heart Failure [118]

This is a machine-generated summary of:

Faulkenberg, Kathleen D.; Williams, J. Bradley; Isaacs, Diana M.; West, Lucianne M.: Practical Considerations and Opportunities for SGLT2 Inhibitor Prescription in Heart Failure [118].

Published in: Current Treatment Options in Cardiovascular Medicine (2020).

Link to original: https://doi.org/10.1007/s11936-020-00825-x

If you want to cite the papers, please refer to the original.

For technical reasons we could not place the page where the original quote is coming from.

Abstract-Summary "Although emerging evidence supports the use of sodium-glucose co-transporter 2 (SGLT2) inhibitors for heart failure patients with or without diabetes, barriers to prescribing these agents still exist."

"This comprehensive review will focus on evidence supporting SGLT2 inhibitors for patients with heart failure and practical considerations when prescribing these agents in clinical practice."

"Based on evidence of improved cardiovascular outcomes for patients initiated on SGLT2 inhibitors, guidelines recommend the use of these agents for people with type 2 diabetes mellitus and cardiovascular disease, or at high cardiovascular risk, to reduce cardiovascular events and lower risk of heart failure hospitalization, independent of hemoglobin A1c."

"Innovative models, such as pharmacist-led cardio-endocrinology and heart failure medication optimization clinics, can be implemented to ensure safe prescribing and monitoring of SGLT2 inhibitors."

Introduction

"The glucagon-like peptide-1 (GLP-1) receptor agonists and sodium-glucose co-transporter 2 (SGLT2) inhibitors have specifically shown improved cardiovascular outcomes compared with placebo in people with or at high risk for CVD [119]."

"Appropriate selection of anti-hyperglycemic agents that are both safe and effective is critical to improve outcomes for individuals with heart failure."

"Guidelines on the management of diabetes recommend the use of SGLT2 inhibitors for people with type 2 diabetes mellitus and CVD or at high cardiovascular risk, to reduce cardiovascular events and lower risk of hospitalization for heart failure (HHF) [120, 121] irrespective of A1c [97]."

"Several studies now have been conducted or are underway to assess the effect of SGLT2 inhibitors on outcomes in individuals with established heart failure with or without diabetes."

"The mechanisms by which these agents reduce the risk of heart failure and other cardiovascular outcomes are less clear."

SGLT2 Inhibitor Cardiovascular Outcome Trials in Type 2 Diabetes Mellitus: Focus on Heart Failure

"A subgroup analysis of 706 patients with HF enrolled in the EMPA-REG OUTCOME trial demonstrated a significant reduction in the composite outcome of HHF or cardiovascular death [5.7% vs. 8.5%; HR: 0.66 (95% CI: 0.55–0.79); $p < 0.001$] in patients treated with empagliflozin vs. placebo."

"Patients in the canagliflozin group had a significant reduction in the composite outcome of cardiovascular death or HHF [16.3% vs. 20.8% per 1000 patient-years; HR: 0.78 (95% CI: 0.67–0.91); $p = 0.002$]."

"There was a significant difference in the composite endpoint of HHF or cardiovascular death for patients randomized to the dapagliflozin group [4.9% vs. 5.8%; HR: 0.83 (95% CI: 0.73–0.95); $p = 0.005$], which was largely driven by a reduction in HHF [39]."

Evidence for Use of SGLT2 Inhibitor in Heart Failure Without Diabetes Mellitus

"This trial was designed to evaluate dual primary endpoints of average of 6- and 12-week adjusted mean NT-proBNP, and the proportion of patients with a Kansas City Cardiomyopathy Questionnaire overall score (KCCQ-OS) increase of ≥ 5 points or a $\geq 20\%$ reduction in NT-proBNP (average of 6 and 12 weeks for both) in those who received dapagliflozin vs. placebo."

"While there was no difference in the average adjusted NT-proBNP between the groups, a significantly greater proportion of patients had ≥ 5 point increase in KCCQ-OS or $\geq 20\%$ reduction in NT-proBNP averaged over 6 and 12 weeks (61.5% vs. 50.4%)."

"Similar to DEFINE-HF, patients receiving dapagliflozin also experienced improvements in KCCQ scores: 58.3% vs. 50.9% had an increase of ≥ 5 points in the total score ($p < 0.001$), and fewer of them experienced significant deterioration (25.3% vs. 32.9%, $p < 0.001$)."

Practical Considerations for Use of SGLT2 Inhibitors in Clinical Practice

"Given the substantial mortality benefit, it is imperative that clinicians adopt SGLT2 inhibitors into the armamentarium of agents used to manage patients with HFrEF, with or without type 2 diabetes."

"There were numerically higher rates of events consistent with volume depletion in all of the trials previously discussed; however, only a significantly higher rate of events with use the of SGLT2 inhibitors was seen in the CANVAS Program (26 vs. 18 event per 1000 patient-years; p = 0.009) [6, 38–41, 122]."

"Discussed trials did not demonstrate a higher rate of AKI with SGLT2 inhibitors but instead, observed a lower rate of renal adverse events in all treatment groups compared with placebo [6, 38, 39, 122]."

"To correcting volume depletion, antihypertensive agents without specific benefit in heart failure should be discontinued prior to SGLT2 inhibitor initiation to reduce the risk of hypotension."

Barriers to Prescribing and Using SGLT2 Inhibitors

"With the new FDA approval for use in patients with heart failure without diabetes mellitus, dapagliflozin is the preferred SGLT2 inhibitor."

"Berg and colleagues recently sought to determine independent risk factors in patients with type 2 diabetes mellitus that would benefit the greatest from an SGLT2 inhibitor to reduce HHF [123]."

"The TIMI Risk Score for Heart Failure in Diabetes (TRS-HF_{DM}) was developed by selecting 25 candidate risk indicators from the placebo arm of the Saxagliptin Assessment of Vascular Outcomes Recorded in Patients with Diabetes Mellitus-Thrombosis in Myocardial Infarction 53 (SAVOR-TIMI 53) trial."

"This tool can easily be employed by practitioners to aid as a decision tool to determine the risk for HHF and absolute risk reduction for treatment with an SGLT2 inhibitor for people with diabetes mellitus."

"For patients with and without type 2 diabetes mellitus, shared decision-making between the patient and provider is critical, and discussions should include factors such as cost, risk profiling, and potential benefits."

Conclusion

"The growing prevalence of heart failure and diabetes mellitus in the USA, and the increased morbidity and mortality rates for patients with these concurrent conditions, makes it critical to select medication regimens aimed at improving outcomes."

"With the complexity of medication management and access related to prescription of SGLT2 inhibitors, innovative models that engage key players of the multidisciplinary team are imperative to ensure optimal patient outcomes."

"The goal of this joint pharmacist-led clinic was to optimize medication management and increase access to novel heart failure therapies, including SGLT2 inhibitors."

"With the FDA approval of dapagliflozin for patients with heart failure, patients without diabetes mellitus are also seen in the pharmacist-led heart failure medication optimization clinic for consideration of initiation and follow-up."

"Pharmacists are uniquely positioned to enhance patient care through the provision of pharmacist-led clinics for medication optimization and follow-up."

Sodium-Glucose Co-transporter 2 Inhibitors and Heart Failure—The Present and the Future [124]

This is a machine-generated summary of:

Nana, Melanie; Morgan, Holly; Bondugulapati, L. N. Rao: Sodium-glucose co-transporter 2 inhibitors and heart failure—the present and the future [124].

Published in: Heart Failure Reviews (2020).

Link to original: https://doi.org/10.1007/s10741-020-09925-z

If you want to cite the papers, please refer to the original.

For technical reasons we could not place the page where the original quote is coming from.

Abstract-Summary "Type 2 diabetes mellitus is associated with an increased risk of heart failure."

"Recent cardiovascular outcome trials have demonstrated that sodium-glucose co-transporter 2 inhibitors, which were introduced to the market in 2013, can incur a clinically significant risk reduction in heart failure outcomes in such patients."

"We discuss the epidemiology and pathophysiology of heart failure in diabetes and explore the landmark trials, the potential mechanisms of benefit of SGLT-2 inhibitors in heart failure, how the trials have led to major changes in treatment guidelines, and future potential directions for use of these drugs, including in those without diabetes."

Introduction

"It is well acknowledged that patients with type 2 diabetes mellitus (T2DM) have a 2- to 4-fold higher risk of heart failure (HF) than those without diabetes mellitus (DM) [125]."

"Morbidity and mortality in heart failure are recognised to be higher in patients with T2DM as opposed to without [126]."

"Recent cardiovascular (CV) outcomes trials have demonstrated that treatment with SGLT-2 inhibitors can improve major adverse cardiovascular events (MACE) in patients with T2DM at high risk of CV events, including a clinically significant risk reduction in HF-related outcomes [127]."

"We discuss the current understanding and evidence supporting this beneficial effect when used in heart failure patients with T2DM and also touch upon their potential use in those without diabetes."

Epidemiology

"The prevalence of diabetes in patients with heart failure has been consistently reported to be between 25 and 40% in both population-based cohorts and clinical trials [128]."

"Studies indicate that > 40% patients hospitalised with heart failure have T2DM [129]."

"It is difficult to establish the exact prevalence of systolic heart failure in T2DM patients, but it is estimated to range between 11 and 28% [130, 131]."

"The Framingham Heart Study reported that in patients with known DM, men had a twofold higher risk and women a fourfold higher risk of HF compared with age-matched controls [99]."

"A significant proportion of patients with T2DM develop HF in the absence of coronary heart disease (CHD) and yet carry comparable mortality risk [132]."

Pathophysiology of Heart Failure in Type 2 Diabetes Mellitus

"The increased frequency of HF in T2DM patients is attributable to a variety of factors including comorbidities such as hypertension, obesity, dyslipidaemia, and ischaemic heart disease."

"Treatment with angiotensin-converting enzyme inhibitors and β-blockers has been demonstrated to reverse remodelling and improve cardiac function in people with heart failure with reduced ejection fraction (HFrEF) [133, 134]."

"In patients with heart failure with preserved ejection fraction (HFpEF), aggressive risk factor management is the only approach which has been shown to provide any improvement [135]."

"Some of the aforementioned pathophysiological pathways might be amenable to pharmacological therapy to reduce the risk of HF in the context of T2DM."

Sodium-Glucose Co-transporter-2 Inhibitors and Cardiovascular Outcome Trials

"This benefit was independent from improvements in glycaemic control as demonstrated by the Empagliflozin Cardiovascular Outcome Event trial in Type 2 Diabetes Mellitus Patients (EMPA-REG OUTCOME) and Canagliflozin Cardiovascular Assessment Study (CANVAS) trials [136, 137]."

"The primary outcome was a composite of death from CV causes, nonfatal MI, or nonfatal stroke, and was lower with canagliflozin than placebo (occurring in 26.9 vs. 31.5 participants per 1000 patient-years; hazard ratio 0.86; $p = 0.02$ for superiority)."

"A recent meta-analysis of the three published CV outcome trials included a total of 34,322 patients with T2DM, with 20,650 patients having established ASCVD, and 13,672 patients with multiple risk factors but no clinically apparent ASCVD."

"This prospective, randomised, placebo-controlled trial aimed to evaluate the effect of dapagliflozin compared with placebo in 4500 patients with HF and reduced ejection fraction (HFrEF)."

Side Effects and Limitations of Sodium-Glucose Co-transporter-2 Inhibitors

"A small increase in the risk of diabetic ketoacidosis, bone fracture, foot and leg amputation, and Fournier's gangrene has also been recognised [127, 137, 138]."

"Following a review by the European Medicines Agency, a safety notice was issued which highlighted to prescribers this rare but not insignificant risk of both diabetic ketoacidosis and Fournier's gangrene [139]."

"Current prescribing guidelines recommend that this class of drugs should be reserved for patients with an estimated glomerular filtration rate (eGFR) of > 60 mL/min/1.73 m^2; thus, this represents the most significant barrier to prescribing these drugs in clinical practice."

"Key trials including DAPA-HF, however, only excluded patients with an eGFR < 30 mL/min/1.73 m^2 without deleterious effects."

Potential Mechanisms of Benefits in Heart Failure Patients Treated with SGLT-2i

"Animal studies to date exploring SGLT1 inhibition have demonstrated detrimental effects on myocardial function [140, 141]."

"SGLT2 co-transporters also modulate myocardial metabolism by shifting from glucose and lipid oxidation to the utilisation of ketone bodies, which is more energy efficient and ultimately improves cardiac contractility."

"The study of DAPAgliflozin on CARDiac substrate uptake, myocardial efficiency, and myocardial contractile work in type 2 diabetes patients (DAPACARD) explores the possible effects of dapagliflozin on cardiac work, metabolism, and biomarker levels [142]."

"DAPACARD is an international, randomised, double-blind trial that aims to examine the effects of dapagliflozin versus matching placebo in 52 patients with T2DM that are on stable metformin therapy prior to and during the 6 weeks of treatment."

"The DAPACARD study is an extensive investigation of cardiac function and metabolism, by advanced imaging with PET and MRI, as well as biomarkers, performed in order to further explore how the SGLT2 inhibitor dapagliflozin influences cardiovascular outcomes in patients with T2DM [142]."

How Does the Evidence Relate to Day-to-Day Practice?

"The Heart Failure Association of the European Society of Cardiology has published a clinical practice update on HF wherein authors reinforced the message that empagliflozin should be considered in patients with T2DM in order to prevent or delay the onset of heart failure or prolong life and also suggested that the other two SGLT-2i (namely canagliflozin and dapagliflozin) should be considered for patients with T2DM and either established CV disease or at high CV risk in order to prevent or delay the onset of and hospitalisations for HF [143]."

"In a scientific statement issued recently by American Heart Association and Heart Failure Society of America, authors acknowledged the beneficial effects of SGLT-2i in T2DM patients with established HF as well as in those T2DM patients who are at higher risk for HF [144]."

Potential Use of Sodium-Glucose Co-transporter-2 Inhibitors in Patients Without Diabetes

"The benefit of adding SGLT-2is in patients with worsening heart failure with ejection fraction of < 50% is also being studied with Sotagliflozin in the SOLOIST trial [145]."

"The DELIVER trial (Dapagliflozin Evaluation to improve the Lives of Patients With Preserved Ejection Fraction Heart Failure) is designed to explore the benefits of Dapagliflozin in patients with HFpEF [146]"

"is a randomised, double-blind, placebo-controlled trial comparing the efficacy and safety of empagliflozin versus placebo on top of guidelines-directed medical therapy in heart failure patients without diabetes to determine whether it improves cardiac function and heart failure parameters [48]."

"These trials will hopefully enable us to understand the mechanisms behind the possible beneficial effects of SGLT-2i in heart failure patients with and without T2DM and as well as in T2DM patients with HFpEF and HFrEF."

Summary

"The mechanisms underlying the beneficial effects of SGLT-2i in HF are not entirely understood; however, their benefit in reducing mortality and morbidity in those with heart failure and T2DM is now well established."

"This class of oral hypoglycaemic drugs have now been persistently demonstrated to provide positive effects on myocardial pump failure."

"There are several studies exploring the potential mechanisms of action which may support the use of these drugs in patients without T2DM in the future."

Sodium-Glucose Cotransporter 2 Inhibitors and Heart Failure: The Best Timing for the Right Patient [147]

This is a machine-generated summary of:

Severino, Paolo; D'Amato, Andrea; Prosperi, Silvia; Costi, Bettina; Angotti, Danilo; Birtolo, Lucia Ilaria; Chimenti, Cristina; Lavalle, Carlo; Maestrini, Viviana; Mancone, Massimo; Fedele, Francesco: Sodium-glucose cotransporter 2 inhibitors and heart failure: the best timing for the right patient [147].

Published in: Heart Failure Reviews (2021).

Link to original: https://doi.org/10.1007/s10741-021-10170-1

If you want to cite the papers, please refer to the original.

For technical reasons we could not place the page where the original quote is coming from.

Abstract-Summary "Sodium-glucose cotransporter 2 inhibitors (SGLT2i), initially born as anti-diabetic drugs, have shown many beneficial effects on the cardiovascular system, in particular against heart failure (HF)."

"Exploiting their pleiotropic effects, SGLT2i are a very valid tool for HF treatment."

"Beyond the indication to reduce HF hospitalization and death risk, in patients with diabetes mellitus at high cardiovascular risk or with established cardiovascular event, SGLT2i administration reported beneficial effects regarding the wide spectrum of HF manifestations and stages, independently by diabetes mellitus presence."

"Given the recent finding about the SGLT2i usefulness in HF patients, further studies are needed to define the best administration timing to maximize the SGLT2i-derived beneficial effects."

Introduction

"SGLT2i use was restricted to diabetic patients with established CVD or at high cardiovascular (CV) risk."

"Many benefits deriving from SGLT2i administration have been observed in HF patients."

"Given the recent findings about the SGLT2i usefulness, also in patients with HF, an important issue concerning the SGLT2i best timing administration is currently ongoing."

"The aim of this review is to discuss the latest findings regarding SGLT2i use, both in HF and in diabetic patients at risk to develop HF, to provide a better comprehension of the best administration timing, according to patient clinical profile."

The Pleiotropic Effects of Sodium-Glucose Cotransporter 2 Inhibitors: Molecular and Pathophysiological Insights

"SGLTs are ubiquitous proteins and, for this reason, SGLT2i show metabolic and hemodynamic effects, which justify their efficacy in T2DM and HF treatment."

"Since diabetic patients have micro- and macrovascular disease, the increased arterial stiffness and afterload promote a vicious circle, through which, the hemodynamic stress, induced by hypertension and reduced arterial blood pressure (BP) variability, causes organ damage."

"This marks another important difference between SGLT2i and other diuretics: the latter are responsible for RAAS hyperactivation, uric acid blood levels increase, electrolytes loss and, above all, metabolic disorders."

"Stimulating magnesium blood level increase, SGLT2i have an anti-arrhythmic and cardioprotective effect [148, 149]."

"SGLT2i can restore a better heart oxygenation through hematocrit and hemoglobin levels increase, stopping the vicious cardio-renal involvement, seen in HF [150]."

"By decreasing the blood glucose values through the glycosuric mechanism, SGLT2i reduce the production of insulin increasing glucagon synthesis, responsible for ketones production, through lipid oxidation [151]."

Type 2 Diabetes Mellitus and Heart Failure: Role of Sodium-Glucose Cotransporter 2 Inhibitors

"Many studies and observations underline the effectiveness of SGLT2i use in patients with T2DM, without previous CV events and HF [152]."

"These observations opened the possibility to use SGLT2i as CV preventive drug, before HF onset, in patients with T2DM."

"New evidences underline that SGLT2i act also on other CV risk factors, beyond T2DM, improving patient's prognosis and reducing the risk of subsequent HF."

"SGLT2i reduce arterial blood pressure, in patients with T2DM and hypertension, providing benefits in terms of CV risk prevention."

"Empagliflozin reduces HF hospitalization, CV and all-cause mortality, independently by baseline CV risk factors, as well as the presence of prior myocardial infarction and ischemic stroke, in T2DM patients with ASCVD."

"Empagliflozin, Dapagliflozin, and Canagliflozin beneficial effect is mainly demonstrated in diabetic patients with high CV risk and regardless of HF, in terms of HF hospitalization prevention."

Heart Failure and Sodium-Glucose Cotransporter 2 Inhibitors: What Is the Best Time of Administration?

"In HF patients, SGLT2i have demonstrated to significantly reduce rehospitalization, all-cause death, and CV death."

"SGLT2i may demonstrate beneficial effects also in HF patients without an overt systemic involvement, slowing down the systemic disease's progression and contrasting heart and systemic alterations, that are already present in the early, preclinical phases of HF."

"Early SGLT2i administration beneficial effect on HF-related adverse events reduction have been identified by the Empagliflozin Outcome Trial in Patients with Chronic Heart Failure and a Reduced Ejection Fraction (EMPEROR-Reduced) trial [153]."

"Their effectiveness according with disease duration, as well as the effect in HF outpatients and the combined effectiveness of SGLT2i with other drugs administered in HF patients."

"In these patients, both the HF worsening, requiring therapy management, and hospitalization events, are significantly reduced by Dapagliflozin administration."

Conclusions

"SGLT2i beneficial effects have been observed at different HF stages, both in acute and chronic HF patients."

"When SGLT2i were administered in patients with recent acute HF and decompensation episode, they demonstrated to significantly modify the disease's progression, reducing HF rehospitalization, CV, and all-cause death."

"SGLT2i significantly impact the prognosis of patients with T2DM and across the wide CV risk factors spectrum, in terms of HF prevention."

"Starting from the concept that, similarly to a cancer, HF should be treated in order to avoid the progressive involvement and dysfunction of systemic organs, regardless of symptoms presence, we are proposing that SGLT2i administration should be started as soon as possible, when clinical conditions allow it, regardless of HF hospitalization, mostly for their cardio- and nephroprotective effects."

"Although actual SGLT2i indication regards patients with symptomatic chronic HFrEF, SGLT2i may represent a further treatment option to contrast left ventricular remodeling and the progressive systemic involvement seen in HF, in addition to first line therapy."

SGLT2 Inhibitors and Their Mode of Action in Heart Failure—Has the Mystery Been Unravelled? [154]

This is a machine-generated summary of:

Pabel, Steffen; Hamdani, Nazha; Luedde, Mark; Sossalla, Samuel: SGLT2 Inhibitors and Their Mode of Action in Heart Failure—Has the Mystery Been Unravelled? [154].

Published in: Current Heart Failure Reports (2021).

Link to original: https://doi.org/10.1007/s11897-021-00529-8

If you want to cite the papers, please refer to the original.

For technical reasons we could not place the page where the original quote is coming from.

Abstract-Summary "The mechanisms of SGLT2i in HF remain elusive."

"This article discusses the current clinical evidence for using SGLT2i in different types of heart failure and provides an overview about the possible underlying mechanisms."

"Clinical and basic data strongly support and extend the use of SGLT2i in HF."

"Further translational studies are needed to determine the mechanisms of SGLT2i in HF."

Introduction: Clinical Background

"The DAPA-HF trial was the first one studying the efficacy of dapagliflozin in patients who suffer from HF with reduced ejection fraction (HFrEF, ejection fraction (EF) ≤ 40%, NYHA II–IV) with and without T2DM with respect to cardiovascular death or worsening HF [41]."

"In 4744 HF patients, dapagliflozin reduced the primary composite outcome of worsening HF (hospitalisation or urgent intravenous therapy for HF) and death from cardiovascular causes by 26% as well as each component of the primary endpoint alone."

"In the EMPEROR-reduced trial enrolling 3730 patients with HFrEF (EF≤ 40%, NYHA II–IV) with and without T2DM, empagliflozin reduced the primary composite outcome of death from cardiovascular cause and hospitalisation for HF [42]."

"Further evidence of the favourable impact of SGLT2i in HF is given by the DEFINE-HF trial, which showed improvement in HF symptoms (based on the KCCQ) over 12 weeks in 263 patients with HF (EF≤ 40%, NYHA II–III) treated with dapagliflozin, irrespective of T2DM [40]."

Mechanisms of SGLT2 Inhibitors in HF

"It is important to distinguish between systemic and myocardial effects when investigating the possible mechanisms of SGLT2i in HF, as direct myocardial mechanisms cannot really be elucidated in a systemic setting where secondary factors (i.e. altered blood pressure) influence the cardiac function."

"In these patients, it was shown that taking SGLT2i not only significantly improved the prognosis of important renal parameters with respect to renal endpoints (eGFR decline above 50%, end-stage chronic kidney disease or death from renal causes), but also reduced the combined risk of death from cardiovascular causes or hospitalisation for HF by 29% in these patients."

"Since glycaemic control has no significant influence on the prognostic effects of SGLT2i, at least in the DAPA-HF and the EMPEROR-Reduced trials, it is unlikely that improvement of T2DM and hyperglycaemia-related metabolic abnormalities significantly contribute to the positive HF outcomes."

"Compelling evidence indicates that SGLT2i favourably affect LV remodelling in T2DM patients and in HF patients, which could be a central mechanism of the beneficial cardiac effects of SGLT2i."

Conclusion

"A plethora of multidirectional mechanisms of SGLT2i, which could underlie the favourable HF outcomes, has been proposed."

"While many theories about the favourable mechanisms of SGLT2i in HF have been postulated, further experimental research is clearly warranted."

"Translational studies i.e. utilising human samples could help to better elucidate the mechanisms of SGLT2i in HF."

Sodium Glucose Cotransporter 2 Inhibitors: Mechanisms of Action in Heart Failure [155]

This is a machine-generated summary of:

Dutka, Mieczysław; Bobiński, Rafał; Ulman-Włodarz, Izabela; Hajduga, Maciej; Bujok, Jan; Pająk, Celina; Ćwiertnia, Michał: Sodium glucose cotransporter 2 inhibitors: mechanisms of action in heart failure [155].

Published in: Heart Failure Reviews (2020).

Link to original: https://doi.org/10.1007/s10741-020-10041-1

If you want to cite the papers, please refer to the original.

For technical reasons we could not place the page where the original quote is coming from.

Abstract-Summary "HF remains the primary cause of hospitalisation for diabetics and, as previous studies have shown, when HF occurs in these patients, intensive glycaemic control does not directly improve the prognosis."

"Patients treated with SGLT2is had a significant decrease in both cardiovascular (CV) and all-cause mortality and less hospitalisations due to HF compared to those given a placebo."

"These groundbreaking clinical trials' results have already changed clinical practice in the management of patients with diabetes at high CV risk."

"This article presents the current state of knowledge about the mechanisms of action of SGLT2is developed for the treatment of diabetes and which, thanks to their cardioprotective effects, may, in the future, become a treatment for patients with HF."

Introduction

"A new group of antidiabetic drugs, sodium-glucose cotransporter 2 inhibitors (SGLT2is), has recently been shown to significantly improve the prognosis in high-risk cardiovascular (CV) patients with type 2 diabetes."

"The unique mechanism of action of this drug, whereby it inhibits SGLT2, also results in certain haemodynamic effects, which are beneficial from the point of view of CV diseases."

"Even if these beneficial haemodynamic effects of SGLT2is are taken into account, it does not fully explain the beneficial CV effects of using these drugs."

"A lot of research is underway to explain the beneficial mechanisms of action of this group of drugs on the CV system."

"It is fascinating that, for the first time in history, an antidiabetic drug has been shown to reduce CV mortality and the number of hospitalisations due to HF, while the mechanisms of such action are not fully understood."

Diabetes and CV Risk

"Type 2 diabetes is associated with a significantly higher risk of CV events such as myocardial infarction and stroke compared to people without diabetes."

"CV incidents account for 80% of deaths among patients with type 2 diabetes [156]."

"The clinical characteristics of patients with type 2 diabetes indicate the frequent coexistence of other significant CV risk factors."

"This combination of CV risk factors is known as metabolic syndrome, which is associated with a significant increase in CV events in type 2 diabetes [156]."

"Data confirms that obese people with insulin resistance but without diabetes have an increased CV risk similar to that in patients with type 2 diabetes [156]."

"This means that in type 2 diabetes, hyperglycaemia is not an independent or major risk factor in the development of atherosclerotic CVD."

Diabetes and HF

"Clinical trials registries show that in patients with type 2 diabetes, HF is almost as common as atherosclerotic CVD."

"Although we have data confirming that the control of classic CV risk factors reduces ischaemic events, in the case of HF in patients with diabetes, intensive glycaemic control does not translate into a significant clinical benefit."

"This is confirmed by interventional studies focused on intensive normalisation of glycaemia in patients with diabetes, in which there was not only no improvement in prognosis in HF but sometimes even an increase in the number of CV incidents with such treatment."

"Recent clinical studies assessing a new class of antidiabetic drug, SGLT2is (empagliflozin, canagliflozin and dapagliflozin), showed a significant decrease in both CV and all-cause mortality, as well as a reduction in the number of hospitalisations due to HF in patients with type 2 diabetes treated with these drugs compared to those given a placebo."

The Target and Mechanisms of Action of SGLT2is

"The fundamental activity of SGLT2is is to inhibit the active reverse transport of glucose by SGLT2 in the luminal surface of the S1 segment of the proximal renal tubule, which is linked to Na^+ transport maintained by Na^+ active extrusion."

"It has also been confirmed that SMIT1 is closely related to glucose uptake in the heart."

"The activation of NOX2 by SMIT1 can modulate glucose sensitisation, which in turn can release ion signals (Na^+ and Ca^{2+}) into cells depending on extracellular glucose concentration."

"As for SGLT1, its increased expression and activity in the hearts of patients with diabetes has been confirmed [157]."

"This is also one of the causes of a significantly increased concentration of sodium ions (Na^+) in the cytoplasm of cardiomyocytes in a failing heart."

"Other causes of this sodium overload of cardiomyocytes in an inefficient heart include increased Na^+ influx through late Na^+ current (INa) and increased sarcolemmal Na^+/H^+ exchanger (NHE) activity."

SGLT2 Inhibition and Clinical Outcomes

"Patients with type 2 diabetes and previously diagnosed CVD took part in the EMPA-REG OUTCOME trial in which empagliflozin was studied."

"Further disparities between these studies may also result from different clinical characteristics of the patient populations studied (in the EMPA-REG OUTCOME trial only patients with confirmed CVD, and in other studies patients both with and without confirmed CVD) [158]."

"In other health economic studies based on the EMPA-REG OUTCOME trial, it has also been confirmed that empagliflozin therapy is cost-effective in patients with both diabetes and confirmed CVD [159–161]."

"In this large real-world study, in which both patients with and those without CV diagnosis participated, it was shown that treatment with SGLT2is versus treatment with another antidiabetic drug resulted in a 39% RRR of hospitalisation due to HF, a 51% reduction in all-cause mortality and a 46% reduction in HF hospitalisation [162]."

The Postulated Mechanisms of the Beneficial Effects of SGLT2is in HF

"In another study with diabetic mice, it was confirmed that, compared to the control group, they had a very significant decrease in ATP production in the heart, which was associated with a significant reduction in the level of glucose and fatty acid oxidation and a particularly large reduction in the oxidation of ketone bodies."

"It was thought that this significant reduction in the number of hospitalisations due to HF and the reduction in CV mortality resulted mainly from the effects of empagliflozin achieved in a group of patients with impaired left ventricular systolic function and HF."

"The results of this study confirm that empagliflozin can significantly reduce increased oxidative stress by intensifying the expression of antioxidant enzymes and reducing ROS production, thus limiting the adverse effects of oxidative stress."

The Importance of SGLT2is as Cardiological Drugs Now and in the Future

"In history, based on this strong evidence from randomised clinical trials, guidelines recommend the use of a specific group of drugs in a specific group of patients with type 2 diabetes to prevent CV incidents."

"Using this mechanism of action of SGLT2is is becoming an attractive, potential therapeutic strategy in HF, which, in the future, may be useful not only for patients with diabetes, but others too."

"An additional effect of empagliflozin demonstrated in this study is the reduction of myocardial fibrosis by inhibiting the TGF-Beta1/Smad3 signalling pathway."

"It has been confirmed in the HF animal model that the severity of myocardial inflammation is significantly reduced by inhibiting the TGF-Beta1/Smad3 signalling pathway [163]."

"This SGLT2i mechanism of action is particularly interesting, as it has been well documented in animal studies, that inhibition of the TGF-Beta1/Smad3 signalling pathway significantly inhibits myocardial fibrosis and left ventricular remodelling in HF regardless of the presence of diabetes."

Conclusions

"A new group of antidiabetic drugs, SGLT2is, have various mechanisms of action that go beyond the hypoglycaemic effect."

"In history, it has been demonstrated that an antidiabetic drug used in patients with type 2 diabetes and high CV risk significantly reduces CV mortality, all-cause mortality and the number of hospitalisations due to HF."

"This became a catalyst for a number of studies aimed at understanding the mechanisms of action of this group of drugs that would be able to explain such favourable CV outcomes."

"Other recently recognised mechanisms of SGLT2is action not only allow a better understanding of these drugs' cardioprotective actions, but, in addition, could be, in the future, a potential therapeutic goal in HF in patients with and without diabetes."

"The basic mechanism of action of these drugs also provides the basis for considering this group of antidiabetic drugs as therapy for cardiological indications in patients without diabetes."

What Makes Sodium-Glucose Co-transporter-2 Inhibitors Stand Out in Heart Failure? [164]

This is a machine-generated summary of:

Khan, Muhammad Shahzeb; Vaduganathan, Muthiah: What Makes Sodium-Glucose Co-Transporter-2 Inhibitors Stand out in Heart Failure? [164].

Published in: Current Diabetes Reports (2020).

Link to original: https://doi.org/10.1007/s11892-020-01347-3

If you want to cite the papers, please refer to the original.

For technical reasons we could not place the page where the original quote is coming from.

Abstract-Summary "We highlight the unique properties of the sodium-glucose cotransporter-2 (SGLT-2 inhibitors) which may lend favorably to their efficient integration in the background of other heart failure (HF) therapies."

"All SGLT-2 inhibitors are once daily medications with minimal drug-drug interactions and do not require titration (for HF treatment) unlike other HF medications."

"SGLT-2 inhibitors offer modest weight loss and blood pressure reduction without major adverse effects of hyperkalemia, making it ideal for near-simultaneous initiation with other HF medications, and use in high-risk populations (including older adults)."

"SGLT-2 inhibitors are the latest class of therapies to demonstrate important clinical benefits among patients with HFrEF, and their pharmacological properties favor ease of use and integration in multi-drug disease-modifying regimens."

Introduction

"In the landmark DAPA-HF trial (Dapagliflozin and Prevention of Adverse Outcomes in Heart Failure), dapagliflozin reduced the composite endpoint of worsening HF events or cardiovascular death by 26% compared with placebo among patients with chronic HF with reduced ejection fraction (HFrEF), irrespective of T2DM status [41]."

"Consistent benefits were observed with a second SGLT-2 inhibitor, empagliflozin, in the EMPEROR-Reduced (Empagliflozin Outcome Trial in Patients With Chronic Heart Failure With Reduced Ejection Fraction) trial among patients with chronic HFrEF with or without T2DM."

"Among over 2000 patients in the contemporary CHAMP-HF (Change the Management of Patients with Heart Failure) registry with HFrEF and comorbid T2DM, the use of SGLT2 inhibitors (2.4%) was low, suggesting a large potential for therapeutic optimization [165]."

"Core therapies, including β-blockers, mineralocorticoid receptor antagonists, renin-angiotensin-aldosterone system (RAAS) inhibitors, and angiotensin-receptor neprilysin inhibitors, have been shown to reduce mortality in HFrEF patients [166]."

Use of SGLT-2 Inhibitors After Worsening HF Events

"A post-hoc analysis of the EMPA-REG OUTCOME (Empagliflozin Cardiovascular Outcome Event Trial in Type 2 Diabetes Mellitus Patients) trial showed that the proportion of patients with a second HF readmission within 45, 60, and 90 days was almost 2 times higher in individuals treated with placebo compared with empagliflozin [167]."

"The proportions of patients with HF re-hospitalization or cardiovascular death and HF re-hospitalization or all-cause death were significantly higher in the placebo group versus empagliflozin at all time points."

"Initial data from the EMPA-RESPONSE-AHF (Effects of Empagliflozin on Clinical Outcomes in Patients with Acute Decompensated Heart Failure) trial showed that empagliflozin reduces a combined endpoint of worsening HF, rehospitalization for HF, or death at 60 days in patients with acute HF [109]."

"The large SOLOIST WHF (Effect of Sotagliflozin on Cardiovascular Events in Patients With Type 2 Diabetes Post Worsening Heart Failure, NCT03521934), which was evaluating the novel combination SGLT-1/2 inhibitor sotagliflozin, was terminated early by the sponsor due to complexities with coronavirus disease 2019 (COVID-19)."

Use of SGLT-2 Inhibitors in Older Patients with HF

"SGLT-2 inhibitors pose a low risk of hypoglycemia (< 1%) in older adults, which is considerably lower than sulfonylureas and incretin-based therapies [168]."

"Older individuals typically have arterial stiffness leading to isolated systolic hypertension."

"SGLT-2 inhibitors have been shown to reduce oxidative stress and improve endothelial function leading to improvement in arterial stiffness [49, 50]."

"It is possible that SGLT-2 inhibitors may also have a favorable effect on blood pressure in patients with hypertension, leading to decreased polypharmacy."

SGLT-2 Inhibitor Dosing and Lack of Need for Titration

"It is important to that note that while higher SGLT-2 inhibitor doses may offer greater glycemic control, large cardiovascular outcomes trials have shown little evidence exists for dose heterogeneity with respect to cardiovascular benefits in T2DM."

"Completed and ongoing HF trials have tested fixed doses of SGLT-2 inhibitors without need for titration."

"Although the SGLT-2:SGLT-1 relative receptor affinity varies among the different agents, all CVOTs with SGLT-2 inhibitors have shown consistent benefit in preventing HF events among patients with at-risk populations with T2DM."

"The cardiovascular outcomes trial testing ertugliflozin has completed [169]."

SGLT-2 Inhibitors and Diuretic Activity

"SGLT-2 inhibitors are associated with osmotic diuresis and natriuresis, which may be synergistic when used in combination with a loop diuretic [170]."

"Distinct from the widely used loop diuretics, SGLT-2 inhibitors may preferentially result in reduction in interstitial volume compared with intravascular volume, thus resulting in less compensatory RAAS activation [170, 171]."

"In DAPA-HF, dosing of concomitant loop diuretics was only modestly lowered during the trial."

"It is suggested that clinicians actively monitor volume status after SGLT-2 initiation and consider decreasing loop diuretic dosing, especially if dizziness or orthostatic hypotension is encountered [108]."

SGLT-2 Inhibitors and Kidney Function

"The recent CARMELINA trial (Cardiovascular and Renal Microvascular Outcome Study with Linagliptin) showed that a substantially higher risk of HF hospitalization was observed in patients with estimated glomerular filtration rate (eGFR) < 60 mL/min per 1.73 m^2 compared with those with eGFR > 60 mL/min per 1.73 m^2 [76]."

"The reduction in HF hospitalization was higher in patients with worse baseline kidney function; a 40% reduction in HF hospitalization was observed among patients with eGFR < 60 mL/min per 1.73 m^2 compared with 31% and 12% reductions in patients with eGFR ≥ 60 to < 90 mL/min per 1.73 m^2 and eGFR ≥ 90 mL/min per 1.73 m^2, respectively [172]."

"Pre-initiation kidney function is encouraged to be > 30 mL/min per 1.73 m^2 for dapagliflozin when used for HF treatment as tested in the DAPA-HF trial."

SGLT-2 Inhibitors and Other HF Therapies

"While the optimal sequence of HFrEF therapies is uncertain, near-simultaneous or clustered initiation of drugs may be feasible for many patients."

"One of the common reasons why guideline-directed medical therapy is not started in clustered fashion by specialists is because of fears of hyperkalemia (due to RAAS inhibition) and low blood pressure."

"Therapies which do not offer cardiovascular risk reduction or mortality benefit in HF, such as calcium channel blockers, should be de-prescribed if low blood pressure with SGLT-2 initiation is a concern."

"As SGLT-2 inhibitors exert a diuretic effect, a dose adjustment in concomitant loop diuretics may be necessary based on clinical signs and symptoms during follow-up."

SGLT-2 Inhibitors and Adjustment of Other Antihyperglycemic Therapies

"Among the large group of patients with HFrEF without concomitant T2DM, dapagliflozin did not appear to lower hemoglobin A1c compared with placebo [41]."

"When initiating SGLT-2 inhibitors in HFrEF and T2DM, certain antihyperglycemic therapies (such as sulfonylureas or dipeptidyl-peptidase-4 inhibitors) may be stopped or dose reduced."

"While metformin has represented a foundational therapy for T2DM, about half of patients enrolled in the DAPA-HF trial were not on background metformin; these patients still derived significant clinical benefits."

"When treating HFrEF, the staged introduction of metformin prior to SGLT-2 inhibitors is likely not required for cardiovascular benefit."

Side Effects of SGLT-2 Inhibitors

"SGLT-2 inhibitors are generally well tolerated, including among patients with HF [46]."

"In 2018, the FDA released a warning related to 12 cases of Fournier's gangrene, a rare but serious and potentially disfiguring perineal infection associated with SGLT-2 inhibitors [173]."

"Rare, euglycemic diabetic ketoacidosis has also been associated with SGLT-2 inhibitors among patients with T2DM."

"It is noteworthy that among patients with HF without T2DM, diabetic ketoacidosis does not appear to be a concern, and no cases were observed in the large DAPA-HF trial in this subset."

Unanswered Questions

"The ongoing DELIVER (Dapagliflozin Evaluation to Improve the Lives of Patients with Preserved Ejection Fraction Heart Failure) and EMPEROR-Preserved (Empagliflozin Outcome Trial in Patients with Chronic Heart Failure with Preserved Ejection Fraction) will provide further insights regarding the role of SGLT-2 inhibitors for this high-risk entity without current effective treatment options."

"SGLT-2 inhibitors may play a role in reversing adverse cardiac remodeling as observed in the EMPA-HEART (Effects of Empagliflozin on Cardiac Structure, Function, and Circulating Biomarkers in Patients with Type 2 Diabetes) CardioLink 6 trial in which patients treated with empagliflozin experienced early and significant reduction in left ventricular mass regression [174]."

"The ongoing PRESERVED-HF (Effects of Dapagliflozin on Biomarkers, Symptoms, and Functional Status in Patients with Preserved Ejection Fraction Heart Failure) and EMBRACE-HF (Empagliflozin Evaluation by Measuring Impact on Hemodynamics in Patients with Heart Failure) will give further information regarding the effect of SGLT-2 inhibitors on cardiac biomarkers, structure, and hemodynamics."

Conclusion

"SGLT-2 inhibitors represent the most recent class of therapies that have been shown to modify clinical course and improve life expectancy among patients with HFrEF."

"Fixed-dose, once daily dosing without need for titration or frequent electrolyte/kidney function monitoring all favor its safe and feasible introduction in multi-drug regimens across a broad range of HFrEF patients."

"Ongoing trials will evaluate if other patients with HF, including those with HFpEF and who are hospitalized for worsening HF, may similarly benefit from this class of therapies."

Bibliography

1. Udell JA, Jones WS, Petrie MC, Harrington J, Anker SD, Bhatt DL, Hernandez AF, Butler J (2022 May 24) Sodium glucose cotransporter-2 inhibition for acute myocardial infarction: JACC review topic of the week. J Am Coll Cardiol 79(20):2058–2068
2. Wu Y-J, Wang S-B, Wang L-S (2022) SGLT2 inhibitors: new hope for the treatment of acute myocardial infarction? Am J Cardiovas Drugs 22:601–613. https://doi.org/10.1007/s40256-022-00545-6
3. Castro-Dominguez Y, Dharmarajan K, McNamara RL (2018) Predicting death after acute myocardial infarction. Trends Cardiovasc Med 28(2):102–109

4. Shimizu W, Kubota Y, Hoshika Y et al (2020) Effects of empagliflozin versus placebo on cardiac sympathetic activity in acute myocardial infarction patients with type 2 diabetes mellitus: the EMBODY trial. Cardiovasc Diabetol 19(1):148
5. Zhao Y, Xu L, Tian D et al (2018) Effects of sodium-glucose co-transporter 2 (SGLT2) inhibitors on serum uric acid level: a meta-analysis of randomized controlled trials. Diabetes Obes Metab 20(2):458–462
6. Neal B, Perkovic V, Mahaffey KW, De Zeeuw D, Fulcher G, Erondu N et al (2017) Canagliflozin and cardiovascular and renal events in type 2 diabetes. N Engl J Med 377(7):644–657
7. Jabbour SA, Hardy E, Sugg J et al (2014) Dapagliflozin is effective as add-on therapy to sitagliptin with or without metformin: a 24-week, multicenter, randomized, double-blind, placebo-controlled study. Diabetes Care 37(3):740–750
8. Bode B, Stenlof K, Harris S, Sullivan D, Fung A, Usiskin K et al (2015) Long-term efficacy and safety of canagliflozin over 104 weeks in patients aged 55–80 years with type 2 diabetes. Diabetes Obes Metab 17(3):294–303
9. Häring HU, Merker L, Seewaldt-Becker E et al (2013) Empagliflozin as add-on to metformin plus sulfonylurea in patients with type 2 diabetes: a 24-week, randomized, double-blind, placebo-controlled trial. Diabetes Care 36(11):3396–3404
10. Sun Z, Chai Q, Zhang Z et al (2021) Inhibition of SGLT1 protects against glycemic variability-induced cardiac damage and pyroptosis of cardiomyocytes in diabetic mice. Life Sci 271:119116
11. Wu W, Chai Q, Zhang Z (2021) Glucose fluctuation accelerates cardiac injury of diabetic mice via sodium-dependent glucose cotransporter 1 (SGLT1). Arch Biochem Biophys 709:108968
12. Lim VG, Bell RM, Arjun S et al (2019) SGLT2 inhibitor, canagliflozin, attenuates myocardial infarction in the diabetic and nondiabetic heart. JACC Basic Transl Sci 4(1):15–26
13. Marfella R, Sardu C, D'Onofrio N, Fumagalli C, Scisciola L, Sasso FC, Siniscalchi M, Marfella LV, D'Andrea D, Minicucci F, Signoriello G, Cesaro A, Trotta MC, Frigé C, Prattichizzo F, Balestrieri ML, Ceriello A, Calabrò P, Mauro C, del Viscovo L, Paolisso G (2023) SGLT-2 inhibitors and in-stent restenosis-related events after acute myocardial infarction: an observational study in patients with type 2 diabetes. BMC Med 21:71. https://doi.org/10.1186/s12916-023-02781-2
14. Paramasivam G, Devasia T, Jayaram A, Rao MS, Vijayvergiya R, Nayak K (2020) In-stent restenosis of drug-eluting stents in patients with diabetes mellitus: clinical presentation, angiographic features, and outcomes. Anatol J Cardiol 23(1):28–34
15. Zhao L, Zhu W, Zhang X, He D, Guo C (2017) Effect of diabetes mellitus on long-term outcomes after repeat drug-eluting stent implantation for in-stent restenosis. BMC Cardiovasc Disord 17(1):16
16. Marfella R, Sasso FC, Siniscalchi M, Paolisso P, Rizzo MR, Ferraro F, Stabile E, Sorropago G, Calabrò P, Carbonara O, Cinquegrana G, Piscione F, Ruocco A, D'Andrea D, Rapacciuolo A, Petronella P, Bresciani A, Rubino P, Mauro C, Paolisso G (2012) Peri-procedural tight glycemic control during early percutaneous coronary intervention is associated with a lower rate of in-stent restenosis in patients with acute ST-elevation myocardial infarction. J Clin Endocrinol Metab 97(8):2862–2871
17. Mone P, Gambardella J, Minicucci F, Lombardi A, Mauro C, Santulli G (2021) Hyperglycemia drives stent restenosis in STEMI patients. Diabetes Care 44(11):e192–e193
18. Vaduganathan M, Docherty KF, Claggett BL, Jhund PS, de Boer RA, Hernandez AF, Inzucchi SE, Kosiborod MN, Lam CSP, Martinez F, Shah SJ, Desai AS, McMurray JJV, Solomon SD (2022) SGLT-2 inhibitors in patients with heart failure: a comprehensive meta-analysis of five randomised controlled trials. Lancet 400(10354):757–767
19. D'Onofrio N, Sardu C, Trotta MC, Scisciola L, Turriziani F, Ferraraccio F, Panarese I, Petrella L, Fanelli M, Modugno P, Massetti M, Marfella LV, Sasso FC, Rizzo MR, Barbieri M, Furbatto F, Minicucci F, Mauro C, Federici M, Balestrieri ML, Paolisso G, Marfella R (2021) Sodium-glucose co-transporter2 expression and inflammatory activity in diabetic atherosclerotic plaques: effects of sodium-glucose co-transporter2 inhibitor treatment. Mol Metab 54:101337

20. Scisciola L, Cataldo V, Taktaz F, Fontanella RA, Pesapane A, Ghosh P, Franzese M, Puocci A, De Angelis A, Sportiello L, Marfella R, Barbieri M (2022) Anti-inflammatory role of SGLT2 inhibitors as part of their anti-atherosclerotic activity: data from basic science and clinical trials. Front Cardiovasc Med 9:1008922
21. Prattichizzo F, de Candia P, Ceriello A (2021) Diabetes and kidney disease: emphasis on treatment with SGLT-2 inhibitors and GLP-1 receptor agonists. Metabolism 120:154799
22. Pitt B, Steg G, Leiter LA, Bhatt DL (2021) The role of combined SGLT1/SGLT2 inhibition in reducing the incidence of stroke and myocardial infarction in patients with type 2 diabetes mellitus. Cardiovasc Drugs Ther 36:561–567. https://doi.org/10.1007/s10557-021-07291-y
23. Bhatt DL, Szarek M, Pitt B et al (2021) Sotagliflozin in patients with diabetes and chronic kidney disease. N Engl J Med 384:129–139
24. Bhatt DL, Szarek M, Steg PG et al (2021) Sotagliflozin in patients with diabetes and worsening heart failure. N Engl J Med 384:117–128
25. Benedikt M, Mangge H, Aziz F, Curcic P, Pailer S, Herrmann M, Kolesnik E, Tripolt NJ, Pferschy PN, Wallner M, Zirlik A, Sourij H, von Lewinski D (2023) Impact of the SGLT2-inhibitor empagliflozin on inflammatory biomarkers after acute myocardial infarction—a post-hoc analysis of the EMMY trial. Cardiovasc Diabetol 22:166. https://doi.org/10.1186/s12933-023-01904-6
26. Dogan I, Karaman K, Sonmez B, Celik S, Turker O (2009) Relationship between serum neutrophil count and infarct size in patients with acute myocardial infarction. Nucl Med Commun 30(10):797–801
27. Chia S, Nagurney JT, Brown DFM, Raffel OC, Bamberg F, Senatore F et al (2009) Association of leukocyte and neutrophil counts with infarct size, left ventricular function and outcomes after percutaneous coronary intervention for ST-elevation myocardial infarction. Am J Cardiol 103(3):333–337
28. Dharma S, Hapsari R, Siswanto BB, van der Laarse A, Jukema JW (2015) Blood leukocyte count on admission predicts cardiovascular events in patients with acute non-ST elevation myocardial infarction. Int J Angiol 24(2):127–132
29. von Lewinski D, Kolesnik E, Tripolt NJ, Pferschy PN, Benedikt M, Wallner M et al (2022) Empagliflozin in acute myocardial infarction: the EMMY trial. Eur Heart J 1(41):4421–4432
30. Paolisso P, Bergamaschi L, Santulli G et al (2022) Infarct size, inflammatory burden, and admission hyperglycemia in diabetic patients with acute myocardial infarction treated with SGLT2-inhibitors: a multicenter international registry. Cardiovasc Diabetol 21(1):77
31. Kologrivova I, Shtatolkina M, Suslova T, Ryabov V (2021) Cells of the immune system in cardiac remodeling: main players in resolution of inflammation and repair after myocardial infarction. Front Immunol 12:664457
32. Wang J, Wang M, Lu X, Zhang Y, Zeng S, Pan X et al (2022) IL-6 inhibitors effectively reverse post-infarction cardiac injury and ischemic myocardial remodeling via the TGF-β1/Smad3 signaling pathway. Exp Ther Med 24(3):576
33. Anzai T (2018 Feb 23) Inflammatory mechanisms of cardiovascular remodeling. Circ J 82(3):629–635
34. Huang M, Yang D, Xiang M, Wang J (2015 Jan) Role of interleukin-6 in regulation of immune responses to remodeling after myocardial infarction. Heart Fail Rev 20(1):25–38
35. Fonseca FA, Izar MC (2022) Role of inflammation in cardiac remodeling after acute myocardial infarction. Front Physiol 13:927163
36. Sayour AA, Oláh A, Ruppert M, Barta BA, Horváth EM, Benke K, Pólos M, Hartyánszky I, Merkely B, Radovits T (2020) Characterization of left ventricular myocardial sodium-glucose cotransporter 1 expression in patients with end-stage heart failure. Cardiovasc Diabetol 19(1):159. https://doi.org/10.1186/s12933-020-01141-1
37. Tripolt NJ, Kolesnik E, Pferschy PN et al (2020) Impact of EMpagliflozin on cardiac function and biomarkers of heart failure in patients with acute MYocardial infarction—the EMMY trial. Am Heart J 221:39–47

38. Zinman B, Wanner C, Lachin JM, Fitchett D, Bluhmki E, Hantel S et al (2015) Empagliflozin, cardiovascular outcomes, and mortality in type 2 diabetes. N Engl J Med 373(22):2117–2128
39. Wiviott SD, Raz I, Bonaca MP, Mosenzon O, Kato ET, Cahn A et al (2019) Dapagliflozin and cardiovascular outcomes in type 2 diabetes. N Engl J Med 380(4):347–357
40. Nassif ME, Sindsor SL, Tang F et al (2019) Dapagliflozin effects on biomarkers, symptoms, and functional status in patients with heart failure with reduced ejection fraction: the DEFINE-HF trial. Circulation 140:1463–1476
41. McMurray JJV, Solomon SD, Inzucchi SE, Køber L, Kosiborod MN, Martinez FA et al (2019) Dapagliflozin in patients with heart failure and reduced ejection fraction. N Engl J Med 381(21):1995–2008
42. Packer M, Anker SD, Butler J, Filippatos G, Pocock SJ, Carson P et al (2020) Cardiovascular and renal outcomes with empagliflozin in heart failure. N Engl J Med 383(15):1413–1424
43. Polidori D, Sha S, Mudaliar S, Ciaraldi TP, Ghosh A, Vaccaro N et al (2013) Canagliflozin lowers postprandial glucose and insulin by delaying intestinal glucose absorption in addition to increasing urinary glucose excretion: results of a randomized, placebo-controlled study. Diabetes Care 36(8):2154–2161
44. Ohgaki R, Wei L, Yamada K et al (2016) Interaction of the sodium/glucose cotransporter (SGLT) 2 inhibitor canagliflozin with SGLT1 and SGLT2. J Pharmacol Exp Ther 358:94–102
45. Cefalo CMA, Cinti F, Moffa S, Impronta F, Sorice GP, Mezza T et al (2019) Sotagliflozin, the first dual SGLT inhibitor: current outlook and perspectives. Cardiovasc Diabetol 18(1):20
46. Lam CSP, Chandramouli C, Ahooja V, Verma S (2019) SGLT-2 inhibitors in heart failure: current management, unmet needs, and therapeutic prospects. J Am Heart Assoc 8(20):e013389
47. Baker HE, Kiel AM, Luebbe ST, Simon BR, Earl CC, Regmi A, Roell WC, Mather KJ, Tune JD, Goodwill AG (2019) Inhibition of sodium–glucose cotransporter-2 preserves cardiac function during regional myocardial ischemia independent of alterations in myocardial substrate utilization. Basic Res Cardiol 114:25. https://doi.org/10.1007/s00395-019-0733-2
48. Santos-Gallego CG, Garcia-Ropero A, Mancini D, Pinney SP, Contreras JP, Fergus I, Abascal V, Moreno P, Atallah-Lajam F, Tamler R, Lala A, Sanz J, Fuster V, Badimon JJ (2019) Rationale and design of the EMPA-TROPISM trial (ATRU-4): are the "cardiac benefits" of empagliflozin independent of its hypoglycemic activity? Cardiovasc Drugs Ther 33:87–95. https://doi.org/10.1007/s10557-018-06850-0
49. Cherney DZ, Perkins BA, Soleymanlou N, Har R, Fagan N, Johansen OE et al (2014) The effect of empagliflozin on arterial stiffness and heart rate variability in subjects with uncomplicated type 1 diabetes mellitus. Cardiovasc Diabetol 13:28
50. Chilton R, Tikkanen I, Cannon CP, Crowe S, Woerle HJ, Broedl UC et al (2015) Effects of empagliflozin on blood pressure and markers of arterial stiffness and vascular resistance in patients with type 2 diabetes. Diabetes Obes Metab 17(12):1180–1193
51. Ferrannini E, Mark M, Mayoux E (2016) CV protection in the EMPA-REG OUTCOME trial: a "thrifty substrate" hypothesis. Diabetes Care 39(7):1108–1114
52. Garcia-Dorado D, Theroux P, Elizaga J, Galinanes M, Solares J, Riesgo M, Gomez MJ, Garcia-Dorado A, Fernandez Aviles F (1987) Myocardial reperfusion in the pig heart model: infarct size and duration of coronary occlusion. Cardiovasc Res 21:537–544
53. Gent S, Skyschally A, Kleinbongard P, Heusch G (2017) Lschemic preconditioning in pigs: a causal role for signal transducer and activator of transcription 3. Am J Physiol Heart Circ Physiol 312:H478–H484. https://doi.org/10.1152/ajpheart.00749.2016
54. Custodio JS, Duraes AR, Abreu M, Albuquerque Rocha N, Roever L (2018) SGLT2 inhibition and heart failure—current concepts. Heart Fail Rev 23:409–418. https://doi.org/10.1007/s10741-018-9703-2
55. Gerstein HC (2008) The hemoglobin A1c level as a progressive risk factor for cardiovascular death, hospitalization for heart failure, or death in patients with chronic heart failure: an analysis of the Candesartan in Heart Failure: Assessment of Reduction in Mortality and Morbidity (CHARM) program. Arch Intern Med 168:1699–1704. https://doi.org/10.1001/archinte.168.15.1699

56. Lavalle-González FJ, Januszewicz A, Davidson J, Tong C, Qiu R, Canovatchel W et al (2013) Efficacy and safety of canagliflozin compared with placebo and sitagliptin in patients with type 2 diabetes on background metformin monotherapy: a randomised trial. Diabetologia 56(12):2582–2592
57. Schernthaner G, Gross J, Rosenstock J, Guarisco M, Fu M, Yee J et al (2013) Canagliflozin compared with sitagliptin for patients with type 2 diabetes who do not have adequate glycemic control with metformin plus sulfonylurea: a 52-week randomized trial. Diabetes Care 36(9):2508–2515
58. Despa S (2002) Intracellular Na+ concentration is elevated in heart failure but Na/K pump function is unchanged. Circulation 105:2543–2548. https://doi.org/10.1161/01.CIR.0000016701.85760.97
59. Wojcik C, Warden BA (2019) Mechanisms and evidence for heart failure benefits from SGLT2 inhibitors. Curr Cardiol Rep 21(10):130. https://doi.org/10.1007/s11886-019-1219-4
60. Zinman B, Wanner C, Lachin JM et al (2015) Empagliflozin, cardiovascular outcomes, and mortality in type 2 diabetes. N Engl J Med 373:2117–2128. EMPAREG-OUTCOMES trial reporting the CV outcomes of empagliflozin
61. Mather A, Pollock C (2011) Glucose handling by the kidney. Kidney Int Suppl 79:S1–S6
62. Rieg T, Vallon V (2018) Development of SGLT1 and SGLT2 inhibitors. Diabetologia 61:2079–2086
63. Zelniker TA, Wiviott SD, Raz I, Im K, Goodrich EL, Bonaca MP et al (2019) SGLT2 inhibitors for primary and secondary prevention of cardiovascular and renal outcomes in type 2 diabetes: a systematic review and meta-analysis of cardiovascular outcome trials. Lancet 393:31–39
64. Sato T, Aizawa Y, Yuasa S, Kishi S, Fuse K, Fujita S et al (2018) The effect of dapagliflozin treatment on epicardial adipose tissue volume. Cardiovasc Diabetol 17:6
65. Bouchi R, Terashima M, Sasahara Y, Asakawa M, Fukuda T, Takeuchi T et al (2017) Luseogliflozin reduces epicardial fat accumulation in patients with type 2 diabetes: a pilot study. Cardiovasc Diabetol 16:32
66. Yagi S, Hirata Y, Ise T, Kusunose K, Yamada H, Fukuda D et al (2017) Canagliflozin reduces epicardial fat in patients with type 2 diabetes mellitus. Diabetol Metab Syndr 9:78
67. Sano M, Takei M, Shiraishi Y, Suzuki Y (2016) Increased hematocrit during sodium-glucose cotransporter 2 inhibitor therapy indicates recovery of tubulointerstitial function in diabetic kidneys. J Clin Med Res 8:844–847
68. Kato ET, Silverman MG, Mosenzon O et al (2019) Effect of dapagliflozin on heart failure and mortality in type 2 diabetes mellitus. Circulation 139:2528–2536
69. Furtado RHM, Bonaca MP, Raz I, Zelniker TA, Mosenzon O, Cahn A et al (2019) Dapagliflozin and cardiovascular outcomes in patients with type 2 diabetes mellitus and previous myocardial infarction. Circulation 139(22):2516–2527
70. Tanaka A, Node K (2020) Promising roles of sodium–glucose cotransporter 2 inhibitors in heart failure prevention and treatment. Diabetol Int 11(3):252–260. https://doi.org/10.1007/s13340-020-00445-7
71. Boonman-de Winter LJ, Rutten FH, Cramer MJ, Landman MJ, Liem AH, Rutten GE et al (2012) High prevalence of previously unknown heart failure and left ventricular dysfunction in patients with type 2 diabetes. Diabetologia 55(8):2154–2162
72. Khan SS, Butler J, Gheorghiade M (2014) Management of comorbid diabetes mellitus and worsening heart failure. JAMA 311(23):2379–2380
73. Eurich DT, Weir DL, Majumdar SR, Tsuyuki RT, Johnson JA, Tjosvold L et al (2013) Comparative safety and effectiveness of metformin in patients with diabetes mellitus and heart failure: systematic review of observational studies involving 34,000 patients. Circ Heart Fail 6(3):395–402
74. Crowley MJ, Diamantidis CJ, McDuffie JR, Cameron CB, Stanifer JW, Mock CK et al (2017) Clinical outcomes of metformin use in populations with chronic kidney disease, congestive heart failure, or chronic liver disease: a systematic review. Ann Intern Med 166(3):191–200

75. White WB, Cannon CP, Heller SR, Nissen SE, Bergenstal RM, Bakris GL et al (2013) Alogliptin after acute coronary syndrome in patients with type 2 diabetes. N Engl J Med 369(14):1327–1335
76. McGuire DK, Alexander JH, Johansen OE, Perkovic V, Rosenstock J, Cooper ME et al (2019) Linagliptin effects on heart failure and related outcomes in individuals with type 2 diabetes mellitus at high cardiovascular and renal risk in CARMELINA. Circulation 139(3):351–361
77. Zinman B, Wanner C, Lachin JM, Fitchett D, Bluhmki E, Hantel S et al (2015) Empagliflozin, cardiovascular outcomes, and mortality in type 2 diabetes. N Engl J Med 373(22):2117–2288
78. Mahaffey KW, Neal B, Perkovic V, de Zeeuw D, Fulcher G, Erondu N et al (2018) Canagliflozin for primary and secondary prevention of cardiovascular events: results from the CANVAS program (Canagliflozin Cardiovascular Assessment Study). Circulation 137(4):323–334
79. Radholm K, Figtree G, Perkovic V, Solomon SD, Mahaffey KW, de Zeeuw D et al (2018) Canagliflozin and heart failure in type 2 diabetes mellitus. Circulation 138(5):458–468
80. Tsutsui H, Isobe M, Ito H, Ito H, Okumura K, Ono M et al (2019) JCS 2017/JHFS 2017 guideline on diagnosis and treatment of acute and chronic heart failure-digest version. Circ J 83(10):2084–2184
81. Januzzi JL Jr, Butler J, Jarolim P, Sattar N, Vijapurkar U, Desai M et al (2017) Effects of canagliflozin on cardiovascular biomarkers in older adults with type 2 diabetes. J Am Coll Cardiol 70(6):704–712
82. Verma S, Garg A, Yan AT, Gupta AK, Al-Omran M, Sabongui A et al (2016) Effect of empagliflozin on left ventricular mass and diastolic function in individuals with diabetes: an important clue to the EMPA-REG OUTCOME trial? Diabetes Care 39(12):e212–e213213
83. Nassif ME, Windsor SL, Tang F, Khariton Y, Husain M, Inzucchi SE et al (2019) Dapagliflozin effects on biomarkers, symptoms, and functional status in patients with heart failure with reduced ejection fraction: the DEFINE-HF trial. Circulation 140(18):1463–1476
84. Butler J, Hamo CE, Filippatos G, Pocock SJ, Bernstein RA, Brueckmann M et al (2017) The potential role and rationale for treatment of heart failure with sodium-glucose co-transporter 2 inhibitors. Eur J Heart Fail 19(11):1390–1400
85. Garla VV, Butler J, Lien LF (2021) SGLT-2 inhibitors in heart failure: guide for prescribing and future perspectives. Curr Cardiol Rep 23:59. https://doi.org/10.1007/s11886-021-01486-3
86. Savarese G, Lund LH (2017) Global public health burden of heart failure. Card Fail Rev 3:7–11
87. Kannel WB, McGee DL (1979) Diabetes and cardiovascular disease. The Framingham study. JAMA 241:2035–2038
88. Preiss D, Zetterstrand S, McMurray JJ, Ostergren J, Michelson EL, Granger CB, Sattar N, Candesartan in Heart Failure Assessment of Reduction in Mortality and Morbidity Investigators et al (2009) Predictors of development of diabetes in patients with chronic heart failure in the Candesartan in Heart Failure Assessment of Reduction in Mortality and Morbidity (CHARM) program. Diabetes Care 32:915–920
89. Scheen AJ (2020) Sodium-glucose cotransporter type 2 inhibitors for the treatment of type 2 diabetes mellitus. Nat Rev Endocrinol 16(10):556–577
90. Butler J, Hamo CE, Filippatos G et al (2017) The potential role and rationale for treatment of heart failure with sodium-glucose co-transporter 2 inhibitors. Eur J Heart Fail 19(11):1390–1400
91. Packer M (2018) Do sodium-glucose co-transporter-2 inhibitors prevent heart failure with a preserved ejection fraction by counterbalancing the effects of leptin? A novel hypothesis. Diabetes Obes Metab 20(6):1361–1366
92. Garvey WT, Van Gaal L, Leiter LA, Vijapurkar U, List J, Cuddihy R et al (2018) Effects of canagliflozin versus glimepiride on adipokines and inflammatory biomarkers in type 2 diabetes. Metabolism 85:32–37
93. Yaribeygi H, Katsiki N, Butler AE, Sahebkar A (2019) Effects of antidiabetic drugs on NLRP3 inflammasome activity, with a focus on diabetic kidneys. Drug Discov Today 24(1):256–262

94. Ryan PB, Buse JB, Schuemie MJ, DeFalco F, Yuan Z, Stang PE et al (2018) Comparative effectiveness of canagliflozin, SGLT2 inhibitors and non-SGLT2 inhibitors on the risk of hospitalization for heart failure and amputation in patients with type 2 diabetes mellitus: a real-world meta-analysis of 4 observational databases (OBSERVE-4D). Diabetes Obes Metab 20(11):2585–2597
95. Khouri C, Cracowski JL, Roustit M (2018) SGLT-2 inhibitors and the risk of lower-limb amputation: is this a class effect? Diabetes Obes Metab 20(6):1531–1534
96. Bersoff-Matcha SJ, Chamberlain C, Cao C, Kortepeter C, Chong WH (2019) Fournier gangrene associated with sodium-glucose cotransporter-2 inhibitors: a review of spontaneous postmarketing cases. Ann Intern Med 170(11):764–769
97. American Diabetes Association (2020) 9. Pharmacologic approaches to glycemic treatment: standards of medical care in diabetes-2020. Diabetes Care 43(Suppl 1):S98–S110
98. Brito D, Bettencourt P, Carvalho D, Ferreira J, Fontes-Carvalho R, Franco F, Moura B, Silva-Cardoso JC, de Melo RT, Fonseca C (2020) Sodium-glucose co-transporter 2 inhibitors in the failing heart: a growing potential. Cardiovasc Drugs Ther 34:419–436. https://doi.org/10.1007/s10557-020-06973-3
99. Kannel WB, Hjortland M, Castelli WP (1974) Role of diabetes in congestive heart failure: the Framingham study. Am J Cardiol 34:29–34. https://doi.org/10.1016/0002-9149(74)90089-7
100. Benjamin EJ, Blaha MJ, Chiuve SE, Cushman M, Das SR, Deo R, de Ferranti SD, Floyd J, Fornage M, Gillespie C, Isasi CR, Jiménez MC, Jordan LC, Judd SE, Lackland D, Lichtman JH, Lisabeth L, Liu S, Longenecker CT, Mackey RH, Matsushita K, Mozaffarian D, Mussolino ME, Nasir K, Neumar RW, Palaniappan L, Pandey DK, Thiagarajan RR, Reeves MJ, Ritchey M, Rodriguez CJ, Roth GA, Rosamond WD, Sasson C, Towfighi A, Tsao CW, Turner MB, Virani SS, Voeks JH, Willey JZ, Wilkins JT, Wu JH, Alger HM, Wong SS, Muntner P, American Heart Association Statistics Committee, Stroke Statistics Subcommittee (2017) Heart disease and stroke statistics—2017 update: a report from the American Heart Association. Circulation 135:e146–e603. https://doi.org/10.1161/CIR.0000000000000485
101. Bogner HR, Miller SD, de Vries HF et al (2010) Assessment of cost and health resource utilization for elderly patients with heart failure and diabetes mellitus. J Card Fail 16:454–460. https://doi.org/10.1016/j.cardfail.2010.01.007
102. Cavender MA, Steg PG, Smith SC et al (2015) Impact of diabetes mellitus on hospitalization for heart failure, cardiovascular events, and death: outcomes at 4 years from the reduction of atherothrombosis for continued health (REACH) registry. Circulation 132:923–931. https://doi.org/10.1161/CIRCULATIONAHA.114.014796
103. Fitchett D, Butler J, van de Borne P, Zinman B, Lachin JM, Wanner C et al (2018) Effects of empagliflozin on risk for cardiovascular death and heart failure hospitalization across the spectrum of heart failure risk in the EMPA-REG OUTCOME(R) trial. Eur Heart J 39(5):363–370
104. Mudaliar S, Alloju S, Henry RR (2016) Can a shift in fuel energetics explain the beneficial cardiorenal outcomes in the EMPA-REG OUTCOME study? A unifying hypothesis. Diabetes Care 39:1115–1122. https://doi.org/10.2337/dc16-0542
105. Monami M, Dicembrini I, Mannucci E (2017) Effects of SGLT-2 inhibitors on mortality and cardiovascular events: a comprehensive meta-analysis of randomized controlled trials. Acta Diabetol 54(1):19–36
106. Wende AR, Brahma MK, McGinnis GR, Young ME (2017) Metabolic origins of heart failure. JACC Basic to Transl Sci. 2(3):297–310. https://doi.org/10.1016/J.JACBTS.2016.11.009
107. Wilcox CS, Shen W, Boulton DW et al (2018) Interaction between the sodium-glucose-linked transporter 2 inhibitor dapagliflozin and the loop diuretic bumetanide in normal human subjects. J Am Heart Assoc 7(4):e007046. https://doi.org/10.1161/JAHA.117.007046
108. Cherney DZI, Udell JA (2016) Use of sodium glucose cotransporter 2 inhibitors in the hands of cardiologists: with great power comes great responsibility. Circulation 134(24):1915–1917. https://doi.org/10.1161/CIRCULATIONAHA.116.024764

109. Damman K, Beusekamp JC, Boorsma EM et al (2020) Randomized, double-blind, placebo-controlled, multicentre pilot study on the effects of empagliflozin on clinical outcomes in patients with acute decompensated heart failure (EMPA-RESPONSE-AHF). Eur J Heart Fail 22:713–722. https://doi.org/10.1002/ejhf.1713
110. Evans M, Morgan AR, Yousef Z, Ellis G, Dashora U, Patel DC, Brown P, Hanif W, Townend JN, Kanumilli N, Moore J, Wilding JPH, Bain SC (2021) Optimising the heart failure treatment pathway: the role of SGLT2 inhibitors. Drugs 81:1243–1255. https://doi.org/10.1007/s40265-021-01538-6
111. Ghosh RK, Ghosh GC, Gupta M, Bandyopadhyay D, Akhtar T, Deedwania P et al (2019) Sodium glucose co-transporter 2 inhibitors and heart failure. Am J Cardiol 124(11):1790–1796. https://doi.org/10.1016/j.amjcard.2019.08.038
112. Berg DD, Jhund PS, Docherty KF, Murphy SA, Verma S, Inzucchi SE et al (2021) Time to clinical benefit of dapagliflozin and significance of prior heart failure hospitalization in patients with heart failure with reduced ejection fraction. JAMA Cardiol 6:499–507. https://doi.org/10.1001/jamacardio.2020.7585
113. Willenheimer R, van Veldhuisen DJ, Silke B, Erdmann E, Follath F, Krum H et al (2005) Effect on survival and hospitalization of initiating treatment for chronic heart failure with bisoprolol followed by enalapril, as compared with the opposite sequence: results of the randomized Cardiac Insufficiency Bisoprolol Study (CIBIS) III. Circulation 112(16):2426–2435. https://doi.org/10.1161/circulationaha.105.582320
114. Sliwa K, Norton GR, Kone N, Candy G, Kachope J, Woodiwiss AJ et al (2004) Impact of initiating carvedilol before angiotensin-converting enzyme inhibitor therapy on cardiac function in newly diagnosed heart failure. J Am Coll Cardiol 44(9):1825–1830. https://doi.org/10.1016/j.jacc.2004.05.087
115. National Institute for Health and Care Excellence (2014) Clinical guideline [CG187]: acute heart failure: diagnosis and management. https://www.nice.org.uk/guidance/cg187/. Accessed 1 Dec 2020
116. Bhatt DL, Szarek M, Steg PG et al (2021) Sotagliflozin in patients with diabetes and recent worsening heart failure. N Engl J Med 384:117–128
117. Bhatt DL, Szarek M, Pitt B, Cannon CP, Leiter LA, McGuire DK et al (2021) Sotagliflozin in patients with diabetes and chronic kidney disease. N Engl J Med 384(2):129–139
118. Faulkenberg KD, Williams JB, Isaacs DM, West LM (2020) Practical considerations and opportunities for SGLT2 inhibitor prescription in heart failure. Curr Treat Options Cardiovasc Med 22. https://doi.org/10.1007/s11936-020-00825-x
119. Cefalu WT et al (2018) Cardiovascular outcomes trials in type 2 diabetes: where do we go from here? Reflections from a diabetes care editors' expert forum. Diabetes Care 41(1):14–31
120. Cosentino F, Grant PJ, Aboyans V et al (2020) 2019 ESC guidelines on diabetes, prediabetes, and cardiovascular diseases developed in collaboration with the EASD. Eur Heart J 41:255–32323
121. Das SR, Everett BM, Birtcher KK et al (2018) 2018 ACC expert consensus decision pathway on novel therapies for cardiovascular risk reduction in patients with type 2 diabetes and atherosclerotic cardiovascular disease: a report of the American College of Cardiology task force on expert consensus decision pathways. J Am Coll Cardiol 72:3200–3223
122. Cannon CP (2020) The VERTIS CV trial: cardiovascular outcomes following ertugliflozin treatment in patients with type 2 diabetes mellitus and atherosclerotic cardiovascular disease. Presented at the American Diabetes Association Virtual Scientific Sessions
123. Berg DD et al (2019) Heart failure risk stratification and efficacy of sodium-glucose cotransporter-2 inhibitors in patients with type 2 diabetes mellitus. Circulation 140(19):1569–1577
124. Nana M, Morgan H, Bondugulapati LNR (2020) Sodium-glucose co-transporter 2 inhibitors and heart failure—the present and the future. Heart Fail Rev 26:953–960. https://doi.org/10.1007/s10741-020-09925-z
125. Rosano GM, Vitale C, Seferovic P (2017) Heart failure in patients with diabetes mellitus. Card Fail Rev 3(1):52–55

126. MacDonald MR, Petrie MC, Varyani F, Ostergren J, Michelson EL, Young JB, Solomon SD, Granger CB, Swedberg K, Yusuf S, Pfeffer MA, McMurray J, CHARM Investigators (2008) Impact of diabetes on outcomes in patients with low and preserved ejection fraction heart failure: an analysis of the Candesartan in Heart failure: Assessment of Reduction in Mortality and morbidity (CHARM) programme. Eur Heart J 29(11):1377–1385
127. Zelniker TA, Wiviott SD, Raz I, Im K, Goodrich EL, Bonaca MP, Mosenzon O, Kato ET, Cahn A, Furtado RHM, Bhatt DL, Leiter LA, McGuire D, Wilding JPH, Sabatine MS (2019) SGLT2 inhibitors for primary and secondary prevention of cardiovascular and renal outcomes in type 2 diabetes: a systematic review and meta-analysis of cardiovascular outcome trials. Lancet 393(10166):31–39
128. Kristensen SL, Preiss D, Jhund PS, Squire I, Cardoso JS, Merkely B et al (2016) Risk related to pre-diabetes mellitus and diabetes mellitus in heart failure with reduced ejection fraction: insights from prospective comparison of ARNI with ACEI to determine impact on Global Mortality and Morbidity in Heart Failure Trial. Circ Heart Fail 9(1):e002560. https://doi.org/10.1161/CIRCHEARTFAILURE.115.002560
129. Greenberg BH, Abraham WT, Albert NM, Chiswell K, Clare R, Stough WG et al (2007) Influence of diabetes on characteristics and outcomes in patients hospitalized with heart failure: a report from the Organized Program to Initiate Lifesaving Treatment in Hospitalized Patients with Heart Failure (OPTIMIZE-HF). Am Heart J 154(2):277.e1–277.e8
130. Boonman-de Winter LJ, Rutten FH, Cramer MJ, Landman MJ, Liem AH, Rutten GE, Hoes AW (2012) High prevalence of previously unknown heart failure and left ventricular dysfunction in patients with type 2 diabetes. Diabetologia 55(8):2154–2162
131. Thrainsdottir IS, Aspelund T, Thorgeirsson G, Gudnason V, Hardarson T, Malmberg K, Sigurdsson G, Rydén L (2005) The association between glucose abnormalities and heart failure in the population-based Reykjavik study. Diabetes Care 28(3):612–616
132. Khan H, Anker SD, Januzzi JL, McGuire DK, Sattar N, Woerle HJ et al (2019) Heart failure epidemiology in patients with diabetes mellitus without coronary heart disease. J Card Fail 25(2):78–86
133. Group CTS (1987) Effects of enalapril on mortality in severe congestive heart failure. Results of the Cooperative North Scandinavian Enalapril Survival Study (CONSENSUS). N Engl J Med 316(23):1429–1435
134. (1999) The cardiac insufficiency bisoprolol study II (CIBIS-II): a randomised trial. Lancet 353(9146):9–13
135. Borlaug BA, Paulus WJ (2011) Heart failure with preserved ejection fraction: pathophysiology, diagnosis, and treatment. Eur Heart J 32(6):670–679
136. Zinman B, Wanner C, Lachin JM, Fitchett D, Bluhmki E, Hantel S, Mattheus M, Devins T, Johansen OE, Woerle HJ, Broedl UC, Inzucchi SE, EMPA-REG OUTCOME Investigators (2015) Empagliflozin, cardiovascular outcomes, and mortality in type 2 diabetes. N Engl J Med 373(22):2117–2128
137. Neal B, Perkovic V, Mahaffey KW, de Zeeuw D, Fulcher G, Erondu N, Shaw W, Law G, Desai M, Matthews DR, CANVAS Program Collaborative Group (2017) Canagliflozin and cardiovascular and renal events in type 2 diabetes. N Engl J Med 377(7):644–657
138. Wiviott SD, Raz I, Bonaca MP, Mosenzon O, Kato ET, Cahn A, Silverman MG, Zelniker TA, Kuder JF, Murphy SA, Bhatt DL, Leiter LA, McGuire D, Wilding JPH, Ruff CT, Gause-Nilsson IAM, Fredriksson M, Johansson PA, Langkilde AM, Sabatine MS, DECLARE–TIMI 58 Investigators (2019) Dapagliflozin and cardiovascular outcomes in type 2 diabetes. N Engl J Med 380(4):347–357
139. Agency EM (2016) EMA confirms recommendations to minimise ketoacidosis risk with SGLT2 inhibitors for diabetes. https://www.ema.europa.eu/en/medicines/human/referrals/sglt2-inhibitors
140. Kashiwagi Y, Nagoshi T, Yoshino T, Tanaka TD, Ito K, Harada T, Takahashi H, Ikegami M, Anzawa R, Yoshimura M (2015) Expression of SGLT1 in human hearts and impairment of cardiac glucose uptake by phlorizin during ischemia-reperfusion injury in mice. PLoS One 10(6):e0130605

141. Connelly KA, Zhang Y, Desjardins JF, Thai K, Gilbert RE (2018) Dual inhibition of sodium-glucose linked cotransporters 1 and 2 exacerbates cardiac dysfunction following experimental myocardial infarction. Cardiovasc Diabetol 17(1):99
142. Åkerblom A, Oldgren J, Latva-Rasku A, Johansson L, Lisovskaja V, Karlsson C, Oscarsson J, Nuutila P (2019) Effects of DAPAgliflozin on CARDiac substrate uptake, myocardial efficiency, and myocardial contractile work in type 2 diabetes patients-a description of the DAPACARD study. Ups J Med Sci 124(1):59–64
143. Seferović PM, Seferović JP, Polovina MM (2019) Diving into the unknown: sodium-glucose cotransporter-2 inhibitors in heart failure without diabetes. Eur J Heart Fail 20(5):853–872
144. Dunlay SM, Givertz MM, Aguilar D, Allen LA, Chan M, Desai AS et al (2019) Type 2 diabetes mellitus and heart failure, a scientific statement from the American Heart Association and Heart Failure Society of America. J Card Fail 25(8):584–619
145. Medicine NUSNLo (2018) Effect of Sotagliflozin on Cardiovascular Events in Patients With Type 2 Diabetes Post Worsening Heart Failure (SOLOIST-WHF Trial). https://clinicaltrials.gov/ct2/show/NCT03521934
146. Nana M, Morgan H, Bondugulapati LR (2021) Sodium-glucose co-transporter 2 inhibitors and heart failure—the present and the future. Heart Fail Rev (4):953–60.
147. Severino P, D'Amato A, Prosperi S, Costi B, Angotti D, Birtolo LI, Chimenti C, Lavalle C, Maestrini V, Mancone M, Fedele F (2021) Sodium-glucose cotransporter 2 inhibitors and heart failure: the best timing for the right patient. Heart Fail Rev 28:709–721. https://doi.org/10.1007/s10741-021-10170-1
148. Ray EC (2020) Evolving understanding of cardiovascular protection by SGLT2 inhibitors: focus on renal protection myocardial effects uric acid and magnesium balance. Curr Opin Pharmacol 54:11–17. https://doi.org/10.1016/j.coph.2020.06.001
149. Severino P, Netti L, Mariani MV, Maraone A, D'Amato A, Scarpati R, Infusino F, Pucci M, Lavalle C, Maestrini V, Mancone M, Fedele F (2019) Prevention of cardiovascular disease: screening for magnesium deficiency. Cardiol Res Pract 2019:4874921. https://doi.org/10.1155/2019/4874921
150. Ghanim H, Abuaysheh S, Hejna J, Green K, Batra M, Makdissi A, Chaudhuri A, Dandona P (2020) Dapagliflozin suppresses hepcidin and increases erythropoiesis. J Clin Endocrinol Metab 105(4):dgaa057. https://doi.org/10.1210/clinem/dgaa057
151. Bonora BM, Avogaro A, Fadini GP (2020) Euglycemic ketoacidosis. Curr Diab Rep 20(7):25. https://doi.org/10.1007/s11892-020-01307-x
152. Seferović PM, Fragasso G, Petrie M, Mullens W, Ferrari R, Thum T, Bauersachs J, Anker SD, Ray R, Çavuşoğlu Y, Polovina M, Metra M, Ambrosio G, Prasad K, Seferović J, Jhund PS, Dattilo G, Čelutkiene J, Piepoli M, Moura B, Chioncel O, Ben Gal T, Heymans S, Jaarsma T, Hill L, Lopatin Y, Lyon AR, Ponikowski P, Lainščak M, Jankowska E, Mueller C, Cosentino F, Lund LH, Filippatos GS, Ruschitzka F, Coats AJS, Rosano GMC (2020) Heart Failure Association of the European Society of Cardiology update on sodium-glucose co-transporter 2 inhibitors in heart failure. Eur J Heart Fail 22(11):1984–1986. https://doi.org/10.1002/ejhf.2026
153. Packer M, Anker SD, Butler J et al (2021) Effect of empagliflozin on the clinical stability of patients with heart failure and a reduced ejection fraction: the EMPEROR-reduced trial. Circulation 143(4):326–336
154. Pabel S, Hamdani N, Luedde M, Sossalla S (2021) SGLT2 inhibitors and their mode of action in heart failure—has the mystery been unravelled? Curr Heart Fail Rep 18:315–328. https://doi.org/10.1007/s11897-021-00529-8
155. Dutka M, Bobiński R, Ulman-Włodarz I, Hajduga M, Bujok J, Pająk C, Ćwiertnia M (2020) Sodium glucose cotransporter 2 inhibitors: mechanisms of action in heart failure. Heart Fail Rev 26:603–622. https://doi.org/10.1007/s10741-020-10041-1
156. Abdul-Ghani M, Del Prato S, Chilton R, DeFronzo RA (2016) SGLT2 inhibitors and cardiovascular risk: lessons learned from the EMPA-REG OUTCOME study. Diab Care 39:717–725

157. Maejima Y (2020) SGLT2 inhibitors play a salutary role in heart failure via modulation of the mitochondrial function. Front Cardiovasc Med. 6:186
158. Mannucci E, Dicembrini I, Nreu B, Monami M (2019) Exploring the heterogeneity of the effects of SGLT-2 inhibitors in cardiovascular outcome trials. Nutr Metab Cardiovasc Dis 30(1):71–76. https://doi.org/10.1016/j.numecd.2019.07.018
159. Ramos M, Foos V, Ustyugova A, Hau N, Gandhi P et al (2019) Cost–effectiveness analysis of empagliflozin in comparison to sitagliptinand saxagliptin based on cardiovascular outcome trials in patients with type II diabetes and established cardiovascular disease. Diabetes Ther 10(6):2153–2167
160. Daacke I, Kandaswamy P, Tebboth A, Kansal A, Reifsnider O (2016) Cost–effectiveness of empagliflozin (Jardiance) in the treatment of patients with type II diabetes mellitus (T2DM) in the UK based on EMPA-REG OUTCOME data. Value Health 19(7):A673
161. Iannazzo S, Mannucci E, Reifsnider O, Maggioni AP (2017) Cost–effectiveness analysis of empagliflozin in the treatment of patients with type II diabetes and established cardiovascular disease in Italy, based on the results of the EMPA-REG OUTCOME study. Farmeconomia Health Econ Ther Pathw 18(1). https://doi.org/10.7175/fe.v18i1.1332
162. Kosiborod M, Cavender MA, Fu AZ, Wilding JP, Khunti K, Holl RW et al (2017) Lower risk of heart failure and death in patients initiated on sodium–glucose cotransporter-2 inhibitors versus other glucose-lowering drugs: the CVD-REAL study (comparative effectiveness of cardiovascular outcomes in new users of sodium–glucose cotransporter-2 inhibitors). Circulation 136:249–259
163. Chen K, Chen W, Liu SL, Wu TS, Yu KF et al (2018) Epigallocatechingallate attenuates myocardial injury in a mouse model of heart failure through TGFβ1/Smad3 signaling pathway. Mol Med Rep 17:7652–7660. https://doi.org/10.3892/mmr.2018.8825
164. Khan MS, Vaduganathan M (2020) What makes sodium-glucose co-transporter-2 inhibitors stand out in heart failure? Curr Diab Rep 20:63. https://doi.org/10.1007/s11892-020-01347-3
165. Vaduganathan M et al (2018) Prescriber patterns of SGLT2i after expansions of U.S. Food and Drug Administration labeling. J Am Coll Cardiol 72(25):3370–3372
166. Ponikowski P, Voors AA, Anker SD, Bueno H, Cleland JGF, Coats AJS, Falk V, González-Juanatey JR, Harjola VP, Jankowska EA, Jessup M, Linde C, Nihoyannopoulos P, Parissis JT, Pieske B, Riley JP, Rosano GMC, Ruilope LM, Ruschitzka F, Rutten FH, van der Meer P, Authors/Task Force Members, Document Reviewers (2016) 2016 ESC guidelines for the diagnosis and treatment of acute and chronic heart failure: the task force for the diagnosis and treatment of acute and chronic heart failure of the European Society of Cardiology (ESC). Developed with the spec. Eur J Heart Fail 18:891–975. https://doi.org/10.1002/ejhf.592
167. Savarese G, Sattar N, Januzzi J, Verma S, Lund LH, Fitchett D, Zeller C, George JT, Brueckmann M, Ofstad AP, Inzucchi SE, Wanner C, Zinman B, Butler J (2019) Empagliflozin is associated with a lower risk of post-acute heart failure rehospitalization and mortality. Circulation 139(11):1458–1460. https://doi.org/10.1161/CIRCULATIONAHA.118.038339
168. Cintra R, Moura FA, Carvalho LSF et al (2019) Inhibition of the sodium-glucose co-transporter 2 in the elderly: clinical and mechanistic insights into safety and efficacy. Rev Assoc Med Bras 65:70–86
169. https://investors.merck.com/news/press-release-details/2020/Merck-Announces-First-Quarter-2020-Financial-Results/default.aspx. Accessed 25 May 2020
170. Griffin M, Rao VS, Ivey-Miranda J, Fleming J, Mahoney D, Maulion C, Suda N, Siwakoti K, Ahmad T, Jacoby D, Riello R, Bellumkonda L, Cox Z, Collins S, Jeon S, Turner JM, Wilson FP, Butler J, Inzucchi SE, Testani JM (2020) Empagliflozin in heart failure: diuretic and cardio-renal effects. Circulation 142:1028–1039. https://doi.org/10.1161/CIRCULATIONAHA.120.045691
171. Hallow KM, Helmlinger G, Greasley PJ, McMurray JJV, Boulton DW (2018) Why do SGLT2 inhibitors reduce heart failure hospitalization? A differential volume regulation hypothesis. Diabetes Obes Metab 20(3):479–487

172. Zelniker TA, Wiviott SD, Raz I, Im K, Goodrich EL, Bonaca MP et al (2019) SGLT2 inhibitors for primary and secondary prevention of cardiovascular and renal outcomes in type 2 diabetes: a systematic review and meta-analysis of cardiovascular outcome trials. Lancet 393(10166):31–39. https://doi.org/10.1016/S0140-6736(18)32590-X. Erratum in: Lancet. 2019 Jan 5;393(10166):30
173. https://www.fda.gov/drugs/drug-safety-and-availability/fda-warns-about-rare-occurrences-serious-infection-genital-area-sglt2-inhibitors-diabetes
174. Verma S, Mazer CD, Yan AT et al (2019) Effect of empagliflozin on left ventricular mass in patients with type 2 diabetes and coronary artery disease: the EMPA-HEART CardioLink-6 randomized clinical trial. Circulation 140:1693–1702. https://doi.org/10.1161/CIRCULATIONAHA.119.042375
175. Ogurtsova K, da Rocha Fernandes JD, Huang Y, Linnenkamp U, Guariguata L, Cho NH, Cavan D, Shaw JE, Makaroff LE (2017) IDF diabetes atlas: global estimates for the prevalence of diabetes for 2015 and 2040. Diabetes Res Clin Pract 128:40–50. https://doi.org/10.1016/j.diabres.2017.03.024

Chapter 5
Potential Role of SGLT2 Inhibitors in the Treatment and Prevention of Diabetic Cardiomyopathy

Mukesh Nandave

Introduction by the Editor

Diabetes cardiomyopathy is a condition that causes heart failure and is significantly linked to an increased incidence of death in diabetes individuals. It is characterized by independent systolic and diastolic dysfunction in hypertension and coronary heart disease. SGLT2i are anti-diabetic medications that promote salt and glucose excretion in urine. They have demonstrated outstanding results in preventing cardiovascular disease in diabetic and nondiabetic individuals based on big randomized clinical trials, including EMPA-REG OUTCOME, the CANVAS program, and the DECLARE-TIMI experiment. It is exciting to note that the EMPA-REG clinical study showed that empagliflozin significantly decreased the relative risk of cardiovascular (CV) mortality and hospitalization for heart failure (HHF) in individuals with T2DM with CV illness (CVD). In T2D individuals with and without a history of CVD receiving standard treatment, the EMPRISE study demonstrated that empagliflozin reduced the incidence of HHF. These positive effects of SGLT2i could not be attributable to their ability to reduce blood sugar or function as natriuresis. SGLT2i may directly contribute to cardioprotection through several pathways. An experiment and clinical data have proven the effectiveness of SGLT2i in cardiac dysfunction. SGLT2i plays a significant role in the treatment of cardiomyopathy by providing beneficial outcomes to metabolism, autophagy, mitochondrial function, oxidative stress, microcirculation, fibrosis, programmed cell death, and intestinal flora shown in Fig. 5.1.

In light of the current issues surrounding SGLT2i, we reviewed a few concepts and provided some insight into probable plans. The use of SGLT2i is recommended for patients with HFrEF (Heart failure with decreased ejection fraction) and T2D,

M. Nandave (✉)
Department of Pharmacology and Pharmaceutical Biotechnology, Delhi Pharmaceutical Sciences and Research University (DPSRU), New Delhi, Delhi, India

M. Nandave (ed.), *Sodium-glucose Cotransporter-2 (SGLT2) Inhibitors in Heart Failure*, https://doi.org/10.1007/978-981-97-7568-2_5

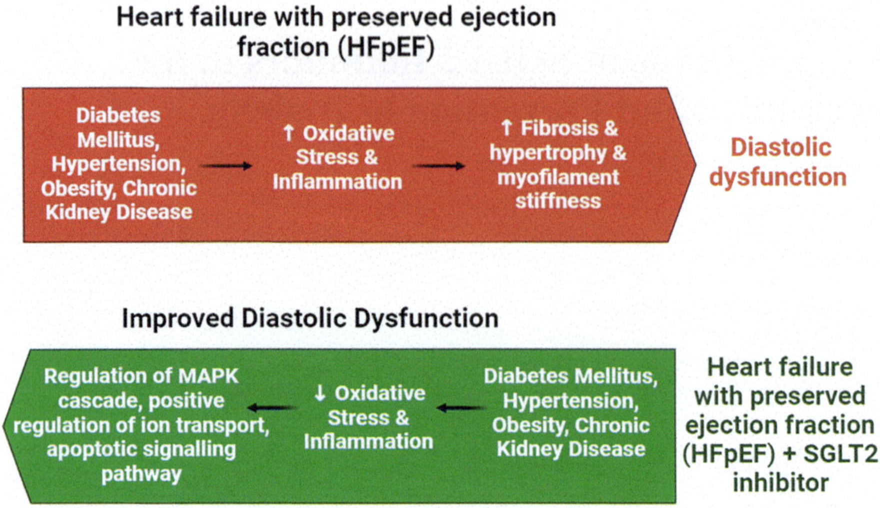

Fig. 5.1 Effect of SGLT2i for the treatment of T2D in patients with HFpEF or HFrEF: The use of SGLT2i has shown improvement in diastolic dysfunction in patients with HFrEF or HF and reduced oxidative stress, inflammation, fibrosis, and myofilament stiffness when compared with patients not using SGLT2i

T2D and coronary heart disease, T2DM and risk factors for coronary heart disease over 50, and albuminuric renal disease with or without T2DM. The benefits of SGLT2i for these individuals have been well demonstrated, and they reduce the risk of hospitalization for HF. Additionally, with the help of customized drugs and timely periodic exams, we may prevent certain potential issues [1].

This chapter focuses on the most recent research on how SGLT2i affects DCM in preclinical investigations. Relevant molecular processes relating to the potential advantages of SGLT2i for DCM are identified to provide a fresh method of avoiding DCM. About few clinical trials have been reported for the role of SGLT2i in the treatment of diabetic cardiomyopathy, As such, an extensive list of all SGLT2i clinical trials necessary for the management of diabetic cardiomyopathy may be seen in Table 5.1. The protective role of SGLT2i in diabetic cardiomyopathy has been questioned in less-reported studies. Dapagliflozin had the highest number of clinical studies that were a significant predictor of protection against diabetic cardiomyopathy.

Machine Generated Summaries

Disclaimer: The summaries in this chapter were generated from Springer Nature publications using extractive AI auto-summarization: An extraction-based summarizer aims to identify the most important sentences of a text using an algorithm and

Table 5.1 An overview of the SGLT2i clinical studies that address diabetic cardiomyopathy

	Purpose	Intervention	Clinical Trials. gov ID	Phase	Brief summary
Based on safeguarding properties of Dapagliflozin in diabetic patient with cardiomyopathy	Determine the clinical benefits of SGLT2i based on a mechanistic approach	Dapagliflozin	NCT04200586	Phase IV	Provide cardiovascular outcomes amongst T2D patients. Moreover, the observational approach is used to magnify the mechanistic visions of the drug
	Evaluation of cardiovascular cardiomyopathy, mortality, and morbidity in T2D patients via SGLT2i (Dapagliflozin)	Dapagliflozin + Placebo	NCT04304560	Phase II	Research indicates that the medication lowers the overabundance of liberated fatty acids, diacylglycerol (DAG), ceramides, and reactive oxygen species (ROS), which might impact cardiac contractility and insulin sensitivity
	Determine the myocardial calcium handling of Dapagliflozin in patients with heart failure with and without diabetes	Dapaglifloz [Farxiga] + Placebo	NCT04591639	Not applicable	Cardiomyopathy and heart failure individuals with diabetes mellitus have different ways of managing calcium in the heart.
Prevention of cardiomyopathy in diabetic patients through polypill process	Using the WATCH-DM risk score, to determine the effectiveness of a polypill-based approach for individuals who have T2D who are at elevated risk of HF	Polypill	NCT06143566	Phase I & II	When compared to patients receiving standard treatment, the usage of a polypill is economical and enhances peak oxygen consumption and medication adherence

uses those original sentences to create the auto-summary (unlike generative AI). As the constituted sentences are machine selected, they may not fully reflect the body of the work, so we strongly advise that the original content is read and cited. The auto generated summaries were curated by the editor to meet Springer Nature publication standards. To cite this content, please refer to the original papers.

Machine generated keywords: cardiomyopathy, diabetic cardiomyopathy, dcm, fibrosis, mouse, dysfunction, tdm, rat, attenuate, inflammation, mitochondrial, calcium, cardiomyocyte, dapa, cardiomyopathy dcm.

Insights into SGLT2 Inhibitor Treatment of Diabetic Cardiomyopathy: Focus on the Mechanisms [2]

This is a machine-generated summary of:

Huang, Keming; Luo, Xianling; Liao, Bin; Li, Guang; Feng, Jian: Insights into SGLT2 inhibitor treatment of diabetic cardiomyopathy: focus on the mechanisms [2].

Published in: Cardiovascular Diabetology (2023).

Link to original: https://doi.org/10.1186/s12933-023-01816-5

If you want to cite the papers, please refer to the original.

For technical reasons we could not place the page where the original quote is coming from.

Abstract-Summary "SGLT2i treatment benefits metabolism, microcirculation, mitochondrial function, fibrosis, oxidative stress, endoplasmic reticulum stress, programmed cell death, autophagy, and the intestinal flora, which are involved in diabetic cardiomyopathy."

"This review summarizes the current knowledge of the mechanisms of SGLT2i for the treatment of diabetic cardiomyopathy."

Introduction

"Diabetes may have been recognized more than 3000 years ago [3], and the incidence and prevalence of this ancient disease have increased with improvements in living and health standards."

"The pathology of diabetic cardiomyopathy includes abnormal carbohydrate and fatty acid metabolism, microvascular disease, endothelial dysfunction, mitochondrial dysfunction, myocardial diastolic dysfunction and fibrosis, excessive cardiomyocyte programmed cell death, increased oxidative stress, endoplasmic reticulum (ER) stress, and glycotoxicity [4–6]."

"Diabetic cardiomyopathy is known to significantly increase the risk of heart failure and can lead to a preserved or reduced ejection fraction [7]."

"In a randomized controlled trial, dapagliflozin reduced heart failure by 27% in T2DM (type 2 diabetes mellitus) patients with cardiovascular disease."

SGLT2i and Improved Heart Function

"The aromatic O-glycoside sergliflozin and the aromatic C-glycoside dapagliflozin officially opened the era of selective SGLT inhibitors [8]."

"Empagliflozin, dapagliflozin, and canagliflozin are 2600, 1200, and 150 times more selective for SGLT2 than for SGLT1 [9]."

"SGLT1 is expressed by cardiomyocytes and may be a target of SGLT2i that improves heart failure [10]."

"Inhibiting SGLT1 with canagliflozin was shown to reduce nicotinamide adenine dinucleotide phosphate (NADPH) oxidase activity in cardiomyocytes, thereby inhibiting the production of superoxide and decreasing inflammation [10]."

"Dapagliflozin and canagliflozin were reported to directly inhibit Na^+/H^+ exchanger-1 (NHE1) and abrogate the increase in cytosolic Na^+ in cardiomyocytes."

"Other studies have shown that the cardiac sodium channel Nav1.5 was a target of SGLT2i and that inhibiting sodium channels ameliorated dysfunctional sodium and calcium homeostasis, improved calcium overload, and decreased the incidence of malignant arrhythmias [11]."

SGLT2i and the Regulation of Heart Metabolism

"Although each molecule of fatty acid produces more ATP than glucose, complete oxidation requires more oxygen."

"Compared with the absence of diabetes, oxidative metabolism in cardiomyocytes under diabetic conditions consumes a higher percentage of fatty acids and a lower percentage of glucose [12], and there is an increase in the use of ketone bodies [13]."

"Empagliflozin has been shown to increase glucose uptake in the human and murine myocardium that was associated with increased GLUT1 expression [14]."

"Increased fatty acid utilization increases the oxygen requirements of cardiomyocytes."

"The mRNA and protein expression of CPT1b was reduced by subcutaneous injection of empagliflozin [15], which indicates that SGLT2i improved cardiomyocyte energy metabolism by reducing fatty acid utilization."

"Adiponectin is a peptide that is secreted by adipocytes, and its effects on lipid metabolism are reflected by a negative correlation with serum TG and association with increased utilization of glucose and fatty acids by muscle tissue [16]."

SGLT2i and Myocardial Mitochondria

"Mitochondrial biogenesis and the growth and division of preexisting mitochondria are regulated by AMPK, peroxisome-proliferator-activated receptor γ coactivator-1α (PGC-1α), and nuclear respiratory factors (NRF)-1 and -2 [17]."

"AMPK activation was shown to increase the transcription of the PGC-1α gene in rat cell nuclei, which then induced the expression of the transcription factor NRF-1 [18]."

"Activation of PGC-1α, NRF-1, and mtTFA increases the transcription and replication of mitochondrial DNA."

"Secker and others [19] found that canagliflozin inhibited the activity of mitochondrial respiratory complex I and promoted complex II activity, and empagliflozin and dapagliflozin increased the activity of complex I. Improvements in mitochondrial function by SGLT2i may be related to a decrease in O-GlcNAcylation."

"Dapagliflozin and other SGLT2i may improve the function of the mitochondrial respiratory chain by directly reducing O-GlcNAc transferase activity and O-GlcNAcylation [20]."

SGLT2i Improve Cardiovascular Disease and Microcirculation

"Primary cultures of rat aortic endothelial cells transduced with an adenovirus encoding a dominant-negative Drp1K38A mutant showed significant inhibition of TNF-α-induced NF-κB-driven promoter activity and VCAM-1 induction."

"SGLT2i were reported to improve endothelial function in mice with STZ-induced diabetes by inhibiting abnormal mitochondrial fission and endothelial inflammation [21]."

"Uric acid concentrations higher than physiological levels inhibit NO synthesis, reduce NO activity and induce NF-κB, leading to the induction of monocyte chemoattractant protein 1 and cyclooxygenase 2 (COX-2), which mediate inflammation and atherosclerosis [22]."

"Uthman and others [23] reported that dapagliflozin and empagliflozin inhibited TNFα-induced ROS generation in human coronary arterial endothelial cells, and the subsequent decrease in NO consumption was responsible for improved blood vessel dilatation."

"Canagliflozin also inhibited angiogenesis in the lower limbs of mice with diabetes and lower limb ischaemia by inhibiting the secretion of vascular endothelial growth factor A by bone marrow-derived mesenchymal stem cells and reducing the proliferation and migration of mesenchymal stem cells [24]."

SGLT2i Improve Ventricular Compliance and Myocardial Fibrosis

"Myocardial fibrosis occurs in cardiomyopathy associated with diabetes, and it involves the accumulation of advanced glycation end products (AGEs) [25] and increased myocardial stiffness that interferes with ventricular diastole."

"Activation of the receptor for AGE (RAGE) by AGEs promotes the proliferation, function, and migration of cardiac fibroblasts, which exacerbates myocardial fibrosis and accelerates cardiac ageing [25–27]."

"In a mouse model of type 2 diabetes, myocardial expression of collagen I and collagen III proteins and connective tissue fraction was increased compared with that in nondiabetic mice and was partially reversed by empagliflozin [28]."

"The effect of SGLT2i on this pathway was demonstrated by Lee and others [29], who found that dapagliflozin induced macrophage polarization to the M2 phenotype and inhibited the M1 phenotype by stimulating signal transducer and activator of transcription 3 (STAT3) signalling in mice with myocardial infarction and attenuated the increase in collagen after infarction."

SGLT2i Inhibit Oxidative Stress

"In an isoprenaline (ISO)-induced oxidative stress model, the phosphorylation of eNOS was significantly inhibited in the heart and kidney and was reversed by canagliflozin [30, 31]."

"In an ISO-induced oxidative stress model, myocardial expression of iNOS was upregulated more than 3 times, but canagliflozin significantly reduced iNOS levels, which also decreased superoxide and nitrate [30]."

"Myocardial oxidative stress caused by ISO manifested as increased levels of MDA, advanced protein oxidation products, and myeloperoxidase and decreased levels of catalase, SOD, and GSH in the myocardium and plasma."

"SIRT1 could decrease oxidative stress in diabetic cardiomyopathy [32, 33]."

"SGLT2i activate SIRT1 and its downstream signals [34, 35], which helps to explain how SGLT2i decrease oxidative stress in diabetic cardiomyopathy."

"The antioxidant effect induced by the activation of SIRT1 in T1DM diabetic cardiomyopathy mainly includes the SIRT1/Nrf2 signalling pathway [32], while in T2DM, it includes the Sirt1/forkhead box class O1 (FOXO1) signalling pathway [33]."

In Diabetes Patients, SGLT2i Rescue Cardiomyocytes from Programmed Cell Death

"Recent studies reported that SGLT2i inhibited caspase-1 and that the mechanism involved a pathway including AMPK/NLRP3/apoptosis-associated speck-like protein containing a CARD (ASC) [36–39]."

"The mRNA expression of NLRP3, ASC, IL-1β, and caspase-1 in cardiomyocytes did not increase significantly in wild-type mice but did so in the myocardia of type 2 diabetic (BTBR ob/ob) mice [40]."

"Dapagliflozin was not associated with the expression of NLRP3, ASC, IL-1β, or caspase-1 in normal wild-type mice but did reverse these factors in BTBR mice."

"LPS increased the mRNA expression of NLRP3 and caspase-1 and decreased the P-AMPK/total-AMPK ratio in cardiac fibroblasts in wild-type and BTBR mice."

"Preincubation of cardiac fibroblasts with dapagliflozin attenuated the changes in the mRNA expression of NLRP3 and caspase-1 and the ratio of P-AMPK/total AMPK induced by LPS in wild-type and BTBR mice [40]."

SGLT2i and Autophagy in the Myocardium

"Empagliflozin has been reported to increase autophagy in the atrial tissue of ZDF rats."

"Li and others [41] reported that empagliflozin decreased the protein expression of CD36, which was associated with an increase in p-AMPK, which activated the AMPK/Unc-51-like kinase 1 (Ulk1)/Beclin1 pathway, increased Ulk1 and Beclin1 expression, and promoted autophagy."

"The difference might be related to nutritional status in the two models because AMPK activates Ulk1 to promote autophagy during glucose starvation."

"Jiang and others [42] reported that in T1DM or T2DM and myocardial infarction, cardiomyocyte survival benefitted from the inhibition of enhanced autophagy by empagliflozin, which depended on the downregulation of NHE1 and NHE1-related genes that induce autophagy, such as Beclin 1 and autophagy-related protein 5."

"Empagliflozin was shown to inhibit the increase in autophagy caused by myocardial infarction with acute hyperglycaemia."

"Empagliflozin can also reverse the increase in the autophagy-related protein LC3II/I and decrease in P62 in cardiomyocytes induced by Tat-beclin1."

SGLT2i Reverse ER Stress in Diabetic Cardiomyopathy

"ER stress involves disturbances in Ca^{2+} or redox balance and the accumulation of misfolded or unfolded proteins that cannot be processed, which initiates an unfolded protein response (UPR) that leads to apoptosis [43]."

"PERK/eIF2α/ATF4/C/EBP-homologous protein (CHOP) are signalling pathways involved in ER stress."

"In these ER stress models induced by heart pressure overload or I/R injury, dapagliflozin and empagliflozin inhibited the increase in p-PERK and its downstream molecules associated with ER stress due to pressure overload by activating SIRT1 and preventing GRP78 detachment [44, 45]."

"SGLT2i have been shown to inhibit ER stress through similar downstream pathways in various organs."

SGLT2i Improve Diabetic Cardiomyopathy by Regulating the Intestinal Microbiota

"Dapagliflozin has been associated with changes in the gut microbiota, the function of extraintestinal blood vessels, and improvements in cardiovascular dysfunction caused by diabetes."

"Eight weeks of dapagliflozin treatment significantly increased Akkermansia muciniphila in the gut microbiota and improved generalized vascular dysfunction in mice with T2DM [46]."

"An increase in the abundance of A. muciniphila and improvements in glucose tolerance and blood glucose levels have been confirmed and correlated with induction of Foxp3-positive regulatory T cells [47]."

"An increase in A. muciniphila was also shown to reduce endotoxaemia and inflammation and prevent atherosclerosis by inducing the expression of tight junction proteins in the gut [48]."

"Empagliflozin has been associated with an increase in the population of SCFA-producing bacteria and improvements in diabetes and cardiovascular function [49]."

"These findings suggest that inhibition of SGLT1 reduces glucose uptake, while unabsorbed glucose temporarily reaches the lower small intestine [50], resulting in an altered glucose load and a possibly altered gut microbiota composition."

SGLT2i in Clinical Treatment

"SGLT2i improves myocardial metabolism in diabetic patients."

"SGLT2i (dapagliflozin, empagliflozin, canagliflozin) reduce the expression of PPAR-γ in the hearts of patients."

"In a clinical randomized controlled trial, the SGLT2i empagliflozin significantly reduced the left ventricular mass relative to body surface area [51]."

"A randomized controlled trial of dapagliflozin demonstrated a significant reduction in left ventricular mass (LVM) in patients with T2DM and left ventricular hypertrophy (LVH) [52]."

"In diabetes patients with atherosclerotic disease, endothelial changes occur in the microvasculature and macrovasculature, and 12 weeks of dapagliflozin treatment resulted in a significant increase in FMD [53]."

"In a 12 week double-blind randomized trial, significant changes in gut microbiota diversity or composition were not observed in T2DM patients after dapagliflozin treatment [54]."

"In patients with HFpEF, especially those with stage A-B heart failure, the effect of SGLT2i treatment is not significant."

Current Challenges and Future Therapeutic Strategies

"The use of SGLT2i has been reported to increase the risk of urinary and genital tract infections by more than 3 times [55]."

"The use of SGLT2i is strongly recommended in patients with HFrEF and with or without T2DM, patients with T2DM and coronary heart disease, patients with T2DM were over 50 years old who had risk factors associated with coronary heart disease, and patients with albuminuric renal disease with or without T2DM."

"For patients with suspected ketoacidosis symptoms such as nausea, vomiting, abdominal pain, and dyspnoea during SGLT2i use, blood and urine ketone body analysis should be performed in time."

"For patients with urinary tract infection during medication use, SGLT2i administration should be paused, and anti-infective therapy should be given."

"SGLT2i should be discontinued in patients with recurrent urinary tract infections."

"Patients taking SGLT2i and diuretics together need to monitor their blood pressure."

Conclusions

"We mainly focused on basic studies to elucidate the pharmacological mechanism of SGLT2i and related signalling pathways or targets for the treatment of diabetic cardiomyopathy."

"Studies have shown that SGLT2i can improve diabetic cardiomyopathy by improving myocardial metabolism, restoring mitochondrial function, improving microcirculatory disorders, reducing myocardial fibrosis, reducing oxidative stress, inhibiting programmed death, regulating autophagy, inhibiting ER stress and regulating the intestinal flora."

"Our aim was to arouse more attention from readers through this review to further explore the potential mechanisms and targets of SGLT2i in the treatment of diabetic cardiomyopathy in the clinic and lay a solid foundation for the reasonable use of SGLT2i; SGLT2i can save more patients with diabetic cardiomyopathy."

Sodium–Glucose Cotransporter 2 Inhibitor Dapagliflozin Attenuates Diabetic Cardiomyopathy [56]

This is a machine-generated summary of:

Arow, M.; Waldman, M.; Yadin, D.; Nudelman, V.; Shainberg, A.; Abraham, N. G.; Freimark, D.; Kornowski, R.; Aravot, D.; Hochhauser, E.; Arad, M.: Sodium–glucose cotransporter 2 inhibitor Dapagliflozin attenuates diabetic cardiomyopathy [56].

Published in: Cardiovascular Diabetology (2020).

Link to original: https://doi.org/10.1186/s12933-019-0980-4

If you want to cite the papers, please refer to the original.

For technical reasons we could not place the page where the original quote is coming from.

Abstract-Summary "Sodium glucose transporter 2 inhibitors (SGLT2I) are recently developed diabetic drugs that primarily work on the kidney."

"We investigated the effect of Dapagliflozin—SGLT2I, on diabetic cardiomyopathy in a mouse model of DM2."

"Cardiomyopathy was induced in diabetic mice (db/db) by subcutaneous infusion of angiotensin II (ATII) for 30 days using an osmotic pump."

"Isolated cardiomyocytes were exposed to glucose (17.5–33 mM) and treated with Dapagliflozin in vitro."

"Angiotensin II infusion induced cardiomyopathy in db/db mice, manifested by cardiac hypertrophy, myocardial fibrosis and inflammation (TNFα, TLR4)."

"Dapagliflozin decreased blood glucose (874 ± 111 to 556 ± 57 mg/dl, $p < 0.05$)."

"It attenuated fibrosis and inflammation and increased the left ventricular fractional shortening in ATII treated db/db mice."

"In isolated cardiomyocytes Dapagliflozin decreased intracellular calcium transients, inflammation and ROS production."

"Voltage-dependent L-type calcium channel (CACNA1C), the sodium–calcium exchanger (NCX) and the sodium–hydrogen exchanger 1 (NHE) membrane transporters expression was reduced following Dapagliflozin treatment."

"Dapagliflozin was cardioprotective in ATII-stressed diabetic mice."

"The cardioprotective effect manifested by decreased fibrosis, reduced inflammation and improved systolic function."

Background

"Patients with diabetes are two to three times more likely to develop cardiovascular disease and are at an increased risk of having a myocardial infarction, stroke or develop heart failure [57, 58]."

"The expression of TNF-α and NF-κB along with collagen were elevated and accompanied by an increase in oxidative stress in the diabetic heart [59]."

"There is no established therapy for diabetic heart disease."

"Classical glucose-lowering therapies reduced the number of coronary events but generally had a neutral effect on cardiovascular mortality and sometimes resulted in heart failure exacerbation [60]."

"A study on the effect Dapagliflozin (DAPA) on cardiovascular events (DECLARE-TIMI 58) reported a lower rate of both cardiovascular death or heart failure (HF) hospitalizations after treating high-risk diabetes [61]."

"The purpose of this study was to investigate the effect of SGLT2I- DAPA on the diabetic heart in a mouse model of DM2."

Methods

"Male homozygous WT or db/db mice (n = 4–8/group), 12–14 weeks old, were used for the experiments."

"Angiotensin II: 12–14 week-old male mice were anesthetized with 2% isoflurane and an ALZET osmotic pump (Durect Corp., Cupertino, CA, USA) was subcutaneously implanted into each mouse."

"Neonatal rat hearts (Sprague-Dawley 1–2 days old) were removed under sterile conditions and washed three times in phosphate-buffered saline (PBS) to remove excess blood cells."

"Cells grown on coverslips were treated with ATII (1 μM) for 2 h and then DAPA (5 μM) was added."

"Oxidative stress was measured in cultured rat neonatal cardiomyocytes exposed to high or normal glucose concentration (33 mM or 17.5 mM) using a 2′,7′-dichlorofluorescin diacetate (DCF-DA) reagent (Sigma-Aldrich, St. Louis, MO, USA)."

"Cardiomyocytes were incubated with DAPA for 2 h; ATII was added to the cells and stand for another 2 h than the cells were loaded with 10 μM DCF-DA for 30 min at 37 °C [62]."

Results

"DAPA had no significant hemodynamic effect in db/db mice in the absence of ATII stress."

"While ATII increases the collagen content in both wt/wt and db/db hearts ($p < 0.05$), DAPA tends to reduce it in ATII treated diabetic hearts."

"Cumulatively we conclude that diabetic heart is highly susceptible to ATII stress inducing changes in cardiac structure such as myocardial hypertrophy and fibrosis."

"The effect of Dapagliflozin was manifest in the ATII-stressed diabetic heart reducing myocardial fibrosis and improving the systolic function."

"Adding DAPA prior to ATII markedly reduced the oxidative stress."

"Cumulatively, our in-vitro experiments suggest a mechanism where DAPA reduces calcium entry and attenuates oxidative stress associated with high glucose and angiotensin and which appears to be independent of glycemic control."

Discussion

"Increases in $[Na^+]$c and $[Ca^{2+}]$ c induce signaling cascades that lead to dysregulation of mitochondrial homeostasis, including impaired energetics, elevated ROS production, cardiac hypertrophy and remodeling [63]."

"The increase in $[Na^+]$c and $[Ca^{2+}]$c is caused by perturbed ion fluxes due to the altered activity of ion channels and/or transporters, including the sodium–calcium exchanger (NCX), the sodium–hydrogen exchanger 1 (NHE-1), L-type calcium channel, the ryanodine receptor regulating SR-calcium release and the sodium–potassium ATPase (Na/K ATPase) [64]."

"The reduction in intracellular calcium appears to be driven by a direct effect of DAPA on the expression of ion channels in the heart i.e. NHE1, NCX and L-type calcium channel."

"Despite these mechanistic insights linking intracellular calcium to cardiac dysfunction, the use of both NHE-1 inhibition and calcium channel blockers proved detrimental and should be avoided in patients with heart failure with reduced ejection fraction (HFrEF) [65]."

Conclusion

"We suggest that DAPA reduced intracellular calcium overload thereby reducing ROS production in the diabetic model of cardiomyopathy."

"Protecting the mitochondria, attenuating inflammation and preventing fibrosis would be consecutive to reducing ROS."

"Since all the pathological pathways in the diabetic heart are augmented in the presence of angiotensin, the effect of DAPA should be most pronounced in ATII stressed diabetic heart."

"Our preclinical observations provide novel insights into the possible mechanisms by which DAPA reduces cardiovascular mortality in humans."

SGLT-2 Inhibition with Dapagliflozin Reduces the Activation of the Nlrp3/ASC Inflammasome and Attenuates the Development of Diabetic Cardiomyopathy in Mice with Type 2 Diabetes. Further Augmentation of the Effects with Saxagliptin, a DPP4 Inhibitor [66]

This is a machine-generated summary of:

Ye, Yumei; Bajaj, Mandeep; Yang, Hsiu-Chiung; Perez-Polo, Jose R.; Birnbaum, Yochai: SGLT-2 Inhibition with Dapagliflozin Reduces the Activation of the Nlrp3/ASC Inflammasome and Attenuates the Development of Diabetic Cardiomyopathy in Mice with Type 2 Diabetes. Further Augmentation of the Effects with Saxagliptin, a DPP4 Inhibitor [66].

Published in: Cardiovascular Drugs and Therapy (2017).

Link to original: https://doi.org/10.1007/s10557-017-6725-2

If you want to cite the papers, please refer to the original.

For technical reasons we could not place the page where the original quote is coming from.

Abstract-Summary "We assessed whether (1) dapagliflozin (Dapa, an SGLT2-inhibitor) attenuates the deterioration of heart function Nlrp3 and inflammasome activation in diabetic mice. (2) The effects can be augmented with saxagliptin (Saxa), a DDP4-inhibitor. (3) Dapa effect is possibly SGLT2-independent on cardiofibroblasts in vitro."

"Type 2 diabetic (BTBR ob/ob) and wild-type (WT) mice received vehicle, Dapa, or Dapa + Saxa for 8 weeks."

"Dapa and Dapa + Saxa improved LVEF to 68 ± 1 and 74.6 ± 1% in the BTBR mice ($p < 0.001$)."

"The mRNA levels of NALP3, ASC, IL-1β, IL-6, caspase-1, and TNFα were significantly higher in the BTBR compared to the WT hearts; and Dapa and Dapa + Saxa significantly attenuated these levels."

"Protein levels of NLRP3, TNFα, and caspase-1 were higher in the BTBR compared to the WT hearts and Dapa, and to a greater extent Dapa+Saxa, attenuated the increase in the BTBR mice."

"Collagen-1 and collagen-3 mRNA levels significantly increased in the BTBR mice and these increases were attenuated by Dapa and Dapa+Saxa."

"Dapa and Dapa + Saxa equally increased the ratio in the BTBR mice."

"This in vitro study showed that NALP3, ASC, IL-1β, and caspase-1 mRNA levels were higher in the BTBR cardiofibroblasts and attenuated with Dapa."

"Dapa attenuated the activation of the inflammasome, fibrosis, and deterioration of LVEF in BTBR mice."

"Adding Saxa to Dapa did not result in a greater effect on myocardial fibrosis and collagen levels."

Introduction

"We showed that DPP4 inhibition attenuated diabetes-induced Nlrp3 inflammasome activation in the kidney and adipose tissue, and the progression of diabetic nephropathy in mice with T2DM (DBDR), as well as type-1 diabetes (Akita) mice [67]."

"The effects of SGLT2 inhibitors treatment on the activation of the Nlrp3 inflammasome and the progression of diabetic cardiomyopathy in a T2DM model have not been reported."

"We assessed whether the SGLT2 inhibitor, dapagliflozin (Dapa), attenuates the activation of the NLRP3 inflammasome and the progression of diabetic cardiomyopathy in mice with T2DM."

"As we found that Dapa protects the heart, reduces activation of the inflammasome, attenuates fibrosis, and attenuates remodeling in the diabetic heart while it has been reported that SGLT2 is not expressed in the heart (at least in non-diabetic animals) [68, 69], we conducted in vitro experiments to see if Dapa attenuated lipopolysaccharide (LPS)-induced inflammasome activation in adult mice cardiofibroblasts to see whether these effects are independent from the glucose-lowering effect of Dapa."

Methods

"For the quantification of fibrosis, samples of left ventricular tissue from all groups were fixed and embedded in paraffin."

"Percent fibrosis area was analyzed using Image J analysis software, expressed as percentage of fibrosis area to the total area of each microscopic field."

"Cells were exposed for 16 h to Dapa (0.4 μM), AMPK activator [A769662 (10 μM), Sigma-Aldrich], AMPK inhibitor [compound C (CC),(10 μM), Sigma-Aldrich], an SGLT1 + SGLT2 inhibitor [phlorizin (PZ), (100 μM), Sigma-Aldrich],

Dapa + CC, or Dapa + PZ, and then stimulated with LPS (10 ng/ml) for 3 h. Control groups (without and with LPS stimulation) were cultured in 1% DMSO."

"After blocking, membranes were incubated with primary antibodies anti-TNFα, anti-ASC1, anti-caspase-1 (Santa Cruz Biotechnology), anti-P-AMPK, anti-T-AMPK (Cell Signaling Technology), anti-NLRP3, or anti-β-actin (Sigma-Aldrich) overnight at 4 °C."

"The differences in glucose and insulin levels during glucose tolerance test were compared using two-way repeated measures ANOVA with Holm-Sidak multiple comparison procedures."

Results

"Dapa alone, and to a greater extent Dapa + Saxa, significantly attenuated the decrease in FS and LVEF in the BTBR mice but did not reach WT levels."

"Dapa and Dapa + Saxa had no effect on the myocardial expression of NLRP3, TNFα, and caspase-1 in the WT mice, yet Dapa, and to a greater extent Dapa + Saxa, attenuated the increase in the BTBR mice."

"Dapa + Saxa completely normalized TNFα levels; however, levels of NLRP3 and caspase-1 were still significantly higher in the BTBR mice receiving Dapa + Saxa than the WT mice."

"As we found a significant effect of Dapa on diabetes-induced activation of the inflammasome, fibrosis, and remodeling, despite the fact that SGLT2 is not expressed in the heart, we conducted in vitro experiments to assess whether Dapa had glucose-lowering- and SGLT2- independent effects using cardiofibroblasts generated from WT and BTBR mice after stimulation with LPS."

Discussion

"We show direct effects of Dapa on attenuation of diabetes-induced activation of the inflammasome, fibrosis, and remodeling in the heart in vivo and on mouse cardiofibroblasts in vitro."

"The in vitro experiment clearly showed that phlorizin, a dual SGLT1 and SGLT2 inhibitor [70–72], does not replicate the effect of Dapa and does not modify the effects of Dapa on AMPK phosphorylation and the attenuation of the inflammasome activation, suggesting that the effects of Dapa are not medicated via SGLT1 inhibition."

"Hawley and others (41) reported that canagliflozin activates AMPK by inhibiting mitochondrial function and increasing cellular AMP in the mouse liver, whereas Dapa and empagliflozin had a significant effect on AMPK phosphorylation at a concentration of 100 μM and only a small effect at 30 μM [73]."

"We report that the effect of Dapa on the LPS-induced inflammasome activation was completely blocked with compound C, an AMPK inhibitor, and these results could be replicated by A769662, an AMPK activator."

Limitations

"Trimenstein and others reported that the half-maximal inhibitory concentration (IC_{50}) of Dapa for SGLT1 in the mouse is 0.3 ± 0.02 μM, a value that is much lower than the IC_50 in humans (1.4 ± 0.007 μM), although the IC_{50} for SGLT2 inhibition was comparable (1.12 ± 0.065 nM in humans and 2.3 ± 0.6 nM in the mouse) [74]."

"We used Dapa at 0.3, 0.4, and 0.5 μM. These concentrations are lower than reported in previous studies [73–75]; however, they are much higher than the IC_{50} of Dapa for SGLT2 in the human kidney and much higher than the concentration of free drug achieved in the clinical setting with oral 5 mg dose (0.015 μM)."

"We report a direct effect of Dapa on the attenuation of LPS-induced activation of the Nlrp3 inflammasome in cardiofibroblasts."

Association of Type 2 Diabetes Mellitus with the Development of New-Onset Atrial Fibrillation in Patients with Non-ischemic Dilated Cardiomyopathy: Impact of SGLT2 Inhibitors [76]

This is a machine-generated summary of:

Tanaka, Hidekazu; Tatsumi, Kazuhiro; Matsuzoe, Hiroki; Soga, Fumitaka; Matsumoto, Kensuke; Hirata, Ken-ichi: Association of type 2 diabetes mellitus with the development of new-onset atrial fibrillation in patients with non-ischemic dilated cardiomyopathy: impact of SGLT2 inhibitors [76].

Published in: The International Journal of Cardiovascular Imaging (2021).

Link to original: https://doi.org/10.1007/s10554-020-02122-x

If you want to cite the papers, please refer to the original.

For technical reasons we could not place the page where the original quote is coming from.

Abstract-Summary "The aim of this study was to investigate the association of type 2 diabetes mellitus (T2DM) with the development of new-onset atrial fibrillation (AF) for non-ischemic dilated cardiomyopathy (DCM) patients."

"We also tested the hypothesis that sodium glucose cotransporter type 2 (SGLT2) inhibitors reduce the risk of development of new-onset AF for non-ischemic DCM patients."

"Kaplan–Meier curve analysis showed that non-ischemic DCM patients without T2DM experienced fewer occurrences of the development of new-onset AF compared with those with T2DM (log-rank $p = 0.0003$)."

"Of the 60 non-ischemic DCM patients with T2DM, those treated with SGLT2 inhibitors experienced fewer occurrences of the development of new-onset AF than did those not treated with SGLT2 inhibitors (log-rank $p = 0.040$)."

"T2DM is associated with the development of new-onset AF in non-ischemic DCM patients, and treatment with SGLT2 inhibitors can significantly reduce the development of new-onset AF."

"Our findings may thus offer a new insight into the management of non-ischemic DCM patients with T2DM."

Introduction

"T2DM is reportedly associated with an increased risk of development of new-onset AF, while findings of a previously reported meta-analysis of cohort and case–control studies indicated that patients with T2DM had an approximate 40% greater risk of developing new-onset AF compared to patients without [77]."

"Dapagliflozin also was found to reduce by 19% the risk of development of new-onset AF for 17,160 T2DM patients without HF by significantly lowering the time to the first AF event during follow-up [78]."

"The association of T2DM with the development of new-onset AF in non-ischemic DCM patients, or the impact of SGLT2 inhibitors on the development of new-onset AF for such patients remains unclear."

"The aim of this study was thus to investigate the association of T2DM with the development of new-onset AF in non-ischemic DCM patients."

"We also tested the hypothesis that SGLT2 inhibitors could reduce the risk of the development of new-onset AF for non-ischemic DCM patients."

Materials and Methods

"Patients were excluded from enrolment in this study if they met any of the following criteria: (1) history or suspicion of coronary artery disease; (2) previous history of open-heart surgery and congenital heart disease; (3) undeniable secondary cardiomyopathy; (4) serious renal dysfunction defined as glomerular filtration rate < 30 mL/min/1.73 m^2; (5) uncontrolled hypertension > 180/100 mmHg; (6) more than moderate primary valvular heart disease other than functional mitral regurgitation; (7) a previous history of electrocardiographically confirmed AF or atrial flutter."

"Eight patients (3.7%) were excluded from all subsequent analyses because of poor echocardiographic image quality to analyze speckle-tracking strain, so that eventually 210 patients with DCM were enrolled in this study."

"Speckle-tracking strain analysis was performed for each patient with the aid of a single dedicated software to evaluate LV longitudinal function, which was assessed in terms of global longitudinal strain (GLS) (AutoSTRAIN, TOMTEC-ARENA: TOMTEC Imaging Systems GmbH, Munich, Germany)."

"GLS was then determined as the averaged peak longitudinal strain of 18 LV segments, and was expressed as an absolute value in accordance with current guidelines [79]."

Results

"Non-ischemic DCM patients with T2DM were more likely to be older and have a lower blood pressure than did those without T2DM."

"New-onset AF occurred in 21 patients (10.0%) over a median follow-up of 6.1 years."

"Non-ischemic DCM patients without T2DM experienced fewer occurrences of the development of new-onset AF compared with those with T2DM (log-rank $p = 0.0003$)."

"Those treated with SGLT2 inhibitors experienced fewer occurrences of the development of new-onset AF compared with those not treated with SGLT2 inhibitors (log-rank $p = 0.040$)."

Discussion

"The findings of our study indicate that the presence of T2DM was associated with the development of new-onset AF in non-ischemic DCM patients."

"Treatment with SGLT2 inhibitors significantly reduced the development of new-onset AF in non-ischemic DCM patients with T2DM."

"This is the first study to show association of T2DM with development of new-onset AF in patients with non-ischemic DCM, and the preventive effect of SGLT2 inhibitors."

"To previous studies using T2DM patients without HF, we demonstrated for the first time the association of T2DM with the development of new-onset AF in non-ischemic DCM patients (LVEF < 45%)."

"Since previous studies also indicated that low GLS was strongly associated with poor outcome in patients with HFrEF [80, 81], treatment with SGLT2 inhibitors may have a significant impact on outcome by reducing the risk of development of new-onset AF in non-ischemic DCM patients with T2DM."

Conclusions

"T2DM is associated with the development of new-onset AF in non-ischemic DCM patients, and treatment with SGLT2 inhibitors can significantly reduce the development of new-onset AF."

"Our findings may thus offer a new insight into the management of non-ischemic DCM patients with T2DM."

Renal Denervation Ameliorates Cardiac Metabolic Remodeling in Diabetic Cardiomyopathy Rats by Suppressing Renal SGLT2 Expression [82]

This is a machine-generated summary of:

Huo, Jun-Yu; Jiang, Wan-Ying; Zhang, Shi-Geng; Lyu, Yi-Ting; Geng, Jie; Chen, Meng; Chen, Yuan-Yuan; Jiang, Zhi-Xin; Shan, Qi-Jun: Renal denervation ameliorates cardiac metabolic remodeling in diabetic cardiomyopathy rats by suppressing renal SGLT2 expression [82].

Published in: Laboratory Investigation (2021).

Link to original: https://doi.org/10.1038/s41374-021-00696-1

If you want to cite the papers, please refer to the original.

For technical reasons we could not place the page where the original quote is coming from.

Abstract-Summary "This study aimed to investigate the effects of renal denervation (RDN) on diabetic cardiomyopathy (DCM) and explore the related mechanisms."

"The surviving rats were divided into three groups: control group, DCM group and DCM + RDN group."

"In the 13th week, the DCM rats exhibited cardiac hypertrophy and interstitial fibrosis accompanied by diastolic dysfunction."

"RDN ameliorated DCM-induced cardiac dysfunction (E/A ratio: RDN 1.07 ± 0.18 vs. DCM 0.93 ± 0.12, P < 0.05; E/E' ratio: RDN 10.74 ± 2.48 vs. DCM 13.25 ± 1.99, P < 0.05) and pathological remodeling (collagen volume fraction: RDN 5.05 ± 2.05% vs. DCM 10.62 ± 2.68%, P < 0.05)."

"Abnormal myocardial metabolism in DCM rats was characterized by suppressed glucose metabolism and elevated lipid metabolism."

"DCM decreased mitochondrial ATP content, depolarized the membrane potential and inhibited the activity of respiratory chain complexes, but RDN attenuated this mitochondrial damage (ATP: RDN 30.98 ± 7.33 μmol/gprot vs. DCM 22.89 ± 5.90 μmol/gprot, P < 0.05; complexes I, III and IV activity: RDN vs. DCM, P < 0.05)."

"RDN prevented DCM-induced cardiac dysfunction and pathological remodeling, which is related to the improvement of metabolic disorders and mitochondrial dysfunction."

Introduction

"Complications, diabetic cardiomyopathy (DCM) has attracted increasing attention in recent years."

"This type of cardiovascular complication can result in cardiac diastolic and systolic dysfunction and ultimately promote the development of heart failure, which dramatically increases the mortality of diabetic patients [83]."

"Any approach to alleviate DCM has the potential to reduce mortality in patients with diabetes."

"Clinical trials have proven that inhibition of renal SGLT2 by inhibitors of SGLT2, such as dapagliflozin, can improve glycemic control and alleviate myocardial inflammation and oxidative stress and is therefore used for the treatment of DCM [84, 85]."

"We established a rat DCM model to explore the effect of RDN on the diabetic heart, explained the related mechanisms from the perspective of myocardial energy metabolism, and then compared its effect with that of an SGLT2 inhibitor in DCM rats."

Materials and Methods

"After a one-week adaptation period, 24 rats were fed a high-fat diet (HFD) for 4 weeks and then given a single intraperitoneal (i.p.) injection of streptozotocin (STZ, 35 mg/kg) to induce type 2 diabetes (T2D), while six rats received standard commercial rat chow and an i.p."

"After successful induction of T2D, the 24 diabetic rats were randomly divided into two groups by a random number method: the RDN group (n = 12), which received real RDN surgery and HFD for another 8 weeks; the DCM group (n = 12), which received sham RDN surgery and HFD for another 8 weeks; and the six rats in the control group, which received sham RDN surgery and standard commercial rat chow for 8 weeks."

"One week after STZ injection, rats in all groups were subjected to RDN or sham RDN surgery."

Results

"Consistent with this finding, WB results also showed that RDN effectively attenuated the overexpression of renal SGLT2 induced by T2D. Considering the important role of SGLT2 in urinary glucose reabsorption, we also collected urine samples through a metabolic cage study."

"WB results showed that the expression of sarcolemmal GLUT4 was significantly reduced in the DCM group, while RDN preserved the expression of GLUT4 in the sarcolemma."

"RDN increased the expression and activity of BDH1, as well as the enzyme activity of SCOT, suggesting that RDN could improve DCM-induced inhibition of ketone metabolism."

"The level of mitochondrial ATP was decreased in the DCM group but increased in the RDN group."

"These results collectively verified that the therapeutic effect of RDN on DCM is mediated by the regulation of renal SGLT2 expression."

Discussion

"We established a DCM model to evaluate the effect of RDN on cardiac energy metabolism and mitochondrial function."

"The major findings were as follows: (1) RDN effectively downregulated the expression of renal SGLT2, promoted UGE and decreased blood glucose concentration; (2) RDN improved cardiac diastolic dysfunction and prevented the progression of cardiac remodeling; (3) RDN attenuated cardiac glucose and lipid metabolism disorders, thus reducing cardiac glucotoxicity and lipotoxicity; and (4) RDN protected mitochondria from damage induced by glucotoxicity and lipotoxicity, ameliorated mitochondrial dysfunction and increased mitochondrial ATP production."

"The findings of the present study confirmed that RDN could ameliorate the glucotoxicity and lipotoxicity of the myocardium under diabetic conditions and that the beneficial effect of RDN on mitochondria may be closely related to the improvement of energy metabolism."

Conclusions

"RDN can effectively improve metabolic disturbances and mitochondrial damage in diabetic cardiomyopathy."

"This protective effect of RDN is mediated by regulation of the expression of SGLT2 in the kidney."

Mechanisms of Diabetic Cardiomyopathy and Potential Therapeutic Strategies: Preclinical and Clinical Evidence [86]

This is a machine-generated summary of:

Tan, Yi; Zhang, Zhiguo; Zheng, Chao; Wintergerst, Kupper A.; Keller, Bradley B.; Cai, Lu: Mechanisms of diabetic cardiomyopathy and potential therapeutic strategies: preclinical and clinical evidence [86].

Published in: Nature Reviews Cardiology (2020).

Link to original: https://doi.org/10.1038/s41569-020-0339-2

If you want to cite the papers, please refer to the original.

For technical reasons we could not place the page where the original quote is coming from.

Abstract-Summary "The pathogenesis and clinical features of diabetic cardiomyopathy have been well-studied in the past decade, but effective approaches to prevent and treat this disease are limited."

"Preclinical studies in animal models of diabetes have identified multiple intracellular pathways involved in the pathogenesis of diabetic cardiomyopathy and potential cardioprotective strategies to prevent and treat the disease, including antifibrotic agents, anti-inflammatory agents and antioxidants."

"In this Review, we discuss the mechanisms underlying the development of diabetic cardiomyopathy and heart failure in type 1 and type 2 diabetes mellitus, and we summarize the evidence from preclinical and clinical studies that might provide guidance for the development of targeted strategies."

Introduction

"The risks of diabetic cardiomyopathy and HF are correlated with the level of glycaemic control: patients with T1DM have a 30% increased risk and those with T2DM an 8% increased risk of HF for each 1% increase in glycated haemoglobin (HbA_{1c}) level [87]."

"Treatment with the DPP4 inhibitor saxagliptin in patients with T2DM has been associated with an increased risk of HF-related hospitalization compared with placebo treatment [88]."

"Treatment with sodium–glucose cotransporter 2 (SGLT2) inhibitors [89–91] and glucagon-like peptide 1 (GLP1) receptor antagonists [92–94] has been shown to reduce the risk of cardiovascular disease in patients with T2DM compared with placebo treatment."

"The DAPA-HF trial [95] reported in 2019 showed that treatment with the SGLT2 inhibitor dapagliflozin reduced the risk of worsening HF or cardiovascular death in patients with HF with reduced ejection fraction (HFrEF) with or without T2DM compared with placebo treatment."

"These clinical trials highlight the need to further our understanding of the pathological mechanisms of diabetic cardiomyopathy and HF in patients with T2DM."

Cardiomyopathy in T1DM and T2DM

"The typical clinical features of diabetic cardiomyopathy associated with T2DM include reduced ventricular compliance with increased systemic and pulmonary venous pressures and congestion despite preserved systolic function [96]."

"Symptoms of systolic dysfunction, more typical in patients with T1DM, include classic HF symptoms of reduced exercise capacity, as well as the onset of arrhythmias owing to mitochondrial dysfunction [97], abnormal Ca^{2+} transport [98] and autonomic neuropathy [99, 100]."

"In T2DM-associated diabetic cardiomyopathy, coronary microvascular inflammation and paracrine effects on cardiomyocytes and endothelial cells mediate concentric left ventricular (LV) remodelling and hypertrophy that increase ventricular stiffness and promote diastolic dysfunction [101–103]."

"T1DM-associated diabetic cardiomyopathy is characterized by cardiomyocyte loss, LV remodelling and increased myocardial collagen deposition, which increase LV end-diastolic volume and impair systolic function [87, 96, 104]."

"Rats with T2DM and hyperinsulinaemia showed more pronounced diastolic stiffness and preserved systolic function, a disease profile that is similar to that in patients with T2DM and concomitant HFpEF [105, 106]."

Pathophysiology of Diabetic Cardiomyopathy

"In the setting of STZ-induced T1DM, transgenic mice expressing in the heart a mutated form of the NF-κB inhibitor IκBα that prevents the activation of canonical NF-κB signalling are protected from cardiac dysfunction and oxidative stress [107]."

"Diabetic mice with transgenic overexpression of the potent antioxidant metallothionein in the heart had a morphologically normal heart, improved cardiac contractility and reduced cardiomyocyte cell death compared with wild-type diabetic mice [108–110]."

"The finding that overexpression of mitochondrial aldehyde dehydrogenase prevented the diabetes-mediated increase in PTEN activation and diabetic cardiomyopathy development in mice with STZ-induced diabetes mellitus lends additional support to the importance of PTEN activation in the negative regulation of AKT-mediated glucose metabolism in the heart [111]."

"A rat model of T2DM induced by a high-fat diet and low-dose STZ had severe insulin resistance and features of diabetic cardiomyopathy, including LV dysfunction, cardiac inflammation and myocardial fibrosis, in addition to increased expression of TRB3 compared with control rats [112]."

Potential Therapeutic Strategies

"Rats with STZ-induced T1DM treated with an anti-TNF monoclonal antibody (C432A) had significantly lower levels of TNF and IL-1β in the heart, which were associated with improved LV function and reduced cardiac types I and III collagen levels in the heart, compared with untreated diabetic rats [113]."

"To test the hypothesis that increased fatty acid oxidation in the diabetic heart leads to an increased risk of lipotoxicity and diabetic cardiomyopathy, hearts from rats with T2DM were infused ex vivo with the CD36 inhibitor sulfo-N-succinimidyl oleate (SSO) before inducing hypoxia, which resulted in a 29% reduction in the rate of fatty acid oxidation and a 48% reduction in triglyceride concentration compared with no treatment, restoring fatty acid metabolism to control levels following hypoxia–reoxygenation [114]."

Future Directions

"The current treatment regimens for patients with T1DM or T2DM aim to treat insulin resistance, lower inflammation and reduce oxidative stress, which all contribute to the pathogenesis of diabetic cardiomyopathy."

"Metabolic disturbances, including hyperglycaemia, dyslipidaemia and associated glucotoxicity, lipotoxicity and oxidative stress are the predominant pathological mechanisms driving the development of diabetic cardiomyopathy in both T1DM and T2DM."

"This observation suggests that a greater understanding of protective epigenetic mechanisms might lead to the development of novel therapeutics for diabetic cardiomyopathy that not only restore metabolic homeostasis in the early stage of diabetes but also erase the 'epigenetic memory' associated with metabolic disturbances responsible for triggering diabetic cardiomyopathy."

"Very few studies have investigated the pathophysiology of RV dysfunction in diabetic cardiomyopathy."

"The pathophysiological role of cGMP signalling in the development of diabetic cardiomyopathy with HFpEF has been validated in a preclinical study with ZDF rats to test the long-term preventive effects of the PDE5A inhibitor vardenafil (used to treat erectile dysfunction) on diabetes-associated HFpEF [115]."

Conclusions

"Although diabetic cardiomyopathy has been recognized for >40 years through a broad range of investigations that have identified numerous pathogenic mechanisms and targets for prevention and treatment, effective strategies for diabetic cardiomyopathy prevention and treatment remain elusive."

"Although measures of myocardial performance can be used to assess subclinical systolic and diastolic LV dysfunction, the onset of myocardial injury clearly occurs early and before the onset of measurable cardiac dysfunction."

"Cardiac hypertrophy, fibrosis, increased stiffness and cardiomyocyte loss are all consequences of dysregulated glucose and lipid metabolism that impairs excitation–contraction coupling, triggers oxidative stress and AGE formation, disrupts normal regulation of cardiomyocyte hyperplasia and hypertrophy, and activates multiple inflammatory pathways in the setting of diabetes."

"Sensitive and specific markers for changes in intracellular signalling pathways involved in the pathogenesis of diabetic cardiomyopathy, as well as novel cardioprotective strategies targeting these pathways, will hopefully improve cardiovascular outcomes in patients with diabetes."

Effects of Empagliflozin in Different Phases of Diabetes Mellitus-Related Cardiomyopathy: A Prospective Observational Study [116]

This is a machine-generated summary of:

Oka, Satoshi; Kai, Takahiko; Hoshino, Katsuomi; Watanabe, Kazunori; Nakamura, Jun; Abe, Makoto; Watanabe, Akinori: Effects of empagliflozin in different phases of diabetes mellitus-related cardiomyopathy: a prospective observational study [116].

Published in: BMC Cardiovascular Disorders (2021).

Link to original: https://doi.org/10.1186/s12872-021-02024-3

If you want to cite the papers, please refer to the original.

For technical reasons we could not place the page where the original quote is coming from.

Abstract-Summary "Diabetes mellitus-related cardiomyopathy (DMCMP), defined as left ventricular (LV) dysfunction caused by hyperglycemia in the absence of coronary artery disease, leads to heart failure (HF)."

"The beneficial effects of SGLT2i on HF depend not only on indirect actions such as osmotic diuresis but also on direct actions on the myocardium, leading to improvements in LV function."

"The aim of this observational study was to compare the efficacy of SGLT2i treatment on LV dysfunction between early and advanced DMCMP."

"Thirty-five symptomatic non-ischemic HF patients with LV ejection fraction > 40% and type 2 diabetes mellitus (T2DM) treated with empagliflozin (EMPA group) and 20 controls treated without SGLT2i were enrolled."

"According to the myocardial extracellular volume fraction (ECV), a reliable marker of cardiac fibrosis quantified by cardiac magnetic resonance, the EMPA group was further divided into early DMCMP ($n = 16$, ECV $\leq 30\%$) and advanced DMCMP ($n = 19$, ECV $> 30\%$) groups and followed up prospectively."

"After 12 months, the EMPA group, especially the early DMCMP group, showed remarkable improvements in LVGLS (ΔLVGLS: $2.9 \pm 3.0\%$ (EMPA) vs. $0.6 \pm 2.2\%$ (controls), $p=0.005$, and $4.6 \pm 1.5\%$ (early DMCMP) vs. $1.6 \pm 3.3\%$ (advanced DMCMP), $p=0.003$) and E/e′ (ΔE/e′: -1.5 ± 4.7 vs. -0.3 ± 3.0, $p=0.253$, and -3.4 ± 5.5 vs. -0.1 ± 3.5, $p=0.043$)."

"The positive effects of empagliflozin on LV dysfunction were more remarkable in early than in advanced DMCMP."

"Early intervention of SGLT2i for DMCMP may be preferable."

Background

"Diabetes mellitus-related cardiomyopathy (DMCMP), which manifests as left ventricular (LV) dysfunction that occurs independently of coronary artery disease and hypertension [117], has been attracting attention as a cause of HF."

"Hyperglycemia drives LV dysfunction and remodeling through the progression of microvascular endothelial dysfunction, myocardial injury, and interstitial fibrosis, which lead to DMCMP [118]."

"The beneficial effects of SGLT2i treatment on HF are explained not only by their indirect actions, such as glycemic control or osmotic diuresis, but also by their direct actions on the myocardium, which lead to improvements in LV function [119, 120]."

"The aim of this study was to compare the efficacy of SGLT2i treatment on LV dysfunction between the early and advanced phases of DMCMP."

Methods

"Exclusion criteria were as follows: (1) age < 20 or > 80 years; (2) in-hospital death; (3) New York Heart Association (NYHA) class I or brain natriuretic peptide (BNP) < 100 pg/mL; (4) LVEF ≤ 40%; (5) coronary artery disease, hypertensive heart disease, or other cardiomyopathy; (6) valvular or congenital heart disease; (7) LVGLS within normal range (absolute value ≥ 18%) [121]; (8) type 1 diabetes mellitus or insulin-dependent T2DM with a C-peptide immunoreactivity index < 0.8 [122] or use of insulin; (9) newly diagnosed T2DM (<1 year) or no antidiabetic medications before the start of administration of empagliflozin; (10) previous use of SGLT2i; (11) persistent arrhythmia; (12) pacemaker implantation; (13) contraindication for CMR (implanted metallic objects, allergy to contrast media, or bronchial asthma); (14) estimated glomerular filtration rate (eGFR) ≤ 30 mL/min/1.73 m^2; (15) malignant tumor or inflammatory disease; (16) pregnancy; (17) refusal to provide informed consent, and (18) history of myocardial infarction, cerebral infarction, pancreatitis, or hospitalization for HF."

Results

"A total of 35 DMCMP patients treated with empagliflozin were enrolled as the EMPA group."

"The EMPA group patients were further divided into early DMCMP (n = 16, global ECV: 27.5 ± 1.9%) and advanced DMCMP (n = 19, global ECV: 38.7 ± 5.3%) groups."

"The T2DM duration of the advanced DMCMP group was significantly longer than that of the early DMCMP group (22 [21–30] vs. 99 [77–81, 83–85, 87–115, 117–126] months, $p < 0.001$)."

Discussion

"In animal models, SGLT2i treatment, via the inhibition of NHE-1, reduces myocardial injury and fibrosis, slows the progression of DMCMP, and improves systolic and diastolic function [125–127]."

"The composite of direct and indirect cardiac actions of SGLT2i could improve HF parameters even in patients with advanced DMCMP."

"LV longitudinal myocardial dysfunction and diastolic dysfunction are clinically important markers observed from the preclinical phase of DMCMP [121, 128], leading to HF."

"Treatment with empagliflozin improved LV functional parameters assessed as LVGLS and E/e′, which were more remarkable in the earlier phase of DMCMP."

"We consider that the small study number and population differences, having more advanced DMCMP patients with higher baseline E/e′ and treatment-resistance, might have affected the result."

"If the follow-up period was longer, LV functional parameters might have improved further in the advanced DMCMP group."

Conclusions

"Empagliflozin had positive effects on LV function that were more remarkable in the early DMCMP group with normal ECV values than in the advanced DMCMP group with elevated ECV values."

"The ECV increase was strongly correlated with T2DM duration."

"Early SGLT2i administration for patients with HF and T2DM may be preferable."

Bibliography

1. McDonald M, Virani S, Chan M, Ducharme A, Ezekowitz JA, Giannetti N et al (2021) CCS/CHFS heart failure guidelines update: defining a new pharmacologic standard of care for heart failure with reduced ejection fraction. Can J Cardiol 37:531–546
2. Huang K, Luo X, Liao B, Li G, Feng J (2023) Insights into SGLT2 inhibitor treatment of diabetic cardiomyopathy: focus on the mechanisms. Cardiovasc Diabetol 22:86. https://doi.org/10.1186/s12933-023-01816-5
3. Ahmed AM (2002) History of diabetes mellitus. Saudi Med J 23:373–378
4. Jia G, Whaley-Connell A, Sowers JR (2018) Diabetic cardiomyopathy: a hyperglycaemia- and insulin-resistance-induced heart disease. Diabetologia 61:21–28
5. Isfort M, Stevens SCW, Schaffer S, Jong CJ, Wold LE (2014) Metabolic dysfunction in diabetic cardiomyopathy. Heart Fail Rev 19:35–48. https://doi.org/10.1007/s10741-013-9377-8
6. Bugger H, Abel ED (2014) Molecular mechanisms of diabetic cardiomyopathy. Diabetologia 57:660–671
7. Holscher ME, Bode C, Bugger H (2016) Diabetic cardiomyopathy: does the type of diabetes matter? Int J Mol Sci 17:2136
8. Isaji M (2011) SGLT2 inhibitors: molecular design and potential differences in effect. Kidney Int Suppl 79:S14. https://doi.org/10.1038/ki.2010.511.S14-9
9. Saisho Y (2020) SGLT2 inhibitors: the star in the treatment of type 2 diabetes? Diseases 8. https://doi.org/10.3390/diseases8020014
10. Kondo H, Akoumianakis I, Badi I, Akawi N, Kotanidis CP, Polkinghorne M et al (2021) Effects of canagliflozin on human myocardial redox signalling: clinical implications. Eur Heart J 42:4947–4960
11. Philippaert K, Kalyaanamoorthy S, Fatehi M, Long W, Soni S, Byrne NJ et al (2021) Cardiac late sodium channel current is a molecular target for the sodium/glucose cotransporter 2 inhibitor empagliflozin. Circulation 143(22):2188–2204. https://doi.org/10.1161/CIRCULATIONAHA.121.053350
12. Dakhili SAT, Greenwell AA, Ussher JR (2023) Pyruvate dehydrogenase complex and glucose oxidation as a therapeutic target in diabetic heart disease. J Lipid Atheroscler 12:47–57
13. Mizuno Y, Harada E, Nakagawa H, Morikawa Y, Shono M, Kugimiya F et al (2017) The diabetic heart utilizes ketone bodies as an energy source. Metabolism 77:65–72
14. Mustroph J, Lücht CM, Wagemann O, Sowa T, Hammer KP, Sag CM et al (2019) Empagliflozin enhances human and murine cardiomyocyte glucose uptake by increased expression of GLUT1. Diabetologia 62:726–729
15. Oshima H, Miki T, Kuno A et al (2019) Empagliflozin, an SGLT2 inhibitor, reduced the mortality rate after acute myocardial infarction with modification of cardiac metabolomes and antioxidants in diabetic rats. J Pharmacol Exp Ther 368(3):524–534
16. Yanai H, Yoshida H (2019) Beneficial effects of adiponectin on glucose and lipid metabolism and atherosclerotic progression: mechanisms and perspectives. Int J Mol Sci 20:1190
17. Jornayvaz FR, Shulman GI (2010) Regulation of mitochondrial biogenesis. Essays Biochem 47:69–84
18. Scarpulla RC (2011) Metabolic control of mitochondrial biogenesis through the PGC-1 family regulatory network. Biochim Biophys Acta 1813:1269–1278
19. Secker PF, Beneke S, Schlichenmaier N, Delp J, Gutbier S, Leist M et al (2018) Canagliflozin mediated dual inhibition of mitochondrial glutamate dehydrogenase and complex I: an off-target adverse effect. Cell Death Dis 9:226
20. Hodrea J, Balogh DB, Hosszu A, Lenart L, Besztercei B, Koszegi S et al (2020) Reduced O-GlcNAcylation and tubular hypoxia contribute to the antifibrotic effect of SGLT2 inhibitor dapagliflozin in the diabetic kidney. Am J Physiol Renal Physiol 318:F1017–F1029
21. Zhou H, Wang S, Zhu P, Hu S, Chen Y et al (2018) Empagliflozin rescues diabetic myocardial microvascular injury via AMPKmediated inhibition of mitochondrial fission. Redox Biol 15:335–346. https://doi.org/10.1016/j.redox.2017.12.019

22. Albu A, Para I, Porojan M (2020) Uric acid and arterial stiffness. Ther Clin Risk Manag 16:39–54
23. Uthman L, Homayr A, Juni RP, Spin EL, Kerindongo R, Boomsma M et al (2019) Empagliflozin and dapagliflozin reduce ROS generation and restore NO bioavailability in tumor necrosis factor α-stimulated human coronary arterial endothelial cells. Cell Physiol Biochem 53:865–886
24. Lin Y, Nan J, Shen J, Lv X, Chen X, Lu X et al (2020) Canagliflozin impairs blood reperfusion of ischaemic lower limb partially by inhibiting the retention and paracrine function of bone marrow derived mesenchymal stem cells. EBioMedicine 52:102637
25. Zhao J, Randive R, Stewart JA (2014) Molecular mechanisms of AGE/RAGE-mediated fibrosis in the diabetic heart. World J Diabetes 5:860–867
26. Shamhart PE, Luther DJ, Adapala RK, Bryant JE, Petersen KA, Meszaros JG et al (2014) Hyperglycemia enhances function and differentiation of adult rat cardiac fibroblasts. Can J Physiol Pharmacol 92:598–604
27. Fang M, Wang J, Li S, Guo Y (2016) Advanced glycation end-products accelerate the cardiac aging process through the receptor for advanced glycation end-products/transforming growth factor-β-Smad signaling pathway in cardiac fibroblasts. Geriatr Gerontol Int 16:522–527
28. Li C, Zhang J, Xue M, Li X, Han F, Liu X et al (2019) SGLT2 inhibition with empagliflozin attenuates myocardial oxidative stress and fibrosis in diabetic mice heart. Cardiovasc Diabetol 18(1):15. https://doi.org/10.1186/s12933-019-0816-2
29. Lee T-M, Chang N-C, Lin S-Z (2017) Dapagliflozin, a selective SGLT2 inhibitor, attenuated cardiac fibrosis by regulating the macrophage polarization via STAT3 signaling in infarcted rat hearts. Free Radic Biol Med 104:298–310
30. Hasan R, Lasker S, Hasan A, Zerin F, Zamila M, Chowdhury FI et al (2020) Canagliflozin attenuates isoprenaline-induced cardiac oxidative stress by stimulating multiple antioxidant and anti-inflammatory signaling pathways. Sci Rep 10:14459
31. Hasan R, Lasker S, Hasan A, Zerin F, Zamila M, Parvez F et al (2020) Canagliflozin ameliorates renal oxidative stress and inflammation by stimulating AMPK-Akt-eNOS pathway in the isoprenaline-induced oxidative stress model. Sci Rep 10:14659
32. Zhang B, Zhai M, Li B, Liu Z, Li K, Jiang L et al (2018) Honokiol ameliorates myocardial ischemia/reperfusion injury in type 1 diabetic rats by reducing oxidative stress and apoptosis through activating the SIRT1-Nrf2 signaling pathway. Oxidative Med Cell Longev 2018:3159801
33. Ren BC, Zhang YF, Liu SS, Cheng XJ, Yang X, Cui XG et al (2020) Curcumin alleviates oxidative stress and inhibits apoptosis in diabetic cardiomyopathy via Sirt1-Foxo1 and PI3K-Akt signalling pathways. J Cell Mol Med 24:12355–12367
34. Kim JW, Lee YJ, You YH, Moon MK, Yoon KH, Ahn YB et al (2019) Effect of sodium-glucose cotransporter 2 inhibitor, empagliflozin, and α-glucosidase inhibitor, voglibose, on hepatic steatosis in an animal model of type 2 diabetes. J Cell Biochem 120:8534–8546
35. Mohamed HE, Asker ME, Keshawy MM, Hasan RA, Mahmoud YK (2020) Inhibition of tumor necrosis factor-α enhanced the antifibrotic effect of empagliflozin in an animal model with renal insulin resistance. Mol Cell Biochem 466:45–54
36. Zhang J, Huang L, Shi X, Yang L, Hua F, Ma J et al (2020) Metformin protects against myocardial ischemia-reperfusion injury and cell pyroptosis via AMPK/NLRP3 inflammasome pathway. Aging 12:24270–24287
37. Hu R, Wang MQ, Ni SH, Wang M, Liu LY, You HY et al (2020) Salidroside ameliorates endothelial inflammation and oxidative stress by regulating the AMPK/NF-kappaB/NLRP3 signaling pathway in AGEs-induced HUVECs. Eur J Pharmacol 867:172797
38. Ma C, Wang X, Xu T, Yu X, Zhang S, Liu S et al (2019) Qingkailing injection ameliorates cerebral ischemia-reperfusion injury and modulates the AMPK/NLRP3 inflammasome signalling pathway. BMC Complement Altern Med 19:320

39. Yue RC, Lu SZ, Luo Y, Wang T, Liang H, Zeng J et al (2019) Calpain silencing alleviates myocardial ischemia-reperfusion injury through the NLRP3/ASC/Caspase-1 axis in mice. Life Sci 233:116631
40. Ye Y, Bajaj M, Yang H-C, Perez-Polo JR, Birnbaum Y (2017) SGLT-2 inhibition with dapagliflozin reduces the activation of the Nlrp3/ASC inflammasome and attenuates the development of diabetic cardiomyopathy in mice with type 2 diabetes. Further augmentation of the effects with saxagliptin, a DPP4 inhibitor. Cardiovasc Drugs Ther 31:119–132
41. Li Y, Yang P, Zhao L, Chen Y, Zhang X, Zeng S et al (2019) CD36 plays a negative role in the regulation of lipophagy in hepatocytes through an AMPK-dependent pathway. J Lipid Res 60:844–855
42. Jiang K, Xu Y, Wang D et al (2021) Cardioprotective mechanism of SGLT2 inhibitor against myocardial infarction is through reduction of autosis. Protein Cell 13:336–359
43. Lee WS, Yoo WH, Chae HJ (2015) ER stress and autophagy. Curr Mol Med 15:735–745
44. Ren FF, Xie ZY, Jiang YN, Guan X, Chen QY, Lai TF et al (2022) Dapagliflozin attenuates pressure overload-induced myocardial remodeling in mice via activating SIRT1 and inhibiting endoplasmic reticulum stress. Acta Pharmacol Sin 43:1721–1732
45. Wang CC, Li Y, Qian XQ, Zhao H, Wang D, Zuo GX et al (2022) Empagliflozin alleviates myocardial I/R injury and cardiomyocyte apoptosis via inhibiting ER stress-induced autophagy and the PERK/ATF4/Beclin1 pathway. J Drug Target 30:858–872
46. Lee DM, Battson ML, Jarrell DK et al (2018) SGLT2 inhibition via dapagliflozin improves generalized vascular dysfunction and alters the gut microbiota in type 2 diabetic mice. Cardiovasc Diabetol 17:62. https://doi.org/10.1186/s12933-018-0708-x
47. Shin NR, Lee JC, Lee HY, Kim MS, Whon TW, Lee MS et al (2014) An increase in the Akkermansia spp. population induced by metformin treatment improves glucose homeostasis in diet-induced obese mice. Gut 63:727–735
48. Li J, Lin S, Vanhoutte PM, Woo CW, Xu A (2016) Akkermansia muciniphila protects against atherosclerosis by preventing metabolic endotoxemia-induced inflammation in Apoe-/- mice. Circulation 133:2434–2446
49. Deng X, Zhang C, Wang P, Wei W, Shi X, Wang P et al (2022) Cardiovascular benefits of empagliflozin are associated with gut microbiota and plasma metabolites in type 2 diabetes. J Clin Endocrinol Metab 107:1888–1896
50. Röder PV, Geillinger KE, Zietek TS, Thorens B, Koepsell H, Daniel H (2014) The role of SGLT1 and GLUT2 in intestinal glucose transport and sensing. PLoS One 9:e89977
51. Verma S, Mazer CD, Yan AT et al (2019) Effect of empagliflozin on left ventricular mass in patients with type 2 diabetes and coronary artery disease: the EMPA-HEART CardioLink-6 randomized clinical trial. Circulation 140:1693–1702. https://doi.org/10.1161/CIRCULATIONAHA.119.042375
52. Brown AJM, Gandy S, McCrimmon R, Houston JG, Struthers AD, Lang CC (2020) A randomized controlled trial of dapagliflozin on left ventricular hypertrophy in people with type two diabetes: the DAPA-LVH trial. Eur Heart J 41(36):3421–3432. https://doi.org/10.1093/eurheartj/ehaa419
53. Sposito AC, Breder I, Soares AAS, Kimura-Medorima ST, Munhoz DB, Cintra RMR et al (2021) Dapagliflozin effect on endothelial dysfunction in diabetic patients with atherosclerotic disease: a randomized active-controlled trial. Cardiovasc Diabetol 20:74
54. van Bommel EJM, Herrema H, Davids M, Kramer MHH, Nieuwdorp M, van Raalte DH (2020) Effects of 12-week treatment with dapagliflozin and gliclazide on faecal microbiome: results of a double-blind randomized trial in patients with type 2 diabetes. Diabetes Metab 46:164–168
55. Dave CV, Schneeweiss S, Patorno E (2019) Comparative risk of genital infections associated with sodium-glucose co-transporter-2 inhibitors. Diabetes Obes Metab 21:434–438
56. Arow M, Waldman M, Yadin D, Nudelman V, Shainberg A, Abraham NG, Freimark D, Kornowski R, Aravot D, Hochhauser E, Arad M (2020) Sodium–glucose cotransporter

2 inhibitor Dapagliflozin attenuates diabetic cardiomyopathy. Cardiovasc Diabetol 19:7. https://doi.org/10.1186/s12933-019-0980-4
57. Di Angelantonio E, Kaptoge S, Wormser D, Willeit P, Butterworth AS, Bansal N, O'Keeffe LM, Gao P, Wood AM, Burgess S et al (2015) Association of cardiometabolic multimorbidity with mortality. JAMA 314(1):52–60
58. Boudina S, Abel ED (2010) Diabetic cardiomyopathy, causes and effects. Rev Endocr Metab Disord 11(1):31–39
59. Suzuki H, Kayama Y, Sakamoto M, Iuchi H, Shimizu I, Yoshino T, Katoh D, Nagoshi T, Tojo K, Minamino T et al (2015) Arachidonate 12/15-lipoxygenase-induced inflammation and oxidative stress are involved in the development of diabetic cardiomyopathy. Diabetes 64(2):618–630
60. Udell JA, Cavender MA, Bhatt DL, Chatterjee S, Farkouh ME, Scirica BM (2015) Glucose-lowering drugs or strategies and cardiovascular outcomes in patients with or at risk for type 2 diabetes: a meta-analysis of randomised controlled trials. Lancet Diabetes Endocrinol 3(5):356–366
61. Wiviott SD, Raz I, Sabatine MS (2019) Dapagliflozin and cardiovascular outcomes in type 2 diabetes. Reply. N Engl J Med 380(19):1881–1882
62. Waldman M, Nudelman V, Shainberg A, Abraham NG, Kornwoski R, Aravot D, Arad M, Hochhauser E (2018) PARP-1 inhibition protects the diabetic heart through activation of SIRT1-PGC-1alpha axis. Exp Cell Res 373(1–2):112–118. https://doi.org/10.1016/j.yexcr.2018.10.003
63. Uthman L, Baartscheer A, Schumacher CA, Fiolet JWT, Kuschma MC, Hollmann MW et al (2018) Direct cardiac actions of sodium glucose cotransporter 2 inhibitors target pathogenic mechanisms underlying heart failure in diabetic patients. Front Physiol 9:1575
64. Munzel T, Gori T, Keaney JF Jr, Maack C, Daiber A (2015) Pathophysiological role of oxidative stress in systolic and diastolic heart failure and its therapeutic implications. Eur Heart J 36(38):2555–2564
65. Yancy CW, Jessup M, Bozkurt B, Butler J, Casey DE Jr, Drazner MH, Fonarow GC, Geraci SA, Horwich T, Januzzi JL et al (2013) 2013 ACCF/AHA guideline for the management of heart failure: a report of the American College of Cardiology Foundation/American Heart Association task force on practice guidelines. J Am Coll Cardiol 62(16):e147–e239
66. Ye Y, Bajaj M, Yang H-C, Perez-Polo JR, Birnbaum Y (2017) SGLT-2 inhibition with dapagliflozin reduces the activation of the Nlrp3/ASC inflammasome and attenuates the development of diabetic cardiomyopathy in mice with type 2 diabetes. Further augmentation of the effects with saxagliptin, a DPP4 inhibitor. Cardiovasc Drugs Ther 31(2):119–132. https://doi.org/10.1007/s10557-017-6725-2
67. Birnbaum Y, Bajaj M, Qian J, Ye Y (2016) Dipeptidyl peptidase-4 inhibition by saxagliptin prevents inflammation and renal injury by targeting the Nlrp3/ASC inflammasome. BMJ Open Diabetes Res Care 4:e000227
68. Zhou L, Cryan EV, D'Andrea MR, Belkowski S, Conway BR, Demarest KT (2003) Human cardiomyocytes express high level of Na+/glucose cotransporter 1 (SGLT1). J Cell Biochem 90:339–346
69. Vrhovac I, Balen Eror D, Klessen D, Burger C, Breljak D, Kraus O et al (2015) Localizations of Na(+)-d-glucose cotransporters SGLT1 and SGLT2 in human kidney and of SGLT1 in human small intestine, liver, lung, and heart. Pflugers Arch 467:1881–1898
70. Saito T, Okada S, Yamada E, Shimoda Y, Osaki A, Tagaya Y et al (2015) Effect of dapagliflozin on colon cancer cell [rapid communication]. Endocr J 62:1133–1137
71. Kashiwagi Y, Nagoshi T, Yoshino T et al (2015) Expression of SGLT1 in human hearts and impairment of cardiac glucose uptake by phlorizin during ischemia-reperfusion injury in mice. PLoS One 10(6):e0130605
72. Ehrenkranz JR, Lewis NG, Kahn CR, Roth J (2005) Phlorizin: a review. Diabetes Metab Res Rev 21:31–38

73. Hawley SA, Ford RJ, Smith BK et al (2016) The Na+/glucose cotransporter inhibitor canagliflozin activates AMPK by inhibiting mitochondrial function and increasing cellular AMP levels. Diabetes 65:2784–2794
74. Tirmenstein M, Dorr TE, Janovitz EB, Hagan D, Abell LM, Onorato JM et al (2013) Nonclinical toxicology assessments support the chronic safety of dapagliflozin, a first-in-class sodium-glucose cotransporter 2 inhibitor. Int J Toxicol 32:336–350
75. Chang YK, Choi H, Jeong JY, Na KR, Lee KW, Lim BJ et al (2016) Dapagliflozin, SGLT2 inhibitor, attenuates renal ischemia-reperfusion injury. PLoS One 11:e0158810
76. Tanaka H, Tatsumi K, Matsuzoe H, Soga F, Matsumoto K, Hirata K-i (2021) Association of type 2 diabetes mellitus with the development of new-onset atrial fibrillation in patients with non-ischemic dilated cardiomyopathy: impact of SGLT2 inhibitors. Int J Cardiovasc Imaging 37:1333. https://doi.org/10.1007/s10554-020-02122-x
77. Huxley RR, Filion KB, Konety S, Alonso A (2011) Meta-analysis of cohort and case–control studies of type 2 diabetes mellitus and risk of atrial fibrillation. Am J Cardiol 108:56–62
78. Zelniker TA, Bonaca MP, Furtado RHM, Mosenzon O, Kuder JF, Murphy SA, Bhatt DL, Leiter LA, McGuire DK, Wilding JPH, Budaj A, Kiss RG, Padilla F, Gause-Nilsson I, Langkilde AM, Raz I, Sabatine MS, Wiviott SD (2020) Effect of dapagliflozin on atrial fibrillation in patients with type 2 diabetes mellitus: insights from the DECLARE-TIMI 58 trial. Circulation 141:1227–1234
79. Lang RM, Badano LP, Mor-Avi V, Afilalo J, Armstrong A, Ernande L, Flachskampf FA, Foster E, Goldstein SA, Kuznetsova T, Lancellotti P, Muraru D, Picard MH, Rietzschel ER, Rudski L, Spencer KT, Tsang W, Voigt JU (2015) Recommendations for cardiac chamber quantification by echocardiography in adults: an update from the American Society of Echocardiography and the European Association of Cardiovascular Imaging. J Am Soc Echocardiogr 28(1–39):e14
80. Chimura M, Onishi T, Tsukishiro Y, Sawada T, Kiuchi K, Shimane A, Okajima K, Yamada S, Taniguchi Y, Yasaka Y, Kawai H (2017) Longitudinal strain combined with delayed-enhancement magnetic resonance improves risk stratification in patients with dilated cardiomyopathy. Heart 103:679–686
81. Mignot A, Donal E, Zaroui A, Reant P, Salem A, Hamon C, Monzy S, Roudaut R, Habib G, Lafitte S (2010) Global longitudinal strain as a major predictor of cardiac events in patients with depressed left ventricular function: a multicenter study. J Am Soc Echocardiogr 23:1019–1024
82. Huo J-Y, Jiang W-Y, Zhang S-G, Lyu Y-T, Geng J, Chen M, Chen Y-Y, Jiang Z-X, Shan Q-J (2021) Renal denervation ameliorates cardiac metabolic remodeling in diabetic cardiomyopathy rats by suppressing renal SGLT2 expression. Lab Investig 102:341. https://doi.org/10.1038/s41374-021-00696-1
83. Kenny HC, Abel ED (2019) Heart failure in type 2 diabetes mellitus. Circ Res 124:121–141
84. Hussein AM et al (2020) Comparative study of the effects of GLP1 analog and SGLT2 inhibitor against diabetic cardiomyopathy in type 2 diabetic rats: possible underlying mechanisms. Biomedicines 8:43
85. Arow M et al (2020) Sodium-glucose cotransporter 2 inhibitor Dapagliflozin attenuates diabetic cardiomyopathy. Cardiovasc Diabetol 19:7
86. Tan Y, Zhang Z, Zheng C, Wintergerst KA, Keller BB, Cai L (2020) Mechanisms of diabetic cardiomyopathy and potential therapeutic strategies: preclinical and clinical evidence. Nat Rev Cardiol 17:585. https://doi.org/10.1038/s41569-020-0339-2
87. Jia G, Hill MA, Sowers JR (2018) Diabetic cardiomyopathy: an update of mechanisms contributing to this clinical entity. Circ Res 122:624–638
88. Scirica BM et al (2014) Heart failure, saxagliptin, and diabetes mellitus: observations from the SAVOR-TIMI 53 randomized trial. Circulation 130:1579–1588
89. Wiviott SD et al (2019) Dapagliflozin and cardiovascular outcomes in type 2 diabetes. N Engl J Med 380:347–357

90. Kato ET et al (2019) Effect of dapagliflozin on heart failure and mortality in type 2 diabetes mellitus. Circulation 139:2528–2536
91. Furtado RHM et al (2019) Dapagliflozin and cardiovascular outcomes in patients with type 2 diabetes mellitus and previous myocardial infarction. Circulation 139:2516–2527
92. Bethel MA et al (2018) Cardiovascular outcomes with glucagon-like peptide-1 receptor agonists in patients with type 2 diabetes: a meta-analysis. Lancet Diabetes Endocrinol 6:105–113
93. Svanstrom H et al (2019) Use of liraglutide and risk of major cardiovascular events: a register-based cohort study in Denmark and Sweden. Lancet Diabetes Endocrinol 7:106–114
94. Bizino MB et al (2019) Effect of liraglutide on cardiac function in patients with type 2 diabetes mellitus: randomized placebo-controlled trial. Cardiovasc Diabetol 18:55
95. McMurray JJV et al (2019) Dapagliflozin in patients with heart failure and reduced ejection fraction. N Engl J Med 381:1995–2008
96. Holscher ME, Bode C, Bugger H (2016) Diabetic cardiomyopathy: does the type of diabetes matter? Int J Mol Sci 17:E2136
97. Duncan JG (2011) Mitochondrial dysfunction in diabetic cardiomyopathy. Biochim Biophys Acta 1813:1351–1359
98. Lebeche D, Davidoff AJ, Hajjar RJ (2008) Interplay between impaired calcium regulation and insulin signaling abnormalities in diabetic cardiomyopathy. Nat Clin Pract Cardiovasc Med 5:715–724
99. Vinik AI, Casellini C, Parson HK, Colberg SR, Nevoret ML (2018) Cardiac autonomic neuropathy in diabetes: a predictor of cardiometabolic events. Front Neurosci 12:591
100. Goldberger JJ, Arora R, Buckley U, Shivkumar K (2019) Autonomic nervous system dysfunction: JACC focus seminar. J Am Coll Cardiol 73:1189–1206
101. van Heerebeek L et al (2008) Diastolic stiffness of the failing diabetic heart: importance of fibrosis, advanced glycation end products, and myocyte resting tension. Circulation 117:43–51
102. Vulesevic B et al (2016) Methylglyoxal-induced endothelial cell loss and inflammation contribute to the development of diabetic cardiomyopathy. Diabetes 65:1699–1713
103. Wan A, Rodrigues B (2016) Endothelial cell-cardiomyocyte crosstalk in diabetic cardiomyopathy. Cardiovasc Res 111:172–183
104. Raev DC (1994) Which left ventricular function is impaired earlier in the evolution of diabetic cardiomyopathy? An echocardiographic study of young type I diabetic patients. Diabetes Care 17:633–639
105. Radovits T et al (2009) Comparative investigation of the left ventricular pressure-volume relationship in rat models of type 1 and type 2 diabetes mellitus. Am J Physiol Heart Circ Physiol 297:H125–H133
106. Matyas C et al (2018) Comparison of speckle-tracking echocardiography with invasive hemodynamics for the detection of characteristic cardiac dysfunction in type-1 and type-2 diabetic rat models. Cardiovasc Diabetol 17:13
107. Thomas CM et al (2014) Cardiac-specific suppression of NF-κB signaling prevents diabetic cardiomyopathy via inhibition of the renin-angiotensin system. Am J Physiol Heart Circ Physiol 307:H1036–H1045
108. Cai L et al (2005) Inhibition of superoxide generation and associated nitrosative damage is involved in metallothionein prevention of diabetic cardiomyopathy. Diabetes 54:1829–1837
109. Liang Q et al (2002) Overexpression of metallothionein reduces diabetic cardiomyopathy. Diabetes 51:174–181
110. Cai L et al (2006) Attenuation by metallothionein of early cardiac cell death via suppression of mitochondrial oxidative stress results in a prevention of diabetic cardiomyopathy. J Am Coll Cardiol 48:1688–1697
111. Zhang Y et al (2012) Mitochondrial aldehyde dehydrogenase (ALDH2) protects against streptozotocin-induced diabetic cardiomyopathy: role of GSK3β and mitochondrial function. BMC Med 10:40
112. Ti Y et al (2011) TRB3 gene silencing alleviates diabetic cardiomyopathy in a type 2 diabetic rat model. Diabetes 60:2963–2974

113. Westermann D et al (2007) Tumor necrosis factor-alpha antagonism protects from myocardial inflammation and fibrosis in experimental diabetic cardiomyopathy. Basic Res Cardiol 102:500–507
114. Mansor LS et al (2017) Inhibition of sarcolemmal FAT/CD36 by sulfo-N-succinimidyl oleate rapidly corrects metabolism and restores function in the diabetic heart following hypoxia/reoxygenation. Cardiovasc Res 113:737–748
115. Matyas C et al (2017) Prevention of the development of heart failure with preserved ejection fraction by the phosphodiesterase-5A inhibitor vardenafil in rats with type 2 diabetes. Eur J Heart Fail 19:326–336
116. Oka S, Kai T, Hoshino K, Watanabe K, Nakamura J, Abe M, Watanabe A (2021) Effects of empagliflozin in different phases of diabetes mellitus-related cardiomyopathy: a prospective observational study. BMC Cardiovasc Disord 21:217. https://doi.org/10.1186/s12872-021-02024-3
117. Boudina S, Abel ED (2007) Diabetic cardiomyopathy revisited. Circulation 115(25):3213–3223
118. Seferović PM, Paulus WJ (2015) Clinical diabetic cardiomyopathy: a two-faced disease with restrictive and dilated phenotypes. Eur Heart J 36(27):1718–1727. https://doi.org/10.1093/eurheartj/ehv134
119. Soga F, Tanaka H, Tatsumi K et al (2018) Impact of dapagliflozin on left ventricular diastolic function of patients with type 2 diabetic mellitus with chronic heart failure. Cardiovasc Diabetol 17:132. https://doi.org/10.1186/s12933-018-0775-z
120. Tanaka H, Soga F, Tatsumi K, Mochizuki Y, Sano H, Toki H, Matsumoto K, Shite J, Takaoka H, Doi T, Hirata KI (2020) Positive effect of dapagliflozin on left ventricular longitudinal function for type 2 diabetic mellitus patients with chronic heart failure. Cardiovasc Diabetol 19:6
121. Ernande L, Bergerot C, Girerd N, Thibault H, Davidsen ES, Pignon-Blanc PG et al (2014) Longitudinal myocardial strain alteration is associated with left ventricular remodeling in asymptomatic patients with type 2 diabetes mellitus. J Am Soc Echocardiogr 27(5):479–488
122. Iwata M, Matsushita Y, Fukuda K, Wakura T, Okabe K, Koshimizu Y et al (2014) Secretory units of islets in transplantation index is a useful predictor of insulin requirement in Japanese type 2 diabetic patients. J Diabetes Investig 5(5):570–580
123. Tan Y, Zhang Z (2020) Mechanisms of diabetic cardiomyopathy and potential therapeutic strategies: preclinical and clinical evidence. Nat Rev Cardiol 17:585–607
124. Lang RM, Badano LP, Mor-Avi V, Afilalo J, Armstrong A, Ernande L et al (2015) Recommendations for cardiac chamber quantification by echocardiography in adults: an update from the American Society of Echocardiography and the European Association of Cardiovascular Imaging. Eur Heart J Cardiovasc Imaging 16(3):233–270
125. Baartscheer A, Schumacher CA, Wüst RCI, Fiolet JWT, Stienen GJM, Coronel R et al (2017) Empagliflozin decreases myocardial cytoplasmic Na(+) through inhibition of the cardiac Na(+)/H(+) exchanger in rats and rabbits. Diabetologia 60:568–573
126. Lin B, Koibuchi N, Hasegawa Y, Sueta D, Toyama K, Uekawa K et al (2014) Glycemic control with empagliflozin, a novel selective SGLT2 inhibitor, ameliorates cardiovascular injury and cognitive dysfunction in obese and type 2 diabetic mice. Cardiovasc Diabetol 13:148
127. Habibi J, Aroor AR, Sowers JR, Jia G, Hayden MR, Garro M et al (2017) Sodium glucose transporter 2 (SGLT2) inhibition with empagliflozin improves cardiac diastolic function in a female rodent model of diabetes. Cardiovasc Diabetol 16:9
128. Chavali V, Tyagi SC, Mishra PK (2013) Predictors and prevention of diabetic cardiomyopathy. Diabetes Metab Syndr Obes 6:151–160

Chapter 6
Role of Therapeutic Potential, Contemporary Management, Unmet needs of SGLT2 Inhibitors in Congestive Heart Failure

Mukesh Nandave

Introduction by the Editor

A significant public health concern is congestive heart failure, which has affected millions globally via tragic circumstances. Offering diagnosis and therapy at the earliest stages and fostering smoothness with appropriate recommendations for the course of treatment about up and down stages of treatments may serve as an unmet need for the early prevention of CHF. Figure 6.1 summarizes the rationale for the invention of SGLT2i in patients having heart failure in diabetic and nondiabetic patients.

This chapter describes the data from cohort studies and clinical trials that suggested SGLT2i might prevent CHF. Researchers provide explanations for the striking outcomes of clinical studies on the prevention of CHF in individuals with and without diabetes. Research on HF indivituals was done to test the working hypothesis of cardiac shield further after the initial encouraging results in cardiovascular outcome studies. In patients with HF with a reduced Left ventricular ejection fraction (LVEF), the Dapagliflozin and Prevention of Adverse Outcomes in Heart Failure (DAPA-HF) research demonstrated a decreased risk of worsening HF or cardiovascular death unrelated to DM status. In the second EMPEROR-REDUCED trial, which examined a similar patient group, the empagliflozin arm had lower cardiovascular mortality and HF hospitalization rates than the placebo arm, independent of DM.

In the difficult-to-treat HF population with preserved LVEF, where only symptomatic treatment was previously authorized, SGLT2i is beneficial. Starting sotagliflozin after an episode of worsening HF reduced the incidence of cardiovascular mortality, HF hospitalizations, or urgent consultations, according to the

M. Nandave (✉)
Department of Pharmacology and Pharmaceutical Biotechnology, Delhi Pharmaceutical Sciences and Research University (DPSRU), New Delhi, Delhi, India

M. Nandave (ed.), *Sodium-glucose Cotransporter-2 (SGLT2) Inhibitors in Heart Failure*, https://doi.org/10.1007/978-981-97-7568-2_6

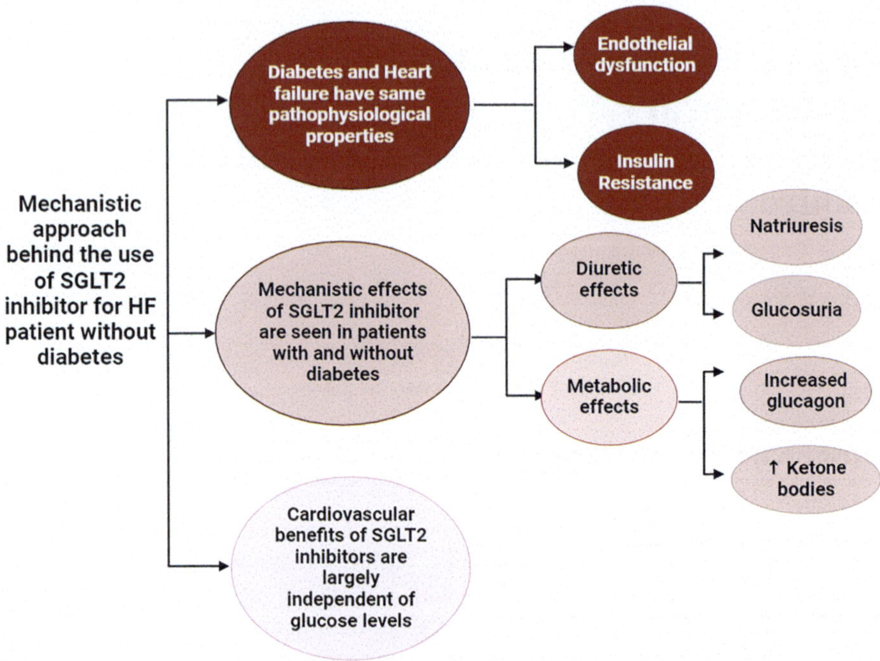

Fig. 6.1 Mechanistic rationale for investigating SGLT-2i in HF beyond T2D. *CV* cardiovascular, *HF* heart failure, *SGLT-2* sodium-glucose cotransporter-2, *T2D* type 2 diabetes mellitus

SOLOIST-WHF research. The results of the EMPEROR-PRESERVED study supported the effectiveness of SGLT2 inhibition for treating heart failure (HF) with LVEF > 40% by showing a 29% decrease in HF hospitalizations along with an increase in patients' quality of life, independent of the presence of DM. People with heart failure with mid-range ejection fraction (HFmrEF) or Heart failure with preserved ejection fraction (HFpEF) who received the intervention in the dapagliflozin DELIVER study had lower endpoint rates than those who received a placebo.

The necessity of using SGLT2i in real clinical practice to lessen the burden of both illnesses is shown by their success in treating heart failure at different degrees of left ventricular ejection fraction. To treat diabetes, diabetic medication in particular has been created. Few clinical trials have been reported for SGLT2i providing benefits to the treatment of congestive heart failure that have been shown below given Table 6.1. Empagiflozin was found to have a major protective effect against heart failure and renal disease based on clinical studies; however, other trials, such as NCT05965934, NCT03560323, and NCT04633005, are being carried out to lower the risk of cardiovascular death and decrease the likelihood of heart failure hospitalisation.

Machine Generated Summaries

Disclaimer: The summaries in this chapter were generated from Springer Nature publications using extractive AI auto-summarization: An extraction-based

Table 6.1 A compilation of all pertinent SGLT2i clinical studies that are helpful in the management of congestive heart failure

	Aim	Sponsor ID	Intervention	Phase	Description
Based on the effect of SGLT2i on diabetic patient with renal diseases which increases the risk of heart failure.	Evaluation of safety and efficacs of DSR therapy in diuretic-resistant patients with chronic volume overload and heart failure (HF) using the Infusate 2.0 peritoneal solution (30% icodextrin, 10% dextrose)	NCT05965934	Direct Sodium Removal Infusate 2.0	Phase I and Phase II	Presented the effectiveness and tolerability of the treatment, the amount of infusate and the length of the dwell period will be changed
	Positron emission tomography (PET) is utilized to measure the myocardial glucose update, while cardiac magnetic resonance imaging is used to analyze left ventricular systolic and diastolic function	NCT03560323	Beta-hydroxy-butyrate	Phase I	Empagliflozin-induced SGLT2i significantly decreased heart failure hospitalization and cardiovascular (CV) death
	The research team will investigate the consequences of high plasma ketones in individuals with T2DM and HF following a 12-week course of SGLT2i (empagliflozin) medication	NCT05057806	Empagliflozin + Placebo	Early Phase I	Increased plasma ketones resulting from a 12-week course of SGLT2i (empagliflozin) medication in individuals diagnosed with T2D and heart failure
	A practical single-center randomized study is recommended to examine the feasibility and effectiveness of a polypill-based approach for the management of HFrEF in a people with low incomes and ethnically mixed population	NCT04633005	Polypill + Control Rx	Early Phase I	Decrease the morbidity and mortality associated with heart failure, moreover, as a means of encouraging the adoption of approved heart failure therapies
	Through a randomized, double-blind, placebo-controlled mechanistic experiment, empagliflozin evaluated the survival rate of patients with worsening heart failure who had T2D	NCT05553938	Empagliflozin + Placebo	Phase I	Not available
	This study aims to investigate the safety of empagliflozin in dialysis patients to get ready for a larger clinical trial in the future	NCT05687058	Empagliflozin (25 mg thrice-weekly post-hemodialysis dosing) + Empagliflozin 10 mg daily dosing	Phase I & Phase II	Empagliflozin could directly improve the heart and may protect significant residual renal function in some dialysis patients
	Investigate the short- and long-term effects, as well as the cardio-renal processes, of SGLT2i in heart failure patients. Examine the impact of long-term combined exposure to SGLT2 and loop diuretics in heart failure patients	NCT03027960	Empagliflozin + Placebo	Phase I	Not available
	The current investigation aims to evaluate whether enhanced cardiac and functional testing determined on 2D-speckle tracking echocardiography or cardiopulmonary functional testing at 6 months is connected with metabolomic alterations generated by SGLT2i	NCT05719714	Dapagliflozin	Phase I and Phase II	illustrated impacts on blood metabolite levels—which are produced when the body breaks down food, drugs, or its own tissues—as well as heart and lung function

summarizer aims to identify the most important sentences of a text using an algorithm and uses those original sentences to create the auto-summary (unlike generative AI). As the constituted sentences are machine selected, they may not fully reflect the body of the work, so we strongly advise that the original content is read and cited. The auto generated summaries were curated by the editor to meet Springer Nature publication standards. To cite this content, please refer to the original papers.

Machine generated keywords: sodiumglucose transporter, hfpef, hfref, transporter sglt, diabetic patient, transport, blocker, initial, benefit sglti, preserve ejection, diuretic, transporter, sglti, prevention, tubular.

SGLT-2 Inhibitors: Potential Novel Strategy to Prevent Congestive Heart Failure in Diabetes? [1]

This is a machine-generated summary of:

Verbrugge, Frederik H.; Vangoitsenhoven, Roman; Mullens, Wilfried; Van der Schueren, Bart; Mathieu, Chantal; Tang, W. H. Wilson: SGLT-2 Inhibitors: Potential Novel Strategy to Prevent Congestive Heart Failure in Diabetes? [1].

Published in: Current Cardiovascular Risk Reports (2015).

Link to original: https://doi.org/10.1007/s12170-015-0467-0

If you want to cite the papers, please refer to the original.

For technical reasons we could not place the page where the original quote is coming from.

Abstract-Summary "Sodium-glucose transporter-2 (SGLT-2) inhibitors have emerged as novel oral glucose-lowering agents for type 2 diabetes."

"SGLT-2 inhibitors improve glycemic control by blocking sodium-glucose cotransport in the renal proximal tubules, thereby promoting glycosuria."

"On a daily base, SGLT-2 inhibitors block ~330–495 mEq sodium reabsorbed in the proximal tubules, although substantial amounts can be reabsorbed more distally in the nephron."

Introduction

"Randomized clinical trials have established the safety and efficacy of SGLT-2 inhibitors to improve glycemic control in type 2 diabetes, and three pharmacological agents (i.e., canagliflozin, empagliflozin, and dapagliflozin) are currently approved for this indication by the Food and Drug Administration and the European Medicines Agency [2, 3]."

"The inherent natriuretic effect of SGLT-2 inhibitors makes this drug class of particular interest for potential use in patients with or at high risk for heart failure."

"This may be especially relevant in heart failure with preserved ejection fraction (which is common and often overlooked in patients with type 2 diabetes), where no pharmacological therapy has been shown to consistently improve clinical outcomes."

"This review critically examines the potential drug mechanisms of SGLT-2 inhibition that are relevant in the setting of heart failure and puts forward the rationale for further explorations with this drug class as a potential novel therapeutic target in heart failure patients with diabetes and even beyond."

Discovery of Sodium-Glucose Transporters

"Dr. Robert Crane discovered in mucosal cells of the gut what is now known as the sodium-glucose transporter-1 (SGLT-1) and demonstrated for the first time the principle of secondary active transport, whereby energy from sodium transport down its concentration gradient into cells is used to absorb hexose sugars [4]."

"At least six sodium-glucose transporters have been identified since, with different affinity for glucose and distribution throughout the body [5, 6]."

Genetics of Sodium-Glucose Transporters

"Inactivating SLC5A1 mutations that render SGLT-1 dysfunctional lead to a phenotype of glucose-galactose malabsorption and may cause fatal diarrhea [7]."

"SGLT-1 is the predominant glucose transporter in the small intestines [8]."

"Patients with mutations inactivating SGLT-2 have persistent glycosuria but are otherwise asymptomatic [9–11]."

Renal Glucose Transport in Health and Diabetes

"Averaged blood glucose levels of 100 mg/dL and a normal glomerular filtration rate (GFR ~ 125 mL/min/1.73 m^2 or ~ 180 L/day), ~180 g glucose is offered to the renal tubular system on a daily base."

"Renal tubular glucose transport undergoes important adaption, and both SGLT-1 and SGLT-2 are upregulated in uncontrolled diabetes, increasing the threshold for glycosuria [12, 13]."

"The exact mechanisms for SGLT-1 and SGLT-2 upregulation in diabetes are incompletely understood but seem to track better with glycemia than insulin levels, suggesting that the trigger might be increased glucose exposure of proximal tubular cells in the nephron [13]."

"As the SGLT-2 receptor is rapidly downregulated when glycemia is adequately controlled, SGLT-2 inhibitors produce a glycosuric effect that is dependent on blood glucose levels, explaining their relatively low risk for hypoglycemia."

Natriuretic Effects of Sodium-Glucose Transporter-2 Inhibitors

"Available SGLT-2 inhibitors (i.e., canagliflozin, dapagliflozin, and empagliflozin) induce 60–90 g (330–495 mmol) glycosuria per day in patients with type 2 diabetes."

"As the glucose/sodium transport ratio of SGLT-2 is 1:1, this implies that a corresponding 330–495 mEq of tubular sodium is prevented from reabsorption by the proximal renal tubules."

"Further evidence supporting the concept that SGLT-2 inhibitors may contribute to meaningful inhibition of proximal tubular sodium transport comes from genetic studies showing that homozygous SLC5A2 mutation carriers—with complete defective SGLT-2 function—have significantly elevated plasma renin activity and aldosterone levels to prevent volume depletion [14]."

"Reassuring, events of dehydration, hypotension or pre-renal azotemia were uncommon (<1%) in phase III trials of SGLT-2 inhibitors in patients with diabetes [2, 15, 16]."

Rationale for Sodium-Glucose Transport Inhibition in Heart Failure

"Decreased renal blood flow (RBF) is a likely underlying pathophysiological culprit and may lead to increased proximal tubular sodium reabsorption through intrinsic renal autoregulation mechanisms, further enhanced by neurohumoral activation through the sympathetic nerve system and angiotensin II [17]."

"This suggests that SGLT-2, in case of poor RBF and renin-angiotensin system activation, might directly contribute to increased proximal sodium reabsorption in heart failure."

"It has been proposed that increased sodium reabsorption in the proximal renal tubules in diabetes, caused by SGLT-2 upregulation, leads to lower sodium and chloride delivery to the macula densa, which is a potent stimulus for afferent arteriolar vasodilation [18, 19]."

"As SGLT-2 upregulation is also promoted by angiotensin II and increased proximal sodium reabsorption represents a characteristic feature of congestive heart failure, SGLT-2 inhibitors might similarly protect the nephron from hyperfiltration in heart failure too [17, 20]."

Sodium-Glucose-2 Inhibition as a Novel Target in Heart Failure with Preserved Ejection Fraction?

"The exact pathophysiological mechanisms underlying heart failure with preserved in contrast to reduced ejection fraction still remain elusive, but the condition is characterized by increased ventricular stiffness, high cardiac filling pressures, impaired ventriculo-arterial coupling, and often a limited capacity to increase cardiac output during exercise, while the impact of neurohumoral activation is less clear [21]."

"Diabetes patients treated with SGLT-2 inhibitors demonstrate a ~ 1–2 kg/m^2 reduction in body mass index on average [22]."

"A consistent 3–6-mmHg decrease in systolic blood pressure is found in patients treated with SGLT-2 inhibitors [23]."

"A recent study in 13 patients with hypertensive heart failure and preserved ejection fraction showed that by adhering to the sodium-restricted DASH diet, favorable changes in diastolic function, arterial elastance, and ventriculo-arterial coupling were observed already after 3 weeks [24]."

"Restoring natriuretic capacity with SGLT-2 inhibitors in heart failure with preserved ejection fraction warrants further investigation through mechanistic studies."

Potential Adverse Effects of Sodium-Glucose Transporter Inhibitors

"SGLT-2 drugs have emerged as relatively safe drugs in patients with type 2 diabetes, at least after medium-term follow-up."

"One phase II study did report a case of severe volume depletion and pre-renal azotemia in a patient that was randomized to dapagliflozin 10 mg once daily and concomitantly treated with multiple antihypertensive drugs including furosemide [25]."

"Clinicians should be alert to decrease diuretic dosages and monitor the development of dehydration in patients taking SGLT-2 inhibitors, especially when there are no clinical signs or symptoms of congestion and in combination with loop diuretic treatment."

"Excess urinary glucose excretion through SGLT-2 inhibition might increase the risk of genito-urinary infections, especially in women."

"Genital mycotic infections were 11–14% in women and 7–8% in men using canagliflozin versus 2 and 1%, respectively, in patients treated with placebo [15]."

Conclusions

"SGLT-2 inhibitors are approved for improving glycemic control in diabetes and have emerged as relatively safe drugs although results of large studies powered for cardiovascular end point evaluation are still pending."

"SGLT-2 inhibition impacts on several potential pathways implied in the pathophysiology of heart failure and might constitute a novel therapeutic option for this condition."

"Mechanistic studies of SGLT-2 inhibitors in heart failure patients with diabetes are warranted to see whether they are useful to prevent or treat congestion, preserve renal function, and reverse or slow down the progression of diabetic cardiomyopathy."

"The latter is currently under investigation in the Research into the Effect of SGLT2 Inhibition on Left Ventricular Remodeling in Patients with Heart Failure and Diabetes Mellitus (REFORM) study (NCT02397421), which may pave the way for more dedicated heart failure studies with SGLT-2 inhibitors."

Diabetes, Heart Failure and Beyond: Elucidating the Cardioprotective Mechanisms of Sodium Glucose Cotransporter 2 (SGLT2) Inhibitors [26]

This is a machine-generated summary of:

Ojha, Utkarsh; Reyes, Lenisse; Eyenga, Florence; Oumbe, Diane; Watkowska, Justyna; Saint-Jacques, Henock: Diabetes, Heart Failure and Beyond: Elucidating the Cardioprotective Mechanisms of Sodium Glucose Cotransporter 2 (SGLT2) Inhibitors [26].

Published in: American Journal of Cardiovascular Drugs (2021).

Link to original: https://doi.org/10.1007/s40256-021-00486-6

If you want to cite the papers, please refer to the original.

For technical reasons we could not place the page where the original quote is coming from.

Abstract-Summary "The sodium glucose cotransporter 2 (SGLT2) inhibitors are a class of drug that have been widely used in the management of type 2 diabetes mellitus that work by inhibiting the reabsorption of glucose in the proximal convoluted tubule."

"Since the EMPA-REG OUTCOME trial, several studies have demonstrated the benefits of SGLT2 inhibitors in reducing cardiovascular risk related to heart failure."

"While the cardiovascular benefits could be explained by their ability to reduce weight, improve glycemic index and lower blood pressure, several recent trials have suggested that SGLT2 inhibitors exhibit pleiotropic effects that underlie their cardioprotective properties."

"These findings have led to an expansion in preclinical and clinical research aiming to understand the mechanisms by which SGLT2 inhibitors improve heart failure outcomes."

Introduction

"The hypothesis that SGLT2 inhibitors induce weight loss, increase insulin sensitivity and reduce blood glucose levels, thus improving heart failure outcomes, may seem logical; however, the role of weight loss in improving heart failure mortality has been contentious."

"These studies support the hypothesis that SGLT2 inhibitors may exert their therapeutic effects in heart failure patients via inhibition of NHE1."

"While the data from these studies came from murine models, they provide novel insight into the different mechanisms by which SGLT2 inhibitors may downregulate inflammation in the heart, leading to improved heart failure outcomes."

"Commandeering the exact mechanisms by which SGLT2 inhibitors reduce cardiovascular risks can open new therapeutic avenues for managing T2DM and heart failure patients."

Intersection Between Diabetes and Heart Failure: Is SGLT2i the "One Stone for Two Birds" Approach? [27]

This is a machine-generated summary of:

Zhang, Qing; Kang, Yu; Tang, Siqi; Yu, Cheuk-Man: Intersection Between Diabetes and Heart Failure: Is SGLT2i the "One Stone for Two Birds" Approach? [27].

Published in: Current Cardiology Reports (2021).

Link to original: https://doi.org/10.1007/s11886-021-01591-3

If you want to cite the papers, please refer to the original.

For technical reasons we could not place the page where the original quote is coming from.

Abstract-Summary "Comparing the similarities and differences in disease characteristics and treatment between the HF patients with and without DM, this review was to investigate whether and how the novel class of sodium-glucose transport protein 2 inhibitors (SGLT2i) would benefit both populations."

"Despite the obviously different clinical profiles, patients of HF with reduced ejection fraction (HFrEF) should be treated the same with guideline directed medical therapy, irrespective of DM status."

"Upon the mounting evidence that supported its use in diabetic patients at high risk of HF, recent large clinical trials demonstrated that SGLT2i could further reduce HF hospitalization or cardiovascular mortality and improve quality of life in diabetic and non-diabetic HFrEF patients who were optimally managed."

Introduction

"Diabetes mellitus (DM) is a common comorbidity in heart failure (HF) patients, occurring in 20–40% of patients with HF with reduced ejection fraction (HFrEF) and more frequently in HF with preserved ejection fraction (HFpEF) [28–30]."

"Besides diabetic cardiomyopathy which displays two distinct phenotypes as metabolism-mediated restrictive HFpEF phenotype and autoimmune-mediated dilated HFrEF phenotype [31], DM drives a fourfold higher prevalence of HF via its combined atherogenic effect with hypertension and dyslipidemia [32]."

"HF patients are predisposed to DM through dysregulated neurohormonal system [33], HF medication, and reduced physical activity [34]."

"This review will focus on the special patient population of HF with DM and compare to the HF population without DM for similarities and differences in terms of disease profile, clinical impact, as well as the implication of medical therapy by the novel class of anti-diabetic drugs, the sodium-glucose transport protein 2 inhibitors (SGLT2i)."

HF Patients with or Without DM: Are They Different?

"HF patients with DM are younger, have higher body mass index (BMI), experience worse symptoms, and have a prevalent background of ischemic heart disease both in HFrEF and HFpEF [29, 35–37]."

"The Prospective Comparison of ARNI With ACEI to Determine Impact on Global Mortality and Morbidity in Heart Failure (PARADIGM-HF) trial found a significantly higher N-terminal pro-brain natriuretic peptide (NT-proBNP) level in HFrEF patients with undiagnosed DM at baseline, compared to the prediabetic and normoglycemic group, but not in those with diagnosed DM [38]."

"Candesartan in Heart failure-Assessment of Reduction in Mortality and Morbidity (CHARM) study showed that DM conferred more adverse effects on patients with HFpEF by increasing the risk of the combined outcome of CV death and HF hospitalization [35]."

"Ather and others also demonstrated that DM was associated with a similarly increased risk of all-cause mortality in HFrEF and HFpEF patients [30]."

HF Patients with or Without DM: Shall Treatment Be Different?

"In a secondary analysis from the Action to Control Cardiovascular Risk in Diabetes (ACCORD) trial, a relative 10% increase or decrease in HbA_{1c} was associated with 32% and 55% higher risks of HF in patients with DM [39]."

"Two large observational studies, however, demonstrated that metformin significantly reduced the risk of death and hospitalization compared to sulfonylurea monotherapy in patients with HF, without causing additional metabolic acidosis."

"A systematic review involving 9 observational studies and 34,000 patients with HF and DM further confirmed its efficacy and safety, showing decreased risks of mortality and all-cause hospitalization and a similar risk of lactic acidosis when compared with the control group (mostly treated with sulfonylurea) [40]."

"ADA/EASD still advocates metformin for its established pharmacological effects and safety profile, whereas SGLT2i (empagliflozin, canagliflozin, and dapagliflozin) is included in the add-on regimen for diabetic patients with HF or chronic kidney disease irrespective of HbA_{1c} [41–43]."

HF Patients With or Without DM: Not Different in the Era of SGLT2i?

"Effects of Empagliflozin on Clinical Outcomes in Patients With Acute Decompensated Heart Failure (EMPA-RESPONSE-AHF) was the first randomized, double-blind, placebo-controlled, multicenter pilot study on the effects of empagliflozin in acute HF (AHF) patients irrespective of LVEF classification and comorbid DM (n = 80) [44]."

"Other SGLT2i trials in AHF are underway, which include Efficacy and Safety of Dapagliflozin in Acute Heart Failure (DICTATE-AHF), Ertugliflozin in Acute Heart Failure, A Study to Test the Effect of Empagliflozin in Patients Who Are in Hospital for Acute Heart Failure (EMPULSE), Effects of Empagliflozin on Diuresis and Renal Function in Patients With Acute Decompensated Heart Failure (EMPAG-HF), and Effect of Empagliflozin on Cardiac Output in Patients With Acute Heart Failure (EMPA Acute Heart Failure)."

[Section 5]

"The Comparative Effectiveness of Cardiovascular Outcomes in New Users of SGLT-2 Inhibitors (CVD-REAL) study enrolled more than 300,000 patients with DM and newly initiated on any SGLT2i or other glucose-lowering drugs from six countries in the USA or Europe."

"The CVD-REAL2 study conducted in over 400,000 patients from Asia Pacific (South Korea, Japan, Singapore, and Australia), Middle East (Israel), and North America (Canada) demonstrated the benefits of SGLT2i over other oral glucose-lowering drugs, with a 49% relative risk reduction in death, 36% in HHF, 19% in myocardial infarction and 32% in stroke."

"Another real-world use of new agents with CV benefits was examined in a cohort of 21,173 patients with DM and CVD [45], which revealed a slow increase in SGLT2i initiation (5 new prescriptions in the first half of 2014 to 83 new prescriptions in the first half of 2019) and a very low prescription rate of SGLT2i (in 1.4% patients only)."

Conclusion

"HF and DM are the two apparently separate disease entities from pathophysiology, diagnosis, and treatment."

"The cumulating evidence supports the reduction of HHF for DM patients treated with SGLT2i and recently extended late-breaking evidence of reducing HHF and improving quality of life by SGLT2i in HFrEF patients with and without DM."

"Such findings not only shifted the paradigm for the foundation of HFrEF therapy, but also pushing into revision of the HF treatment guidelines."

Benefits of SGLT2i for the Treatment of Heart Failure Irrespective of Diabetes Diagnosis: A State-of-the-Art Review [46]

This is a machine-generated summary of:

Delgado, Elías; Jódar, Esteban; Mezquita-Raya, Pedro; Moreno-Pérez, Óscar: Benefits of SGLT2i for the Treatment of Heart Failure Irrespective of Diabetes Diagnosis: A State-of-the-Art Review [46].

Published in: Diabetes Therapy (2022).

Link to original: https://doi.org/10.1007/s13300-022-01278-0

If you want to cite the papers, please refer to the original.

For technical reasons we could not place the page where the original quote is coming from.

Abstract-Summary "HF-associated risk in patients with type 2 diabetes mellitus (T2D) is even higher than in patients without T2D owing to the strong reciprocal relationship between conditions."

"Until recently, no therapy to treat patients with diabetes also reduced cardiovascular risks related to HF."

"Recent clinical studies (DAPA-HF, EMPEROR-Reduced and EMPEROR-Preserved, SOLOIST-WHF trial) and meta-analysis have demonstrated that sodium–glucose cotransporter-2 inhibitors (SGLT2i) are among the first antidiabetic drugs capable of reducing cardiovascular risks related to HF and improving the prognosis of patients with and without diabetes."

Introduction

"In patients with HF, morbidity and mortality remain high despite advances in therapy."

"Patients with type 2 diabetes mellitus (T2D) who had five risk-factor variables within target ranges [glycated hemoglobin level, low-density lipoprotein cholesterol level (LDLc), albuminuria, smoking, and blood pressure] appeared to have little or no excess risk of death, myocardial infarction, or stroke compared with the general population."

"The overall hazard ratio for hospitalization for HF among patients with no risk-factor variables outside the target ranges, compared with controls, was 1.45 [95% confidence interval (CI) 1.34–1.57] [47]."

"Several HF risk scores have been published, and most of them have reported a remarkably consistent list of the principal risk factors, including age, sex, coronary artery disease (CAD), myocardial infarction (MI), hypertension, obesity, and diabetes mellitus (DM), particularly T2D [48]."

General Mechanisms of Heart Failure (Preserved and Reduced)

"Of worsening LV remodeling and cardiac decompensation, patients transition from asymptomatic to symptomatic HF [49]."

"HF with reduced ejection fraction (HFrEF) is considered in patients with an LVEF $\leq$ 40%, with or without signs of clinical HF."

"Those patients with an LVEF between 41% and 49% have HF with mildly reduced EF (HFmrEF), and those with an LVEF $\geq$ 50% and symptoms and signs of HF, with evidence of structural and/or functional cardiac abnormalities and/or raised natriuretic peptides (NPs), have HF with preserved ejection fraction (HFpEF)."

"The definition of pre-HFpEF is taking shape as presenting in an asymptomatic patient (absence of signs or symptoms of HF) with preserved LVEF, structural heart abnormalities (similar to those reported for HFpEF), and elevated biomarker surrogates of cardiac dysfunction (mainly natriuretic peptides, with cut-point values similar to those reported for HFpEF)."

Heart Failure in Patients with and Without T2DM, Current Understanding and Clinical Practice Consequences

"T2D is an independent risk factor for HF in many hospital-based and population-based cardiovascular studies, and in particular, it has been estimated that, compared with patients without diabetes, the risk of HF is fivefold and twofold higher in women and men with diabetes, respectively [50]."

"The presence of diabetes markedly increases the risk of 1-year adverse clinical outcomes in outpatients with HF independent of multiple common risk factors."

"Patients with T2D have an increased risk of developing HF, but also those with HF are at higher risk for the development of T2D and a worse prognosis when both pathologies are present [51]."

"The development of HF in these patients produces an increased mortality risk and worse evolution."

Description of the Pathological Mechanisms That Link T2D with Heart Failure: Direct and Indirect Effects of SGLT2i on Myocardial Function

"T2D can lead to the development of HFrEF and HFpEF through diverse mechanisms."

"The available evidence suggests that T2D can promote the development of HFrEF by two main mechanisms: (1) by activating the sodium–hydrogen exchanger and undermining cardiomyocyte survival [52] and (2) by suppressing nutrient deprivation signaling autophagy and thereby promoting cardiomyocyte stress and dysfunction [52]."

"T2D can promote the development of HFpEF by enhancing the expansion of visceral (and especially epicardial) adipose tissue depots, which can promote cardiac inflammation, fibrosis, and microcirculatory dysfunction."

SGLT2i in Clinical Trials and Meta-Analyses in Heart Failure

"The main outcome (cardiovascular death or hospitalization for heart failure) event was significantly reduced in the empagliflozin (19.4%) group compared with the placebo (24.7%) group (HR 0.75, 95% CI 0.65–0.86, $P < 0.001$; NNT 19), and this reduction was consistent in patients regardless of their diabetes status."

"In the EMPEROR-Preserved Trial carried out in 5988 patients with HF and EF > 40%, empagliflozin was also demonstrated to reduce the combined risk of cardiovascular death or hospitalization for HF in patients with HFpEF (HR 0.79, 95% CI 0.69–0.90, $P < 0.001$), regardless of the presence or absence of diabetes, with an NNT of 31."

"In these patients with T2D with newly diagnosed, worsening heart failure, sotagliflozin therapy started before or shortly after discharge resulted in a significantly lower total number of deaths from cardiovascular causes and hospitalizations and urgent visits for HF than placebo (HR 0.67, 95% CI 0.52–0.85, $P < 0.001$)."

New Guidelines: Moving Towards an Intensive and Multidimensional Approach for HF Treatment

"On the basis of this clinical evidence, several HF guidelines have introduced SGLT2i as a first-line HF treatment [53–55]."

"The Canadian guidelines [55] recommend that, in the absence of contraindications, patients with HFrEF be treated with combination therapy from the beginning, including one evidenced-based medication from each of the categories (ARNI, B-blocker, MRA, and SGLT2i) (strong recommendation; moderate level of evidence)."

Future Perspectives in the Treatment of HF for Patients with and Without T2D

"On the basis of these promising findings in patients with chronic HF, it would be interesting to develop studies that assess the early use of SGLT2i in the acute phase of admission for HF and personalize treatment for the most significant benefit."

"The EMPULSE-HF study has shown that, among patients with acute decompensated HF, empagliflozin versus placebo is associated with significant clinical benefits at 90 days."

"Some authors suggest the importance of evaluating the clinical efficacy and safety of the SGLT2i in nondiabetic patients with acute decompensated HF [56]."

"In the DARE-19 trial, treatment with dapagliflozin did not result in a statistically significant risk reduction in organ dysfunction, death, or improvement in clinical recovery in patients with coronavirus disease 2019 (COVID-19) [57]."

Conclusions

"In HF, morbidity and mortality remain high despite advances in therapy, and new therapies are needed to improve the prognosis of these patients, mainly when T2D is also present."

"Several recent clinical studies (DAPA-HF, EMPEROR-Reduced, EMPEROR-Preserved, SOLOIST-WHF trial) and meta-analyses have demonstrated that SGLT2i reduce the risk of HF hospitalization, improve QOL, and increase survival in HF across the whole LVEF spectrum."

"In light of the favorable results obtained in the studies as mentioned above, SGLT2i are among the first antidiabetic drugs capable of reducing cardiovascular risks related to HF and consistently improving the prognosis in different populations and settings."

"On the basis of this clinical evidence, several HF guidelines have introduced SGLT2i as a first-line treatment for HF from the start, and several studies are underway to specify the role of SGLT2i with regard to HF outcomes in different vulnerable populations, including the hospital setting."

Promise of SGLT2 Inhibitors in Heart Failure: Diabetes and Beyond [58]

This is a machine-generated summary of:

Martens, Pieter; Mathieu, Chantal; Verbrugge, Frederik H.: Promise of SGLT2 Inhibitors in Heart Failure: Diabetes and Beyond [58].

Published in: Current Treatment Options in Cardiovascular Medicine (2017).

Link to original: https://doi.org/10.1007/s11936-017-0522-x

If you want to cite the papers, please refer to the original.

For technical reasons we could not place the page where the original quote is coming from.

Abstract-Summary "This review provides mechanistic insight in the pleiotropic effects of sodium-glucose transporter-2 (SGLT-2) inhibitors with particular interest to the pathophysiology of heart failure."

"The SGLT-2 inhibitor empagliflozin has recently demonstrated an unprecedented 38% reduction in cardiovascular mortality in patients with diabetes."

"Despite modest effects on long-term glycemic control, highly significant reductions in heart failure admissions and end-stage kidney disease were observed."

"SGLT-2 inhibitors are the latest approved class of glucose-lowering agents."

"Treatment with SGLT-2 inhibitors in diabetes leads to a sustained ~1% reduction in glycated hemoglobin levels, with favorable reductions in both arterial blood pressure (~3–6 mmHg) and body weight (~2–4 kg/m^2)."

"SGLT-2 inhibitors decrease proximal tubular sodium and chloride reabsorption, leading to a reset of the tubuloglomerular feedback."

"Decreased vascular stiffness and improved endothelial function are observed with the use of SGLT-2 inhibitors in diabetes."

"Those multiple nonglycemic effects reinforce SGLT-2 inhibitors as the preferred glucose-lowering drug to treat diabetic patients with heart failure."

Introduction

"In the Framingham cohort, diabetic men and women had a 2.4- and 5-fold increased risk to develop HF, respectively [59]."

"The presence of diabetes confers a 30% greater risk for hospital admissions due to HF [60]."

"Disturbingly, however, an increased incidence of HF hospitalizations has been observed with peroxisome proliferator-activated receptor gamma (PPARγ) agonists and the dipeptidyl peptidase-4 (DPP-4) inhibitor saxagliptin [61–63]."

"This review article provides essential mechanistic insight in the pleiotropic effects of SGLT-2 inhibitors, with a particular interest to the pathophysiology of HF."

Mechanism of Action of Sodium-Glucose Transporter-2 Inhibitors

"The remaining glucose is reabsorbed by a related transporter that is predominant in the S3 segment of the proximal tubules, i.e., the sodium-glucose transporter-1 (SGLT-1), which has lower capacity but higher affinity for glucose."

"There is marked upregulation of the SGLT-2 in the case of hyperglycemia, explaining the much higher threshold of approximately 300-g filtered glucose before occurrence of glycosuria in diabetes [12, 13]."

"SGLT-2 hyperactivity also implies increased proximal tubular reabsorption of sodium as well as chloride—the latter is following sodium, driven by the lumen-negative potential present in the S1 and S2 segments of the proximal tubules."

"SGLT-2 inhibitors, at commercially available doses in patients with normal or elevated GFR, induce glycosuria of approximately 60–90 g/day by blocking SGLT-2-mediated proximal tubular glucose reabsorption [64]."

"The efficacy of SGLT-2 inhibitors to induce glycosuria decreases with lower plasma glucose levels or a drop in GFR, explaining their inherent low risk for development of hypoglycemia."

Glucose-Lowering Drugs in Diabetes and Cardiovascular Risk

"The United Kingdom Prospective Diabetes Study (UKPDS) was the first large trial that assessed the impact of glycemic control on cardiovascular endpoints."

"UKPDS demonstrated a highly significant 25% reduction in microvascular complications of diabetes after 10 years, yet no significant reduction in cardiovascular endpoints was observed [65]."

"Results of a subsequent 10-year post-interventional follow-up of the UKPDS survivor cohort did show a significant reduction of all-cause mortality and myocardial infarction in the original intervention group, despite similar glycemic control compared to the control group during the post-intervention period [66]."

"The Action to Control Cardiovascular Risk in Diabetes (ACCORD) trial was subsequently designed to determine whether a strategy of targeting normal HbA1c levels <6.0% compared to <7.5% would reduce the cardiovascular risk even further."

Glucose-Lowering Drugs in Diabetes and Heart Failure Risk

"It should not be surprising that their use in diabetes is associated with a 42% increased risk for HF admissions [67, 68]."

"The risk for worsening HF with DPP-4 inhibitors is less consistent, not readily explained, and might depend on the specific agent used [67]."

"There is concern that any glucose-lowering drug that induces weight gain (i.e., insulin, sulphonylurea, and PPARγ agonists) may thereby contribute to worsening HF, as every 1 kg of weight gain in diabetes is associated with a 7% increased risk for HF readmissions [67]."

Sodium-Glucose Transporter-2 Inhibitors and Heart Failure Risk

"The BI 10773 (Empagliflozin) Cardiovascular Outcome Event Trial in Type 2 Diabetes Mellitus Patients (EMPA-REG OUTCOME) randomized 7020 patients with type 2 diabetes, an estimated GFR > 30 mL/min/1.73 m^2, and established cardiovascular disease (11% were previously admitted for HF and 47% had a myocardial infarction) to receive placebo, empagliflozin 10 mg, or empagliflozin 25 mg on top of usual glucose-lowering care [69]."

"More evidence supporting a class effect of SGLT-2 inhibitors will arise when the results of the CANagliflozin cardiovascular Assessment Study (CANVAS) with canagliflozin (NCT01032629), the Multicenter Trial to Evaluate the Effect of Dapagliflozin on the incidence of Cardiovascular Events (DECLARE-TIMI58) with dapagliflozin (NCT01730534), and the Cardiovascular Outcomes Following Ertugliflozin Treatment in Type 2 Diabetes Mellitus Participants With Vascular Disease (VERTIS CV) study with ertugliflozin (NCT01986881) become available."

Nonglycemic Effects of Sodium-Glucose Transporter-2 Inhibitors

"Although erythropoietin concentration—stimulating red blood cell mass and thus hematocrit—also rises following initiation of SGLT-2 inhibitors, this effect dissipates quickly within 6–8 weeks and is unlikely to explain the observed drop in plasma volume [70]."

"Because SGLT-2 inhibitors reduce the afferent arteriolar tone by means of the tubulo-glomerular feedback as explained above, blood flow in the renal medulla is decreased."

"Because the tubulo-glomerular feedback is reset with SGLT-2 inhibitors, there is a lack of sympathetic nerve system activation, despite a potent reduction in plasma volume, which is especially attractive in HF from a pathophysiological perspective [71]."

"In chronic kidney disease whereas the number of functional nephrons is rapidly declining, this increase in efferent arteriolar vasoconstriction augments filtration in the remaining nephrons to preserve total GFR, but does so at the cost of elevated hydrostatic pressure inside the glomerular capillaries."

"Just like renin-angiotensin system blockers, SGLT-2 inhibitors decrease the intra-glomerular hydrostatic pressure."

Potential Adverse Effects of Sodium-Glucose Transporter-2 Inhibitors

"A clear link has been shown between glycosuria induced by SGLT-2 inhibitors and an increased risk for urinary, but especially genital infections, mainly due to Candida species [72]."

"A large meta-analysis of more than 35,000 patients has illustrated a relative risk of 15% (HR 1.15, 95%CI 1.06–1.26) for urinary tract infections, while the risk for genital infections was nearly five times increased with SGLT-2 inhibitors (HR 4.75, 95%CI 4.00–5.63)."

"Besides, volume depletion secondary to natriuresis and osmotic diuresis may occur in patients at risk including older patients, patients using diuretics or suffering from preexisting chronic kidney disease [72]."

"Larger meta-analyses do not confirm early reports of an enhanced risk for bladder cancer, bone fraction due to accelerated osteoporosis, venous thrombosis or keto-acidosis—at least when prescribed on label for type 2 diabetes [72]."

The Prospect of Sodium-Glucose Transporter-2 Inhibitors in Heart Failure

"The beneficial pleiotropic effects of SGLT-2 inhibitors within the cardiovascular system, together with their favorable safety profile, make this medication class attractive for the treatment of diabetes in patients with HF as well as cardiovascular diseases in general."

"As the risk for hypoglycemic episodes is low, SGLT-2 inhibitors might even benefit HF patients in the absence of diabetes because they reduce plasma volume expansion, improve natriuretic and diuretic responses, as well as shift the myocardial metabolism toward more favorable energetics [73, 74]."

"In patient with impaired GFR < 30 mL/min/1.73 m^2, SGLT-2 inhibitors exhibit a blunted or complete loss of glycosuric effects, yet presumably without complete loss of influence on the tubulo-glomerular feedback system, which then remains an attractive target to protect the glomerulus against hyper-filtration."

"This hypothesis is further reinforced by the beneficial effects that are observed with SGLT-2 inhibitors on endothelial function which is believed to be a pathophysiological culprit in HF with preserved ejection fraction."

Different Effects of SGLT2 Inhibitors According to the Presence and Types of Heart Failure in Type 2 Diabetic Patients [75]

This is a machine-generated summary of:

Hwang, In-Chang; Cho, Goo-Yeong; Yoon, Yeonyee E.; Park, Jin Joo; Park, Jun-Bean; Lee, Seung-Pyo; Kim, Hyung-Kwan; Kim, Yong-Jin; Sohn, Dae-Won: Different effects of SGLT2 inhibitors according to the presence and types of heart failure in type 2 diabetic patients [75].

Published in: Cardiovascular Diabetology (2020).

Link to original: https://doi.org/10.1186/s12933-020-01042-3

If you want to cite the papers, please refer to the original.

For technical reasons we could not place the page where the original quote is coming from.

Abstract-Summary "We investigated the changes in cardiac function in diabetic patients according to the presence and types of heart failure (HF)."

"After a median 13 months of follow-up, HF patients with SGLT2i showed a significant decrease in left ventricular end-diastolic dimension (LV-EDD; from 57.4 mm [50.0–64.9] to 53.0 mm [48.0–60.0]; $p < 0.001$) and improvement in LV-EF (from 36.1% [25.6–47.5] to 45.0% [34.8–56.3]; $p < 0.001$)."

"LV mass index and diastolic parameters also showed improvements in HF patients with SGLT2i."

"The SGLT2i-induced improvements in cardiac function were more prominent in HF patients than those without HF, and in HFrEF patients than HFpEF patients."

"Use of SGLT2i improved cardiac function in diabetic patients, regardless of the presence of HF."

"The improvements were more prominent in HF patients, especially in those with HFrEF."

Background

"The SGLT2 inhibitors (SGLT2i) have demonstrated robust benefits in terms of the prevention of heart failure (HF) and the reduction in cardiovascular mortality, which was the first evidence for prevention of major cardiovascular events by anti-diabetic medications."

"These hypotheses were further supported by the recently published trial of dapagliflozin, the Dapagliflozin and Prevention of Adverse-outcomes in Heart Failure (DAPA-HF) trial, which extended the benefits of SGLT2i to those with HF with reduced ejection fraction (HFrEF) even in the absence of diabetes."

"It is unclear whether the cardiovascular benefits of SGLT2i would be similar between the diabetic patients with versus without HF, and between those with HFrEF versus HFpEF."

"We aimed to compare the SGLT2i-induced changes in cardiac function and geometry assessed by echocardiography in type 2 diabetic patients according to the presence and types of HF, using a retrospective cohort."

Methods

"For the patients with SGLT2i prescription, those with all echocardiograms performed before, but not after, the initial SGLT2i prescription were excluded."

"Patients with all echocardiograms performed after, but not before, the initial SGLT2i prescriptions were also excluded."

"Patients with no echocardiography performed 6–24 months after the initial SGLT2i prescription were excluded."

"After exclusion, 202 diabetic patients for whom SGLT2i were prescribed, and for whom the baseline echocardiography was performed before the initial SGLT2i prescription and the follow-up echocardiography was performed at 6–24 months after the initial SGLT2i prescription were identified."

"As a sensitivity analysis, we compared the changes in echocardiographic parameters according to the use of SGLT2i between patients with HF with reduced EF (LV-EF $< 40\%$ at baseline) and those with HF with preserved EF (HFpEF) (LV-EF $\geq 40\%$ at baseline)."

Results

"Use of angiotensin converting enzyme inhibitors (ACEi), angiotensin receptor blocker (ARB), beta-blockers, mineralocorticoid antagonists (MRA), and diuretics were more frequent in patients with HF (groups 3 and 4) compared to those without HF (groups 1 and 2), but were not different according to the use of SGLT2i (groups 1 vs. 2; groups 3 vs. 4)."

"In the HF patients, those with SGLT2i treatment (group 4) showed a prominent improvement in LV-EF (from 36.1 [25.6–47.5] to 45.0% [34.8–56.3]; $p < 0.001$) as well as LV-GLS (from 10.3 [7.3–12.5] to 11.4% [8.4–14.3]; $p = 0.001$)."

"The changes in LV-EF and LV-GLS did not show different according to the SGLT2i treatment in HFpEF patients."

Discussion

"Several studies that showed improvements in LV diastolic function and reduction in LV-MI by SGLT2i in diabetic patients without overt HF [76, 77]."

"Our findings are consistent with these studies that the use of SGLT2i resulted in small but significant improvements in LV geometry and diastolic function in diabetic patients without overt HF."

"We observed more prominent improvements in LV function by SGLT2i in diabetic patients with HF compared to those without, which was independent of the use of cardioprotective medications for HF (ACEi, ARB, beta-blockers, and MRA)."

"Beneficial effect of SGLT2i has also been suggested in patients with HFpEF: in an echocardiographic study by Soga and others the mitral E/e' ratio, LV-MI, and LAVI were decreased with dapagliflozin treatment among diabetic patients with high prevalence of HFpEF (69%) and HFmrEF (17%), whereas the improvement in LV systolic function and the reduction in BNP levels were minimal [78]."

Conclusion

"In this retrospective cohort study, the use of SGLT2i improved LV systolic and diastolic function, as well as LV geometry, in diabetic patients regardless of the presence of HF."

"The improvement in LV function was more prominent in those with HFrEF patients compared to those with HFpEF or those without HF."

"These effects of SGLT2i may contribute to the reduction in HF morbidity and mortality in diabetic patients."

Use of Sodium-Glucose Cotransporter-2 Inhibitors in Clinical Practice for Heart Failure Prevention and Treatment: Beyond Type 2 Diabetes. A Narrative Review [79]

This is a machine-generated summary of:

Rao, Shaline: Use of Sodium-Glucose Cotransporter-2 Inhibitors in Clinical Practice for Heart Failure Prevention and Treatment: Beyond Type 2 Diabetes. A Narrative Review [79].

Published in: Advances in Therapy (2021).

Link to original: https://doi.org/10.1007/s12325-021-01989-z

If you want to cite the papers, please refer to the original.

For technical reasons we could not place the page where the original quote is coming from.

Abstract-Summary "An established treatment for T2D, sodium-glucose cotransporter-2 inhibitors (SGLT-2is; canagliflozin, dapagliflozin, empagliflozin, and ertugliflozin) have demonstrated beneficial effects on CV outcomes in long-term studies of patients with T2D with established CV disease and/or a broad range of CV risk factors."

"Recent studies have extended these findings to patients with HF, with and without T2D, finding that SGLT-2is (particularly dapagliflozin and empagliflozin) are effective therapeutic interventions for the treatment and prevention of HF."

"This narrative review article discusses the use of SGLT-2is in the treatment and prevention of HF in patients with and without T2D. Dapagliflozin was the first SGLT-2i to receive US Food and Drug Administration (FDA) approval for treatment of HF, to reduce the risk of CV death and hospitalization for HF in adults with HF with reduced ejection fraction (HFrEF) with and without T2D. Recently, the FDA also approved empagliflozin for this indication."

"Given the new HFrEF indications for dapagliflozin and empagliflozin, and the likelihood of similar approvals for other SGLT-2is, cardiology guidelines are beginning to integrate SGLT-2is into a standard-of-care treatment regimen for patients with HFrEF."

"Further clinical trial evidence may lead to more widespread use and further integration of SGLT-2is into standard-of-care regimens for the treatment and management of HF in patients with and without T2D."

Introduction

"SGLT-2is have been shown to have beneficial effects on both CV and renal outcomes in patients with T2D [80–87], and SGLT-2is are the first class of antidiabetic drugs to have demonstrated beneficial effects on HF outcomes and, thus, may serve as a novel treatment option for patients without T2D with or at risk of HF."

"As with general CV and renal effects, the beneficial effects of SGLT-2is on HF outcomes specifically are thought to be due to nonglycemic mechanisms [80, 82]."

"This narrative review examines the role of SGLT-2is for the prevention and treatment of HF in individuals with T2D but also as a novel approach to HF treatment in patients without T2D. An assessment of important SGLT-2i CV outcome trials (CVOTs) will provide guidance on the use of SGLT-2is in routine clinical practice, specifically their placement in the T2D-specific and general HF treatment paradigm."

Methods

"The topic of this narrative review article is the use of SGLT-2is in the prevention and treatment of HF in patients with or without T2D. To identify key studies relevant to this topic, non-systematic literature searches were conducted in the PubMed database using search terms associated with SGLT-2is (i.e., "SGLT-2 inhibitor," "sodium-glucose cotransporter 2 inhibitor," "canagliflozin," "dapagliflozin," "empagliflozin," "ertugliflozin," "sotagliflozin") and heart failure."

"The PubMed literature searches were limited to recent publications in English, published between July 2015 and October 2021, and to those reporting clinical trials and meta-analyses of SGLT-2is."

"Publications identified through the literature search results were reviewed, and studies reporting CV and/or renal outcomes for SGLT-2is were included in the review."

"Although applying a date range to the search excluded studies published before July 2015, it is unlikely to affect the content of this review because HF is a new indication for SGLT-2is."

SGLT-2i Effects on Cardiovascular Outcomes

"A meta-analysis of three of these CVOTs (DECLARE-TIMI 58, CANVAS, and EMPA-REG OUTCOME) showed significant reductions in the risk of CV death or HHF by 23% and the risk of HHF by 31% with SGLT-2is across patients, regardless of the presence of CVD or HF at baseline [88]."

"DAPA-CKD demonstrated a significantly reduced risk of the primary composite outcome (i.e., sustained decline in eGFR $\geq$ 50%, end-stage renal disease [ESRD], or death from renal or CV causes; HR, 0.61; $P < 0.001$) with dapagliflozin versus placebo [89]."

"In the CREDENCE study with a patient population at high risk of kidney failure, canagliflozin was associated with significant reductions in the risk of HHF (39%; $P < 0.001$), the risk of CV death or HHF (31%; $P < 0.001$), and the risk of the composite renal outcome (ESRD, doubling of serum creatinine level, or death from renal or CV causes; 30%; $P = 0.00001$) [86]."

SGLT-2is and HF Outcomes

"Additional findings pertaining to the beneficial effects of an SGLT-2i in patients with HFrEF were reported by the Empagliflozin Outcome Trial in Patients with Chronic Heart Failure and a Reduced Ejection Fraction (EMPEROR-Reduced) study [90]."

"Sotagliflozin reduced the risk of the revised primary endpoint of total number of deaths from CV causes and HHF and urgent visits for HF by 33% (HR, 0.67 [95% CI 0.52–0.85]; $P < 0.001$)."

"A significant reduction in the first hierarchical secondary outcome of the number of HHF/urgent visits for HF was also seen (HR, 0.64; $P < 0.001$), but there were no significant effects on other secondary endpoints, including all-cause deaths."

"The primary composite endpoint of death from CV causes or HHF was significantly reduced with empagliflozin compared with placebo by 21% (HR, 0.79 [95% CI 0.69–0.90]; $P < 0.001$) [91]."

Knowledge Gaps Regarding the Use of SGLT-2is for HF in Clinical Practice

"Despite mounting evidence of the cardioprotective effects of SGLT-2is in patients with and without T2D, there are several knowledge gaps associated with their use in clinical practice for the prevention and treatment of HF [92]."

"The differential effects of SGLT-2is on HF outcomes in patients with HFpEF versus HFrEF are only just being clarified."

"The Dapagliflozin Evaluation to Improve the Lives of Patients with Preserved Ejection Fraction Heart Failure (DELIVER) study is investigating the effects of SGLT-2is on CV and HF outcomes in patients with HFpEF [93]."

"It is hoped that data from ongoing and future studies will provide additional evidence regarding the beneficial effects of SGLT-2is on outcomes in patients with HF irrespective of T2D status as well as demonstrating that SGLT-2is are safe and effective in both patients with HFpEF and HFrEF and those with acute HF."

Clinical Ramifications of SGLT-2is for HF Prevention and Treatment

"In 2019, the European Society of Cardiology (ESC) guidelines recommended SGLT-2is (canagliflozin, dapagliflozin, and empagliflozin) to reduce the risk of HHF in patients with T2D and risk of CKD progression [94]."

"This was followed by two position papers in 2020 by the Heart Failure Association (HFA) of the ESC recommending the use of SGLT-2is (empagliflozin, canagliflozin, dapagliflozin, and ertugliflozin) to reduce the risk of HHF in patients with T2D with either established CVD or high CV risk [95, 96]."

"The 2021 ESC guidelines recommended SGLT-2is (canagliflozin, dapagliflozin, empagliflozin, ertugliflozin, and sotagliflozin) for the reduction of HHF, major CV events, end-stage renal dysfunction, and CV death in patients with T2D at risk of CV events [53]."

"In patients with HFrEF and T2D, the SGLT-2is dapagliflozin, empagliflozin, and sotagliflozin were recommended to reduce HHF and CV death by the 2021 ESC guidelines [97]."

Physicians' Perspectives Regarding the Role of SGLT-2is in Treating HF

"To optimize CV outcomes, an important consideration may be the use of SGLT-2i therapy as part of the initial therapeutic approach in patients with T2D at risk of CVD [98]."

"The following serious AEs, although rare, have been associated with SGLT-2i therapy and should be taken into consideration in patients with underlying comorbidities and concomitant medications: diabetic ketoacidosis (DKA), renal injury, volume depletion, and lower-limb amputation [99]."

"Healthcare professionals can reduce the potential for serious or severe AEs among their patients through risk assessment and identification of patients who are at a lower risk of AEs before initiating SGLT-2i therapy, ongoing monitoring through regular clinic visits, and by being aware of and educating their patients to recognize early signs and symptoms associated with possible development of complications and the need to seek medical attention should these occur."

Conclusions

"Additional studies are providing clinical evidence on the role of SGLT-2is in the treatment of patients with HFpEF with or without T2D. The EMPEROR-Preserved study results of empagliflozin in HFpEF are encouraging, and the ongoing DELIVER study will also provide data on dapagliflozin use in HFpEF."

"The increasing amount of evidence for SGLT-2i therapy in patients with HF who do not have T2D will likely lead to increased use in cardiology practice."

"Given their favorable benefit-risk profile and wide-ranging effects, it is hoped that SGLT-2is will provide a useful treatment option to help reduce the significant disease burden associated with HF in patients without T2D as well as in those with T2D."

SGLT2 Inhibitors Break the Vicious Circle Between Heart Failure and Insulin Resistance: Targeting Energy Metabolism [100]

This is a machine-generated summary of:

Wang, Xiaodan; Ni, Jingyu; Guo, Rui; Li, Lan; Su, Jing; He, Feng; Fan, Guanwei: SGLT2 inhibitors break the vicious circle between heart failure and insulin resistance: targeting energy metabolism [100].

Published in: Heart Failure Reviews (2021).

Link to original: https://doi.org/10.1007/s10741-021-10096-8

Copyright of the summarized publication:

If you want to cite the papers, please refer to the original.

For technical reasons we could not place the page where the original quote is coming from.

Abstract-Summary "A number of mechanisms ascribe to the progression of cardiac IR, in which the main factors are the shift of myocardial substrate metabolism."

"Studies have found that SGLT2 inhibitors, an anti-diabetic drug, can improve the cardiac prognosis of patients with T2DM, which may be at least partially due to the relief of cardiac IR."

"Basic and clinical studies have revealed the important role of cardiac IR in the pathogenesis and progression of HF, and studies suggest that energy metabolism plays an important role in the pathogenesis of cardiac IR and HF."

"The regulation of SGLT2 inhibitors on cardiac energy status including carbohydrates, fatty acids (FA), amino acids and ketones, ATP transfer to the cytoplasm, and mitochondrial functional status have received extensive attention in HF, but its specific mechanism of action is still unclear."

Introduction

"The prevalence of IR in heart failure patients is no less than 30%, indicating a strong association exists between HF and IR [101]."

"Several large-scale clinical trials and real-world studies revealed that diabetes has a very high prevalence, morbidity, and mortality of heart failure."

"Excluding previous coronary or rheumatic heart disease, diabetic men developed congestive heart failure twice as often as the non-diabetic cohort, while diabetic women had a five-fold increase in risk [59]."

"SGLT2 inhibitors are promising therapeutic targets for cardiovascular disease with IR based on their robust positive effect on CV risk."

"We emphasize that the regulation of myocardial metabolic elasticity is the primary mechanism for SGLT2 inhibitors to improve HF and IR [102–104], which may have a transformative impact on clinical medicine."

The Interaction Between Heart Failure and Insulin Resistance

"The decrease of FA metabolism in heart failure energetic status results from insulin, which inhibits FA oxidation by activating acetyl CoA carboxylase (ACC), thereby enhancing the tissue level of malonyl CoA results in the declining of FA uptake."

"While in advanced HF, IR develops in the myocardium, leading to the down-regulation of glucose metabolism whereas stimulating cardiac FA uptake which contribute to entire ATP production via CD36 and the compensatory increase of AMP-activated protein kinase (AMPK) [105]."

"By increasing the level of baseline protein phosphorylation associated with insulin signaling such as ACC, Akt, and AMPK, mutant cells may increase the uptake and decrease the oxidation of FA, therefore supported insulin resistant as well as impaired glucose responsiveness [106]."

"Post-translational modifications could cause heart failure by impaired myocardial energy metabolism; therefore, the upregulation of ketone oxidation and acetyl-CoA pool has been assumed to increase the lysine acetylation of substrate, eventually lead to hyperacetylated status and partially conferred IR [107]."

SGLT2 Inhibitor Improve HF and IR by Regulating Energy Metabolism

"Speaking, the mechanism of SGLT2 inhibitors to improve cardiovascular effects mainly involves inhibiting of sodium and hydrogen exchange, osmotic diuresis, lowering blood pressure and weight, increasing erythropoietin levels, improving inflammation, oxidative stress and arteriosclerosis, and reducing left ventricular load, relieving cardiac fibrosis, and improving myocardial energy production [108]."

"Studies also confirmed that SGLT2 inhibitors may increase the heart energy production of diabetic mice by increasing the heart oxidation rate of glucose and fatty acids [109]."

"During IRI, the dependence of cardiac function and energy metabolism recovery on SGLT1 increases in the drug-resistant diabetic phenotype [110], while empagliflozin treatment will significantly reduce blood glucose levels without lowering serum insulin levels."

"Hiroto Oshima, and others explored the effect of SGLT2 inhibitors on the oxidation of fatty acids and ketone bodies and found that treatment with empagliflozin before myocardial infarction can increase glucose oxidation and ketone utilization, improve glucose and elevate blood and myocardial β-OHB levels."

Clinical Evidences of SGLT2 Inhibitors in Heart Failure with Diabetes

"In view of the increasing clinical evidence of the beneficial cardiovascular events (a combination of cardiovascular death, non-fatal myocardial infarction, and non-fatal stroke) of SGLT2 inhibitors in patients with type 2 diabetes, the American Diabetes Association (ADA), the European Association for the Study of Diabetes (EASD), and the European Society of Cardiology (ESC) strongly recommends that SGLT2 inhibitors be used in patients with type 2 diabetes who have a high cardiovascular risk or patients with type 2 diabetes and heart failure, especially in patients with reduced ejection fraction, to reduce the HF, major adverse cardiovascular events and progression of chronic kidney disease in 2019."

"Another large international observational study enrolled more than 386,000 patients with type 2 diabetes in 13 countries/regions in four geographic regions confirmed that compared with DPP-4 inhibitors, the initiation of SGLT2 inhibitors reduced heart failure, death, myocardial infarction, and stroke, and improves the composite outcome of death or hospitalization due to heart failure."

Conclusion

"SGLT2 inhibitors can increase the utilization of glucose and fatty acid, and shift the myocardial fuel utilization from glucose to ketone bodies, free fatty acids, and BCAAs."

"This transformation can increase the energy production of the diabetic heart, along with the improvement of heart remodeling, showing the therapeutic potential of SGLT2 inhibitors for heart failure and IR."

"Most of the clinical trials are limited to patients with HFrEF; therefore, it is necessary to conduct research on the application of SGLT2 inhibitors in HFpEF patients to provide more evidence in this field."

"Research studies on the mechanism of SGLT2 inhibitors regulating energy metabolism are still in progress to further reveal the improvement effect of SGLT2 inhibitors on HF and cardiac IR and provide a better prognosis for patients with HF."

Role of SGLT2 Inhibitors in Patients with Diabetes Mellitus and Heart Failure [111]

This is a machine-generated summary of:

Verbrugge, Frederik H.: Role of SGLT2 Inhibitors in Patients with Diabetes Mellitus and Heart Failure [111].

Published in: Current Heart Failure Reports (2017).

Link to original: https://doi.org/10.1007/s11897-017-0340-1

If you want to cite the papers, please refer to the original.

For technical reasons we could not place the page where the original quote is coming from.

Abstract-Summary "This review aims to summarize the evidence on cardiovascular risks and benefits of glucose-lowering drugs in diabetic patients, with a particular focus on the role of sodium-glucose transporter-2 (SGLT-2) inhibitors and their promising potential as a heart failure treatment."

"The SGLT-2 inhibitor empagliflozin has emerged as the first glucose-lowering drug to lower cardiovascular mortality in diabetes with an unprecedented 38% relative risk reduction."

"SGLT-2 inhibitors should be considered as a first-line drug to achieve glycemic control in diabetic patients at high risk for cardiovascular diseases and heart failure in particular."

Introduction

"The rate of hospital admissions due to heart failure was 35% lower with empagliflozin compared to placebo in the BI 10773 (Empagliflozin) Cardiovascular Outcome Event Trial in Type 2 Diabetes Mellitus Patients (EMPA-REG OUTCOME)."

"SGLT-2 inhibitors are already an important therapeutic option to achieve glycemic control in patients with diabetes at high risk for heart failure development."

"A position statement is defended that SGLT-2 inhibitors should be the first-line drug to treat diabetes in heart failure."

"Further, potential pathophysiological pathways targeted by SGLT-2 inhibitors are discussed, which provides the rationale to test these drugs outside of their current indication for glycemic control, in the broader population of patients with heart failure."

Glucose Handling by the Nephron

"Because glucose is freely filtered by the renal glomeruli, approximately 180 g is presented to the renal tubules on a daily basis, assuming an average blood glucose level of 100 mg/dL and glomerular filtration rate (GFR) of 125 mL/min/1.73 m^2."

"The remainder of glucose is reabsorbed in the third and last segment of the proximal tubules by the high-affinity, low-capacity sodium-glucose transporter-1 (SGLT-1)."

"Both SGLT-2 and SGLT-1 operate through an electrochemical sodium gradient that is created by sodium/potassium ATPases located on the basolateral membrane of tubular cells."

"On the basolateral side, facilitated glucose transport is orchestrated by the glucose transporters 2 and 1, respectively."

Working Mechanism of Sodium-Glucose Transporter-2 Inhibitors in Diabetes

"The threshold for occurrence of glycosuria is therefore increased to blood glucose levels of approximately 180 mg/dL, corresponding to >300 g of filtered glucose [12, 13]."

"Abundancy of the SGLT-2 and SGLT-1 in proximal tubular cells seems to track better with glycaemia than insulin levels, suggesting that increased glucose exposure of the nephron is the direct trigger for upregulation [13]."

"As the SGLT-2 is rapidly down-regulated again when glycaemia is adequately controlled, SGLT-2 inhibitors produce a glycosuric effect that is dependent of blood glucose levels, explaining their inherently low risk for hypoglycemia development."

"SGLT-2 inhibitors at commercially available doses in diabetic patients with normal or elevated GFR induce glycosuria of approximately 60–90 g per day [64]."

The EMPA-REG Outcome Trial with Empagliflozin

"The combined primary endpoint in EMPA-REG OUTCOME was death from cardiovascular causes, non-fatal myocardial infarction, or non-fatal stroke, and the primary hypothesis was non-inferiority of empagliflozin compared to placebo [112]."

"Occurrence of the primary endpoint was 10.5% in the pooled empagliflozin and 12.1% in the placebo group (HR (95%CI) = 0.86 (0.74–0.99); $p < 0.001$ for non-inferiority; $p = 0.04$ for superiority) [69]."

"The main driver of superiority with empagliflozin was a spectacular 38% reduction in cardiovascular mortality (HR (95%CI) = 0.62 (0.49–0.77)), while the risk of non-fatal myocardial infarction was more modestly reduced (HR (95%CI) = 0.87 (0.70–1.09)), and the risk of non-fatal stroke even slightly increased (HR (95%CI) = 1.24 (0.92–1.67))."

"Treatment with empagliflozin reduced the risk for heart failure readmissions by 35% from 4.1 to 2.7% (HR (95%CI) = 0.65 (0.50–0.85)), corresponding to a number needed to treat of 73 to prevent one readmission."

Cardiovascular Risk Reduction Through Glycemic Control

"As glycemic control was improved with empagliflozin compared to placebo in the EMPA-REG OUTCOME, the question arises to what extent this explains the observed reduction in cardiovascular risk."

"The first evidence that better glycemic control contributes to cardiovascular risk reduction came from the UK Prospective Diabetes Study (UKPDS)."

"The difference in HbA1c levels with the intervention arm was roughly double in UKPDS compared to EMPA-REG OUTCOME, with follow-up and thus time exposed to better glycemic control also three times longer in the former trial."

"This suggests that factors other than glycemic control must have contributed to the cardiovascular risk reduction observed in EMPA-REG OUTCOME."

"The American Diabetes Association recommends stringent glycemic control with HbA1c levels <7.0% only when achievable without increased risk for hypoglycemia in patients with low co-morbidity burden who are expected to survive long enough for benefits to accrue [113]."

Comparison of Empagliflozin with Other Glucose-Lowering Medications

"Although EMPA-REG OUTCOME was the first randomized clinical trial demonstrating compelling cardiovascular risk reduction with a glucose-lowering drug, extensive evidence is available for other pharmacological agents as well."

"Concerns that the increased mortality risk with intensive glycemic control in ACCORD was due to a higher use of the peroxisome proliferator-activated receptor gamma (PPARγ) agonist rosiglitazone let the Food and Drug Administration and European Medicines Agency to decide that new diabetes drugs should demonstrate cardiovascular safety using a primary endpoint of major adverse cardiovascular events [114]."

"Three large randomized clinical trials have convincingly demonstrated the neutral impact of DPP-4 inhibitors on cardiovascular risk [63, 115, 116]."

"Both liraglutide and semaglutide have demonstrated a significantly reduced risk of major cardiovascular events, when compared to placebo in patients with diabetes at high cardiovascular risk [117, 118]."

Adverse Effects with Sodium-Glucose Transporter-2 Inhibitors

"As explained, SGLT-2 inhibitors are very safe drugs with a low risk of hypoglycemia development."

"When combining SGLT-2 inhibitors with sulfonylurea or insulin, decreasing the dose of these latter medications should be considered."

"The most prominent adverse effect observed with SGLT-2 inhibitors is an increased risk of genital infections, mainly due to Candida species."

"In a large meta-analysis including more than 35,000 patients, this risk was nearly five times increased [72]."

Sodium-Glucose Transporter-2 Inhibitors as the First-Line Treatment for Diabetes in Heart Failure

"When comparing different glucose-lowering agents, SGLT-2 inhibitors seem to be the obvious choice in diabetes patients at high risk for or with established heart failure."

"Considering the quality of evidence provided by the EMPA-REG OUTCOME, one might defend that empagliflozin should be the preferred first-line agent to achieve glycemic control in such patients."

"The potential synergistic effects of SGLT-2 inhibitors with GLP-1 agonists and possibly also pioglitazone deserve attention and should be the topic of further study."

"The latter medications probably offer stronger protection against atherosclerosis progression and may be of greatest benefit in patients with cerebrovascular or ischemic heart disease."

Sodium-Glucose Transporter-2 Inhibitors as a Treatment for Heart Failure Without Diabetes?

"As the unique pharmacological profile of SGLT-2 inhibitors puts them at the crossroads of important hemodynamic, neurohumoral, renal, metabolic, and vascular endothelial pathways implied in heart failure, it has been suggested that they may benefit even patients without diabetes [73]."

"Further, increased hematocrit levels observed with SGLT-2 inhibitors due to hemoconcentration and increased endogenous erythropoietin release may improve oxygen delivery to tissues [70, 119]."

"Besides, SGLT-2 inhibitors may improve diuretic efficacy, which is emerging as an important prognostic factor independently from renal function in heart failure [120]."

"Further, an intriguing hypothesis is that SGLT-2 inhibitors may improve the efficiency of myocardial energy metabolism through offering of an increased fuel load of ketone bodies such as β-hydroxybutyrate [119]."

"Treatment with SGLT-2 inhibitors is associated with significant improvements in markers of arterial stiffness and endothelial function such as pulse wave velocity and pulse pressure difference [71]."

Conclusions

"SGLT-2 inhibitors are an exciting new therapeutic option to achieve glycemic control in diabetes."

"The SGLT-2 inhibitor empagliflozin reduces cardiovascular risk, especially with regards to heart failure, making it the preferred agent to treat diabetes in patients with or at high risk for this condition."

"Results of cardiovascular endpoint evaluation with other SGLT-2 inhibitors will soon be available and might confirm a class effect."

"As SGLT-2 inhibitors may target underlying pathways implied in heart failure disease progression, they might even emerge as a dedicated treatment for patients without diabetes in the near future."

Bibliography

1. Verbrugge FH, Vangoitsenhoven R, Mullens W, Van der Schueren B, Mathieu C, Tang WH (2015) Wilson SGLT-2 inhibitors: potential novel strategy to prevent congestive heart failure in diabetes? Curr Cardiovasc Risk Rep 9(8):38. https://doi.org/10.1007/s12170-015-0467-0
2. Bailey C, Gross JL, Pieters A, Bastien A, List JF (2010) Effect of dapagliflozin in patients with type 2 diabetes who have inadequate glycaemic control with metformin: a randomised, double-blind, placebo-controlled trial. Lancet 375(9733):2223–2233

3. Forst T, Guthrie R, Goldenberg R, Yee J, Vijapurkar U, Meininger G, Stein P (2014) Efficacy and safety of canagliflozin over 52 weeks in patients with type 2 diabetes on background metformin and pioglitazone. Diabetes Obes Metab 16(5):467–477
4. Crane RK (1960) Intestinal absorption of sugars. Physiol Rev 40:789–825
5. Hediger MA, Rhoads DB (1994) Molecular physiology of sodium-glucose cotransporters. Physiol Rev 74:993–1026
6. Wright EM, Loo DD, Hirayama BA (2011) Biology of human sodium glucose transporters. Physiol Rev 91:733–794
7. Martin MG, Turk E, Lostao MP, Kerner C, Wright EM (1996) Defects in Na+/glucose cotransporter (SGLT1) trafficking and function cause glucose-galactose malabsorption. Nat Genet 12:216–220
8. Zhou L, Cryan EV, D'Andrea MR, Belkowski S, Conway BR, Demarest KT (2003) Human cardiomyocytes express high level of Na+/glucose cotransporter 1 (SGLT1). J Cell Biochem 90:339–346
9. Elsas LJ, Rosenberg LE (1969) Familial renal glycosuria: a genetic reappraisal of hexose transport by kidney and intestine. J Clin Invest 48:1845–1854
10. van den Heuvel LP, Assink K, Willemsen M, Monnens L (2002) Autosomal recessive renal glucosuria attributable to a mutation in the sodium glucose cotransporter (SGLT2). Hum Genet 111:544–547
11. Santer R, Kinner M, Lassen CL, Schneppenheim R, Eggert P, Bald M et al (2003) Molecular analysis of the SGLT2 gene in patients with renal glucosuria. J Am Soc Nephrol 14:2873–2882
12. Vidotti DB, Arnoni CP, Maquigussa E, Boim MA (2008) Effect of long-term type 1 diabetes on renal sodium and water transporters in rats. Am J Nephrol 28:107–114
13. Freitas HS, Anhe GF, Melo KF, Okamoto MM, Oliveira-Souza M, Bordin S et al (2008) Na(+)-glucose transporter-2 messenger ribonucleic acid expression in kidney of diabetic rats correlates with glycemic levels: involvement of hepatocyte nuclear factor-1alpha expression and activity. Endocrinology 149:717–724
14. Calado J, Sznajer Y, Metzger D, Rita A, Hogan MC, Kattamis A et al (2008) Twenty-one additional cases of familial renal glucosuria: absence of genetic heterogeneity, high prevalence of private mutations and further evidence of volume depletion. Nephrol Dial Transplant 23:3874–3879
15. Cefalu WT, Leiter LA, Yoon KH, Arias P, Niskanen L, Xie J et al (2013) Efficacy and safety of canagliflozin versus glimepiride in patients with type 2 diabetes inadequately controlled with metformin (CANTATA-SU): 52 week results from a randomised, double-blind, phase 3 non-inferiority trial. Lancet 382(9896):941–950
16. Roden M, Weng J, Eilbracht J, Delafont B, Kim G, Woerle HJ et al (2013) Empagliflozin monotherapy with sitagliptin as an active comparator in patients with type 2 diabetes: a randomised, double-blind, placebo-controlled, phase 3 trial. Lancet Diab Endo 1(3):208–219
17. Verbrugge FH, Dupont M, Steels P, Grieten L, Swennen Q, Tang WH et al (2014) The kidney in congestive heart failure: 'are natriuresis, sodium, and diuretics really the good, the bad and the ugly? Eur J Heart Fail 16:133–142. This manuscript reviews the alterations in renal sodium handling that occur in heart failure and highlights the potentially important role for inhibition of proximal sodium transport to cease neurohumoral activation and improve natriuresis in heart failure
18. Schnermann J (1998) Juxtaglomerular cell complex in the regulation of renal salt excretion. Am J Phys 274:R263–R279
19. Vallon V, Richter K, Blantz RC, Thomson S, Osswald H (1999) Glomerular hyperfiltration in experimental diabetes mellitus: potential role of tubular reabsorption. J Am Soc Nephrol 10:2569–2576
20. Bautista R, Manning R, Martinez F, Avila-Casado Mdel C, Soto V, Medina A et al (2004) Angiotensin II-dependent increased expression of Na+-glucose cotransporter in hypertension. Am J Physiol Renal Physiol 286:F127–F133

21. Aurigemma GP, Gaasch WH (2004) Clinical practice. Diastolic heart failure. N Engl J Med 351:1097–1105
22. Monami M, Nardini C, Mannucci E (2014) Efficacy and safety of sodium glucose co-transport-2 inhibitors in type 2 diabetes: a meta-analysis of randomized clinical trials. Diabetes Obes Metab 16:457–466
23. Oliva RV, Bakris GL (2014) Blood pressure effects of sodium-glucose co-transport 2 (SGLT2) inhibitors. J Am Soc Hypertens 8:330–339
24. Hummel SL, Seymour EM, Brook RD, Sheth SS, Ghosh E, Zhu S et al (2013) Low-sodium DASH diet improves diastolic function and ventricular-arterial coupling in hypertensive heart failure with preserved ejection fraction. Circ Heart Fail 6:1165–1171
25. Wilding JP, Norwood P, T'Joen C, Bastien A, List JF, Fiedorek FT (2009) A study of dapagliflozin in patients with type 2 diabetes receiving high doses of insulin plus insulin sensitizers: applicability of a novel insulin-independent treatment. Diabetes Care 32:1656–1662
26. Ojha U, Reyes L, Eyenga F, Oumbe D, Watkowska J, Saint-Jacques H (2021) Diabetes, heart failure and beyond: elucidating the Cardioprotective mechanisms of Sodium Glucose Cotransporter 2 (SGLT2) inhibitors. Am J Cardiovas Drugs 22:35–46. https://doi.org/10.1007/s40256-021-00486-6
27. Zhang Q, Kang Y, Tang S, Yu C-M (2021) Intersection between diabetes and heart failure: is SGLT2i the "one stone for two birds" approach? Curr Cardiol Rep 23:171. https://doi.org/10.1007/s11886-021-01591-3
28. Echouffo-Tcheugui JB, Xu H, DeVore AD et al (2016) Temporal trends and factors associated with diabetes mellitus among patients hospitalized with heart failure: findings from Get With The Guidelines-Heart Failure registry. Am Heart J 182:9–20
29. Yap J, Tay WT, Teng TK et al (2019) Association of diabetes mellitus on cardiac remodeling, quality of life, and clinical outcomes in heart failure with reduced and preserved ejection fraction. J Am Heart Assoc 8(17):e013114
30. Ather S, Chan W, Bozkurt B, Aguilar D, Ramasubbu K, Zachariah AA et al (2012) Impact of noncardiac comorbidities on morbidity and mortality in a predominantly male population with heart failure and preserved versus reduced ejection fraction. J Am Coll Cardiol 59:998–1005
31. Seferovic PM, Paulus WJ (2015) Clinical diabetic cardiomyopathy: a two-faced disease with restrictive and dilated phenotypes. Eur Heart J 36(27):1718–1727, 1727a–1727c
32. Dei Cas A, Khan SS, Butler J, Mentz RJ, Bonow RO, Avogaro A et al (2015) Impact of diabetes on epidemiology, treatment, and outcomes of patients with heart failure. JACC Heart Fail 3(2):136–145. https://doi.org/10.1016/j.jchf.2014.08.004
33. Paolillo S, Rengo G, Pellegrino T et al (2015) Insulin resistance is associated with impaired cardiac sympathetic innervation in patients with heart failure. Eur Heart J Cardiovasc Imaging 16(10):1148–1153
34. Preiss D, van Veldhuisen DJ, Sattar N et al (2012) Eplerenone and new-onset diabetes in patients with mild heart failure: results from the Eplerenone in Mild Patients Hospitalization and Survival Study in Heart Failure (EMPHASIS-HF). Eur J Heart Fail 14(8):909–915
35. MacDonald MR, Petrie MC, Varyani F et al (2008) Impact of diabetes on outcomes in patients with low and preserved ejection fraction heart failure: an analysis of the Candesartan in Heart failure: Assessment of Reduction in Mortality and morbidity (CHARM) programme. Eur Heart J 29(11):1377–1385
36. Kristensen SL, Mogensen UM, Jhund PS et al (2017) Clinical and echocardiographic characteristics and cardiovascular outcomes according to diabetes status in patients with heart failure and preserved ejection fraction: a report from the I-Preserve Trial (Irbesartan in Heart Failure With Preserved Ejection Fraction). Circulation 135(8):724–735
37. Aguilar D, Deswal A, Ramasubbu K, Mann DL, Bozkurt B (2010) Comparison of patients with heart failure and preserved left ventricular ejection fraction among those with versus without diabetes mellitus. Am J Cardiol 105(3):373–377

38. Kristensen SL, Preiss D, Jhund PS et al (2016) Risk related to pre-diabetes mellitus and diabetes mellitus in heart failure with reduced ejection fraction: insights from prospective comparison of ARNI with ACEI to determine impact on global mortality and morbidity in heart failure trial. Circ Heart Fail 9(1):e002560
39. Segar MW, Patel KV, Vaduganathan M et al (2020) Association of long-term change and variability in glycemia with risk of incident heart failure among patients with type 2 diabetes: a secondary analysis of the ACCORD trial. Diabetes Care 43(8):1920–1928
40. Eurich DT, Weir DL, Majumdar SR et al (2013) Comparative safety and effectiveness of metformin in patients with diabetes mellitus and heart failure: systematic review of observational studies involving 34,000 patients. Circ Heart Fail 6(3):395–402
41. Davies MJ, D'Alessio DA, Fradkin J et al (2018) Management of hyperglycemia in type 2 diabetes, 2018. A consensus report by the American Diabetes Association (ADA) and the European Association for the Study of Diabetes (EASD). Diabetes Care 41(12):2669–2701
42. Buse JB, Wexler DJ, Tsapas A et al (2020) 2019 Update to: management of hyperglycemia in type 2 diabetes, 2018. A consensus report by the American Diabetes Association (ADA) and the European Association for the Study of Diabetes (EASD). Diabetes Care 43(2):487–493
43. American Diabetes Association (2021) Pharmacologic approaches to glycemic treatment. Standards of medical care in diabetes-2021. Diabetes Care 44(Suppl 1):S111–s124
44. Damman K, Beusekamp JC, Boorsma EM et al (2020) Randomized, double-blind, placebo-controlled, multicentre pilot study on the effects of empagliflozin on clinical outcomes in patients with acute decompensated heart failure (EMPA-RESPONSE-AHF). Eur J Heart Fail 22:713–722. https://doi.org/10.1002/ejhf.1713
45. Hamid A, Vaduganathan M, Oshunbade AA et al (2020) Antihyperglycemic therapies with expansions of US Food and Drug Administration indications to reduce cardiovascular events: prescribing patterns within an academic medical center. J Cardiovasc Pharmacol 76(3):313–320
46. Delgado E, Jódar E, Mezquita-Raya P, Moreno-Pérez Ó (2022) Benefits of SGLT2i for the treatment of heart failure irrespective of diabetes diagnosis: a state-of-the-art review. Diabetes Therapy 13:19–34. https://doi.org/10.1007/s13300-022-01278-0
47. Rawshani A, Rawshani A, Franzén S et al (2018) Risk factors, mortality, and cardiovascular outcomes in patients with type 2 diabetes. N Engl J Med 379(7):633–644
48. Echouffo-Tcheugui JB, Greene SJ, Papadimitriou L et al (2015) Population risk prediction models for incident heart failure. Circ Heart Fail 8:438–447
49. Kemp CD, John V, Conte JV (2012) The pathophysiology of heart failure. Cardiovasc Pathol 21(5):365–371
50. American Diabetes Association (2018) Pharmacologic approaches to glycemic treatment: standards of medical care in diabetes-2018. Diabetes Care 41:S73–S85
51. De Couto G, Ouzounian M, Liu PP (2010) Early detection of myocardial dysfunction and heart failure. Nat Rev Cardiol 7(6):334–344
52. Packer M (2021) Critical examination of mechanisms underlying the reduction in heart failure events with SGLT2 inhibitors: identification of a molecular link between their actions to stimulate erythrocytosis and to alleviate cellular stress. Cardiovasc Res 117(1):74–84
53. McDonagh TA, Metra M, Adamo M et al (2021) 2021 ESC guidelines for the diagnosis and treatment of acute and chronic heart failure. Eur Heart J 42(36):3599–3726
54. Maddox TM, Januzzi JL Jr et al (2021) Update to the 2017 ACC expert consensus decision pathway for optimization of heart failure treatment: answers to 10 pivotal issues about heart failure with reduced ejection fraction: a report of the American College of Cardiology solution set oversight committee. J Am Coll Cardiol 77(6):772–810
55. McDonald M, Virani S, Chan M et al (2021) CCS/CHFS heart failure guidelines update: defining a new pharmacologic standard of care for heart failure with reduced ejection fraction. Can J Cardiol 37(4):531–546

56. Tromp J, Ponikowski P, Salsali A et al (2021) Sodium–glucose co-transporter 2 inhibition in patients hospitalized for acute decompensated heart failure: rationale for and design of the EMPULSE trial. Eur J Heart Fail 23:826–834
57. Kosiborod MN, Esterline R, Furtado RHM et al (2021) Dapagliflozin in patients with cardiometabolic risk factors hospitalised with COVID-19 (DARE-19): a randomised, double-blind, placebo-controlled, phase 3 trial. Lancet Diabetes Endocrinol 9(9):586–594
58. Martens P, Mathieu C, Verbrugge FH (2017) Promise of SGLT2 inhibitors in heart failure: diabetes and beyond. Curr Treat Options Cardiovasc Med 19:23. https://doi.org/10.1007/s11936-017-0522-x
59. Kannel WB, Hjortland M, Castelli WP (1974) Role of diabetes in congestive heart failure: the Framingham study. Am J Cardiol 34:29–34. https://doi.org/10.1016/0002-9149(74)90089-7
60. Cubbon RM, Woolston A, Adams B, Gale CP, Gilthorpe MS, Baxter PD et al (2014) Prospective development and validation of a model to predict heart failure hospitalisation. Heart 100(12):923–929
61. Dormandy JA, Charbonnel B, Eckland DJ et al (2005) Secondary prevention of macrovascular events in patients with type 2 diabetes in the PROactive study (prospective pioglitazone clinical trial in macrovascular events): a randomised controlled trial. Lancet 366:1279–1289. https://doi.org/10.1016/S0140-6736(05)67528-9
62. Komajda M, McMurray JJV, Beck-Nielsen H, Gomis R, Hanefeld M, Pocock SJ et al (2010) Heart failure events with rosiglitazone in type 2 diabetes: data from the RECORD clinical trial. Eur Heart J 31:824–831
63. Scirica BM, Bhatt DL, Braunwald E, Steg PG, Davidson J, Hirshberg B, Ohman P, Frederich R, Wiviott SD, Hoffman EB, Cavender MA, Udell JA, Desai NR, Mosenzon O, McGuire D, Ray KK, Leiter LA, Raz I, SAVOR-TIMI 53 Steering Committee and Investigators (2013) Saxagliptin and cardiovascular outcomes in patients with type 2 diabetes mellitus. N Engl J Med 369:1317–1326. https://doi.org/10.1056/NEJMoa1307684
64. Tahrani AA, Barnett AH, Bailey CJ (2013) SGLT inhibitors in management of diabetes. Lancet Diabetes Endocrinol 1:140–151
65. (1998) Intensive blood-glucose control with sulphonylureas or insulin compared with conventional treatment and risk of complications in patients with type 2 diabetes (UKPDS 33). UK Prospective Diabetes Study (UKPDS) Group. Lancet 352(9131):837–853
66. Holman RR, Paul SK, Bethel MA, Matthews DR, Neil HA (2008) 10-year follow-up of intensive glucose control in type 2 diabetes. N Engl J Med 359(15):1577–1589
67. Udell JA, Cavender MA, Bhatt DL, Chatterjee S, Farkouh ME, Scirica BM (2015) Glucose-lowering drugs or strategies and cardiovascular outcomes in patients with or at risk for type 2 diabetes: a meta-analysis of randomised controlled trials. Lancet Diabetes Endocrinol 3(5):356–366
68. Nesto RW, Bell D, Bonow RO, Fonseca V, Grundy SM, Horton ES et al (2004) Thiazolidinedione use, fluid retention, and congestive heart failure: a consensus statement from the American Heart Association and American Diabetes Association. Diabetes Care 27(1):256–263
69. Zinman B, Wanner C, Lachin JM, Fitchett D, Bluhmki E, Hantel S et al (2015) Empagliflozin, cardiovascular outcomes, and mortality in type 2 diabetes. N Engl J Med 373(22):2117–2128
70. Lambers Heerspink HJ, de Zeeuw D, Wie L, Leslie B, List J (2013) Dapagliflozin a glucose-regulating drug with diuretic properties in subjects with type 2 diabetes. Diabetes Obes Metab 15(9):853–862
71. Cherney DZ, Scholey JW, Jiang S, Har R, Lai V, Sochett EB et al (2012) The effect of direct renin inhibition alone and in combination with ACE inhibition on endothelial function, arterial stiffness, and renal function in type 1 diabetes. Diabetes Care 35(11):2324–2330. Insightful study demonstrating that the sodium-glucose transporter-2 inhibitor empagliflozin was able to reverse glomerular hyperfiltration in diabetes

72. Wu JHY, Foote C, Blomster J et al (2016) Effects of sodium-glucose cotransporter-2 inhibitors on cardiovascular events, death, and major safety outcomes in adults with type 2 diabetes: a systematic review and meta-analysis. Lancet Diabetes Endocrinol 4(5):411–419
73. Verbrugge FH, Vangoitsenhoven R, Mullens W, Van der Schueren BJ, Mathieu C, Tang WH (2015) SGLT-2 inhibitors: potential novel strategy to prevent congestive heart failure in diabetes? Curr Cardiovasc Risk Rep 9:38
74. Heerspink HJ, Perkins BA, Fitchett DH, Husain M, Cherney DZ (2016) Sodium glucose cotransporter 2 inhibitors in the treatment of diabetes mellitus: cardiovascular and kidney effects, potential mechanisms, and clinical applications. Circulation 134(10):752–772
75. Hwang I-C, Cho G-Y, Yoon YE, Park JJ, Park J-B, Lee S-P, Kim H-K, Kim Y-J, Sohn D-W (2020) Different effects of SGLT2 inhibitors according to the presence and types of heart failure in type 2 diabetic patients. Cardiovasc Diabetol 19:69. https://doi.org/10.1186/s12933-020-01042-3
76. Matsutani D, Sakamoto M, Kayama Y, Takeda N, Horiuchi R, Utsunomiya K (2018) Effect of canagliflozin on left ventricular diastolic function in patients with type 2 diabetes. Cardiovasc Diabetol 17(1):73. https://doi.org/10.1186/s12933-018-0717-9
77. Otagaki M, Matsumura K, Kin H, Fujii K, Shibutani H, Matsumoto H, Takahashi H, Park H, Yamamoto Y, Sugiura T et al (2019) Effect of tofogliflozin on systolic and diastolic cardiac function in type 2 diabetic patients. Cardiovasc Drugs Ther 33(4):435–442
78. Soga F, Tanaka H, Tatsumi K et al (2018) Impact of dapagliflozin on left ventricular diastolic function of patients with type 2 diabetic mellitus with chronic heart failure. Cardiovasc Diabetol 17:132. https://doi.org/10.1186/s12933-018-0775-z
79. Rao S (2021) Use of sodium-glucose cotransporter-2 inhibitors in clinical practice for heart failure prevention and treatment: beyond type 2 diabetes. A narrative review. Adv Ther 39:845–861. https://doi.org/10.1007/s12325-021-01989-z
80. Fitchett D, Zinman B, Wanner C et al (2016) Heart failure outcomes with empagliflozin in patients with type 2 diabetes at high cardiovascular risk: results of the EMPA-REG OUTCOME® trial. Eur Heart J 37:1526–1534
81. Neal B, Perkovic V, Mahaffey KW et al (2017) Canagliflozin and cardiovascular and renal events in type 2 diabetes. N Engl J Med 377:644–657
82. Rådholm K, Figtree G, Perkovic V et al (2018) Canagliflozin and heart failure in type 2 diabetes mellitus: results from the CANVAS program. Circulation 138:458–468
83. Verma S, Wanner C, Zwiener I et al (2019) Influence of microvascular disease on cardiovascular events in type 2 diabetes. J Am Coll Cardiol 73:2780–2782
84. Wiviott SD, Raz I, Bonaca MP et al (2019) Dapagliflozin and cardiovascular outcomes in type 2 diabetes. N Engl J Med 380:347–357
85. Zinman B, Wanner C, Lachin JM et al (2015) Empagliflozin, cardiovascular outcomes, and mortality in type 2 diabetes. N Engl J Med 373:2117–2128
86. Perkovic V, Jardine MJ, Neal B et al (2019) Canagliflozin and renal outcomes in type 2 diabetes and nephropathy. N Engl J Med 380:2295–2306
87. Furtado RHM, Bonaca MP, Raz I et al (2019) Dapagliflozin and cardiovascular outcomes in patients with type 2 diabetes mellitus and previous myocardial infarction. Circulation 139:2516–2527
88. Zelniker TA, Wiviott SD, Raz I et al (2019) SGLT2 inhibitors for primary and secondary prevention of cardiovascular and renal outcomes in type 2 diabetes: a systematic review and meta-analysis of cardiovascular outcome trials. Lancet 393:31–39
89. Heerspink HJL, Stefansson BV, Correa-Rotter R et al (2020) Dapagliflozin in patients with chronic kidney disease. N Engl J Med 383:1436–1446
90. Packer M, Anker SD, Butler J et al (2020) Cardiovascular and renal outcomes with empagliflozin in heart failure. N Engl J Med 383:1413–1424
91. Anker SD, Butler J, Filippatos G et al (2021) Empagliflozin in heart failure with a preserved ejection fraction. N Engl J Med 385:1451–1461

92. O'Meara E, McDonald M, Chan M et al (2020) CCS/CHFS heart failure guidelines: clinical trial update on functional mitral regurgitation, SGLT2 inhibitors, ARNI in HFpEF, and tafamidis in amyloidosis. Can J Cardiol 36:159–169
93. Butler J, Handelsman Y, Bakris G, Verma S (2020) Use of sodium-glucose co-transporter-2 inhibitors in patients with and without type 2 diabetes: implications for incident and prevalent heart failure. Eur J Heart Fail 22:604–617
94. Cosentino F, Grant PJ, Aboyans V et al (2020) 2019 ESC guidelines on diabetes, pre-diabetes, and cardiovascular diseases developed in collaboration with the EASD. Eur Heart J 41:255–323
95. Seferovic PM, Fragasso G, Petrie M et al (2020) Heart Failure Association of the European Society of cardiology update on sodium-glucose co-transporter 2 inhibitors in heart failure. Eur J Heart Fail 22:1984–1986
96. Seferovic PM, Fragasso G, Petrie M et al (2020) Sodium glucose co-transporter-2 inhibitors in heart failure: beyond glycaemic control. A position paper of the heart failure Association of the European Society of cardiology. Eur J Heart Fail 22:1495–1503
97. Ali A, Bain S, Hicks D et al (2019) SGLT2 inhibitors: cardiovascular benefits beyond HbA1c-translating evidence into practice. Diab Ther 10:1595–1622
98. Gonzalez DE, Foresto RD, Ribeiro AB (1992) SGLT-2 inhibitors in diabetes: a focus on renoprotection. Rev Assoc Med Bras 2020(66):s17–s24
99. Vardeny O, Vaduganathan M (2019) Practical guide to prescribing sodium-glucose cotransporter 2 inhibitors for cardiologists. JACC Heart Fail. 7:169–172
100. Wang X, Ni J, Guo R, Li L, Su J, He F, Fan G (2021) SGLT2 inhibitors break the vicious circle between heart failure and insulin resistance: targeting energy metabolism. Heart Fail Rev 27:961–980. https://doi.org/10.1007/s10741-021-10096-8
101. Boonman-de Winter LJ et al (2012) High prevalence of previously unknown heart failure and left ventricular dysfunction in patients with type 2 diabetes. Diabetologia 55(8):2154–2162. https://doi.org/10.1111/1753-0407.12645
102. Aubert G, Martin OJ, Horton JL, Lai L, Vega RB, Leone TC et al (2016) The failing heart relies on ketone bodies as a fuel. Circulation 133:698–705
103. Ferrannini E, Baldi S, Frascerra S, Astiarraga B, Heise T, Bizzotto R et al (2016) Shift to fatty substrate utilization in response to sodium–glucose cotransporter 2 inhibition in subjects without diabetes and patients with type 2 diabetes. Diabetes 65:1190–1195
104. Mizuno Y, Harada E, Nakagawa H, Morikawa Y, Shono M, Kugimiya F et al (2017) The diabetic heart utilizes ketone bodies as an energy source. Metabolism 77:65–72
105. Birkenfeld AL, Jordan J, Dworak M, Merkel T, Burnstock G (2019) Myocardial metabolism in heart failure: purinergic signalling and other metabolic concepts. Pharmacol Ther 194:132–144. https://doi.org/10.1016/j.pharmthera.2018.08.015
106. Hemnes AR et al (2020) BMPR2 dysfunction impairs insulin signaling and glucose homeostasis in cardiomyocytes. Am J Physiol Lung Cell Mol Physiol 318(2):L429–L441. https://doi.org/10.1152/ajplung.00555.2018
107. Taegtmeyer H (2016) Failing heart and starving brain: ketone bodies to the rescue. Circulation 134(4):265–266. https://doi.org/10.1161/CIRCULATIONAHA.116.022141
108. Verma S (2019) Potential mechanisms of sodium-glucose co-transporter 2 inhibitor-related cardiovascular benefits. Am J Cardiol 124(Suppl 1):S36–s44. https://doi.org/10.1016/j.amjcard.2019.10.028
109. Verma S, Rawat S, Ho KL et al (2018) Empagliflozin increases cardiac energy production in diabetes: novel translational insights into the heart failure benefits of SGLT2 inhibitors. JACC Basic Transl Sci 3(5):575–587
110. Yoshii A, Nagoshi T, Kashiwagi Y, Kimura H, Tanaka Y, Oi Y et al (2019) Cardiac ischemia-reperfusion injury under insulin-resistant conditions: SGLT1 but not SGLT2 plays a compensatory protective role in diet-induced obesity. Cardiovasc Diabetol 18(1):85
111. Verbrugge FH (2017) Role of SGLT2 inhibitors in patients with diabetes mellitus and heart failure. Curr Heart Fail Rep 14:275–283. https://doi.org/10.1007/s11897-017-0340-1

112. Zinman B, Inzucchi SE, Lachin JM, Wanner C, Ferrari R, Fitchett D et al (2014) Rationale, design, and baseline characteristics of a randomized, placebo-controlled cardiovascular outcome trial of empagliflozin (EMPA-REG OUTCOME™). Cardiovasc Diabetol 13(1):102
113. American Diabetes Association (2016) Standards of medical care in diabetes-2016 abridged for primary care providers. Clin Diabetes 34(1):3–21
114. Nissen SE, Wolski K (2007) Effect of rosiglitazone on the risk of myocardial infarction and death from cardiovascular causes. N Engl J Med 356(24):2457–2471
115. White WB, Cannon CP, Heller SR, Nissen SE, Bergenstal RM, Bakris GL, Perez AT, Fleck PR, Mehta CR, Kupfer S, Wilson C, Cushman WC, Zannad F, EXAMINE Investigators (2013) Alogliptin after acute coronary syndrome in patients with type 2 diabetes. N Engl J Med 369:1327–1335. https://doi.org/10.1056/NEJMoa1305889
116. Green JB, Bethel MA, Armstrong PW, Buse JB, Engel SS, Garg J, Josse R, Kaufman KD, Koglin J, Korn S, Lachin JM, McGuire D, Pencina MJ, Standl E, Stein PP, Suryawanshi S, van de Werf F, Peterson ED, Holman RR, TECOS Study Group (2015) Effect of sitagliptin on cardiovascular outcomes in type 2 diabetes. N Engl J Med 373:232–242. https://doi.org/10.1056/NEJMoa1501352
117. Marso SP, Daniels GH, Brown-Frandsen K, Kristensen P, Mann JF, Nauck MA et al (2016) Liraglutide and cardiovascular outcomes in type 2 diabetes. N Engl J Med 375(4):311–322
118. Marso SP, Bain SC, Consoli A, Eliaschewitz FG, Jodar E, Leiter LA et al (2016) Semaglutide and cardiovascular outcomes in patients with type 2 diabetes. N Engl J Med 375(19):1834–1844. Randomised clinical trial showing a significant 26% relative reduction in cardiovascular events in patients with diabetes treated with the glucagon-like peptide-1 agonist semaglutide. However, this reduction was completely driven by non-fatal myocardial infarction and non-fatal stroke without impact on cardiovascular mortality
119. Ferrannini E, Mark M, Mayoux E (2016) CV protection in the EMPA-REG OUTCOME trial: a "thrifty substrate" hypothesis. Diabetes Care 39(7):1108–1114
120. Verbrugge FH, Mullens W, Tang WH (2016) Management of cardio-renal syndrome and diuretic resistance. Curr Treat Options Cardiovasc Med 18(2):11

Chapter 7
A comprehensive Review of Preclinical and Clinical Information on the Cardiovascular Advantages of SGLT2 Inhibitors

Mukesh Nandave

Introduction by the Editor

Diabetes is a major global mortality and source of morbidity worldwide. Antidiabetic medications have been observed to occasionally increase the risk of cardiovascular problems, whereas SGLT2i demonstrated promising benefits in clinical trials.

One of the main factors contributing to the severity of heart failure is the unfavorable cardiac remodelling caused by cardiac hypertrophy, fibrosis, and inflammation. Adverse cardiac remodelling may be reversed by SGLT2-inhibitor therapy, according to several pre-clinical and clinical investigations. Patients with heart failure have not shown this impact, despite it being noted in those with type 2 diabetes and left ventricular hypertrophy.

This is especially fascinating considering the majority of its advantages for the cardiovascular system have been related to heart failure outcomes. This suggests that, in addition to ventricular stress and remodelling, SGLT2 inhibition may have new direct cardioprotective benefits in the setting of heart failure (Fig. 7.1).

Nearly 90% of cardiac energy under normal conditions comes from mitochondrial oxidative metabolism; fuel comes mostly from free fatty acids and glucose, with smaller amounts coming from lactate, ketones, and amino acids. Myocardial dysfunction in type 2 diabetes and heart failure is caused by dysregulated fatty acid oxidation and reduced glucose absorption or oxidation. Ketone bodies are a "superfuel," creating ATP more effectively than glucose or free fatty acids in this environment of limited fuel choices and poor energy reserve.

Treatment with SGLT2-inhibitor drugs increases hepatic production and reduces ketones excreted in the urine, resulting in moderate but chronic hyperketonemia. In

M. Nandave (✉)
Department of Pharmacology and Pharmaceutical Biotechnology, Delhi Pharmaceutical Sciences and Research University (DPSRU), New Delhi, Delhi, India

M. Nandave (ed.), *Sodium-glucose Cotransporter-2 (SGLT2) Inhibitors in Heart Failure*, https://doi.org/10.1007/978-981-97-7568-2_7

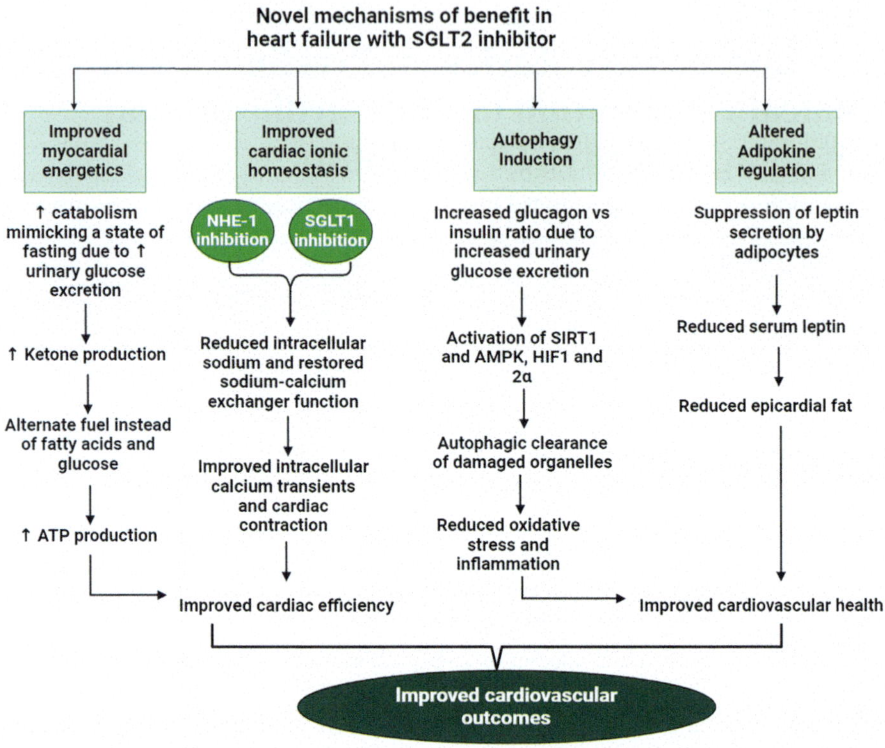

Fig. 7.1 Schematic diagram showing proposed novel mechanisms of action of SGLT2 inhibitors in heart failure. *AMPK* adenosine monophosphate-activated protein kinase, *HIF* hypoxia-inducible factor, *NHE* sodium-hydrogen exchanger, *SGLT* sodium-glucose co-transporter, *SIRT* sirtuin

these circumstances, the heart and kidneys readily absorb beta-hydroxybutyrate or ketones, and preferentially oxidize them over fatty acids and glucose. Beta-hydroxybutyrate improves cardiac efficiency in mouse hearts by increasing external cardiac effort and decreasing oxygen consumption.

Consequently, a theory has been put out suggesting that the cardiovascular advantages of SGLT2-inhibitor medication might be associated with a change in cardiac metabolism from oxidation of glucose and fatty acids to more oxygen-efficient ketone bodies, hence increasing cardiac efficiency [1].

Cardiovascular problems have decreased significantly in recent years due to rosiglitazone, which has shown a significant contrary. Since then, the US FDA and other drug regulatory organizations have required post-marketing cardiovascular outcome study data submission for newer diabetes medicines. This is done to stop any further unfounded claims about the safety or lack of cardiovascular risk from the newest classes. At the moment, SGLT2i, with FDA approval, includes dapagliflozin, canagliflozin, and empagliflozin. We don't have enough information on cardiovascular outcomes for this unique class.

Since 2008, several randomized controlled trials (RCTs) have established the efficacy of SGLT2i as an oral antidiabetic therapy. However, before approval, evidence of the cardiovascular safety of SGLT2i was necessary due to concerns regarding the potential negative impact of thiazolidinedione, the antidiabetic agent, on heart failure. From 2015 to 2020, four randomized controlled trials (RCTs) showed positive results on cardiovascular and renal endpoints, surpassing the threshold of non-inferiority. Following a flurry of pre-clinical and clinical research, SGLT2i was established as the first-line treatment for individuals with any combination of heart failure (HF), chronic kidney disease (CKD), and T2D, regardless of ejection fraction.

Numerous RCTs have examined the effects of SGLT2i on the kidneys and heart (summarised in the preceding chapters). The population selection criteria, cohort size, kind of assessed outcomes, and length of follow-up vary significantly among these trials.

Preclinical Models: SGLT2i's Cardioprotective Effects

Animal models with and without T2D have been used to study the cardioprotective effects of SGLT2i. In HF animals, SGLT2i was shown to enhance systolic activity, and cardiac dilation, and decrease both atrial and ventricular fibrosis in addition to reducing myocardial hypertrophy, fibrosis, and cardiomyocyte apoptosis.

These findings were validated in non-diabetic mice given doxorubicin therapy, which stopped the early LV function metrics, namely geometrical deformation indices, from declining. Additionally, the study revealed the expression of SGLT-1 receptors in the heart for the first time, paving the way for the successful clinical testing of SGLT-1/2 antagonists like sotagliflozin in patients with HF who were neither diabetic nor non-diabetic [2].

Preclinical models have demonstrated how the advantage of SGLT2i treatment may be attributed to a change toward a more effective energy route. Comparable research, however, utilizing P-MRS to assess cardiac PCr/ATP levels during dobutamine stress and at rest, was unable to demonstrate appreciable variations in cardiac energetics in either HFrEF or HFpEF. It's interesting to note that the quantity of epicardial and subcutaneous adipose tissue is dramatically decreased following SGLT2i therapy, and this decrease is correlated with a decrease in circulating inflammatory indicators. As a lipid storage organ, epicardial adipose tissue (EAT) decrease may be a sign in the oblique form of the myocardial fuel switch brought on by SGLT2i. Notably, elevated CV risk is associated with excess or aberrant EAT [3, 4].

Clinical Models: SGLT2i's Cardioprotective Effects

In 9 randomized clinical trials and 1385 patients, a recently published meta-analysis found that SGLT2i therapy substantially reduced LV end-diastolic volume (LVEDV), LV end-systolic volume (LVVESV), LVM, and LVM index. Individuals receiving SGLT2i also saw a notable improvement in LVEF, regardless of the HF phenotype or the duration of follow-up employed. The impact on LVMi in DM2 individuals is also unaffected by the length of diabetes. On the other hand, in a group of non-diabetic individuals with LVH but no HF, SGLT2i did not affect LVM and LVMi. It is still up for discussion whether these changes are largely caused by changes in extracellular volume, cardiomyocyte size, or a mix of the two [5].

The best method to offer non-invasive answers to this topic could be to employ CMR imaging, which can estimate ECV when combined with T1 mapping analysis. In a predetermined analysis of the EMPA-HEART, individuals with diabetes treated with empagliflozin had significantly lower ECV and indexed ECV as compared to placebo. There was no significant difference in intracellular volume (ICV) between the two groups, as determined by calculating (1-ECV) × (LVMi/1.05) [6].

Based on research it was found that 3% rise in ECV in diabetes patients was linked to a 52% increase in the probability of mortality or heart failure hospitalization, a 1.4% decrease in ECV in a very short period (6 months) becomes more pertinent. Another research in non-diabetic individuals supported the decrease in ECV by showing a decrease in cardiomyocyte volume following empagliflozin medication. NCT03782259 and NCT04490681 are ongoing trials that will yield further information on the effect of SGLT2i on ECV.

But in addition to increasing renal glucose excretion, this family of drugs has also shown several non-glycemic benefits, such as decreased weight, management of hypertension, diuretic activity, protection of the kidneys, a reduction in arterial stiffness, and a drop in uric acid levels. Empagliflozin dramatically decreased cardiovascular illness and mortality, according to a newly published EMPA-REG OUTCOME study. An overview of all currently available clinical and preclinical cardiovascular outcome data for SGLT2i is given in this chapter, including important clinical trials that are underway or have just concluded.

Machine Generated Summaries

Disclaimer: The summaries in this chapter were generated from Springer Nature publications using extractive AI auto-summarization: An extraction-based summarizer aims to identify the most important sentences of a text using an algorithm and uses those original sentences to create the auto-summary (unlike generative AI). As the constituted sentences are machine selected, they may not fully reflect the body of the work, so we strongly advise that the original content is read and cited. The auto generated summaries were curated by the editor to meet Springer Nature publication standards. To cite this content, please refer to the original papers.

Machine generated keywords: sglti, canvas, cvot, choice, gliflozin, sgltis, subject, antihyperglycemic, cardiovascular renal, glp, participant, antihyperglycemic drug, among patient, fda, renal outcome.

Significance of SGLT2 Inhibitors: Lessons from Renal Clinical Outcomes in Patients with Type 2 Diabetes and Basic Researches [7]

This is a machine-generated summary of:

Kitada, Munehiro; Hirai, Taro; Koya, Daisuke: Significance of SGLT2 inhibitors: lessons from renal clinical outcomes in patients with type 2 diabetes and basic researches [7].

Published in: Diabetology International (2020).

Link to original: https://doi.org/10.1007/s13340-020-00444-8

If you want to cite the papers, please refer to the original.

For technical reasons we could not place the page where the original quote is coming from.

Abstract-Summary "Despite multifactorial management including the administration of renin–angiotensin system inhibitors, patients often do not experience sufficient suppression of DKD progression and, thus, remain at risk for ESKD."

"Recent studies on cardiovascular outcomes among patients with T2DM have clearly shown that sodium–glucose cotransporter 2 (SGLT2) inhibitors, such as empagliflozin, canagliflozin, and dapagliflozin, have cardiorenal protective effects apart from their glucose-lowering effects."

"SGLT2 inhibitors have been found to improve renal outcomes, including ESKD, by slowing renal function decline and reducing urinary albumin excretion through their class effect."

Introduction

"Diabetic kidney disease (DKD), a microvascular complication of diabetes, has been the leading cause of end-stage kidney disease (ESKD), with patients suffering from DKD also recognized to be at high risk for cardiovascular disease (CVD) [8]."

"Multifactorial management against all cardiorenal disease-related risk factors has been recommended for DKD, with several clinical studies having demonstrated the beneficial effect thereof [9–12]."

"Among the multifactorial management approaches, renin–angiotensin system (RAS) inhibitors have been particularly recommended for suppressing DKD progression based on the evidence provided in several clinical studies [9, 13, 14]."

"Despite multifactorial management including the administration of RAS inhibitors, patient often do not experience sufficient suppression of DKD progression and, thus, remain at risk for ESKD."

Clinical Evidence for SGLT2is on Renoprotection Among Patients with T2DM

"The EMPA-REG OUTCOME trial compared the effects of empagliflozin and placebo on CV outcomes over a period of 192 weeks among patients with T2DM who received standard anti-diabetic therapy, had high CV risk, and had an estimated glomerular filtration rate (eGFR) of 30 mL/min/1.73 m^2 [15]."

"Despite a GFR of 30–45 mL/min/1.73 m^2, a small initial decline in eGFR was observed in the canagliflozin group followed by a return to baseline levels, a result consistent with those observed in patients with normal renal function."

"SGLT2is promoted a 30% reduction in the risk for substantial loss of renal function, ESKD, or death due to kidney disease even among those with a baseline eGFR of 30–45 mL/min/1.73 m^2 and exhibited consistent renoprotective effects across studies irrespective of baseline UACR and usage of RAS inhibitors."

Conclusions

"SGLT2is are a class of glucose-lowering drugs prescribed for patients with diabetes."

"Recent clinical evidence has clearly showed that SGLT2is exert renoprotective effects, such as decelerated decline in renal function, reduced urinary albumin excretion, and suppression of progression to ESKD among patients with T2DM who had CKD, independent of their glucose-lowering effects [16]."

"Clinical evidence presented herein, therefore, positively recommended the use of SGLT2is among indicated patients."

"The detailed mechanism by which SGLT2i exert their cardiorenal effects among patients with T2DM still remain unclear, therefore warranting further basic studies."

Rationale, Design, and Baseline Characteristics of the Utopia Trial for Preventing Diabetic Atherosclerosis Using an SGLT2 Inhibitor: A Prospective, Randomized, Open-Label, Parallel-Group Comparative Study [17]

This is a machine-generated summary of:

Katakami, Naoto; Mita, Tomoya; Yoshii, Hidenori; Shiraiwa, Toshihiko; Yasuda, Tetsuyuki; Okada, Yosuke; Umayahara, Yutaka; Kaneto, Hideaki; Osonoi, Takeshi; Yamamoto, Tsunehiko; Kuribayashi, Nobuichi; Maeda, Kazuhisa; Yokoyama, Hiroki; Kosugi, Keisuke; Ohtoshi, Kentaro; Hayashi, Isao; Sumitani, Satoru; Tsugawa, Mamiko; Ohashi, Makoto; Taki, Hideki; Nakamura, Tadashi; Kawashima, Satoshi; Sato, Yasunori; Watada, Hirotaka; Shimomura, Iichiro; On behalf of the UTOPIA study investigators, None: Rationale, Design, and Baseline Characteristics of the Utopia Trial for Preventing Diabetic Atherosclerosis Using an SGLT2 Inhibitor: A Prospective, Randomized, Open-Label, Parallel-Group Comparative Study [17].

Published in: Diabetes Therapy (2017).

Link to original: https://doi.org/10.1007/s13300-017-0292-1

If you want to cite the papers, please refer to the original.

For technical reasons we could not place the page where the original quote is coming from.

Abstract-Summary "The aim of the ongoing study described herein is to investigate the preventive effects of tofogliflozin, a potent and selective SGLT2 inhibitor, on the progression of atherosclerosis in subjects with type 2 diabetes (T2DM) using carotid intima-media thickness (IMT), an established marker of cardiovascular disease (CVD), as a marker."

"The aim was to recruit a total of 340 subjects with T2DM but no history of apparent CVD at 24 clinical sites and randomly allocate these to a tofogliflozin treatment group or a conventional treatment group using drugs other than SGLT2 inhibitors."

"Secondary outcomes include changes in glycemic control, parameters related to β-cell function and diabetic nephropathy, the occurrence of CVD and adverse events, and biochemical measurements reflecting vascular function."

"This is the first study to address the effects of SGLT2 inhibitors on the progression of carotid IMT in subjects with T2DM without a history of CVD."

Introduction

"The EMPA-REG OUTCOME trial, a clinical trial designed to clarify the effects of the SGLT2 inhibitor empagliflozin on clinical CV outcomes in patients with T2DM and established CV manifestations, showed that this agent markedly reduced the risk of CV mortality compared to placebo [18]."

"A multicenter, placebo-controlled, randomized, double-blind parallel-group study involving 230 Japanese T2DM patients with inadequate glycemic control on diet/exercise therapy demonstrated that tofogliflozin 10, 20, or 40 mg administered orally once daily for 24 weeks significantly decreased glycated hemoglobin (HbA1c), fasting blood glucose, and body weight compared to placebo [19]."

"We initiated a multicenter randomized controlled trial to investigate the preventive effects of tofogliflozin on the progression of atherosclerosis in subjects with T2DM but without a history of apparent CV events, with patients not treated with tofogliflozin as the control group."

Methods

"Primary study outcomes are the changes in mean IMT of the common carotid artery (mean-IMT-CCA) and maximum IMT of the CCA (max-IMT-CCA) during the 104-week treatment period measured by carotid arterial echography."

"In a 2-year observation period, the registration of at least 310 patients is required to obtain 90% power to detect a difference of 0.04 mm in IMT between the two treatment groups, assuming an SD of 0.108 mm for individual differences (which was presumed to be common to both groups), a 10% dropout, and a 0.05 level of significance."

"Analyses of the primary and secondary endpoints are to be performed in the full analysis set, which will include all participants who received at least one treatment dose during the study period and who did not seriously violate the study protocol, such as by not providing informed consent or registering outside the study period."

Conclusion

"The UTOPIA trial is a multicenter, prospective, randomized, investigator-initiated clinical trial with the aim to investigate the preventive effects of tofogliflozin, a potent and selective SGLT2 inhibitor, on the progression of atherosclerosis in subjects with T2DM but without a history of apparent atherosclerotic disease, using common carotid IMT, a widely used surrogate marker of atherosclerosis, as the primary endpoint."

"Several clinical studies have assessed the inhibitory effects of a variety class of anti-diabetic agents (e.g. biguanides, thiazolidinediones, alpha-glucosidase inhibitors, and DPP-4 inhibitors) on carotid IMT progression [20–25]."

"Tanaka and others recently published the protocol of the PROTECT study [26], the only ongoing study to assess the preventive effect of SGLT2 inhibitors on the progression of carotid atherosclerosis using carotid IMT as a surrogate marker."

"The PROTECT study is a 24-month prospective study in 480 Japanese subjects with T2DM, with the aim to assess the preventive effect of ipragliflozin, another SGLT2 inhibitor, on the progression of carotid IMT."

Sodium-Glucose Co-transporter 2 (SGLT2) Inhibitors: Are They All the Same? A Narrative Review of Cardiovascular Outcome Trials [27]

This is a machine-generated summary of:

Williams, David M.; Nawaz, Asif; Evans, Marc: Sodium-Glucose Co-Transporter 2 (SGLT2) Inhibitors: Are They All the Same? A Narrative Review of Cardiovascular Outcome Trials [27].

Published in: Diabetes Therapy (2020).

Link to original: https://doi.org/10.1007/s13300-020-00951-6

If you want to cite the papers, please refer to the original.

For technical reasons we could not place the page where the original quote is coming from.

Abstract-Summary "Important improvements in cardiovascular risk factors and adverse cardiovascular, heart failure and renal outcomes have been observed in numerous cardiovascular outcome trials (CVOTs) investigating the use of sodium-glucose co-transporter 2 (SGLT2) inhibitors over the last 5 years."

"Discussion around the choice of SGLT2 inhibitor has been again revived by the recent publication of results from the VERTIS-CV, EMPEROR-reduced and DAPA-CKD trials investigating cardiovascular, heart failure and renal outcomes associated with various SGLT2 inhibitors."

"This narrative review gives an overview of the mechanism of action and differences in the underlying pharmacology of the various SGLT2 inhibitors and discusses the key cardiovascular, heart failure and renal outcomes from completed CVOTs for SGLT2 inhibitors."

Digital Features

"This article is published with digital features, including a summary slide, to facilitate understanding of the article."

"To view digital features for this article go to https://doi.org/10.6084/m9.figshare.13089386 ."

Background

"Specific cardiovascular outcomes are required to be reported for drug therapies used to treat T2D, including cardiovascular death, non-fatal myocardial infarction (MI) and non-fatal stroke [28], reported as a combined major adverse cardiovascular event (MACE) measure in cardiovascular outcome trials (CVOTs)."

"To address this, the US Food and Drug Administration (FDA) recently suggested minimum numbers of important study participant variables including age and proportion of people with underlying cardiovascular and/or renal disease to minimise confusion when comparing CVOTs and improve trial validity to real-world populations [29]."

"We compare SGLT2 inhibitors with completed CVOT results, illustrating similarities and differences in trial design, and key glycaemic, body weight, cardiovascular, renal and adverse event outcomes to support clinicians when choosing between these drugs."

Mechanisms of Cardiovascular and Renal Benefit with SGLT2 Inhibition

"SGLT2 inhibitors indirectly improve cardiac function by enhancing diuresis and natriuresis to reduce plasma and interstitial fluid volumes thereby reducing cardiac preload [30]."

"The use of SGLT2 inhibitors may be associated with more stable renal function associated with diuresis than that observed with the current use of thiazide or loop diuretics in the treatment of people with heart failure."

"Further indirect mechanisms of SGLT2 inhibitor-mediated cardiovascular benefit include improved myocardial energy efficiency by shifting to ketone metabolism, a more energy efficient substrate than glucose or fatty acids."

"Other putative direct mechanisms of cardiovascular benefit associated with these drugs include improved endothelial function [31], though this is often argued to be an indirect consequence of improved metabolic parameters generally associated with diabetes treatment."

"Further direct mechanisms suggested for the benefits seen with SGLT2 inhibitors include direct myocardial Na/H pump inhibition which improves sensitivity to endogenous natriuretic peptides, and reduces cardiac hypertrophy, fibrosis and remodelling [32]."

SGLT2 Inhibitors: Do They All Work the Same Way?

"Differences in trial outcomes may reflect differences in the mechanism and pharmacology of the various SGLT2 inhibitors, differences in trial design or study populations, or all of these factors."

"Differences in the pharmacology of these drugs including the dose, absorption, distribution, metabolism and excretion of these drugs as well as their relative affinity for the SGLT2 protein versus the sodium-glucose co-transporter 1 (SGLT1) protein are important."

"Drugs which have varying affinity to inhibit SGLT2 and SGLT1 may have differing efficacy with respect to glycaemic control and other metabolic measures."

"Canagliflozin has the least selectivity for the SGLT2 protein versus the SGLT1 protein (~250 fold) whilst empagliflozin has the highest (~2500 fold)."

"Whilst these drugs work by a similar mechanism such pharmacological differences may account for some of the variation in clinical outcomes observed with these drugs."

Cardiovascular Outcome Trials and SGLT2 Inhibitors

"Populations in the heart failure outcome trials (DAPA-HF and EMPEROR-reduced) were quite different as all participants were diagnosed with HFrEF and observed to have lower BMI, systolic blood pressure and mean eGFR, and included participants without T2D. However, there were no significant differences in cardiovascular outcomes in people with or without T2D in either of the heart failure outcome trials."

"Participants in the renal outcome trials (CREDENCE and DAPA-CKD) were observed to have lower mean BMI and eGFR than participants included in previous CVOTs investigating these drugs and demonstrated good cardiovascular and renal outcome results [33, 34]."

"Differences in the proportion of participants with heart failure and specifically HFpEF in the VERTIS-CV trial and the low cardiovascular event rate in the DECLARE-TIMI trial may explain why these trials did not demonstrate superiority for 3-point MACE whilst the EMPA-REG and CANVAS trials did."

Adverse Events

"A previous meta-analysis of randomised controlled trials investigating SGLT2 inhibitors observed significantly higher rates of DKA in those using SGLT2 inhibitors versus control, particularly in people aged over 60 years [35]."

"The use of SGLT2 inhibitors did not increase the rate of hypoglycaemia in any major CVOT, and hypoglycaemia rates were significantly lower in the DECLARE-TIMI trial."

"The reasons for this difference are unclear, though like other SGLT2 inhibitor trials, the DAPA-HF and DAPA-CKD studies did not demonstrate significant changes in hypoglycaemia rates."

"Consistently across each of the trials, the rate of genital tract infection was higher in those using SGLT2 inhibitors and the rate of urinary tract infections was only significantly higher in the VERTIS-CV study."

"There was a significantly lower rate of acute kidney injury (AKI) associated with SGLT2 inhibitor use in the DECLARE-TIMI and EMPA-REG trials, and a trend to reduced AKI incidence in all other CVOTs to date."

Conclusions

"The use of SGLT2 inhibitors in clinical trials consistently results in improved cardiovascular risk factors, renal outcomes, HHF rates and does not lead to cardiovascular harm."

"These differences probably result from variations in the participant characteristics in each study and the subsequent cardiovascular event rate in each trial influencing statistical analysis."

"There are now so many cardiovascular, renal and heart failure outcome trials with different study designs, interventions and outcomes it is increasingly difficult to see the wood from the trees."

Effects of Exenatide and Open-Label SGLT2 Inhibitor Treatment, Given in Parallel or Sequentially, on Mortality and Cardiovascular and Renal Outcomes in Type 2 Diabetes: Insights from the EXSCEL Trial [36]

This is a machine-generated summary of:

Clegg, Lindsay E.; Penland, Robert C.; Bachina, Srinivas; Boulton, David W.; Thuresson, Marcus; Heerspink, Hiddo J. L.; Gustavson, Stephanie; Sjöström, C. David; Ruggles, James A.; Hernandez, Adrian F.; Buse, John B.; Mentz, Robert J.; Holman, Rury R.: Effects of exenatide and open-label SGLT2 inhibitor treatment, given in parallel or sequentially, on mortality and cardiovascular and renal outcomes in type 2 diabetes: insights from the EXSCEL trial [36].

Published in: Cardiovascular Diabetology (2019).

Link to original: https://doi.org/10.1186/s12933-019-0942-x

If you want to cite the papers, please refer to the original.

For technical reasons we could not place the page where the original quote is coming from.

Abstract-Summary "Sodium-glucose cotransporter-2 inhibitors (SGLT2i) and glucagon-like peptide-1 receptor agonists (GLP-1 RA) improve cardiovascular and renal outcomes in patients with type 2 diabetes through distinct mechanisms."

"We aim to provide insight into the effects of open-label SGLT2i use in parallel with or shortly after once-weekly GLP-1 RA exenatide (EQW) on cardiorenal outcomes."

"In the EXSCEL cardiovascular outcomes trial EQW arm, SGLT2i drop-in occurred in 8.7% of participants."

"These EQW + SGLT2i users were propensity-matched to: (1) placebo-arm participants not taking SGLT2i (n=572 per group); and to (2) EQW-arm participants not taking SGLT2i (n=575), based on their last measured characteristics before SGLT2i initiation, and equivalent study visit in comparator groups."

"In adjusted analyses, the risk for MACE with combination EQW + SGLT2i use was numerically lower compared with both placebo (adjusted hazard ratio 0.68, 95% CI 0.39–1.17) and EQW alone (0.85, 0.48–1.49)."

"Combination EQW+SGLT2i use also nominally significantly improved estimated eGFR slope compared with placebo (+1.94, 95% CI 0.94–2.94 mL/min/1.73 m^2/year) and EQW alone (+2.38, 1.40–3.35 mL/min/1.73 m^2/year)."

"This post hoc analysis supports the hypothesis that combinatorial EQW and SGLT2i therapy may provide benefit on cardiovascular outcomes and mortality."

Background

"Members of both the glucagon-like peptide-1 receptor agonist (GLP-1 RA) and sodium-glucose cotransporter-2 inhibitor (SGLT2i) classes of anti-hyperglycemic drugs have demonstrated cardio- and reno-protective effects in cardiovascular outcomes trials (CVOTs) conducted in patients with type 2 diabetes mellitus."

"The 104 week DURATION-8, 24 week AWARD-10, and 30 week SUSTAIN 9 trials demonstrated that simultaneous initiation of GLP-1 RA exenatide and SGLT2i dapagliflozin, or addition of GLP-1 RAs dulaglutide and semaglutide to open-label SGLT2i, durably improved glycemic control and cardiovascular risk factors without increasing the risk of hypoglycemia [37–40]."

"No clinical trial or real world evidence on long-term cardiovascular outcomes, mortality, and renal disease progression with combination GLP-1 RA and SGLT2i treatment have been reported to date."

"The EXenatide Study of Cardiovascular Event Lowering (EXSCEL) was a randomized, placebo-controlled, global pragmatic clinical trial designed to assess the effect of subcutaneous once-weekly GLP-1 RA exenatide (EQW) 2 mg on cardiovascular outcomes in 14,752 participants with type 2 diabetes mellitus and a range of cardiovascular risk [41]."

Methods

"We also generated cohorts matched to only subjects taking exenatide and SGLT2i simultaneously, and performed a sensitivity analysis where we censored subjects in the primary analysis at initiation of open-label GLP-1 RA (in violation of study protocol) to further probe the impact of variation in drug usage patterns within our cohorts."

"Covariates used for propensity matching were: age, sex, ethnicity, smoking status (trial baseline), race, region, duration of diabetes, history of heart failure, history of prior cardiovascular disease (CVD), microalbuminuria, macroalbuminuria, BMI, eGFR, systolic blood pressure, HbA_{1c}, total cholesterol, and use of renin-angiotensin-aldosterone system inhibitors, thiazolidinediones, metformin, dipeptidyl peptidase-4 inhibitors, and insulin."

"eGFR slope vs. time was analyzed in both sets of propensity-matched cohorts using a mixed-model repeated measures (MMRM) analysis to estimate the overall treatment effect on eGFR slope."

Results

"Median follow-up time for ACM in the placebo comparison was 13.3 months (IQR 6.5–23.1) for the combination cohort and 14.2 months (IQR 4.5–27.0) for the placebo cohort."

"MMRM-estimated slopes in the placebo comparison were + 1.21 mL/min/1.73 m^2/year (se 0.37) in the combination cohort and – 0.71 mL/min/1.73 m^2/year (se 0.33) in the placebo cohort, resulting in an estimated treatment effect of + 1.94 mL/min/1.73 m^2/year (95% CI 0.94–2.94, $p < 0.001$)."

"In the EQW comparison, the estimated slope was + 1.27 mL/min/1.73 m^2/year (se 0.38) in the combination cohort, and – 1.11 mL/min/1.73 m^2/year (se 0.32) in the EQW cohort, giving an estimated treatment effect of + 2.38 mL/min/1.73 m^2/year (95% CI 1.40–3.35, $p < 0.001$)."

Discussion

"The similar improvement in eGFR slope in both comparisons in our population suggests the observed eGFR slope improvement may be due primarily to SGLT2i contributions when used on top of GLP-1 RA, consistent with previous GLP-1 RA studies generally showing an effect more so on macroalbuminuria than on eGFR-based endpoints [42]."

"These potentially complementary sets of mechanisms support the hypothesis that combination GLP-1 RA and SGLT2i treatment may results in further CV and renal benefit than observed with either class alone [43–45]."

"The results presented here support a potential added benefit for the combination of EQW and SGLT2i on ACM, at a minimum, an end-point on which both classes alone have shown some effect, and which may reflect a convergence of multiple mechanisms of action by these two drug classes."

Conclusions

"This analysis provides the first insight, from a credible cohort with adjudicated CV events, into long-term cardiorenal outcomes in subjects using EQW and SGLT2i either in parallel or relatively close sequence."

"The results, supporting the hypothesis that this combination may provide additional benefit particularly on mortality, motivate additional, more comprehensive study of combination GLP-1 RA and SGLT2i in the future."

From Skepticism to Hope: The Evolving Concept of the Initiation and Use of Sodium-Glucose Cotransporter 2 Inhibitors in Hospitalized Patients [46]

This is a machine-generated summary of:

Koufakis, Theocharis; Mustafa, Omar G.; Ajjan, Ramzi A.; Garcia-Moll, Xavier; Zebekakis, Pantelis; Dimitriadis, George; Kotsa, Kalliopi: From Skepticism to Hope: The Evolving Concept of the Initiation and Use of Sodium-Glucose Cotransporter 2 Inhibitors in Hospitalized Patients [46].

Published in: Drugs (2022).

Link to original: https://doi.org/10.1007/s40265-022-01730-2

If you want to cite the papers, please refer to the original.

For technical reasons we could not place the page where the original quote is coming from.

Abstract-Summary "The positive and rapid effects of sodium-glucose cotransporter 2 inhibitors (SGLT2i) on cardiorenal outcomes raises the possibility that they might confer benefits to hospitalized patients."

"In recent, well designed, randomized trials (SOLOIST-WHF and EMPULSE) recruiting inpatients with heart failure (HF), SGLT2i demonstrated the potential to improve survival and quality of life and reduce the number of HF events, time to first HF event, hospitalizations, and urgent visits for HF compared with placebo."

"In DARE-19, the administration of dapagliflozin to inpatients with cardiometabolic risk factors and COVID-19 was based on the hypothesis that the anti-inflammatory properties of SGLT2i could alleviate organ damage."

"These promising findings in the field of cardiometabolic medicine set the stage for future research to explore whether the benefits of gliflozins can expand to inpatients with non-cardiometabolic disorders, including sepsis, cirrhotic ascites, and malignancies."

"The concept of inpatient use of SGLT2i has evolved greatly over the past few years."

"The latest evidence suggests that SGLT2i may be effective and safe in the hospital setting, provided patients are carefully selected and closely monitored."

Introduction

"Back in 2020, we speculated on the risk–benefit ratio of administering sodium-glucose cotransporter 2 inhibitors (SGLT2i) to hospitalized patients with diabetes mellitus and concluded that "potential benefits deriving from the use of SGLT2i in the inpatient setting cannot mitigate possible risks, at least until robust evidence on their efficacy in hospitalized individuals become available" [47]."

"Although initially developed as drugs for the management of hyperglycemia, they soon became known to significantly improve outcomes related to heart failure (HF) and chronic kidney disease (CKD), leading to their licensed use in patients with both entities, regardless of diabetes status."

"The rationale behind the use of SGLT2i in hospitals is based on the practical dosing scheme, the low risk of hypoglycemia (if given as antihyperglycemic agents), but mainly to their potential to alleviate the deleterious effects of cardiorenal injury."

Recent Evidence

"In the SOLOIST-WHF (Effect of Sotagliflozin on Cardiovascular Events in Patients With Type 2 Diabetes Post Worsening Heart Failure) trial, 1222 patients with T2D requiring hospitalization due to exacerbation of HF were randomly assigned to either sotagliflozin or placebo [48]."

"In this trial, 530 patients hospitalized with acute HF (47% had diabetes) were randomized to receive empagliflozin 10 mg or placebo in addition to standard treatment [49]."

"A recent meta-analysis that pooled data from five high-quality randomized controlled trials (RCTs) reassuringly demonstrated a similar risk of urinary tract infections (including severe ones, such as urosepsis) among patients with HF assigned to SGLT2i compared with those assigned to placebo (relative risk 1.09, 95% CI 0.94–1.26; $p = 0.24$) [50]."

The Clinician's Perspective

"SGLT2i have been tested as adjunct therapy in patients with inadequately controlled type 1 diabetes (T1D) and proved to be effective in reducing glycated hemoglobin, body weight, and insulin dose [51, 52]."

"DKA is a potentially fatal complication that can be experienced by a certain number of patients, especially when SGLT2i are introduced during hospitalization."

"It can be argued that good clinical practice dictates that selection of patients for various therapies is done with care, while monitoring needs to be intensified in the presence of known side effects, particularly at the initiation phase, to ensure a high benefit/risk ratio."

"It could be said that the renal effects of the inpatient use of SGLT2i should be studied in more detail, considering that so far most studies have focused on safety rather than potential benefits."

Conclusion

"During the past 2 years, the concept of the in-hospital use of SGLT2i evolved through evidence from well-designed randomized trials demonstrating that these drugs might be both effective and well tolerated to start in the inpatient setting, provided that patients are properly selected and closely monitored."

"The promising findings in the field of cardiometabolic medicine set the stage for future research to explore whether the benefits of gliflozins can expand to inpatients with non-cardiometabolic disorders."

"Real-world data are much needed to prove whether the present hope about the inpatient use of gliflozins will transform into future confidence."

Effects of Sodium/Glucose Cotransporter 2 (SGLT2) Inhibitors and Combined SGLT1/2 Inhibitors on Cardiovascular, Metabolic, Renal, and Safety Outcomes in Patients with Diabetes: A Network Meta-Analysis of 111 Randomized Controlled Trials [53]

This is a machine-generated summary of:

Teo, Yao Neng; Ting, Adriel Z. H.; Teo, Yao Hao; Chong, Elliot Yeung; Tan, Joshua Teik Ann; Syn, Nicholas L.; Chia, Alys Z. Q.; Ong, How Ting; Cheong, Alex Jia Yang; Li, Tony Yi-Wei; Poh, Kian Keong; Yeo, Tiong Cheng; Chan, Mark Yan-Yee; Wong, Raymond C. C.; Chai, Ping; Sia, Ching-Hui: Effects of Sodium/Glucose Cotransporter 2 (SGLT2) Inhibitors and Combined SGLT1/2 Inhibitors on Cardiovascular, Metabolic, Renal, and Safety Outcomes in Patients with Diabetes: A Network Meta-Analysis of 111 Randomized Controlled Trials [53].

Published in: American Journal of Cardiovascular Drugs (2022).

Link to original: https://doi.org/10.1007/s40256-022-00528-7

If you want to cite the papers, please refer to the original.

For technical reasons we could not place the page where the original quote is coming from.

Abstract-Summary "This network meta-analysis aimed to compare the treatment effect across various outcomes between pure SGLT2 inhibitors and combined SGLT1/2 inhibitors in patients with diabetes."

"Frequentist network meta-analysis was conducted to summarize the treatment effects reported in individual trials, stratified by type 1 (T1DM) and type 2 diabetes mellitus (T2DM)."

"Frequentist network meta-analysis demonstrated that in T2DM patients, SGLT1/2 inhibitors led to a decreased hazard rate of myocardial infarction (hazard ratio [HR] 0.74, 95% confidence interval [CI] 0.56–0.98) and stroke (HR 0.65, 95% CI 0.47–0.92) compared with SGLT2 inhibitors."

"SGLT2 inhibitors achieved a greater hemoglobin A1c (HbA1c) reduction than SGLT1/2 inhibitors (0.16%, 95% CI 0.06–0.26)."

"In patients with T2DM, the risk of diarrhea (risk ratio [RR] 1.42, 95% CI 1.07–1.88) and severe hypoglycemia (RR 5.89, 95% CI 1.41–24.57) were found to be higher with SGLT1/2 inhibitor use compared with SGLT2 inhibitor use."

"No differences were observed for cardiovascular, metabolic, and safety outcomes between SGLT1/2 inhibitors and SGLT2 inhibitors in patients with T1DM."

"In patients with T2DM, compared with pure SGLT2 inhibitors, combined SGLT1/2 inhibitors demonstrated a lower risk of myocardial infarction and of stroke, but were associated with a higher risk of diarrhea and severe hypoglycemia."

Introduction

"Sodium-glucose cotransporter 2 (SGLT2) inhibitors are a class of anti-hyperglycemic drugs that has been steadily increasing in popularity due to its cardiovascular and renal benefits, which have been demonstrated to be consistent and significant in recent randomized controlled trials [54–58]."

"By inhibiting both SGLT1 and SGLT2, these combined inhibitors are theoretically able to further minimize glucose reabsorption in the kidneys to achieve a greater anti-hyperglycemic effect as compared with pure SGLT2 inhibitors."

"Dual SGLT1/2 inhibitors are a new, promising anti-hyperglycemic treatment for patients with diabetes because they retain the benefits of the well-known SGLT2 inhibitors while having supposedly superior anti-hyperglycemic effects."

"There have been no head-to-head randomized controlled trials comparing the efficacy of combined SGLT1/2 inhibitors against pure SGLT2 inhibitors in patients with diabetes."

"We conducted a systematic review and network meta-analysis comparing the treatment effect across various outcomes between combined SGLT1/2 inhibitors and pure SGLT2 inhibitors in patients with diabetes."

Methodology

"We included randomized controlled trials investigating the clinical outcomes of SGLT2 inhibitors or SGLT1/2 inhibitors used for a minimum duration of 12 weeks in patients with diabetes."

"We excluded all randomized controlled trials that did not report on cardiovascular, metabolic, renal, or safety outcomes in patients with diabetes."

"Apart from cardiovascular, metabolic, renal, and safety outcomes, baseline information of patients was collected for age, sex, smoking status, type and duration of diabetes mellitus, hypertension, hyperlipidemia, atrial fibrillation, previous stroke, and previous myocardial infarction."

"For panel data or longitudinal outcomes, pre-intervention baseline imbalances were corrected using the simple analysis of change scores method [59]."

"For clinical outcomes with little evidence of inconsistency ($p > 0.10$ from Wald test), consistency models were fitted with restricted maximum likelihood models that assumed a common heterogeneity variance τ^2 for all treatment contrasts."

"Treatment estimates were reported as hazard ratios (HRs) or risk ratios (RRs) and mean differences for time-to-event and continuous outcomes, respectively."

Results

"Ten trials recruited patients with type 1 diabetes mellitus (five SGLT1/2 inhibitor trials and five SGLT2 inhibitor trials), and 91 trials recruited patients with type 2 diabetes mellitus."

"Mixed cohorts of patients with and without diabetes mellitus were seen in four included trials, in which data for the subgroup of type 2 diabetes mellitus were reported."

"A total of six SGLT1/2 trials and 89 SGLT2 trials reported outcomes for patients with type 2 diabetes mellitus."

"Two articles, Petrie and others [60] and Serenelli and others [61], reported separate outcomes for the DAPA-HF trial."

"Persson and others [62] and Wheeler and others [63] reported separate outcomes for the DAPA-CKD trial."

"Strojek and others [64] and Strojek and others [65] reported separate outcomes for the trial registered NCT00680745."

"Gause-Nilsson and others [66] and Leiter and others [67] reported separate outcomes for the trial registered NCT01042977."

"Bode and others [68] and Bode and others [69] reported separate outcomes for the trial registered NCT01106651."

"Cardiovascular outcomes could not be analyzed in patients with type 1 diabetes mellitus due to insufficient studies."

Discussion

"In this frequentist network meta-analysis of 111 randomized controlled trials, we demonstrated that in patients with type 2 diabetes, compared with pure SGLT2 inhibitors, combined SGLT1/2 inhibitors demonstrated a lower risk of myocardial infarction and of stroke, but were associated with a higher risk of diarrhea and severe hypoglycemia."

"In patients with type 1 diabetes mellitus, our network meta-analysis found no statistically significant differences in treatment effects between SGLT2 inhibitors and SGLT1/2 inhibitors for the investigated cardiovascular, metabolic, and safety outcomes."

"In the analysis of cardiovascular outcomes including myocardial infarction and stroke, data was available from only one to two SGLT1/2 inhibitor trials, namely the SCORED and SOLOIST-WHF trials, which recruited diabetic patients with chronic kidney disease and worsening heart failure, respectively."

"Data for the SGLT1/2 inhibitor group on the incidence of severe hypoglycemia in patients with type 2 diabetes mellitus were available in only one trial, limiting the reliability of our findings."

Conclusion

"This frequentist network meta-analysis of 111 randomized controlled trials demonstrated that in patients with type 2 diabetes, compared with pure SGLT2 inhibitors, combined SGLT1/2 inhibitors demonstrated a lower risk of myocardial infarction and of stroke, but were associated with a higher risk of diarrhea and severe hypoglycemia."

"Further research comparing SGLT2 inhibitors and SGLT1/2 inhibitors in different patient populations where SGLT2 inhibitors have exhibited beneficial effects, such as patients with heart failure, should be considered to explore the relative efficacy and potential of the combined inhibitor class as an alternative treatment option to SGLT2 inhibitors."

Generalizability of Cardiovascular Safety Trials on SGLT2 Inhibitors to the Real World: Implications for Clinical Practice [70]

This is a machine-generated summary of:

Nicolucci, Antonio; Candido, Riccardo; Cucinotta, Domenico; Graziano, Giusi; Rocca, Alberto; Rossi, Maria C.; Tuccinardi, Franco; Manicardi, Valeria: Generalizability of Cardiovascular Safety Trials on SGLT2 Inhibitors to the Real World: Implications for Clinical Practice [70].

Published in: Advances in Therapy (2019).

Link to original: https://doi.org/10.1007/s12325-019-01043-z

If you want to cite the papers, please refer to the original.

For technical reasons we could not place the page where the original quote is coming from.

Abstract-Summary "The aim of the present study was to investigate the generalizability of CVOTs on SGLT2i to Italian adults with T2DM; we estimated the proportions of this patient population who would be eligible for enrollment in EMPA-REG OUTCOME (empagliflozin), CANVAS (canagliflozin), DECLARE-TIMI 58 (dapagliflozin), and VERTIS-CV (ertugliflozin) studies."

"Data on 455,662 adult patients with T2DM seen during 2016 were analyzed against the published patient eligibility criteria for the four CVOTs."

"The current use of SGLT2i in potentially eligible patients was assessed."

"Among the population identified, the proportion of patients meeting major eligibility criteria was 11.7% for EMPA-REG OUTCOME, 29.4% for CANVAS, 55.9% for DECLARE-TIMI 58, and 12.8% for VERTIS-CV."

"Of the patients eligible for these CVOTs, only a minority (range 4.4–6.8%) was actually prescribed an SGLT2i."

"The percentage of patients potentially eligible for treatment with SGLT2i varies as a reflection of different eligibility criteria applied in the trials."

Introduction

"Following the US Food and Drug Administration (FDA) guidance on the evaluation of novel agents for the treatment of T2DM with respect to major adverse cardiac events [71], a number of cardiovascular outcomes safety trials (CVOTs) have been conducted."

"These differences in study populations may prevent meaningful comparisons between the findings of the different CVOTs, and pose problems when assessing the potential CV safety of a particular treatment in a real-world T2DM population."

"The aim of our study was to estimate the proportions of this patient population who would be eligible for enrollment in each of these studies, and compare the characteristics of the CVOTs populations with those of everyday practice patients potentially eligible for these trials; we also evaluated which proportion of all potentially eligible patients was actually treated with an SGLT2i."

Methods

"This observational, cross-sectional study was conducted in a network of 222 Italian diabetes clinics participating in the last edition of AMD Annals initiative."

"These centers, accounting for approximately one-fourth of all the clinics operating within the national healthcare system, all share the same software for data extraction from electronic medical records."

"Data from participating centers are annually collected and centrally analyzed anonymously."

"The primary aim of the study was to estimate the proportion of adults with T2DM attending diabetes clinics in Italy who would meet the criteria for inclusion in each of the four SGLT2i CVOTs."

"On the basis of Italian regulations, the written informed consent from participants was not required, being extracted data anonymous."

Results

"Patients in the AMD Annals database were less likely to be treated with metformin and secretagogues, and more likely to be treated with DPP-IV inhibitors and insulin."

"Patients in the AMD Annals database were less likely to be treated with metformin and secretagogues, and more likely to be treated with DPP-IV inhibitors."

"Patients in the AMD Annals database were less likely to be treated with metformin and secretagogues, and more likely to be treated with DPP-IV inhibitors and insulin."

"There were 342,205 patients in the AMD Annals database evaluable for eligibility in VERTIS-CV, of whom 51.4% had an HbA1c value between 7.0% and 10.5%, and 23.6% had established CV disease."

"Patients in the AMD Annals database were less likely to be treated with metformin and secretagogues, and more likely to be treated with DPP-IV inhibitors and insulin."

Discussion

"The difference in percentages closely reflects the inclusion of patients with established CV disease only, as in the case of EMPA-REG OUTCOME and VERTIS, or also patients carrying multiple CV risk factors, as in DECLARE-TIMI 58 and CANVAS."

"Compared with a similar study conducted in the USA [72], percentages of patients eligible for the different CVOTs were higher in Italy (DECLARE-TIMI 58: 55.9% vs. 39.8%; EMPA-REG OUTCOME: 11.7% vs. 4.1%; CANVAS: 29.4% vs. 8.8%; VERTIS-CV 12.8% vs. 4.8%)."

"Compared with patients in the CVOTs, eligible patients in the AMD Annals database differed in many aspects, including older age and longer diabetes duration, lower BMI and HbA1c levels, lower prevalence of established cardiovascular and cerebrovascular disease, higher rates of microvascular complications and peripheral arterial disease, and different glucose-lowering and cardiovascular background therapies."

Conclusions

"Our study shows that the percentage of patients potentially eligible for treatment with agents that demonstrated CV risk reduction in recent CVOTs varies as a reflection of different eligibility criteria applied in the trials."

"These differences should be taken into consideration when evaluating the generalizability and applicability of CVOTs to real-world populations."

"A large number of patients that could benefit from SGLT2i in terms of not only CV protection but also renal protection do not receive the treatment."

"Since existing CVOTs targeted high-risk populations, with either established CV disease or multiple CV risk factors, the treatment of choice when low-risk patients require therapy intensification remains to be established."

SGLT2 Inhibitors Through the Windows of EMPA-REG and CANVAS Trials: A Review [73]

This is a machine-generated summary of:

Rastogi, Ashu; Bhansali, Anil: SGLT2 Inhibitors Through the Windows of EMPA-REG and CANVAS Trials: A Review [73].

Published in: Diabetes Therapy (2017).

Link to original: https://doi.org/10.1007/s13300-017-0320-1

If you want to cite the papers, please refer to the original.

For technical reasons we could not place the page where the original quote is coming from.

Abstract-Summary "EMPA-REG OUTCOME and CANVAS trials were designed to study the cardiovascular safety of empagliflozin and canagliflozin, respectively."

"Further, all patients in EMPA-REG had prior CV events (secondary prevention), compared to CANVAS that also included subjects with no prior CV events, indicating the beneficial effects of canagliflozin in primary prevention of CV events as well."

"Increases in lower extremity amputation and fracture incidence were observed with canagliflozin in CANVAS and this needs further substantiation, though these events were not systematically captured in the EMPA-REG study."

Introduction

"The US Food and Drug Administration (FDA) 2008 regulations mandate the sponsors to conduct cardiovascular outcome trials (CVOTs) for ensuring cardiovascular (CV) safety of newly marketed antidiabetes agents [74]."

"CVOTs have been conducted for both empagliflozin and canagliflozin to test for non-inferiority for the prespecified primary CV outcome variables with HR of less than 1.3."

"The CV outcome results of empagliflozin cardiovascular outcomes and mortality in type 2 diabetes trial (EMPA-REG) [18] and canagliflozin cardiovascular assessment study (CANVAS) [56] with empagliflozin and canagliflozin, respectively, have demonstrated tangible benefits beyond the thoughts of the diabetes-treating community."

"The SGLT2i are another class of oral antihyperglycemic drugs (OADs) that have exhibited beneficial CV outcomes independent of glycemic control."

Study Design

"Both CANVAS and EMPA-REG trials had a large sample size, included subjects with high CV risk, had well-defined primary endpoints and predefined criteria for event adjudication."

"All patients in EMPA-REG study had prior CV events compared to CANVAS that also included subjects (33%) with no prior CV events."

"The CANVAS trial included the pooled results of two separate cohorts, i.e., CANVAS primarily aimed for three-point major adverse cardiovascular events (3P-MACE) and CANVAS-R for renal outcomes, which is likely to introduce an inherent bias for the analysis of primary outcomes, as pooled data of two different cohorts with separate aims makes it statistically less robust."

"Both the EMPA-REG and CANVAS trials examined the exploratory variables despite this limitation [18, 56, 75]."

CV Outcome

"Canagliflozin decreased the 3P-MACE by 14% (HR 0.86, 95% CI 0.75–0.97), which is a composite of CV death, non-fatal myocardial infarction and non-fatal stroke in CANVAS, identical to empagliflozin (HR 0.86; 95% CI 0.74–0.99, $p = 0.04$ for superiority) in the EMPA-REG study [18, 56]."

"The individual components of 3P-MACE in the EMPA-REG trial showed a trend for non-inferiority (HR either side of 1.0), except for CV deaths (HR 0.62, 95% CI 0.49–0.77), which was the major driver for 3P-MACE reduction."

"Yes, it is probably true, as subjects with prior CV events in the CANVAS trial had 18% reduction in CV death (HR 0.82, 95% CI 0.72–0.95) compared to only 2% in those without prior CV events (HR 0.98, 95% CI 0.74–1.30)."

Time Point for CV Benefits

"Divergence in the survival curve for MACE was observed at 3 months in the EMPA-REG study (as the curved lines started drifting at 3 months) as opposed to at approximately 1 year in the CANVAS trial [18, 56]."

"An early separation in the survival curve lines with empagliflozin has been attributed to the hemodynamic effects [76], alternate fuel hypothesis [77, 78], favorable lipid profile [18], and improved endothelial function [18]."

"The effect of canagliflozin on MACE was observed after a year, thereby suggesting the predominant favorable effect on atherosclerosis, as the process of atherosclerosis is heralded only in months or years and not within a few weeks of intervention."

"All plausible explanations require further substantiation."

Ethnic Variations in CV Benefits

"There were appreciable ethnic differences in the CV outcomes in both trials."

"Similar geographical variations in all-cause and CV mortality have been observed amongst patients with diabetes from North America and the rest of the world with intensive versus conventional glycemic control across ACCORD, ADVANCE, PROactive, UDGP, and VADT trials [79]."

"There was an increase in all-cause and CV mortality in North America compared with the rest of the world."

Effect on Non-fatal Stroke

"Canagliflozin reduced the risk of non-fatal stroke by 10% (HR 0.90, 95% CI 0.71–1.15), unlike empagliflozin that increased the risk by 24% (HR 1.24, 95% CI 0.92–1.67), though the difference was not statistically significant ($p = 0.16$) [18, 56]."

"Further, the hazard ratio for stroke was similar irrespective of systolic [HR 1.14 (0.77, 1.68 CI)] and diastolic blood pressure control [HR 1.23 (0.82, 1.85 CI)] (> 140/90 versus < 140/90 mmHg, $p = 0.79$ for interaction) with empagliflozin in the EMPA-REG study [18]."

"A higher rate of stroke incidence observed with empagliflozin was in spite of a similar reduction in systolic and diastolic blood pressure with either empagliflozin or canagliflozin in the two trials [18, 56]."

Effect on Renal Outcome

"Both EMPA-REG [80] and CANVAS [56] trials demonstrated significant renal benefits despite renal outcome measures adjudicated in the two trials being broadly dissimilar and annihilating a head-to-head comparison of renal benefits."

"CANVAS participants had a 27% reduction in albuminuria progression (HR 0.73, 95% CI 0.67–0.79) and 40% reduction in the composite renal outcome (HR 0.60, 95% CI 0.47–0.77) [defined as 40% reduction in the estimated glomerular filtration rate (eGFR), the need for renal replacement therapy, or death from renal causes]."

"The EMPA-REG study also showed a 38% reduction (HR 0.62, 95% CI 0.54–0.72) in progression to macroalbuminuria and 39% reduction in incident or worsening nephropathy (HR 0.61, 95% CI 0.53–0.70) (defined as progression to macroalbuminuria, doubling of serum creatinine, requirement for renal replacement therapy, or death due to renal events)."

Adverse Events

"One surprise was the almost twofold increased risk for lower extremity amputations (LEA) with canagliflozin (HR 1.97; 95% CI 1.41–2.75, $p < 0.001$), unlike empagliflozin."

"Further, the US FDA Adverse Event Reporting System (FAERS) analysis exhibited a higher frequency of LEA (including any amputation and toe amputation) with canagliflozin with a proportional reporting ratio (PRR) of 5.33 (95% CI 4.04–7.04, $p < 0.0001$), 0.25 with dapagliflozin, and 2.37 with empagliflozin compared to non-SGLT2i agents for diabetes indication [81]."

"The possible explanations for increased risk of fracture risk include increase in serum phosphate and consequent secondary hyperparathyroidism, postural fall due to volume depletion (HR 1.03 with empagliflozin and HR 1.44 with canagliflozin) [82], decrease in estrogen secretion subsequent to weight loss (predominantly fat), and possible decrease in BMD [83]."

Conclusions

"Both EMPA-REG and CANVAS have provided us an opportunity to tunnel away from the glucocentric approach and think beyond the glycemic benefits of OADs towards improved cardiovascular and renal outcomes."

"The comparison of results between EMA-REG and CANVAS is confounded by the differences in the enrolled subjects, design of the trials, and analytical approach."

"Superiority for CV outcomes is shown by both trials in subjects with prior CVD, but empagliflozin fared better in Asian subjects."

Use of Animal Models for Investigating Cardioprotective Roles of SGLT2 Inhibitors [84]

This is a machine-generated summary of:

Al Thani, Najlaa A.; Hasan, Maram; Yalcin, Huseyin C.: Use of Animal Models for Investigating Cardioprotective Roles of SGLT2 Inhibitors [84].

Published in: Journal of Cardiovascular Translational Research (2023).

Link to original: https://doi.org/10.1007/s12265-023-10379-5

If you want to cite the papers, please refer to the original.

For technical reasons we could not place the page where the original quote is coming from.

Abstract-Summary "A good number of randomized clinical trials revealed that SGLT2is significantly prevented heart failure (HF) and cardiovascular death in T2DM patients."

"Despite ongoing clinical trials in HF patients without T2DM, there have been a limited number of translational studies on the cardioprotective properties of SGLT2is."

"We summarize the animal models constructed to study the cardioprotective mechanisms of SGLT2is to help deliver a more comprehensive understanding of the in vivo work that has been done in this field and to help select the most optimal animal model to use when studying the different cardioprotective effects of SGLT2is."

Introduction

"To SGLT2is' direct benefits in T2DM, studies have witnessed cardiac improvements in patients treated with gliflozins through large randomized clinical trials."

"The most notable major clinical SGLT2i trials include the EMPA Cardiovascular Outcome Event Trial in T2DM Patients (EMPA-REG OUTCOME) [18], the Canagliflozin Cardiovascular Assessment Study (CANVAS) program [56], the Dapagliflozin Effect on Cardiovascular Events–Thrombolysis in Myocardial Infarction 58 (DECLARE-TIMI58) trial [85], and the Dapagliflozin and Prevention of Adverse Outcomes in Heart Failure (DAPA-HF) trial [55]."

"Other hypotheses include whether cardioprotective mechanisms are mediated by SGLT2i binding directly to SGLT2 in cardiac cells or indirectly by upregulating SGLT1 expression in cardiovascular disease [86]."

"Animal models used to study the cardioprotective mechanisms of SGLT2i will be summarized."

"This paper aims to help elucidate the cardioprotective effects of SGLT2is observed in human clinical trials by summarizing the cardioprotective effects studied in SGLT2i animal models in the hopes that this may aid future clinical research of SGLT2is and its usage as a form of cardiac therapy."

Rodent Models

"The following studies that investigated SGLT2is' cardiac remodeling effects in rodent models have also examined and suggested potential mechanisms and pathways involved including anti-metabolic and inflammatory pathways, oxidative stress mechanisms, and possible microbiota involvement."

"In a study using T2DM KK-Ay mice, Li and others (2019) [87] investigated the effect of SGLTi EMPA on myocardial injury (MI) of the left ventricle (LV) and the potential anti-inflammatory mechanism behind observed cardiac remodeling effects."

"In an alternative study looking into relating SGLT2i's cardiac remodeling effects and several potential causative pathways, Lee and others (2019) [88] used a spontaneous hypertensive rat (SHR) model to study the effect of SGLT2i EMPA and subsequent cardiac remodeling effects."

"In a study conducted by Nambu and others (2020) [89], the effects of SGLT2i EMPA were investigated on exercise endurance plus the function of skeletal muscle mitochondria with the oxidation process of fatty acid in male C57BL/6 J mice model with HF after the induction of MI and administration of EMPA."

Pig Models

"Due to the pig model's suitability to elucidate metabolic queries of the human metabolism, the few SGLT2i pig model studies revolve mainly around metabolic alterations following MI and SGLT2i treatment with a focus on the cardiac remodeling of swine hearts."

"Further data from this study demonstrates that CANA preserves cardiac contractile function and efficiency during acute regional MI through acute effects on cardiac volume regulation that cannot be explained by myocardial fuel switching also known as the "thrifty fuel" hypothesis as no changes in myocardial uptake of glucose, lactate, ketones, or free fatty acid were seen in this study; however, since metabolically normal pigs were used, this could have limited the examination of the metabolic remodeling effects."

"In the study conducted by Santos-Gallego and others (2019) [90] using nondiabetic pig specimens, data demonstrated that using SGLT2i EMPA to inhibit SGLT2 chronically improves adverse anatomical LV remodeling, enhances LV systolic function, and decreases neurohormonal activation in a nondiabetic pig model of HF."

Rabbit Models

"Similar to pig models, there is not much research carried out on SGLT2i's cardioprotective effects using rabbits."

"The few studies published focus on the effects of SGLT2i on $[Na^+]$ and $[Ca^{2+}]$ cardiac concentrations and SGLT2i's anti-atherosclerotic and anti-inflammatory effects."

"By using SGLT2i EMPA treatment, NHE flux was directly inhibited, causing a reduction in cytoplasmic $[Na^+]$ and cytoplasmic $[Ca^{2+}]$ and increased mitochondrial $[Ca^{2+}]$ in rabbit cardiomyocytes."

"Another SGLT2i study involving rabbit models looked into the anti-atherosclerotic and anti-inflammatory effects of SGLT2i."

"Lee and others (2020) [91] studied the changes in the polarization of M1 and M2 macrophages and the expression of a number of inflammatory mediators as effective elements in the protective mechanism of SGLT2i DAPA against the progression of atherosclerosis in a normoglycemic atherosclerotic rabbit model."

Zebrafish Models

"Only one zebrafish animal model study of SGLT2i's cardioprotective effects has been conducted."

"Shi and others (2017) [92] examined biomarker changes elicited by SGLT2i EMPA in a validated zebrafish model of heart failure."

"The increase in NPPA (ANP) and NPPB (BNP) expression in zebrafish embryos that were exposed to aristolochic acid (AA) to induce HF was reversed in HF embryos treated with EMPA."

"To further confirm if the effects of EMPA were mediated through SGLT2 inhibition, SGLT2 (slc5a2 gene) morpholino knockdown (MO) zebrafish embryos were created and treated with AA to see if similar results to the EMPA-treated embryos could be produced."

"Their findings showed that the SGLT2 MO zebrafish models have similar upregulated expressions of NPPB as well as reduced the expression of anti-inflammatory genes cox-2 and IL-1β."

Next Steps: Limitations and Future Directions

"The key studies previously mentioned in this review studying SGLT2i's cardioprotective effects in animal models have highlighted potential limitations associated with various animal models that should be considered in future directions."

"In this review, the most popular animal model to study the cardioprotective effects of SGLT2is is the rodent model."

"In regard to their suitability as an animal model for cardiac studies, several critical differences between humans and rodents limit their potential as an ideal model for elucidating the pathogenesis of cardioprotective effects of SGLT2is [93]."

"All metabolites detected in monkeys were also found in humans, further confirming that NHPs provide a more realistic animal model for SGLT2i studies [94]."

"Drosophilae are also fairly easy to manage and have been extensively studied, having been previously used in T2DM and insulin signaling studies, and could pose as a potential animal model for the study of SGLT2i's cardioprotective effects [95]."

Conclusion

"The cardioprotective effects of SGLT2i can be classified into three separate remodeling outcomes: cardiac remodeling, ionic remodeling, and metabolic remodeling."

"Cardiac remodeling is a result of improved cardiac tissue plasticity, elasticity, and overall function that can be attributed to anti-inflammatory properties of SGLT2i."

"Ionic remodeling is a result of improved ionic homeostasis within cardiac tissues following SGLT2i treatment."

"This would be a result of the lack of bioavailable glucose following SGLT2i treatment."

Research into the Effect of SGLT2 Inhibition on Left Ventricular Remodelling in Patients with Heart Failure and Diabetes Mellitus (REFORM) Trial Rationale and Design [96]

This is a machine-generated summary of:

Singh, Jagdeep S. S.; Fathi, Amir; Vickneson, Keeran; Mordi, Ify; Mohan, Mohapradeep; Houston, J. Graeme; Pearson, Ewan R.; Struthers, Allan D.; Lang, Chim C.: Research into the effect Of SGLT2 inhibition on left ventricular remodelling in patients with heart failure and diabetes mellitus (REFORM) trial rationale and design [96].

Published in: Cardiovascular Diabetology (2016).

Link to original: https://doi.org/10.1186/s12933-016-0419-0

If you want to cite the papers, please refer to the original.

For technical reasons we could not place the page where the original quote is coming from.

Abstract-Summary "Heart failure (HF) and diabetes (DM) are a lethal combination."

"The current armamentarium of anti-diabetic agents has been shown to be less efficacious and sometimes even harmful in diabetic patients with concomitant cardiovascular disease, especially HF."

"Sodium glucose linked co-transporter type 2 (SGLT2) inhibitors are a new class of anti-diabetic agent that has shown potentially beneficial cardiovascular effects such as pre-load and after load reduction through osmotic diuresis, blood pressure reduction, reduced arterial stiffness and weight loss."

"This has been supported by the recently published EMPA-REG trial which showed a striking 38 and 35% reduction in cardiovascular death and HF hospitalisation respectively."

"It is designed specifically to test the safety and efficacy of the SLGT2 inhibitor, dapagliflozin, on diabetic patients with known HF."

"This trial will be able to determine if SGLT2 inhibitor therapy produces potentially beneficial effects in patients with DM and HF, thereby replacing current medications as the drug of choice when treating patients with both DM and HF."

Background

"This association can be lethal since DM has consistently been shown to be an independent predictor of increased morbidity and mortality in patients with HF; [97] patients with DM and HF have a median survival of 4 years [98]."

"For most patients, metformin is the first choice anti-diabetic drug in type 2 DM including those with HF."

"Metformin alone is often not enough to keep glycaemia under control and there frequently is a need for a second line anti-diabetic drug in patients with HF and DM."

"The additional natriuretic effect (and resultant osmotic diuresis) of SGLT2 inhibitors could potentially be beneficial in patients with cardiovascular disease, especially those with HF, thereby distinguishing SGLT2-inhibitors from all the other oral anti-diabetic agents."

"The EMPA-REG Outcomes trial had demonstrated a remarkable reduction in CV mortality and HF hospitalisations, by 38 and 35% respectively, among patients with high CV risk who were treated with empagliflozin [18]."

Methods

"The primary outcome is to determine if dapagliflozin induces a change in LV end systolic volume (ESV) or LV end diastolic volume (EDV) in patients with DM associated HF when compared to placebo."

"To determine if there is a change in LV mass, LV ejection fraction (EF), right ventricular (RV) EDV, RV ESV, RV EF, atrial dimensions and volumes, and LV remodelling index (RI) (LV mass/LVEDV) with dapagliflozin in DM associated HF compared with placebo."

"To determine if dapagliflozin can improve exercise tolerance in DM patients with HF as measured by pre and post 6 min walk test and CPEX."

"To determine if dapagliflozin use results in any change in diuretic dose among patients with DM and HF."

"It was also determined that the SD for 10 g mean change in LV mass in the HF population is 9.6 using cardiac MRI, implying 20 patients are required per arm [99]."

Discussion

"This effect of SGLT2 inhibitors on positive LV remodelling will have major implications on morbidity and mortality in patients with DM and HF."

"By ensuring the trial is adequately powered for all three facets of LV remodelling we will, for the first time in humans, determine if treatment with an SGLT2 inhibitor be able to induce positive LV remodelling in diabetic patients with HF."

"By causing weight loss and improving insulin sensitivity, SGLT2 inhibitors could significantly increase the effort tolerance of patients with HF, thereby reducing morbidity and mortality."

"The EMPA-REG Outcomes trial revealed potentially beneficial effects of empagliflozin among patients with HF, however it is unknown if these effects are seen throughout the SGLT2 inhibitor class."

"This study will be able to provide insights into the mechanism of the positive cardiovascular effects conferred by SGLT2 inhibitor therapy and may also help underpin future outcome trials in HF patients involving this drug class."

Limitations

"This is a relatively small, single centre trial."

"The use of cardiac MRI has allowed the power of the trial to be preserved despite the small number of participants."

"This may necessitate dose adjustments during the trial which could confound the final outcome."

Conclusions

"SGLT2 inhibitors could potentially improve LV remodelling and exercise capacity in these patients, thus offering an important new approach to HF management in DM."

"If they improve exercise capacity and LV remodelling in HF by reducing both preload and afterload, a strong case could be made for a larger trial specifically in HF patients with DM to test if SGLT2 inhibitors really do have a mortality benefit in this unique patient group."

"This study will, with careful monitoring, begin to address this combination, and for the reasons given above, it is likely to be more beneficial than harmful in patients with HF."

"If this study shows that SGLT2 inhibitors have the dual effect of being a diuretic and favourably remodelling the LV in HF patients, then they would stand head and shoulders above other potential second line anti-diabetics for use in HF patients."

Informing and Empowering Patients and Clinicians to Make Evidence-Supported Outcome-Based Decisions in Relation to SGLT2 Inhibitor Therapies: The Use of the Novel Years of Drug Administration (YoDa) Concept [100]

This is a machine-generated summary of:

Varadhan, Lakshminarayanan; Saravanan, Ponnusamy; Ali, Sarah N.; Hanif, Wasim; Patel, Vinod: Informing and Empowering Patients and Clinicians to Make Evidence-Supported Outcome-Based Decisions in Relation to SGLT2 Inhibitor Therapies: The Use of the Novel Years of Drug administration (YoDa) Concept [100].

Published in: Clinical Drug Investigation (2022).

Link to original: https://doi.org/10.1007/s40261-021-01105-7

If you want to cite the papers, please refer to the original.

For technical reasons we could not place the page where the original quote is coming from.

Abstract-Summary "The American Diabetes Association guidelines for the management of type 2 diabetes mellitus recommends treating patients with atherosclerotic cardiovascular diseases, heart failure or diabetic kidney disease with sodium-glucose co-transporter-2 inhibitors or glucagon-like peptide-1 receptor agonists, irrespective of the baseline HbA1c, to reduce adverse renal and cardiovascular outcomes."

"We propose using the calculated 'YoDa' (Years of Drug administration) as an easily comparable metric between the drug accrual cost and clinical outcomes."

"YoDa is calculated as a product of numbers needed to treat and the median duration in years that the trial ran over, to accrue the positive clinical outcomes."

"We also propose a series of steps or 'deliberations', which a clinician should consider in making a final choice of sodium-glucose co-transporter-2 inhibitor therapy."

"A comprehensive summary of the sodium-glucose co-transporter-2 inhibitor trials, clinical phenotyping and YoDa calculations for various significant clinical outcomes could assist making evidence-based, patient-individualised and cost-effective management plans for diabetes care."

Introduction

"These studies were primarily conducted to show non-inferiority and cardiovascular (CV) safety to comply with US Food and Drug Administration regulatory requirements for new glucose-lowering agents in T2D. The European Association for the Study of Diabetes-American Diabetes Association (EASD-ADA) consensus guidelines proposed the use of a SGLT2i as a preferred second-line drug, in patients with established atherosclerotic cardiovascular disease (ASCVD), HF with reduced ejection fraction or chronic kidney disease (CKD) with significant proteinuria [101]."

"Individual drug choice should therefore depend on patient preferences for the potential beneficial outcomes; a clinician's informed decision making, comparable cost effectiveness and the evidence base."

"The objective of this article is to provide a clinical summary of the various SGLT2i CVOTs published and discuss how the positive clinical outcomes from the trial data can be applied to specific patient groups with T2D. The EASD-ADA guideline step of considering SGLT2i in patients with established atherosclerotic disease, HF or diabetic kidney disease (DKD) will be examined from a clinical efficacy and cost-efficiency perspective to guide choosing between the drugs [102]."

Years of Drug Administration: YoDa Concept

"This is a useful result, a study of 5 years duration vs 3 years would result in very different years of treatment, which could be translated into potential costs to accrue a benefit."

"The YoDa can then be multiplied by the annual cost of the drug, (which is commonly readily available from sources such as the British National Formulary and ADA Guidelines 2021) to provide an indication of the cost of deferring or saving an event from occurring, at least for the duration equal to the length of the trial from which such evidence is derived [102, 103]."

"The idea may also help compare the cost effectiveness of drugs across various studies; for instance, the MICRO-HOPE study showed that the NNT for ramipril, for MACE prevention, was 22 for 4.5 years."

SGLT2i Trials

"Multiple CVOTs and independent randomised controlled trials have been published on the safety and outcomes of SGLT2i in patients with T2D, specifically looking at MACE (combination of CV death, non-fatal myocardial infarction or non-fatal stroke), but also reporting on benefits with hospitalisation for HF (hHF), CKD progression and all-cause mortality."

"The ADA guidelines advise the initiation of SGLT2i or GLP-1RA in patients with established ASCVD or patients with very high risk of such events [102]."

"The inclusion criteria of many of the trials had an overlap of established or high risk for a CV event labelled under the umbrella of ASCVD."

"The NNT to prevent one event is not often included for all outcomes but can be calculated from the absolute risk reduction data presented in the relevant papers."

Using the SGLT2i Trial Data in Clinical Practice

"EMPA-REG OUTCOME assessed the safety and efficacy of empagliflozin in patients with ASCVD and showed a modest but significant 14% reduction in MACE (largely driven by a 38% reduction in CV deaths), a 32% reduction in all-cause mortality, a 35% reduction in incident HF or hHF, and a 36% reduction in renal endpoints [18]."

"Both these studies showed significant reductions in the combination of CV deaths or hHF, driven by HF protection predominantly, and no heterogeneity in outcomes between patients with ASCVD or risk factors, but the benefit for CV deaths or hHF was generally more in the ASCVD cohort."

"The ADA recommends the use of SGLT2i (or GLP-1RA) with proven CV benefits in this 'clinical phenotype' of patients with CKD (such as an estimated GFR < 60 mL/min/1.73 m^2), irrespective of HbA1c, with a primary treatment intention to reduce CV events and reduce progression to end-stage renal disease."

Discussion

"CVD-REAL, a large database comparative study of SGLT2i with other antidiabetic medications, showed a significant 39% reduction in hHF and a 51% reduction in all-cause mortality, with a large proportion of patients not having ASCVD, and therefore proving that the benefit may also extend to patients with low CV risk [104, 105]."

"A comparative study combining the various published studies amongst these two classes have demonstrated that SGLT2i, as a class, has significant benefits in hHF and CKD progression compared with GLP-1RA [106]."

"A comparison between these two classes also demonstrated that the adverse CV and renal outcomes were fewer with SGLT2i (apart from strokes) compared with GLP-1RA on similar cohorts of patients [107]."

"The YoDa calculation is useful to provide simple clinical guidance to choose between the drugs and is not meant to directly compare or brand a particular drug as less or more effective than the others in the class."

Limitations

"A number of benefits such as overall secondary prevention of MACE and hHF and a reduction in renal outcomes with SGLT2i can be a class effect and might be generalized between the drugs; the trials however had not consistently demonstrated this depending on the patient's inclusion characteristics and choosing a drug within the SGLT2i class can be difficult and challenging [108, 109]."

"A combination of clinical phenotyping, accessible trial data to the patient and clinician, and YoDa can guide an appropriate choice."

"Further, various other factors such as patient characteristics and priorities, individualised clinical outcome targets and other co-morbidities influence decision making."

"A sub-analysis of cohorts in larger trials (such as patients with ASCVD in CANVAS or DECLARE-TIMI 58) may yield a different NNT."

"Using the median duration of a trial, as an equivalent of treatment duration to measure cost effectiveness, has its own limitations."

Conclusions

"The YoDa concept provides a triangulated approach between the evidence base from randomised controlled trials, clinical phenotyping and practical cost consideration to facilitate effective clinical decision making."

"With the latest diabetes management recommendations moving away from using the HbA1c alone as the primary target and instead focusing on CV outcomes, the deliberation-based stepwise approach and YoDa can serve as an effective approach to guide management planning."

"The summaries of key SGLT2i landmark studies and the novel approaches used in this paper would help facilitate the process of informed decision making, with the patient as the centre of focus of care."

"The above deliberations can provide a template to review the risk profile and clinical treatment target of the patient at each consultation to tailor treatment choices."

Bibliography

1. Joshi SS, Singh T, Newby DE, Singh J (2021) Sodium-glucose co-transporter 2 inhibitor therapy: mechanisms of action in heart failure. Heart 107(13):1032–1038
2. Al Thani NA, Hasan M, Yalcin HC (2023) Use of animal models for investigating cardioprotective roles of SGLT2 inhibitors. J Cardiovasc Transl Res 16(5):975–986
3. Chin KL, Ofori-Asenso R, Hopper I, von Lueder TG, Reid CM, Zoungas S, Wang BH, Liew D (2019) Potential mechanisms underlying the cardiovascular benefits of sodium glucose cotransporter 2 inhibitors: a systematic review of data from preclinical studies. Cardiovasc Res 115(2):266–276
4. Frąk W, Hajdys J, Radzioch E, Szlagor M, Młynarska E, Rysz J, Franczyk B (2023) Cardiovascular diseases: therapeutic potential of SGLT-2 inhibitors. Biomedicine 11(7):2085
5. Carluccio E, Biagioli P, Reboldi G, Mengoni A, Lauciello R, Zuchi C, D'Addario S, Bardelli G, Ambrosio G (2023) Left ventricular remodeling response to SGLT2 inhibitors in heart failure: an updated meta-analysis of randomized controlled studies. Cardiovasc Diabetol 22(1):235
6. Verma S, Mazer CD, Yan AT, Mason T, Garg V, Teoh H, Zuo F, Quan A, Farkouh ME, Fitchett DH, Goodman SG (2019) Effect of empagliflozin on left ventricular mass in patients with type 2 diabetes mellitus and coronary artery disease: the EMPA-HEART CardioLink-6 randomized clinical trial. Circulation 140(21):1693–1702
7. Kitada M, Hirai T, Koya D (2020) Significance of SGLT2 inhibitors: lessons from renal clinical outcomes in patients with type 2 diabetes and basic researches. Diabetol Int 11(3):245–251. https://doi.org/10.1007/s13340-020-00444-8
8. Ninomiya T, Perkovic V, de Galan BE et al (2009) Albuminuria and kidney function independently predict cardiovascular and renal outcomes in diabetes. J Am Soc Nephrol 20:1813–1821
9. Kitada M, Kanasaki K, Koya D (2014) Clinical therapeutic strategies for early stage of diabetic kidney disease. World J Diabetes 15(5):342–356
10. Gaede P, Vedel P, Larsen N et al (2003) Multifactorial intervention and cardiovascular disease in patients with type 2 diabetes. N Engl J Med 348:383–393
11. Araki SI (2018) Comprehensive risk management of diabetic kidney disease in patients with type 2 diabetes mellitus. Diabetol Int 9:100–107
12. Yokoyama H, Araki S, Honjo J et al (2013) Association between remission of macroalbuminuria and preservation of renal function in patients with type 2 diabetes with overt proteinuria. Diabetes Care 36:3227–3333
13. Brenner BM, Cooper ME, de Zeeuw D et al (2001) Effects of losartan on renal and cardiovascular outcomes in patients with type 2 diabetes and nephropathy. N Engl J Med 345:861–869
14. Lewis EJ, Hunsicker LG, Clarke WR et al (2001) Renoprotective effect of the angiotensin-receptor antagonist irbesartan in patients with nephropathy due to type 2 diabetes. N Engl J Med 345:851–860
15. Zinman B, Wanner C, Lachin JM et al (2015) Empagliflozin, cardiovascular outcomes, and mortality in type 2 diabetes. N Engl J Med 373:2117–2288
16. Koya D (2019) Diabetic kidney disease: its current trends and future therapeutic perspectives. J Diabetes Investig 10:1174–1176
17. Katakami N, Mita T, Yoshii H, Shiraiwa T, Yasuda T, Okada Y, Umayahara Y, Kaneto H, Osonoi T, Yamamoto T, Kuribayashi N, Maeda K, Yokoyama H, Kosugi K, Ohtoshi K, Hayashi I, Sumitani S, Tsugawa M, Ohashi M, Taki H, Nakamura T, Kawashima S, Sato Y, Watada H, Shimomura I, On behalf of the UTOPIA study investigators (2017) None rationale, design, and baseline characteristics of the Utopia trial for preventing diabetic atherosclerosis using an SGLT2 inhibitor: a prospective, randomized, open-label, parallel-group comparative study. Diabetes Ther 8(5):999–1013. https://doi.org/10.1007/s13300-017-0292-1
18. Zinman B, Wanner C, Lachin JM, Fitchett D, Bluhmki E, Hantel S et al (2015) Empagliflozin, cardiovascular outcomes, and mortality in type 2 diabetes. N Engl J Med 373(22):2117–2128

19. Kaku K, Watada H, Iwamoto Y, Utsunomiya K, Terauchi Y, Tobe K et al (2014) Efficacy and safety of monotherapy with the novel sodium/glucose cotransporter-2 inhibitor tofogliflozin in Japanese patients with type 2 diabetes mellitus: a combined Phase 2 and 3 randomized, placebo-controlled, double-blind, parallel-group comparative study. Cardiovasc Diabetol 13:65
20. Katakami N, Yamasaki Y, Hayaishi-Okano R, Ohtoshi K, Kaneto H, Matsuhisa M et al (2004) Metformin or gliclazide, rather than glibenclamide, attenuate progression of carotid intima-media thickness in subjects with type 2 diabetes. Diabetologia 47:1906–1913
21. Mazzone T, Meyer PM, Feinstein SB, Davidson MH, Kondos GT, D'Agostino RB Sr et al (2006) Effect of pioglitazone compared with glimepiride on carotid intima-media thickness in type 2 diabetes: a randomized trial. JAMA 296:2572–2581
22. Yamasaki Y, Katakami N, Furukado S, Kitagawa K, Nagatsuka K, Kashiwagi A et al (2010) Long term effects of pioglitazone on carotid atherosclerosis in Japanese patients with type 2 diabetes without a recent history of macrovascular morbidity. J Atheroscler Thromb 17:1132–1140
23. Yamasaki Y, Katakami N, Hayaishi-Okano R, Matsuhisa M, Kajimoto Y, Kosugi K et al (2005) Alpha-glucosidase inhibitor reduces the progression of carotid intima-media thickness. Diabetes Res Clin Pract 67:204–210
24. Mita T, Katakami N, Shiraiwa T, Yoshii H, Onuma T, Kuribayashi N et al (2016) Sitagliptin attenuates the progression of carotid intima-media thickening in insulin-treated patients with type 2 diabetes: the sitagliptin preventive study of intima-media thickness evaluation (SPIKE): a randomized controlled trial. Diabetes Care 39(3):455–464
25. Mita T, Katakami N, Yoshii H, Onuma T, Kaneto H, Osonoi T et al (2016) Alogliptin, a dipeptidyl peptidase 4 inhibitor, prevents the progression of carotid atherosclerosis in patients with type 2 diabetes: the study of preventive effects of alogliptin on diabetic atherosclerosis (SPEAD-A). Diabetes Care 39(1):139–148
26. Tanaka A, Murohara R, Taguchi T, Eguchi K, Suzuki M, Kitakaze M, on behalf of the PROTECT Study Investigators et al (2016) Rationale and design of a multicenter randomized controlled study to evaluate the preventive effect of ipragliflozin on carotid atherosclerosis: the PROTECT study. Cardiovasc Diabetol 15:133
27. Williams DM, Nawaz A, Evans M (2020) Sodium-glucose co-transporter 2 (SGLT2) inhibitors: are they all the same? A narrative review of cardiovascular outcome trials. Diab Ther 12(1):55–70. https://doi.org/10.1007/s13300-020-00951-6
28. Food and Drug Administration (FDA) (2008) Guidance for industry: diabetes mellitus—evaluating cardiovascular risk in new antidiabetic therapies to treat type 2 diabetes. www.fda.gov/downloads/Drugs/GuidanceComplianceRegulatoryInformation/Guidances/ucm071627.pdf . Accessed 23 Sept 2020
29. Food and Drug Administration (FDA) (2020) Type 2 diabetes mellitus: evaluating the safety of new drugs for improving glycaemic control. Guidance for industry 2020. https://www.fda.gov/regulatory-information/search-fda-guidance-documents/type-2-diabetes-mellitus-evaluating-safety-new-drugs-improving-glycemic-control-guidance-industry. Accessed 22 Sept 2020
30. Dekkers CCJ, Sjöström CD, Greasley PJ, Cain V, Boulton DW, Heerspink HJL (2019) Effects of the sodium-glucose co-transporter-2 inhibitor dapagliflozin on estimated plasma volume in patients with type 2 diabetes. Diabetes Obes Metab 21:2667–2673
31. Shigiyama F, Kumashiro N, Miyagi M et al (2017) Effectiveness of dapagliflozin on vascular endothelial function and glycemic control in patients with early-stage type 2 diabetes mellitus: DEFENCE study. Cardiovasc Diabetol 16:84
32. Packer M, Anker SD, Butler J, Filippatos G, Zannad F (2017) Effects of sodium-glucose cotransporter 2 inhibitors for the treatment of patients with heart failure: proposal of a novel mechanism of action. JAMA Cardiol 2:1025–1029

33. European Society of Cardiology (2020) DAPA-CKD trial meets primary endpoint in patients with chronic kidney disease. https://www.escardio.org/The-ESC/Press-Office/Press-releases/DAPA . Accessed 23 Sept 2020
34. Perkovic V, Jardine MJ, Neal B et al (2019) Canagliflozin and renal outcomes in type 2 diabetes and nephropathy. N Engl J Med 380:2295–2306
35. Liu J, Li L, Li S et al (2020) Sodium-glucose co-transporter-2 inhibitors and the risk of diabetic ketoacidosis in patients with type 2 diabetes: a systematic review and meta-analysis of randomized controlled trials. Diabetes Obes Metab 22(9):1619–1627
36. Clegg LE, Penland RC, Bachina S, Boulton DW, Thuresson M, Heerspink HJL, Gustavson S, Sjöström CD, Ruggles JA, Hernandez AF, Buse JB, Mentz RJ, Holman RR (2019) Effects of exenatide and open-label SGLT2 inhibitor treatment, given in parallel or sequentially, on mortality and cardiovascular and renal outcomes in type 2 diabetes: insights from the EXSCEL trial. Cardiovasc Diabetol 18(1):138. https://doi.org/10.1186/s12933-019-0942-x
37. Frías J, Guja C, Hardy E, Ahmed A, Dong F, Öhman P, Jabbour SA (2016) Exenatide once weekly plus dapagliflozin once daily versus exenatide or dapagliflozin alone in patients with type 2 diabetes inadequately controlled with metformin monotherapy (DURATION-8): a 28 week, multicentre, double-blind, phase 3, randomised controlled trial. Lancet Diabetes Endocrinol 4(12):1004–1016
38. Ludvik B, Frías JP, Tinahones FJ, Wainstein J, Jiang H, Robertson KE et al (2018) Dulaglutide as add-on therapy to SGLT2 inhibitors in patients with inadequately controlled type 2 diabetes (AWARD-10): a 24-week, randomised, double-blind, placebo-controlled trial. Lancet Diabetes Endocrinol 6(5):370–381. https://doi.org/10.1016/S2213-8587(18)30023-8
39. Zinman B, Bhosekar V, Busch R, Holst I, Ludvik B, Thielke D et al (2019) Semaglutide once weekly as add-on to SGLT-2 inhibitor therapy in type 2 diabetes (SUSTAIN 9): a randomised, placebo-controlled trial. Lancet Diabetes Endocrinol 7(5):356–367. https://doi.org/10.1016/S2213-8587(19)30066-X
40. Hardy E, Öhman P, Jabbour S, Guja C, Frias J, Bhattacharya S (eds) (2018) DURATION-8 randomized controlled trial 104-week results: efficacy and safety of once-weekly exenatide (ExQW) plus once-daily dapagliflozin (DAPA) vs ExQW or DAPA alone. European Association for the Study of Diabetes, Berlin
41. Holman RR, Bethel MA, George J, Sourij H, Doran Z, Keenan J et al (2016) Rationale and design of the EXenatide Study of Cardiovascular Event Lowering (EXSCEL) trial. Am Heart J 174:103–110. https://doi.org/10.1016/j.ahj.2015.12.009
42. Giugliano D, Maiorino MI, Bellastella G, Longo M, Chiodini P, Esposito K (2019) GLP-1 receptor agonists for prevention of cardiorenal outcomes in type 2 diabetes: an updated meta-analysis including the REWIND and PIONEER 6 trials. Diabetes Obes Metab 21(11):2576–2580. https://doi.org/10.1111/dom.13847
43. DeFronzo RA (2017) Combination therapy with GLP-1 receptor agonist and SGLT2 inhibitor. Diabetes Obes Metab 19(10):1353–1362. https://doi.org/10.1111/dom.12982
44. Goncalves E, Bell DSH (2018) Combination treatment of SGLT2 inhibitors and GLP-1 receptor agonists: symbiotic effects on metabolism and cardiorenal risk. Diabetes Ther 9(3):919–926. https://doi.org/10.1007/s13300-018-0420-6
45. Heerspink HJ, Perkins BA, Fitchett DH, Husain M, Cherney DZ (2016) Sodium glucose cotransporter 2 inhibitors in the treatment of diabetes mellitus: cardiovascular and kidney effects, potential mechanisms, and clinical applications. Circulation 134(10):752–772
46. Koufakis T, Mustafa OG, Ajjan RA, Garcia-Moll X, Zebekakis P, Dimitriadis G, Kotsa K (2022) From skepticism to hope: the evolving concept of the initiation and use of sodium-glucose cotransporter 2 inhibitors in hospitalized patients. Drugs 82(9):949–955. https://doi.org/10.1007/s40265-022-01730-2
47. Koufakis T, Mustafa OG, Ajjan RA et al (2020) The use of sodium-glucose co-transporter 2 inhibitors in the inpatient setting: is the risk worth taking? J Clin Pharm Ther 45:883–891
48. Bhatt DL, Szarek M, Steg PG et al (2021) Sotagliflozin in patients with diabetes and recent worsening heart failure. N Engl J Med 384:117–128

49. Voors AA, Angermann CE, Teerlink JR et al (2022) The SGLT2 inhibitor empagliflozin in patients hospitalized for acute heart failure: a multinational randomized trial. Nat Med 28:568–574
50. Borovac JA, Kurir T, Mustapic I et al (2022) SGLT2 inhibitors and the risk of urinary tract infections in patients with heart failure: a pooled analysis examining safety endpoints. Kardiol Pol 80:198–201
51. Mathieu C, Dandona P, Gillard P et al (2018) Efficacy and safety of dapagliflozin in patients with inadequately controlled type 1 diabetes (the DEPICT-2 Study): 24-week results from a randomized controlled trial. Diabetes Care 41:1938–1946
52. Dandona P, Mathieu C, Phillip M et al (2017) Efficacy and safety of dapagliflozin in patients with inadequately controlled type 1 diabetes (DEPICT-1): 24 week results from a multicentre, double-blind, phase 3, randomised controlled trial. Lancet Diabetes Endocrinol 5:864–876
53. Teo YN, Ting AZH, Teo YH, Chong EY, Tan JTA, Syn NL, Chia AZQ, Ong HT, Cheong AJY, Li TY-W, Poh KK, Yeo TC, Chan MY-Y, Wong RCC, Chai P, Sia C-H (2022) Effects of sodium/glucose cotransporter 2 (SGLT2) inhibitors and combined SGLT1/2 inhibitors on cardiovascular, metabolic, renal, and safety outcomes in patients with diabetes: a network meta-analysis of 111 randomized controlled trials. Am J Cardiovas Drugs 22(3):299–323. https://doi.org/10.1007/s40256-022-00528-7
54. Cannon CP, Pratley R, Dagogo-Jack S, Mancuso J, Huyck S, Masiukiewicz U et al (2020) Cardiovascular outcomes with ertugliflozin in type 2 diabetes. N Engl J Med 383(15):1425–1435
55. McMurray JJV, Solomon SD, Inzucchi SE, Køber L, Kosiborod MN, Martinez FA et al (2019) Dapagliflozin in patients with heart failure and reduced ejection fraction. N Engl J Med 381(21):1995–2008
56. Neal B, Perkovic V, Mahaffey KW, De Zeeuw D, Fulcher G, Erondu N et al (2017) Canagliflozin and cardiovascular and renal events in type 2 diabetes. N Engl J Med 377(7):644–657
57. Packer M, Anker SD, Butler J, Filippatos G, Pocock SJ, Carson P et al (2020) Cardiovascular and renal outcomes with empagliflozin in heart failure. N Engl J Med 383(15):1413–1424
58. Teo YH, Teo YN, Syn NL, Kow CS, Yoong CSY, Tan BYQ et al (2021) Effects of sodium/glucose cotransporter 2 (SGLT2) inhibitors on cardiovascular and metabolic outcomes in patients without diabetes mellitus: a systematic review and meta-analysis of randomized-controlled trials. J Am Heart Assoc 10(5):e019463
59. Higgins JPT, Chandler J, Cumpston M, Li T, Page MJ, Welch VA (2019) Cochrane handbook for systematic reviews of interventions. The Cochrane Collaboration, 2nd edn. Wiley, Chichester
60. Petrie MC, Verma S, Docherty KF et al (2020) Effect of dapagliflozin on worsening heart failure and cardiovascular death in patients with heart failure with and without diabetes. JAMA 323:1353–1368
61. Serenelli M, Böhm M, Inzucchi SE, Køber L, Kosiborod MN, Martinez FA et al (2020) Effect of dapagliflozin according to baseline systolic blood pressure in the Dapagliflozin and Prevention of Adverse Outcomes in Heart Failure trial (DAPA-HF). Eur Heart J 41(36):3402–3418. https://doi.org/10.1093/eurheartj/ehaa496
62. Persson F, Rossing P, Vart P, Chertow GM, Hou FF, Jongs N et al (2021) Efficacy and safety of dapagliflozin by baseline glycemic status: a prespecified analysis from the DAPA-CKD trial. Diabetes Care 44(8):1894–1897
63. Wheeler DC, Stefánsson BV, Jongs N, Chertow GM, Greene T, Hou FF et al (2021) Effects of dapagliflozin on major adverse kidney and cardiovascular events in patients with diabetic and non-diabetic chronic kidney disease: a prespecified analysis from the DAPA-CKD trial. Lancet Diabetes Endocrinol 9(1):22–31
64. Strojek K, Yoon KH, Hruba V, Elze M, Langkilde AM, Parikh S (2011) Effect of dapagliflozin in patients with type 2 diabetes who have inadequate glycaemic control with glimepiride: a randomized, 24-week, double-blind, placebo-controlled trial. Diabetes Obes Metab 13:928–938

65. Strojek K, Yoon KH, Hruba V, Sugg J, Langkilde AM, Parikh S (2014) Dapagliflozin added to glimepiride in patients with type 2 diabetes mellitus sustains glycemic control and weight loss over 48 weeks: a randomized, double-blind, parallel-group, placebo-controlled trial. Diabetes Ther 5(1):267–283
66. Gause-Nilsson IDT, Sugg J, Parikh SJ, Johnsson E, Leiter LA (2014) Two-year efficacy and safety of dapagliflozin for patients with type 2 diabetes mellitus and a history of cardiovascular disease. Diabetologia 57(1):S325
67. Leiter LA, Cefalu WT, de Bruin TW, Gause-Nilsson I, Sugg J, Parikh SJ (2014) Dapagliflozin added to usual care in individuals with type 2 diabetes mellitus with preexisting cardiovascular disease: a 24-week, multicenter, randomized, double-blind, placebo-controlled study with a 28-week extension. J Am Geriatr Soc 62(7):1252–1262
68. Bode B, Stenlöf K, Sullivan D, Fung A, Usiskin K (2013) Efficacy and safety of canagliflozin treatment in older subjects with type 2 diabetes mellitus: a randomized trial. Hosp Pract (1995) 41(2):72–84
69. Bode B, Stenlof K, Harris S, Sullivan D, Fung A, Usiskin K et al (2015) Long-term efficacy and safety of canagliflozin over 104 weeks in patients aged 55–80 years with type 2 diabetes. Diabetes Obes Metab 17(3):294–303
70. Nicolucci A, Candido R, Cucinotta D, Graziano G, Rocca A, Rossi MC, Tuccinardi F, Manicardi V (2019) Generalizability of cardiovascular safety trials on SGLT2 inhibitors to the real world: implications for clinical practice. Adv Ther 36(10):2895–2909. https://doi.org/10.1007/s12325-019-01043-z
71. FDA. Guidance for Industry. diabetes mellitus—evaluating cardiovascular risk in new antidiabetic therapies to treat type 2 diabetes. FDA website. https://www.fda.gov/downloads/Drugs/Guidances/ucm071627.pdf. Accessed 4 Apr 2019
72. Wittbrodt ET, Eudicone JM, Bell KF, Enhoffer DM, Latham K, Green JB (2018) Eligibility varies among the 4 sodium-glucose cotransporter-2 inhibitor cardiovascular outcomes trials: implications for the general type 2 diabetes US population. Am J Manag Care 24(8 Suppl):S138–S145
73. Rastogi A, Bhansali A (2017) SGLT2 inhibitors through the windows of EMPA-REG and CANVAS trials: a review. Diabetes Ther 8(6):1245–1251. https://doi.org/10.1007/s13300-017-0320-1
74. FDA (2008) Guidance for industry: diabetes mellitus—evaluating cardiovascular risk in new antidiabetic therapies to treat type 2 diabetes. US Department of Health and Human Resources, Washington, DC
75. Neal B, Perkovic V, Mahaffey KW et al (2017) Optimizing the analysis strategy for the CANVAS Program: a prespecified plan for the integrated analyses of the CANVAS and CANVAS-R trials. Diabetes Obes Metab 19:926–935
76. McMurray J (2015) EMPA-REG—the "diuretic hypothesis". J Diabetes Complications 30:3–4
77. Ferrannini E, Mark M, Mayoux E (2016) CV protection in the EMPA-REG OUTCOME trial: a "thrifty substrate" hypothesis. Diabetes Care 39(7):1108–1114
78. Mudaliar S, Alloju S, Henry RR (2016) Can a shift in fuel energetics explain the beneficial cardiorenal outcomes in the EMPA-REG OUTCOME Study? A unifying hypothesis. Diabetes Care 39:1115–1122. https://doi.org/10.2337/dc16-0542
79. Sardar P, Udell JA, Chatterjee S, Bansilal B, Mukherjee D, Farkouh ME (2015) Effect of intensive versus standard blood glucose control in patients with type 2 diabetes mellitus in different regions of the world: systematic review and meta analysis of randomized controlled trials. JAHA 4(5):e001577. https://doi.org/10.1161/JAHA.114.001577
80. Wanner C, Inzucchi SE, Lachin JM, Fitchett D, von Eynatten M, Mattheus M, Johansen OE, Woerle HJ, Broedl UC, Zinman B (2016) EMPA-REG OUTCOME investigators. Empagliflozin and progression of kidney disease in type 2 diabetes. N Engl J Med 375(4):323–334. https://doi.org/10.1056/NEJMoa1515920
81. Fadini GP, Avogaro A (2017) SGLT2 inhibitors and amputations in the US FDA adverse events reporting system. Lancet Diabetes Endocrinol 5:680–681

82. Watts NB, Bilezikian JP, Usiskin K et al (2016) Effects of canagliflozin on fracture risk in patients with type 2 diabetes mellitus. J Clin Endocrinol Metab 101:157–166
83. Bilezikian JP et al (2016) Evaluation of bone mineral density and bone biomarkers in patients with type 2 diabetes treated with canagliflozin. J Clin Endocrinol Metab 101(1):44–51
84. Al Thani NA, Hasan M, Yalcin HC (2023) Use of animal models for investigating cardioprotective roles of SGLT2 inhibitors. J Cardiovas Transl Res 16:975–986. https://doi.org/10.1007/s12265-023-10379-5
85. Wiviott SD, Raz I, Bonaca MP, Mosenzon O, Kato ET, Cahn A et al (2019) Dapagliflozin and cardiovascular outcomes in type 2 diabetes. N Engl J Med 380(4):347–357
86. Banerjee SK, McGaffin KR, Pastor-Soler NM, Ahmad F (2009) SGLT1 is a novel cardiac glucose transporter that is perturbed in disease states. Cardiovasc Res 84(1):111–118
87. Li C, Zhang J, Xue M, Li X, Han F, Liu X et al (2019) SGLT2 inhibition with empagliflozin attenuates myocardial oxidative stress and fibrosis in diabetic mice heart. Cardiovasc Diabetol 18(1):15. https://doi.org/10.1186/s12933-019-0816-2
88. Lee HC, Shiou YL, Jhuo SJ, Chang CY, Liu PL, Jhuang WJ et al (2019) The sodium-glucose co-transporter 2 inhibitor empagliflozin attenuates cardiac fibrosis and improves ventricular hemodynamics in hypertensive heart failure rats. Cardiovasc Diabetol 18(1):45. https://doi.org/10.1186/s12933-019-0849-6
89. Nambu H, Takada S, Fukushima A, Matsumoto J, Kakutani N, Maekawa S, Shirakawa R, Nakano I, Furihata T, Katayama T (2020) Empagliflozin restores lowered exercise endurance capacity via the activation of skeletal muscle fatty acid oxidation in a murine model of heart failure. Eur J Pharmacol 866:172810
90. Santos-Gallego CG, Requena-Ibanez JA, San Antonio R et al (2019) Empagliflozin ameliorates adverse left ventricular remodeling in nondiabetic heart failure by enhancing myocardial energetics. J Am Coll Cardiol 73(15):1931–1944
91. Lee S-G, Lee S-J, Lee J-J, Kim J-S, Lee O-H, Kim C-K, Kim D, Lee Y-H, Oh J, Park S (2020) Anti-inflammatory effect for atherosclerosis progression by sodium-glucose cotransporter 2 (SGLT-2) inhibitor in a normoglycemic rabbit model. Korean Circ J 50:443
92. Shi X, Verma S, Yun J, Brand-Arzamendi K, Singh KK, Liu X et al (2017) Effect of empagliflozin on cardiac biomarkers in a zebrafish model of heart failure: clues to the EMPA-REG OUTCOME trial? Mol Cell Biochem 433:97–102
93. Wichi R, Malfitano C, Rosa K, De Souza SB, Salemi V, Mostarda C, De Angelis K, Irigoyen MC (2007) Noninvasive and invasive evaluation of cardiac dysfunction in experimental diabetes in rodents. Cardiovasc Diabetol 6:1–7
94. Zhang W, Li X, Ding H, Lu Y, Stilwell GE, Halvorsen Y-D, Welihinda A (2020) Metabolism and disposition of the SGLT2 inhibitor bexagliflozin in rats, monkeys and humans. Xenobiotica 50:559–569
95. Hwangbo DS, Gersham B, Tu M-P, Palmer M, Tatar M (2004) Drosophila dFOXO controls lifespan and regulates insulin signalling in brain and fat body. Nature 429:562–566
96. Singh JSS, Fathi A, Vickneson K, Mordi I, Mohan M, Houston JG, Pearson ER, Struthers AD, Lang CC (2016) Research into the effect Of SGLT2 inhibition on left ventricular remodelling in patients with heart failure and diabetes mellitus (REFORM) trial rationale and design. Cardiovasc Diabetol 15:97. https://doi.org/10.1186/s12933-016-0419-0
97. Murcia AM, Hennekens CH, Lamas GA et al (2004) Impact of diabetes on mortality in patients with myocardial infarction and left ventricular dysfunction. Arch Intern Med 164(20):2273–2279
98. Cubbon RM, Adams B, Rajwani A, Mercer BN, Patel PA, Gherardi G, Gale CP, Batin PD, Ajjan R, Kearney L et al (2013) Diabetes mellitus is associated with adverse prognosis in chronic heart failure of ischaemic and non-ischaemic aetiology. Diab Vasc Dis Res 10:330–336
99. Grothues F, Smith GC, Moon JC, Bellenger NG, Collins P, Klein HU, Pennell DJ (2002) Comparison of interstudy reproducibility of cardiovascular magnetic resonance with

two-dimensional echocardiography in normal subjects and in patients with heart failure or left ventricular hypertrophy. Am J Cardiol 90:29–34

100. Varadhan L, Saravanan P, Ali SN, Hanif W, Patel V (2022) Informing and empowering patients and clinicians to make evidence-supported outcome-based decisions in relation to SGLT2 inhibitor therapies: the use of the novel Years of Drug administration (YoDa) Concept. Clin Drug Investig 42(2):113–125. https://doi.org/10.1007/s40261-021-01105-7
101. Davies MJ, D'Alessio DA, Fradkin J, Kernan WN, Mathieu C, Mingrone G et al (2018) Management of hyperglycemia in type 2 diabetes, 2018: a consensus report by the American Diabetes Association (ADA) and the European Association for the Study of Diabetes (EASD). Diabetes Care 41(12):2669–2701
102. American Diabetes Association (2021) 6. Glycemic targets: standards of medical care in diabetes: 2021. Diabetes Care 44(Suppl. 1):S73–S84
103. Joint Formulary Committee (2020) British National Formulary, 80th edn. BMJ Group and Pharmaceutical Press, London
104. Kosiborod M, Lam CSP, Kohsaka S, Kim DJ, Karasik A, Shaw J et al (2018) Cardiovascular events associated with SGLT-2 inhibitors versus other glucose-lowering drugs: the CVD-REAL 2 study. J Am Coll Cardiol 71(23):2628–2639
105. Kosiborod M, Cavender MA, Fu AZ, Wilding JP, Khunti K, Holl RW et al (2017) Lower risk of heart failure and death in patients initiated on sodium-glucose cotransporter-2 inhibitors versus other glucose-lowering drugs: the CVD-REAL Study (Comparative Effectiveness of Cardiovascular Outcomes in New Users of Sodium-Glucose Cotransporter-2 Inhibitors). Circulation 136(3):249–259
106. Zelniker TA, Wiviott SD, Raz I, Im K, Goodrich EL, Furtado RHM et al (2019) Comparison of the effects of glucagon-like peptide receptor agonists and sodium-glucose cotransporter 2 inhibitors for prevention of major adverse cardiovascular and renal outcomes in type 2 diabetes mellitus. Circulation 139(17):2022–2031
107. Palmer SC, Tendal B, Mustafa RA, Vandvik PO, Li S, Hao Q et al (2021) Sodium-glucose cotransporter protein-2 (SGLT-2) inhibitors and glucagon-like peptide-1 (GLP-1) receptor agonists for type 2 diabetes: systematic review and network meta-analysis of randomised controlled trials. BMJ 372:m4573
108. Zelniker TA, Wiviott SD, Raz I, Im K, Goodrich EL, Bonaca MP et al (2019) SGLT2 inhibitors for primary and secondary prevention of cardiovascular and renal outcomes in type 2 diabetes: a systematic review and meta-analysis of cardiovascular outcome trials. Lancet 393(10166):31–39
109. Lo KB, Gul F, Ram P, Kluger AY, Tecson KM, McCullough PA et al (2020) The effects of SGLT2 inhibitors on cardiovascular and renal outcomes in diabetic patients: a systematic review and meta-analysis. Cardiorenal Med 10(1):1–10
110. Forouzanfar MH, Moran A, Phillips D, Mensah G, Ezzati M, Naghavi M, Murray CJL (2013) Prevalence of heart failure by cause in 21 regions: global burden of diseases, injuries and risk factors-2010 study. J Am Coll Cardiol 61(10_S):E786

Chapter 8
Exploring the Current Selective Drugs of SGLT2 Inhibitors for the Treatment of Cardiovascular Disease in Type 2 Diabetes

Mukesh Nandave

Introduction by the Editor

Applications of SGLT2i in cardiovascular illness are being studied more thoroughly in addition to its efficacy in HF. The current FDA-approved drug has been mentioned in the Fig. 8.1. There is evidence from experimental studies that SGLT2i may have a cardioprotective effect after myocardial infarction. Researchers who conducted randomization 72 h before percutaneous coronary intervention (PCI) found that individuals who received empagliflozin for 26 weeks saw a substantial decrease in blood NT-proBNP levels throughout 26 weeks as compared to placebo. The Empagliflozin on Hospitalisation for Heart Failure and Mortality in Patients with Acute Myocardial Infarction (EMPACT-MI) and the Dapagliflozin Effects on Cardiovascular Events in Patients with an Acute Heart Attack (DAPA-MI), which are both listed in Table 8.1 below, are two trials that are presently being conducted to assess the effects of SGLTi on the outcomes of the cardiovascular system in myocardial infarction patients.

The American Diabetes Association (ADA) recommends using SGLT2i to treat T2D patients with heart failure (HF) or those at high risk of developing HF. SGLT2i (dapagliflozin and empagliflozin) should be used in the treatment of chronic, stable HFrEF (category 1 recommendation for lowering hospitalizations for heart failure and cardiovascular deaths) regardless of baseline diabetes status, according to the most recent heart failure guidelines from the European Society of Cardiology (ESC) and the American Heart Association/American College of Cardiology/Heart Failure Society of America (AHA/ACC/HFSA) (2022). The AHA/ACC/HFSA HF recommendations 2022 present a class 2A recommendation for HFmrEF and HFpEF based on the findings of the EMPEROR-Preserved research; however, later

M. Nandave (✉)
Department of Pharmacology and Pharmaceutical Biotechnology, Delhi Pharmaceutical Sciences and Research University (DPSRU), New Delhi, Delhi, India

M. Nandave (ed.), *Sodium-glucose Cotransporter-2 (SGLT2) Inhibitors in Heart Failure*, https://doi.org/10.1007/978-981-97-7568-2_8

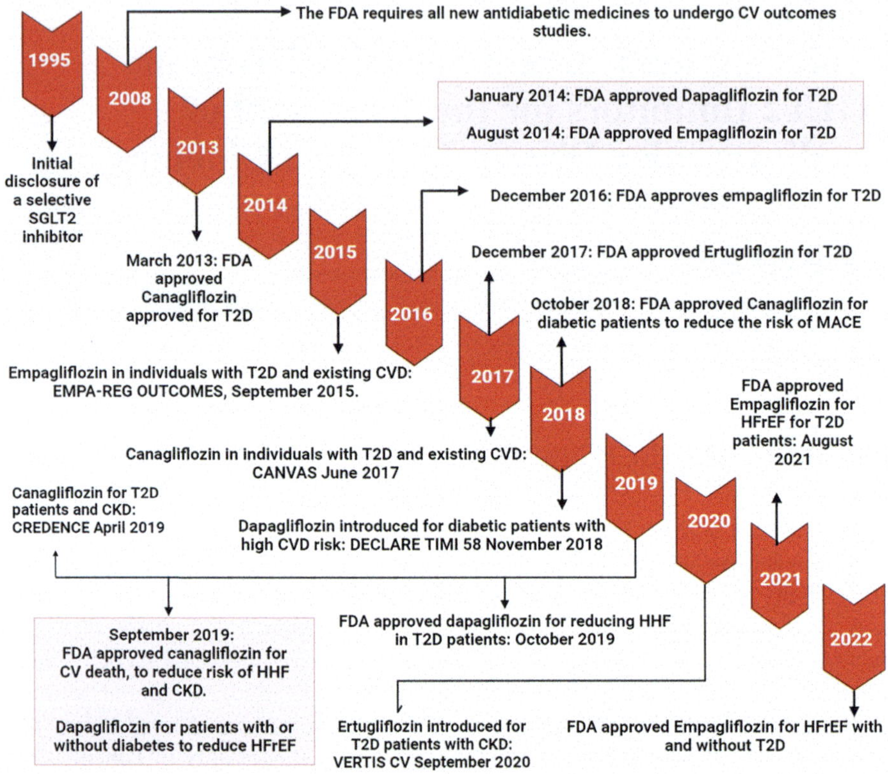

Fig. 8.1 Timeline summarizing the development and approval of SGLT-2is. *CKD* chronic kidney disease, *CV* cardiovascular, *CVD* cardiovascular disease, *FDA* US Food and Drug Administration, *HF* heart failure, *HFpEF* heart failure with preserved ejection fraction, *HFrEF* heart failure with reduced ejection fraction, *HHF* hospitalization for heart failure, *SGLT-2i* sodium-glucose cotransporter-2 inhibitor, *T2D* type 2 diabetes

guidelines may upgrade this recommendation after the publication of the DELIVER trial. The ESC 2021 recommendations do not address the use of SGLT2i in HFmrEF and HFpEF since they were released before the EMPEROR-Preserved and DELIVER studies were published. The medication is administered as a single daily dose (10 mg for dapagliflozin and empagliflozin, respectively) without the requirement for dose titration or regular laboratory testing. Experts advise initiating SGLT2i in patients hospitalized for HF as part of an aggressive strategy of quick, simultaneous optimization of medical therapy since the medication has an advantageous signal in patients with acute WHF and takes less than a month to generate a clinical benefit.

Table 8.1 A succinct explanation of how SGLT2i prevents cardiovascular disease in the context of therapy

	Sponsor	Objective	Intervention	Phase	Outcome
Considering that SGLT2i may have a part in the control of cardiovascular disorders in diabetic individuals facing renal failure	NCT04792190	The goal is to register 25 individuals scheduled for catheter ablation of patients with AF (permanent or paroxysmal)	Dapagliflozin + Placebo	Phase IV	Approximate fraction of time in AF
	NCT04509674	Determine whether the medication empagliflozin reduces the risk of heart failure-related hospitalization as well as the risk of cardiovascular disease-related death	Drug: Empagliflozin + Placebo	Phase III	Aggregate of all-cause mortality or time to initial hospitalisation for heart failure
	NCT04564742	This trial will compare the effects of dapagliflozin against a placebo, administered once daily, on hospitalization for heart failure (HHF), cardiovascular (CV) mortality, and other cardiometabolic outcomes in patients who have experienced myocardial infarction (MI)	Dapagliflozin + Placebo	Phase III	Duration until any one of the elements in this composite first appears: Cardiovascular mortality or hospitalization for heart failure
	NCT04600921	Focused on how ertugliflozin affected ventricular arrhythmias in general and treatment strategies such as implanted devices, coronary artery disease, cardiac failure biomarkers, and changes to physical function, anxiousness, stress, and quality of life	Ertugliflozin + Placebo	Phase III	ventricular fibrillation and supraventricular tachycardia episodes

Machine Generated Summaries

Disclaimer: The summaries in this chapter were generated from Springer Nature publications using extractive AI auto-summarization: An extraction-based summarizer aims to identify the most important sentences of a text using an algorithm and uses those original sentences to create the auto-summary (unlike generative AI). As the constituted sentences are machine selected, they may not fully reflect the body of the work, so we strongly advise that the original content is read and cited. The auto generated summaries were curated by the editor to meet Springer Nature publication standards. To cite this content, please refer to the original papers.

Machine generated keywords: tdm, ami, mouse, cvd, central, metformin, inhibitor dapagliflozin, action sglt, patient tdm, fibrosis, patient ami, glp, obesity, ascvd, placebo.

Transitioning to GLP-1 RAs and SGLT2 Inhibitors as the First Choice for Managing Cardiometabolic Risk in Type 2 Diabetes [1]

This is a machine-generated summary of:

Jha, Kunal K.; Adhikari, Rishav; Tasdighi, Erfan; Osuji, Ngozi; Rajan, Tanuja; Blaha, Michael J.: Transitioning to GLP-1 RAs and SGLT2 Inhibitors as the First Choice for Managing Cardiometabolic Risk in Type 2 Diabetes [1].

Published in: Current Atherosclerosis Reports (2022).

Link to original: https://doi.org/10.1007/s11883-022-01066-y

If you want to cite the papers, please refer to the original.

For technical reasons we could not place the page where the original quote is coming from.

Abstract-Summary "This forward-looking review summarizes existing evidence from cardiovascular outcome trials on cardiometabolic risk-reduction in type 2 diabetes (T2DM) management, with attention to updating and personalizing recommendations from recent diabetes practice guidelines issued by cardiology societies."

"According to large clinical trials, sodium-glucose cotransporter-2 inhibitors showed robust results in reducing heart failure (HF) hospitalization and chronic kidney disease (CKD) progression, while glucagon-like peptide-1 receptor agonists demonstrated the largest effects on HbA1c reduction, weight loss, and atherosclerotic cardiovascular disease outcomes prevention, including stroke."

"Future studies should investigate the addition of obesity-predominant risk, in conjunction with coronary artery disease, stroke, CKD, and HF, as a new influential indicator for choosing the optimal cardiometabolic agent."

Introduction

"Patients with T2DM are at higher risk of coronary artery disease (CAD), stroke, heart failure (HF), and chronic kidney disease (CKD) [2, 3]."

"Glycated hemoglobin (HbA1c) is nearly universally measured in patients with cardiometabolic disease and is a known marker of glycemic status, which helps to establish the diagnosis of T2DM."

"A prospective study among patients with T2DM showed that higher HbA1c was modestly, but not statistically significantly, associated with atherosclerotic cardiovascular events [4], while a meta-analysis comprising 50,000 patients with no history of T2DM and normal fasting blood glucose showed that the risk of CAD was increased 20% per 1% higher HbA1c [5]."

"HbA1c alone cannot explain the majority of cardiometabolic risk, which has resulted in reorientation of T2DM standards of care towards cardiometabolic risk management rather than solely glycemic control."

Metformin: Still a Primary Tool for Effective Diabetes Management?

"Potential cardioprotective benefits of metformin have been suggested by the UKPDS sub-study of overweight patients with newly diagnosed T2DM, randomized to metformin versus insulin/sulfonylurea."

"A 2011 meta-analysis of 35 randomized clinical trials comparing metformin to placebo and other conventional therapy (insulin, sulfonylurea, alpha-glucosidase inhibitor and thiazolidinedione) demonstrated that metformin reduced major adverse cardiovascular events (MACE), MI, stroke, peripheral artery disease, and cardiovascular (CV) death against placebo (OR = 0.79, 95% CI, [0.64–0.98]) but not compared to other conventional therapies (OR = 1.03, 95% CI, [0.72–1.77]) [6], suggest that metformin has potentially modest but uncertain cardioprotective benefits."

"Results of the ongoing VA-IMPACT trial enrolling veterans with prediabetes and atherosclerotic cardiovascular disease will give more clarity regarding the CV benefit of metformin compared to placebo [7]."

"Metformin continues to be the most prescribed medicine in patients with T2DM."

Sodium-Glucose Cotransporter-2 Inhibitors: A Novel Therapy with Unexpected Cardiovascular Benefit

"The anti-glycemic efficacy of SGLT2is varies widely, and depends on medication, dose, baseline eGFR, and concomitant use with other blood glucose-lowering therapies."

"SGLT2is reduce systolic blood pressure by 4–6 mmHg, diastolic blood pressure by 1–2 mmHg [8], and weight by 4–6lbs [9]."

"SGLT2is are safe and well-tolerated but clinicians should be aware of a few adverse events, including genital mycotic infection, volume depletion, dehydration, and orthostatic hypotension."

"Euglycemic DKA can be triggered in patients using SGLT2is in the setting of surgery, infection, trauma, a major illness, reduced food intake, persistent vomiting, gastroparesis, dehydration, and reduced insulin dosages [10, 11]."

"As SGLT2is are filtered by the glomerulus, they are contraindicated in patients with advanced renal disease (eGFR < 20–30 ml/min/1.73 m2)."

"Patients who are already receiving SGLT2is can safely continue them if eGFR ultimately falls below this range."

First-Generation SGLT2i CVOTs

"In the pivotal EMPA-REG OUTCOME trial, empagliflozin (N = 7020, 63 years old, mean HbA1c: 8%, median follow-up: 3.1 years) demonstrated 14% reduction in a 3-point composite MACE (HR = 0.86, 95% CI, [0.754–0.99]) in patients with T2DM and established cardiovascular disease (CVD), primarily driven by a 38% reduction in CV mortality [8]."

"The CANVAS trial (N = 10,142, 63.3 years old, mean HbA1c: 8.2%, mean T2DM duration:13.5 years, mean follow-up: 3.5 years) evaluating canagliflozin showed 14% RRR in MACE, which was driven by HF hospitalization reduction (HR = 0.67, 95% CI, [0.52–0.87])."

"In DECLARE-TIMI58 (N = 17,160, 64 years old, mean HbA1c: 8.3%, median T2DM duration: 11 years, median follow-up: 4.2 years), dapagliflozin reduced a dual endpoint of CV mortality or HF hospitalization, primarily driven by a reduction in HF hospitalization (HR = 0.73, [0.61–0.88]) [12]."

Second-Generation SGLT2i CVOTs (Dedicated Heart Failure) and Chronic Kidney Disease Trials

"The SOLOIST-WHF Trial (N = 1222, 69.5 years old, median follow-up: 9 months) evaluated the effect of sotagliflozin, a novel dual SGLT1 and SGLT2 inhibitor in patients with T2DM who were recently hospitalized for heart failure, showing a 22% RRR in composite of CV death and HF-related hospitalization or urgent care visits [13]."

"The EMPEROR-Preserved trial (N = 5988, 71.9 years old, class II–IV HF, mean EF of 54.3% with median follow-up of 26.2 months) evaluating empagliflozin in patients with heart failure with preserved ejection fraction (HFpEF) was the first trial in the history of any drug to show beneficial CV outcomes in HFpEF patients."

"The DAPA-CKD (N = 4304, 61.8 years old, median follow-up: 2.4 years) trial of dapagliflozin demonstrated similar outcomes; 39% RRR in MARCE, and subgroup analysis revealed that renal benefit was T2DM-independent [14]."

Real-World Evidence and Generic SGLT2i

"Randomized clinical trials often have strict entry criteria and their practical applicability might be limited for the larger real-world population."

"CVD-REAL II evaluated MI and stroke as additional outcomes and strongly suggests that SGLT2is have class effects and their benefits are consistent across geographic regions [15, 16]."

GLP-1RA Therapy—Jointly Tackling Obesity, Diabetes, Metabolism, and ASCVD

"GLP-1RAs are incretin-based therapies for the management of T2DM and obesity, with demonstrated CV risk reduction in patients with T2DM."

"Non-glycemic effects of GLP-1 RAs include significant weight loss, reduced lipid parameters and blood pressure, decreased inflammation, and renal protection."

"Five GLP-1 RAs are FDA-approved for glycemic control: dulaglutide, exenatide, liraglutide, lixisenatide, and semaglutide."

"Two GLP-1RAs are approved for weight loss: injectable liraglutide and semaglutide."

"Most GLP-1 RAs are administered by subcutaneous injections, although oral semaglutide recently became available."

"The main adverse events associated with GLP-1 RAs are GI-related: nausea, vomiting, constipation, and diarrhea."

GLP-1 RA CVOTs

"LEADER, the first CVOT to evaluate a long acting GLP-1 RA, liraglutide, (N = 9340, 64 years old, mean HbA1c 8.7%, mean duration of T2DM 12.8 years, median follow-up of 3.8 years), showed that 3-point MACE (CV death, MI, or nonfatal stroke) incidence decreased by 13%, driven primarily by reduction in CV mortality (HR = 0.78, 95% CI, [0.66–0.93]) [17]."

"In SUSTAIN-6 (N = 3297, 64 years old, mean HbA1c: 8.7%, mean T2DM duration: 13.9 years and median follow-up: 2.1 years), a CVOT of once-weekly injectable semaglutide in patients with T2DM, semaglutide reduced the composite 3-point MACE by 26%, which was largely driven by lower risk of nonfatal stroke (HR = 0.61, 95% CI, [0.38–0.99]) [18]."

Metanalysis of GLP-1RA Trials

"In a recent meta-analysis of eight CVOTs examining the effects of GLP-1RAs on cardiorenal outcomes in T2DM patients, investigators found a 14% reduction in a 3-point MACE (HR = 0.86, 95% CI, [0.79–0.94]) with greatest benefit in participants with established CVD [19]."

"GLP-1RAs also reduced CV mortality by 13%, HF hospitalization by 10%, nonfatal stroke by 16%, all-cause mortality by 12%, and composite renal endpoints by 17% [19]."

"Improvement in renal outcomes was mostly due to reduction of new-onset macroalbuminuria (HR = 0.74, 95% CI, [0.67–0.82], $p < 0.001$) [19], suggesting that GLP-1 RAs have both CV benefits and renal protective effects."

FDA Prescription Label Expansion for SGLT2is and GLP-1RAs

"Based on the EMPA-REG OUTCOME trial, in 2016, empagliflozin became the first antidiabetic to receive an FDA indication for reduction of CV events in adults with T2DM and CVD [20]."

"In 2020, the FDA approved dapagliflozin for reduction in CV death and hospitalization for HF events in adults with heart failure with reduced ejection fraction (HFrEF) irrespective of their T2DM status, the first time an antidiabetic therapy was repurposed to treat HF even in the absence of T2DM [21]."

"In February 2020, the FDA approved dulaglutide for the reduction of MACE in adults with T2DM who have established cardiovascular disease or multiple cardiovascular risk factors, opening the door for using GLP-1 RAs for primary prevention [22]."

Key Takeaways Comparing Various Guidelines and Expert Consensus

"Several society guidelines and expert consensus statements strongly recommend prescribing SGLT2is/GLP-1RAs in patients with T2DM with established CVD or at high CV risk, but each takes a slightly distinct approach to achieve this aim."

"In patients with T2DM who have ASCVD or high/very high CV risk, SGLT2is and GLP-1RAs are the first-line therapies."

"In the ESC 2021 CVD prevention guidelines, for individuals with T2DM and ASCVD or high risk of ASCVD (i.e., no established ASCVD and end organ damage with poor glycemic control or > 10 years of DM), CKD, or HF, the use of SGLT2is or GLP-1RAs are recommended over metformin [23]."

"The recently published American Diabetes Association 2022 Standards of Medical Care for T2DM patients with established ASCVD or CKD endorses prescribing SGLT2is or GLP-1RAs with demonstrated CV benefits as the first-line therapy for comprehensive glycemic control and/or CV risk modification [24]."

Combination Therapy

"Small trials that evaluated the feasibility of co-initiation of SGLT2is and GLP-1RAs revealed that combination therapy was safe, well-tolerated, and provided improved glycemic control."

"A recent 2022 meta-analysis with pooled data from eight CVOTs, evaluating 1895 patients with T2DM, showed that in comparison to monotherapy, the combination of SGLT2is and GLP-1 RAs results in higher reduction of HbA1c (0.77% [95% CI: − 1.03, − 0.50]), SBP (Standardized Mean Difference (SMD) − 0.33 mmHg; [95% CI: − 0.49, − 0.17]), BMI (SMD − 0.96 kg/m^2; [95% CI: − 1.69, − 0.23]), and LDL-C (SMD − 23.41 mmol/L; [95% CI: − 33.74, − 13.08]) [25]."

"Several trials are underway to determine whether a GLP-1RA, SGLT2i, or combination therapy is most effective in reducing CV and renal outcomes [26–28]."

Cardiac Imaging: A Decision Aid Guiding Prioritization of SGLT2is or GLP-1 RA Therapy in Patients with T2DM

"Coronary calcium scores (CAC) and coronary computed tomography angiography (CCTA) improve ASCVD risk stratification in T2DM patients, and can help in precise allocation of cardiometabolic medications [29–33]."

"CCTA could be instrumental as a decision aid in T2DM patients with angina, whereas CAC can be helpful in asymptomatic T2DM patients [29, 33]."

"A pooled analysis of multiple cohorts showed that individuals without overt CVD but with CAC > 100 would benefit from a GLP-1RA, while restricting use in individuals with CAC = 0 may reduce costs with little impact on CV event rates [34]."

"Current ESC guidelines explicitly cite CAC scoring and identification of obstructive disease on CTA as reasons to prioritize selection of CV risk-reducing therapies."

Novel FDA-Approved Cardiometabolic Therapies

"Finerenone, a selective, nonsteroidal mineralocorticoid antagonist, reduced CV outcomes and improved renal parameters in the FIGARIO-DKD [35] and FIDELIO-DKD [36] trials."

"A pooled analysis of these trials (FIDELITY study) demonstrated that finerenone improved CV outcomes by 14% (95% CI, 0.78–0.95; p = 0.0018) and renal outcomes by 23% (95% CI, 0.67–0.88; p = 0.0002) in patients with CKD and T2DM [37]."

"The SURPASS-CVOT of tirzepatide is ongoing and will further clarify the impact on glycemic control and CV outcomes compared to the GLP-1RA dulaglutide."

"The FDA has recently approved tirzepatide to improve glycemic control in adults with T2DM [38]."

Updated Algorithm for Selecting GLP-1 RA Vs. SGLT2i

"A challenge for many clinicians remains the nuanced difficulty in selecting the optimal cardiometabolic therapy for each patient."

"Based on our expert opinion, GLP-1RAs should be considered the superior agent for improvement of glycemic parameters, weight loss, primary ASCVD prevention, secondary stroke reduction, and improvement in obesity-associated comorbidities."

"We anticipate further support for this position from ongoing CVOTs such as SELECT."

"SGLT2is will almost always be the preferred agents later in the disease process (i.e., when HF and CKD has become evident), and older patients with multiple comorbidities."

Conclusion

"Despite the significant CV benefits, strong endorsement by multiple guidelines, and the FDA's expansion of medication indications, therapeutic inertia remains prominent among cardiologists."

"Lack of prescription ownership between physician specialties, frequent changes in the landscape of T2DM therapies, the need for insurance prior-authorization, concerns about adverse effects, and patient specific barriers have engendered therapeutic hesitancy among cardiologists."

"Understanding patient, physician, and healthcare-associated barriers will help alleviate therapeutic inertia to dramatically improve patient outcomes."

Comparison of SGLT2 Inhibitors with DPP-4 Inhibitors Combined with Metformin in Patients with Acute Myocardial Infarction and Diabetes Mellitus [39]

This is a machine-generated summary of:

Lyu, Young Sang; Oh, Seok; Kim, Jin Hwa; Kim, Sang Yong; Jeong, Myung Ho: Comparison of SGLT2 inhibitors with DPP-4 inhibitors combined with metformin in patients with acute myocardial infarction and diabetes mellitus [39].

Published in: Cardiovascular Diabetology (2023).
Link to original: https://doi.org/10.1186/s12933-023-01914-4

If you want to cite the papers, please refer to the original.

For technical reasons we could not place the page where the original quote is coming from.

Abstract-Summary "This study evaluated cardiovascular outcomes by comparing SGLT2i with dipeptidyl peptidase-4 inhibitors (DPP-4i) in combination with metformin in diabetic patients with AMI."

"This study involved 779 diabetic participants with AMI from a Korean nationwide multicenter observational cohort, who were divided into two groups: (1) metformin plus SGLT2i group (SGLT2i group, n = 186) and (2) metformin plus DPP-4i (DPP-4i group, n=593)."

"After IPTW, the rate of MACEs in the SGLT2i group was not significantly lower than that in the DPP-4i group (hazard ratio [HR], 0.99; 95% confidence interval [Cl], 0.46 to 2.14, p=0.983)."

"In our exploratory analysis, the left ventricular ejection fraction showed a significant improvement in the SGLT2i group than in the DPP-4i group before achieving statistical balancing (6.10 ± 8.30 versus 2.95 ± 10.34, p=0.007) and after IPTW adjustment (6.91 ± 8.91 versus 3.13 ± 10.41, p = 0.027)."

"Our findings demonstrated that SGLT2i did not influence the rate of MACEs compared with DPP-4i in combination with metformin in diabetic patients with AMI but did improve left ventricular ejection fraction."

Background

"Cardiovascular disease is the leading cause of mortality in patients with DM [40]."

"Many clinicians use sodium-glucose cotransporter 2 inhibitors (SGLT2i) or dipeptidyl peptidase-4 inhibitors (DPP-4i) in patients with DM as a second-line therapy in combination with metformin (MET) monotherapy."

"In recently published cardiovascular outcome trials (CVOTs), SGLT2i have proven cardiovascular benefits in patients with DM in both primary and secondary prevention [8–38, 40–42], which is driven by a low incidence of cardiovascular death and hospitalization for heart failure (HF)."

"In patients with AMI, the combination of OHAs appears to be an important strategy for achieving glycemic goals and long-term cardiovascular benefits."

"Determining the optimal combination of OHAs is important for the desired clinical outcomes of AMI."

"This study aimed to evaluate cardiovascular outcomes by comparing the use of SGLT2i versus DPP-4i in combination with MET in patients with AMI and concomitant DM."

Methods

"According to the international guidelines [43], AMI is defined as myocardial injury characterized by a rise or fall in cardiac markers and related clinical manifestations as follows: (1) myocardial ischemia-related symptoms and/or signs; (2) new-onset changes in the 12-lead electrocardiogram (ECG), including deviated ST-segments (either elevation or depression), inverted T-waves, or the development of pathological Q-waves; (3) imaging evidence for loss of viable myocardium or regional wall motion abnormalities; or (4) existence of intracoronary thrombi during coronary angiography."

"In IPTW, the propensity score was constructed using multiple logistic regression analysis with the following baseline covariates: age, sex, use of emergency medical services, BMI, Killip classification, medical history, smoking history, family history of CAD, use of thrombolysis, LMCA disease, multivessel CAD, PCI, final diagnosis (STEMI or non-STEMI), initial HbA1c level, post-discharge medications, vascular approach (femoral or non-femoral), use of glycoprotein IIb/IIIa inhibitors, thrombus aspiration, intracoronary imaging guidance, preprocedural TIMI flow grade, ACC/AHA lesion characteristics, treatment strategies, and IRA."

Results

"Prior CAD was more frequent in the DPP-4i group than in the SGLT2i group."

"The SGLT2i group had more instances of STEMI as a final diagnosis than the DPP-4i group."

"Initial HbA1c levels were higher in the SGLT2i group than in the DPP-4i group."

"Among discharge medications, beta-blockers were more frequently prescribed to individuals in the SGLT2i group compared to those in the DPP-4i group."

Discussion

"This study aimed to compare the cardiovascular outcomes of SGLT2i and DPP-4i as add-on therapies in patients with AMI and concomitant DM receiving MET."

"Our study demonstrated the potential benefit of SGLT2i over DPP-4i in improving LVEF, implying that the use of SGLT2i may exert beneficial effects in the clinical setting of AMI, although it did not reduce MACE."

"Only one retrospective observational study evaluated patients with AMI and concomitant type 2 DM, revealing that the use of SGLT2i was related with a reduced risk of adverse cardiovascular events [44]."

"The results of our study were significantly different from those of previous observational [45, 46] and network meta-analyses comparing SGLT2i and DPP-4i [47], demonstrating that SGLT2i have a beneficial effect on cardiovascular disease compared with DPP-4i."

"In our study, LVEF was significantly improved in patients treated with SGLT2i than in patients treated with DPP-4i before achieving statistical balancing and after IPTW adjustment."

Conclusions

"The use of SGLT2i compared with DPP-4i over one year did not demonstrate a statistically significant difference in composite cardiovascular outcomes in patients with AMI and concomitant DM."

"The use of SGLT2i appeared to improve left ventricular systolic function compared with the use of DPP-4i."

Sodium Glucose Transporter 2 (SGLT2) Inhibition with Empagliflozin Improves Cardiac Diastolic Function in a Female Rodent Model of Diabetes [48]

This is a machine-generated summary of:

Habibi, Javad; Aroor, Annayya R.; Sowers, James R.; Jia, Guanghong; Hayden, Melvin R.; Garro, Mona; Barron, Brady; Mayoux, Eric; Rector, R. Scott; Whaley-Connell, Adam; DeMarco, Vincent G.: Sodium glucose transporter 2 (SGLT2) inhibition with empagliflozin improves cardiac diastolic function in a female rodent model of diabetes [48].

Published in: Cardiovascular Diabetology (2017).

Link to original: https://doi.org/10.1186/s12933-016-0489-z

If you want to cite the papers, please refer to the original.
For technical reasons we could not place the page where the original quote is coming from.

Abstract-Summary "Obese and diabetic individuals are at increased risk for impairments in diastolic relaxation and heart failure with preserved ejection fraction."

"To determine whether targeting SGLT2 improves diastolic relaxation, we utilized empagliflozin (EMPA) in female db/db mice."

"EMPA treatment (DbE) improved glycemic indices ($P < 0.05$), but not BP ($P > 0.05$)."

"DbC and DbE had already established impaired diastolic relaxation as indicated by impaired septal wall motion (>tissue Doppler derived E′/A′ ratio) and increased left ventricular (LV) filling pressure (.

"Although these abnormalities persisted throughout the study period in DbC, diastolic function improved with EMPA treatment."

"DbC exhibited eccentric LV hypertrophy that was slightly improved by EMPA, indicated by a reduction in cardiomyocyte cross sectional area."

"EMPA improved glycemic indices along with diastolic relaxation, as well as SGK1/ENaC profibrosis signaling and associated interstitial fibrosis, all of which occurred in the absence of any changes in BP."

Background

"Affected individuals are likely to have one or more CVD complications, such as hypertension and cardiac diastolic dysfunction; indeed, diabetes is often considered a CVD equivalent."

"Diastolic heart failure, a CVD risk factor usually associated with aging, has dramatically increased in incidence in association with the increases in obesity and diabetes."

"We tested whether SGLT2 inhibitor therapy would attenuate the development of the earliest manifestation of diabetic heart disease, diastolic dysfunction, in part, by reducing blood pressure (BP), cardiac oxidative stress and pro-fibrotic factors."

"Diastolic dysfunction is especially pronounced in obese, insulin resistant and diabetic females [49–52]."

"We hypothesized that the SGLT2i, EMPA would blunt the development/progression of diastolic dysfunction and the associated abnormalities in cardiac remodeling in insulin resistant female diabetic db/db mice ($Lepr^{db/db}$)."

"The db/db mouse exhibits a non-dipping BP pattern, diastolic dysfunction and cardiac remodeling; these CVD features of metabolic disease are also observed in obese and insulin resistant humans [53–55]."

Methods

"There were 17 CkC, 19 DbC and 19 DbE. The first and second cohorts consisted of 5–6 mice per group and subsets of these mice were used for cardiac function, urine and plasma biochemistry, histological (light and electron microscopy) and immunological studies."

"At the end of the study mice were anesthetized with 3% isoflurane and a terminal blood sample was drawn immediately from the left ventricle."

"Immediately prior to the start of treatment, in the middle of the treatment period and within 48 h of the end of treatment, mice were placed in metabolic chambers for 24 h urine collection and subsequent determination of concentrations of electrolytes and glucose."

"Samples of the LV free wall were cut into 2 mm squares and placed immediately in primary TEM fixative as previously described."

Results

"At both measuring times, i.e., before treatment began and at the end of the treatment period, DbC and DbE mice had elevated fasting glucose and HbA1c consistent with diabetes, compared to CkC. By the end of the 5 week study period, the fasting glucose and HbA1c of DbC were both elevated compared to pre-treatment levels."

"In the setting of obesity, cardiac output (CO) and stroke volume (SV) were elevated in the DbC and DbE groups compared to the lean CkC mice."

"Measures of LV wall thickness tended to be slightly greater in DbC and DbE and LV lumen diameters were similar among groups."

"Cardiomyocyte cross sectional area was significantly reduced in DbE compared to DbC, although it did not reduce to that of CkC. The increases in CO, LV filling pressure, cardiomyocyte size and LV mass, in the absence of an increase in LV wall thickness, comprise a suite of traits suggestive of eccentric hypertrophy."

Discussion

"The results of this investigation support the hypothesis that treatment with the SGLT2i, EMPA, improves cardiac diastolic function in female mice in the setting of obesity and diabetes, even in the absence of a reduction in BP."

"The improvement in diastolic function was associated, not only with improved glycemia, but with improvements in cardiac structure, including reductions in interstitial myocardial fibrosis and associated pro-fibrotic SGK1/ENaC protein expression levels, cardiomyocyte hypertrophy and cardiomyocyte mitochondrial ultrastructure."

"Others have reported increased LV mass and wall thickness in female diabetic db/db mice of similar age and that remodeling was associated with diastolic dysfunction [53]."

"Further study is needed to determine whether improvement in myocardial insulin sensitivity contributes to improved diastolic function in db/db mice treated with EMPA."

A SGLT2 Inhibitor Dapagliflozin Suppresses Prolonged Ventricular-Repolarization Through Augmentation of Mitochondrial Function in Insulin-Resistant Metabolic Syndrome Rats [56]

This is a machine-generated summary of:

Durak, Aysegul; Olgar, Yusuf; Degirmenci, Sinan; Akkus, Erman; Tuncay, Erkan; Turan, Belma: A SGLT2 inhibitor dapagliflozin suppresses prolonged ventricular-repolarization through augmentation of mitochondrial function in insulin-resistant metabolic syndrome rats [56].

Published in: Cardiovascular Diabetology (2018).

Link to original: https://doi.org/10.1186/s12933-018-0790-0

If you want to cite the papers, please refer to the original.

For technical reasons we could not place the page where the original quote is coming from.

Abstract-Summary "We examined mechanisms of a SGLT2-inhibitor dapagliflozin (DAPA)-related cardioprotection in overweight insulin-resistant MetS-rats comparison with insulin (INSU), behind its glucose-lowering effect."

"DAPA-treatment of MetS-rats significantly augmented the increased blood pressure, prolonged Q–R interval, and low heart rate with depressed left ventricular function and relaxation of the aorta."

"DAPA, more prominently than INSU-treatment, preserved the depolarized mitochondrial membrane potential, and altered mitochondrial protein levels such as Mfn-1, Mfn-2, and Fis-1 as well as provided significant augmentation in cytosolic Ca^{2+}-homeostasis."

"DAPA also induced significant augmentation in voltage-gated Na^{+}-currents and intracellular pH, and the cellular levels of increased oxidative stress, protein-thiol oxidation and ADP/ATP ratio in cardiomyocytes from MetS rats."

"DAPA-treatment normalized the increases in the mRNA level of SGLT2 in MetS-rat heart."

"Our data provided a new insight into DAPA-associated cardioprotection in MetS rats, including suppression of prolonged ventricular-repolarization through augmentation of mitochondrial function and oxidative stress followed by improvement of fusion–fission proteins, out of its glucose-lowering effect."

Introduction

"Epidemiological studies reported that there was an association between higher mortality rates and uncontrolled glycemic control, primarily through the use of insulin, in patients with both T2DM and heart failure [57, 58] via flooding the heart with energy-providing substrates, including fats and sugars with insulin and insulin-sensitizing medications [59]."

"On the basis of these studies, here, we aimed to examine the molecular mechanism of the beneficial effect of an SGLT2 inhibitor on cardiac dysfunction in insulin-resistant overweight MetS rats."

"We also aimed to determine in vivo effects of DAPA on a mitochondrial function by determination of mitochondrial membrane potential, mitofusion-fission proteins, and glucose homeostasis together with any augmentation of cellular oxidative stress under hyperglycemia and insulin resistance in MetS rats."

"Our study provided a mechanism for a complete cardioprotective action of DAPA in vivo in overweight insulin-resistant MetS-rats through not an only augmentation of voltage-gated K^{+}-channel currents but also mitochondrial function and increased oxidative stress, in part, under the control of fusion–fission proteins at the cellular level via insulin-independent pathways."

Methods

"Whole-cell TTX-sensitive voltage-dependent Na^+-channel currents (I_{Na}) in cardiomyocytes were recorded as described, previously [60]."

"Whole-cell voltage-dependent the L-type Ca^{2+}-currents (I_{CaL}) were recorded and calculated as described, previously [61]."

"Isolated cardiomyocytes, following loading with the fluorescent Ca^{2+} indicators Fura-2 AM (4-μM), intracellular transient global free Ca^{2+} changes under electric-field stimulation (Ca^{2+}-transients) were measured at room temperature (21 ± 2 °C), as described, previously [61]."

"Fluorescence recordings were by use of either a PTI Ratiomaster microspectrofluorometer and FELIX software (Photon Technology International) for Ca^{2+} and Na^+ or a laser scanning microscope (confocal microscopy, Leica TCS SP5, Germany) for pH_i, as described previously [60]."

"Measurement of ROS production was performed in CM-H2DCFDA loaded (5 μM with 45-min incubation at 37 °C) cardiomyocytes, as described previously [62]."

Results

"DAPA but not INSU treatment significantly normalized the increased mRNA level of SGLT2 in MetS rat heart."

"In another set of experiments, we also determined the basal level of intracellular H^+ (or intracellular pH, $[pH]_i$ as $\Delta F_{590/640}$ intensity change) in cardiomyocytes from MetS rats comparison to those of control rats."

"Since the previous studies demonstrated a role for mitochondrial redox signaling (showing via both ROS and RNS) in the etiology of MetS and highlighted a potential therapeutic agent to treat MetS in human subjects [63, 64], we determined the effect of DAPA treatment on mitochondrial membrane potential (MMP, as FCCP responses) in isolated JC-1 loaded cardiomyocytes from MetS rats."

"DAPA but not INSU treatment of MetS rats preserved the MMP level, significantly."

"Either DAPA or INSU treatment of MetS rats normalized these values to those of controls."

"Either DAPA or INSU treatment of MetS rats preserved this ratio, significantly."

Discussion

"Our data suggested an important information about the molecular mechanism of an SGLT2-inhibitor DAPA-treatment benefits on cardiovascular function in MetS rats via targeting directly heart, behind its glucose-lowering effect."

"All together, SGLT2 inhibitor DAPA may inhibit a myocardial NHE leading to increased mitochondrial $[Ca^{2+}]$ and decreased cytoplasmic $[Ca^{2+}]_i$ and $[H^+]_i$ through mitochondrial NCX activity in MetS rat heart."

"In support of these findings, some studies have reported that SGLT2 inhibitors, including DAPA, might act as antioxidants by decrease in a cardiac oxidative stress, out of glucose lowering effects [65–67]."

"Those evidences, including our current data with DAPA support the potential role of DAPA in MetS-associated heart dysfunction as antioxidant and inflammatory modulators through suppression of induction of oxidative stress, independent of its SGLT2 and glucose lowering effects."

Limitations

"In this present current study by uses of MetS mimicking rats, we demonstrated that DAPA-treatment of these rats comparison to those of INSU-treatment significantly augmented all systemic parameters, including electrical and mechanical activities of the heart."

"The numbers of animals used i here were relatively small and the duration of treatment was limited to 2 weeks while one DAPA dose was used for the treatment."

"These facts might explain why we observed no effect on body weight and there was small effect on blood glucose and OGTT with DAPA treatment."

"The findings of this study in animal models align well with recent clinical trial outcomes and further suggest a potential clinical utility for DAPA in the treatment of cardiac dysfunction in any type of pathological condition."

Conclusions

"This present study shows that treatment with DAPA led to improvements in the depressed left ventricular function, and prolonged Q–R interval and low heart-rate in a MetS-rat model with slight but significant hyperglycemia and severe insulin resistance."

"The results of this investigation support the hypothesis that treatment with the SGLT2 inhibitor, DAPA, improves cardiac dysfunction function in the setting of MetS, diabetes, or obesity even in the little effect on high blood glucose and insulin resistance."

"This study provides a new insight into DAPA-associated cardioprotection in MetS-rats through augmentation of mitochondrial function and oxidative stress via improvement of fusion–fission proteins, behind its glucose-lowering effect."

The SGLT2 Inhibitor Canagliflozin Reduces Atherosclerosis by Enhancing Macrophage Autophagy [68]

This is a machine-generated summary of:

Chen, Hongping; Teng, Da; Xu, Bowen; Wang, Chunxiao; Wang, Hua; Jia, Wenjuan; Gong, Lei; Dong, Haibin; Zhong, Lin; Yang, Jun: The SGLT2 Inhibitor Canagliflozin Reduces Atherosclerosis by Enhancing Macrophage Autophagy [68].

Published in: Journal of Cardiovascular Translational Research (2023).

Link to original: https://doi.org/10.1007/s12265-023-10390-w

If you want to cite the papers, please refer to the original.

For technical reasons we could not place the page where the original quote is coming from.

Abstract-Summary "Recent studies indicate that autophagy widely participates in atherogenesis."

"This study aimed to assess the effect of canagliflozin (CAN) on atherogenesis via autophagy."

"Macrophages and ApoE − / − mice were used in this study."

"The cholesterol efflux assay demonstrated that CAN enhanced cholesterol efflux from macrophages via autophagy, resulting in lower lipid droplet concentrations in macrophages."

"CAN resulted in increased macrophage autophagy in atherosclerotic plaques of ApoE − / − mice, confirming that CAN could inhibit the progression of AS via promoting macrophage autophagy."

Introduction

"Multiple clinical trials have shown that SGLT2 inhibitors may give benefits beyond the treatment of diabetes, including a reduction in the risk of hospitalization for heart failure or death from cardiovascular causes."

"SGLT2 inhibitors may benefit the cardiovascular system by reducing adipose tissue-mediated inflammation and pro-inflammatory cytokine production, promoting ketone bodies as the metabolic substrate for the heart and kidneys, reducing oxidative stress, lowering serum uric acid levels, reducing glomerular hyperfiltration and albuminuria, and suppressing advanced glycation end-product signaling [69]."

"Xu and others found that empagliflozin reduces obesity-induced inflammation and insulin resistance by promoting the conversion of white fat to brown, increasing fat metabolism, and activating M2 macrophage polarization, which may be an important pathway for the cardiovascular benefits of SGLT2 [70, 71]."

"Since therapeutic SGLT2 leads to substantial loss of energy in the form of glucose via sodium–glucose co-transporter, it is an intriguing possibility that SGLT-2 inhibitors may affect the level of cellular autophagy following the intracellular energy changes."

Methods

"The cells at logarithmic growth phase were treated with phorbol 12-myristate-13-acetate (PMA) (Sigma, USA) for 24 h followed by ox-LDL (80 μg/ml) (Yiyuan Biotechnologies, China) alone for 48 h to become atherosclerotic macrophages for further investigations [72]."

"THP-1 cells were induced into macrophages on a 12-well plate, then transfected with mRFP-GFP-LC3 adenovirus and treated with ox-LDL for 48 h. After 12 h of CAN (10 μM/L) intervention, the cell slides were subjected to the following treatments: The cells were fixed in 4% paraformaldehyde for 30 min in the dark, washed twice with PBS, and then penetrated for 10 min in the dark with 0.1% Triton."

"After washing 3 × with PBS, the frozen slices were fixed in 4% paraformaldehyde for 20 min, followed by being incubated at 37 °C for 30 min with Oil Red O solution (Solarbio, China)."

Results

"To further explore how CAN regulated macrophage autophagy, BAF was used in the in vitro study."

"As an agent that affects glucose transport, CAN is anticipated to modulate the activation of macrophage energy-related pathways."

"Recent investigations have demonstrated that autophagy increases the extracellular transfer of LDs in macrophages [73, 74]."

"To investigate if CAN modulates the extracellular transport of LDs via autophagy, the lipid content of macrophages was evaluated using Oil Red O staining."

"Our data revealed that CAN induced autophagy and enhanced LDs extracellular transport in macrophages."

"To determine if CAN enhanced autophagy upregulation in macrophages, we assessed the expression of LC3II and P62 in plaques via western blot."

"To further visualize autophagy, we calculated the number of autophagic vesicles within macrophages within plaques using TEM."

"As with in vitro research, the foregoing results demonstrated that CAN increase autophagy within plaque macrophages."

Discussion

"We discovered that CAN prevented atherosclerotic plaque development via increasing macrophage autophagy."

"SGLT2 inhibitors down-regulate cellular glucose transport, which may lead to a relative lack of energy in macrophages and thus promote the production of intracellular autophagy."

"Autophagy has been known to improve macrophage lipid transport [75, 76]."

"Several recent studies have revealed that SGLT2 inhibitors lower the volume of atherosclerotic plaques in mice and influence the composition of macrophages, collagen fibers, lipids, and smooth muscle cells [77–81]."

"The animals used in this study were treated for 21 weeks, and we should have used longer durations to better understand CAN's role in plaque autophagy."

"In addition to macrophages, plaques contain smooth muscle cells and endothelial cells, and the control of autophagy by CAN in these two types of cells requires urgent investigation in order to fully assess CAN's regulatory effect on autophagy in plaques."

Conclusion

"It was revealed that CAN prevented the advancement of atherosclerotic plaques by activating macrophage autophagy and regulating macrophage lipid metabolism during the autophagosome formation phase via the AMPK/mTOR/Beclin1 axis."

"These findings expand our knowledge of how SGLT2 inhibitors function to prevent the progression of AS and introduce novel therapeutic approaches for the treatment of atherosclerotic diseases."

Recent Understandings About Hypertension Management in Type 2 Diabetes: What Are the Roles of SGLT2 Inhibitor, GLP-1 Receptor Agonist, and Finerenone? [82]

This is a machine-generated summary of:

Sawami, Kosuke; Tanaka, Atsushi; Node, Koichi: Recent understandings about hypertension management in type 2 diabetes: What are the roles of SGLT2 inhibitor, GLP-1 receptor agonist, and finerenone? [82].

Published in: Hypertension Research (2023).

Link to original: https://doi.org/10.1038/s41440-023-01324-9

If you want to cite the papers, please refer to the original.

For technical reasons we could not place the page where the original quote is coming from.

Abstract-Summary "The risk of cardiovascular disease increases by three to six-fold with the coexistence of diabetes and hypertension; therefore, the management of blood pressure to prevent cardiovascular disease is a particularly important issue in patients with diabetes."

"Clinical trial findings have resulted in recommendations to control blood pressure to <130/80 mmHg in Japanese patients with diabetes."

"The target blood pressure and selection of anti-hypertensive medications should vary depending on the duration of diabetes and comorbidities, and guidelines and clinical trial results should be interpreted flexibly to provide anti-hypertensive treatment tailored to individual patients."

"Beyond considering the thresholds for how far to lower blood pressure, blood pressure management in patients with diabetes will require understanding the additive cardioprotective value of drugs aimed at lowering blood pressure and the quality of blood pressure lowering."

Diabetes and Hypertension

"Hypertension is the most potent risk factor for cardiovascular mortality and was responsible for 10.8 million cardiovascular deaths worldwide in 2021, particularly those due to ischemic heart disease and stroke [83]."

"The risk of cardiovascular disease is increased by three to six-fold in patients with both diabetes and hypertension, compared to people without both conditions [84]."

"Effective therapeutic interventions for both diabetes and hypertension are important because diabetes and hypertension synergistically increase the risk of cardiovascular disease, the leading cause of death in patients with diabetes."

"Hypertension also increases the risk of microvascular complications, including diabetic retinopathy and diabetic nephropathy, by 1.1 to 1.3- and 1.4 to 2.5-fold, respectively."

Pathology of Hypertension in Diabetes

"Blood pressure is defined by circulating plasma volume and peripheral vascular resistance."

"The central pathology of type 2 diabetes is insulin resistance and hyperinsulinemia [85]."

"Insulin resistance is closely related to obesity, leading to the accrual of new vasculature, further increasing circulating plasma volume [86]."

"Insulin resistance is also considered a major cause of vascular endothelial dysfunction, leading to reduced endothelium-dependent vasodilatory responses [86]."

Current Recommendation in Guidelines

"The primary goal of antihypertensive treatment for patients with diabetes is to reduce cardiovascular disease."

"The United Kingdom Prospective Diabetes Study (UKPDS) 36 and 38 was one of the first large clinical trials to report the effect of lowering blood pressure in patients with diabetes, showing that lowering blood pressure reduced macrovascular and microvascular complications [87, 88]."

"While most guidelines recommend controlling systolic blood pressure (SBP) to <130 mmHg including Japanese Society of Hypertension (JSH), the American Diabetes Association (ADA) and the European Society of Cardiology (ESC)/ European Association for the study of Diabetes (EASD) does not recommend targeting SBP at <120 mmHg with mention of a lower limit [89–92]."

"These subtle differences in recommendations are because blood pressure targets to prevent cardiovascular events remain inconsistent [93]."

Implications of Clinical Trials on Blood Pressure Control in Patients with Diabetes

"The event rate in the standard therapy group was lower than expected, possibly due to differences in the use of statins, aspirin, and other medications; however, the ACCORD BP results suggested that controlling SBP < 120 mmHg is less effective in terms of reducing cardiovascular disease except for stroke."

"The results of a meta-analysis of 100,000 patients from 45 trials published in 2015 showed that a 10-mmHg reduction in blood pressure was associated with significant reductions in all-cause mortality, cardiovascular disease events (defined as the composite of myocardial infarction, sudden cardiac death, revascularization, fatal and nonfatal stroke, and fatal and nonfatal heart failure), ischemic heart disease, and stroke in patients with type 2 diabetes [94]."

"The results of the clinical trials and meta-analysis suggested that lowering SBP to <140 mmHg in patients with diabetes reduces all-cause mortality and cardiovascular disease events, as well as albuminuria; however, the effect of lowering SBP to <130 mmHg to prevent cardiovascular disease except for stroke is not clear."

A New Perspective on Blood Pressure Control in Patients with Diabetes

"In this meta-analysis of 51 trials, 103,325 patients with diabetes, and 255,208 patients without diabetes, a 5 mmHg reduction in SBP reduced cardiovascular events (the composite of fatal and non-fatal stroke, fatal and nonfatal ischemic heart disease, and fatal and requiring hospitalization heart failure); however, the effect was slightly attenuated in patients with diabetes (HR 0.94, 95% CI 0.91–0.98 for diabetes, HR 0.89, 95% CI 0.87–0.92 for non-diabetes, p-value for interaction = 0.0013) [95]."

"The practical insight that can be learned from the results of this meta-analysis at this time is that the effect of "blood pressure lowering itself" may attenuate in reducing ischemic heart disease, cardiovascular death, and all-cause mortality in patients with diabetes than in non-diabetes patients."

Moderate Hypotensive but High Cardiorenal Protective Effects of SGLT2i, GLP-1RA, and Finerenone

"Sodium-glucose cotransporter 2 inhibitors (SGLT2i) and glucagon-like peptide-1 receptor agonist (GLP-1RA) have emerged as hypoglycemic agents with superior efficacy in cardiorenal protective effects and are now actively recommended for first-line use in patients with diabetes with established cardiovascular disease or with multiple cardiovascular risks [96]."

"These results suggest that the antihypertensive effect of SGLT2i may be slightly higher than that of GLP-1RA and that the combination of antihypertensive medications and SGLT2i in patients with diabetes improved blood pressure control more than the combination with GLP-1RAs [97]."

"GLP-1RA is characterized by a lack of diastolic blood pressure-lowering effect and a slight increase in heart rate in the early stages of administration [98]."

"Whether this blood pressure change itself contributes to the favorable cardiovascular event reduction is still under debate, but it may suggest that a direct approach to diabetes-related conditions may be more effective than the act of lowering blood pressure itself."

What Is Effective Blood Pressure Lowering in Patients with Diabetes?

"Although remain questions regarding setting a certain threshold and uniformly lowering blood pressure to prevent cardiovascular events, especially ischemic heart disease and cardiovascular death, in patients with diabetes, even a 5-mmHg reduction in blood pressure may reduce the absolute risk of cardiovascular events [95]."

"We believe that individualization of blood pressure management here means focusing on selecting drugs that have been proven to reduce cardiovascular events according to the patient's pathophysiology, rather determining specific target blood pressure values individually."

"The selection of drugs based on the in-depth consideration of scientific evidence and individual patient condition is the first step toward precision medicine [99], and the antihypertensive effect obtained using such an approach may be an effective blood pressure-lowering strategy that improves the prognosis of patients with diabetes."

Conclusion

"The question of the extent to which lowering blood pressure itself may reduce cardiovascular events remains unanswered in patients with type 2 diabetes (Graphical Abstract)."

"Even if the guideline-recommended blood pressure threshold is reached, there may still be residual cardiovascular risk."

"Rather than eliminating that residual risk by further lowering blood pressure strictly, patients may benefit more from cardiorenal protective agents such as SGLT2i, GLP-1RA, and finerenone."

Combining Glucagon-Like Peptide-1 Receptor Agonists (GLP-1RAs) and Sodium-Glucose Cotransporter-2 Inhibitors (SGLT2is) in Patients with Type 2 Diabetes Mellitus (T2DM) [100]

This is a machine-generated summary of:

Gourdy, Pierre; Darmon, Patrice; Dievart, François; Halimi, Jean-Michel; Guerci, Bruno: Combining glucagon-like peptide-1 receptor agonists (GLP-1RAs) and sodium-glucose cotransporter-2 inhibitors (SGLT2is) in patients with type 2 diabetes mellitus (T2DM) [100].

Published in: Cardiovascular Diabetology (2023).

Link to original: https://doi.org/10.1186/s12933-023-01798-4

If you want to cite the papers, please refer to the original.

For technical reasons we could not place the page where the original quote is coming from.

Abstract-Summary "The presented cumulative evidence supports the benefits of GLP-1RA plus SGLT2i combination therapy on metabolic-cardiovascular-renal disease in patients with T2DM, with a low hypoglycemia risk."

"We encourage the adoption of GLP-1RA plus SGLT2i combination therapy in patients with T2DM and established atherosclerotic cardiovascular disease (ASCVD) or multiple risk factors for ASCVD (i.e., age ≥ 55 years, overweight/obesity, dyslipidemia, hypertension, current tobacco use, left ventricular hypertrophy, and/or proteinuria)."

"In case of persistent albuminuria and/or uncontrolled metabolic risks (i.e., inadequate glycemic control, hypertension, overweight/obesity) on SGLT2i therapy, GLP-1RAs should be considered as the preferential add-on therapy in T2DM patients with chronic kidney disease."

"Despite the potential clinical benefits of GLP-1RA plus SGLT2i combination therapy in patients with T2DM, several factors may delay this combination to become a common practice soon, such as reimbursement and costs associated with polypharmacy."

Introduction

"A more modest benefit of GLP-1RAs on HHF has been reported, as highlighted by a meta-analysis of 8 CVOTs of 60,080 patients with T2DM and increased cardiovascular risk or with established cardiovascular disease, in which GLP-1RAs reduced HHF by 11% compared to placebo (HR, 0.89; 95% CI, 0.82–0.98; $p = 0.013$) [101]."

"Another meta-analysis [102], which included a total of 1604 participants with T2DM or obesity, found that combination therapy with SGLT2is and GLP-1RAs significantly decreased the incidence of cardiovascular events (reported in 2 RCTs) compared with active control/placebo (relative risk [RR], 0.19; 95% CI, 0.04–0.96)."

"In three nested case–control studies from England and Wales, involving 440,089 patients with T2DM and without ASCVD treated with non-insulin glucose-lowering medication, combined SGLT2i and GLP-1RA therapy used for primary prevention was associated with 30% lower odds of MACE (defined as myocardial infarction/acute coronary syndrome, stroke/transient ischemic attack, and/or cardiovascular death) compared with other combination regimens (OR, 0.70; 95% CI, 0.50–0.98) [103]."

Impact of Chronic GLP-1 RA and SGLT-2I Therapy on In-Hospital Outcome of Diabetic Patients with Acute Myocardial Infarction [104]

This is a machine-generated summary of:

Trombara, Filippo; Cosentino, Nicola; Bonomi, Alice; Ludergnani, Monica; Poggio, Paolo; Gionti, Luigia; Baviera, Marta; Colacioppo, Pierluca; Roncaglioni, Maria Carla; Leoni, Olivia; Bortolan, Francesco; Agostoni, Piergiuseppe; Genovese, Stefano; Marenzi, Giancarlo: Impact of chronic GLP-1 RA and SGLT-2I therapy on in-hospital outcome of diabetic patients with acute myocardial infarction [104].

Published in: Cardiovascular Diabetology (2023).

Link to original: https://doi.org/10.1186/s12933-023-01758-y

If you want to cite the papers, please refer to the original.

For technical reasons we could not place the page where the original quote is coming from.

Abstract-Summary "Whether their benefits occur also during hospitalization for acute myocardial infarction (AMI) in patients with diabetes mellitus (DM) is not known."

"We evaluated in-hospital outcomes of patients hospitalized with AMI according to their chronic use of GLP-1 RA and/or SGLT-2i."

"They were stratified according to DM status, then grouped into three cohorts using a propensity score matching: non-DM patients; DM patients treated with GLP-1 RA and/or SGLT-2i; DM patients not treated with GLP-1 RA/SGLT-2i."

"The primary endpoint rate was 16% (n = 502) and progressively increased from non-DM patients to DM patients treated with and without GLP-1 RA/SGLT-2i (13%, 16%, and 20%, respectively; $P < 0.0001$)."

"Compared with non-DM patients, DM patients with GLP-1 RA/SGLT-2i had a 30% higher risk of the primary endpoint, while those not treated with GLP-1 RA/SGLT-2i had a 60% higher risk ($P<0.0001$)."

"Chronic therapy with GLP-1 RA and/or SGLT-2i has a favorable impact on the clinical outcome of DM patients hospitalized with AMI."

Introduction

"Diabetes mellitus (DM) is a relevant risk factor and frequent comorbidity in patients hospitalized with acute myocardial infarction (AMI), with a prevalence of 20–30% [105–107]."

"It has been recently demonstrated that the higher in-hospital mortality in DM patients with AMI is mainly driven by their higher rate of cardiac and renal dysfunction [108]."

"While waiting for the results of ongoing randomized clinical trials focusing on the protective role of these drugs in AMI patients [109], the evaluation of in-hospital outcomes in DM patients, chronically treated with these anti-hyperglycemic agents at the time of hospitalization with AMI, represents a good opportunity to explore their potential role in this acute clinical setting."

"We analyzed administrative data from Lombardy, the most populous Italian region, with the aim to evaluate in-hospital outcomes in patients hospitalized with AMI according to their DM status and their anti-hyperglycemic therapy at the time of hospitalization."

Methods

"Our study used connected administrative health databases of the Lombardy region, Italy, which include population registries with demographic data of all residents and detailed information on drug prescriptions, hospital records, and medical exemptions."

"They are compiled by the hospital specialists directly in charge of the patients upon their discharge, and are validated by hospitals against detailed clinical-instrumental data, as they determine reimbursement from the national health system."

"We included in this study patients since 2010 because GLP-1 RA and SGLT-2i were available in the Italian market from 2010 and 2015, respectively."

"Patients with DM were further stratified according to GLP-1 RA/SGLT-2i treatment for at least 3 months before index hospitalization."

"The two non-fatal components of the primary endpoint were retrieved from the clinical conditions (acute heart failure) and procedures (RRT) coded in hospital records."

"Anti-hyperglycemic therapy before hospitalization, not present by definition in patients without DM, was excluded from the propensity score matching."

Results

"Of them, 1030 patients with DM were treated with GLP-1 RA/SGLT-2i (median time of drug administration prior to AMI 19 [108–129] months)."

"A lower risk of each secondary endpoint was observed in DM patients treated with GLP-1 RA/SGLT-2i, when compared with DM patients not treated with these drugs."

"A similar incidence of the primary endpoint was found between patients on GLP-1 RA and those on SGLT-2i (17% vs. 15%; P = 0.46, adjusted OR 1.34 [0.94–1.91])."

"At the sensitivity analysis comparing DM patients treated with GLP-1 RA/SGLT-2i and those treated with DPP-4i, the former showed a significant adjusted lower risk of the primary endpoint (OR 0.45; 95% CI 0.37–0.55)."

Discussion

"The results of the present study showed that patients with DM on chronic GLP-1 RA and/or SGLT-2i therapy have a better clinical outcome during hospitalization for AMI compared to those not treated with these anti-hyperglycemic drugs."

"Recent data from the SWEDEHEART registry confirmed that treatment with GLP-1 RA initiated soon after a first AMI in patients with DM is associated with a lower risk of major cardiovascular events at a median follow-up of 3 years [130]."

"Our study is the first evaluating the potential impact of chronic GLP-1 RA and/or SGLT-2i therapy on in-hospital outcomes of DM patients hospitalized with AMI and treated with current standards of care."

"The finding that DM patients treated with GLP-1 RA and/or SGLT-2i showed a lower risk than those not treated with these drugs for each component of the primary endpoint supports a cardiac and renal protective effect of these drugs also during AMI hospitalization."

Study Limitations

"Administrative databases are a reliable tool to describe outcomes of patient cohorts representing the real clinical care, since they collect data over time in a standardized way and at low cost."

"The small number of events does not allow us to detect a potentially significant difference in the beneficial effect between GLP-1 RA and SGLT-2i or among single agents of the same class of drugs."

"Clinical trials of patients randomized to GLP-1 RA vs. SGLT-2i vs. both together are not currently available."

"One observational study found SGLT-2i to be more effective than GLP-1 RA in improving cardiovascular outcomes of DM patients [131] while another showed the superiority of GLP-1 RA [132], and a third one reported no differences in major cardiovascular events between these two drug classes [133]."

"GLP-1 RA and SGLT-2i can be prescribed in Italy only by diabetes specialists and this can represent a selection bias potentially identifying a population in which control of risk factors is more rigorous."

Conclusions

"Our study indicates that chronic therapy with GLP-1 RA and/or SGLT-2i has a favorable impact on the clinical outcome of DM patients hospitalized with AMI and seems to reduce the prognostic gap still existing between DM and non-DM patients."

"These promising data further support the rationale for the ongoing randomized clinical trials investigating these drugs in patients with AMI."

A Randomised Study of the Impact of the SGLT2 Inhibitor Dapagliflozin on Microvascular and Macrovascular Circulation [134]

This is a machine-generated summary of:

Ott, Christian; Jumar, Agnes; Striepe, Kristina; Friedrich, Stefanie; Karg, Marina V.; Bramlage, Peter; Schmieder, Roland E.: A randomised study of the impact of the SGLT2 inhibitor dapagliflozin on microvascular and macrovascular circulation [134].

Published in: Cardiovascular Diabetology (2017).

Link to original: https://doi.org/10.1186/s12933-017-0510-1

If you want to cite the papers, please refer to the original.

For technical reasons we could not place the page where the original quote is coming from.

Abstract-Summary "The sodium–glucose cotransporter 2 inhibitor, dapagliflozin, has been shown to improve diabetic control and reduce blood pressure in patients with type 2 diabetes mellitus."

"After a 4-week run-in/washout phase, patients (N = 59) received 6 weeks of either dapagliflozin 10 mg or placebo once daily."

"Six weeks of dapagliflozin treatment resulted in improvements in diabetes control, including blood glucose and insulin resistance, and reduced office and 24-h ambulatory blood pressure values."

"RCF decreased from 324 AU at baseline to 308 AU after treatment with dapagliflozin (p = 0.028), while there was little difference after the placebo (318 AU; p = 0.334)."

"The arteriole remodelling that was seen after the placebo phase was not evident after the dapagliflozin phase."

"Central systolic and diastolic blood pressure values were significantly lower after 6 weeks of dapagliflozin, by 3.0 and 2.2 mmHg, respectively (p = 0.035 and 0.020, respectively vs. baseline)."

"Six weeks of dapagliflozin treatment resulted in numerous beneficial effects."

Background

"Early changes to the vasculature in patients with type 2 diabetes are characterised by hyperperfusion of microvessels such as those in the eye and kidney, vascular remodelling, and arterial stiffening [135]."

"This results in an inadequate increase in systolic blood pressure (BP) and a relative decrease in diastolic BP, thus increasing central PP at any given value of mean arterial pressure."

"Ott and others demonstrated that the dipeptidyl peptidase (DPP)-4 inhibitor, saxagliptin, was able to reduce retinal capillary flow (RCF) and improve central haemodynamics compared to placebo during a 6-week treatment period [135]."

"Cherney and others showed that, in patients with type 1 diabetes, empagliflozin resulted in a reduction in arterial stiffness over the course of an 8-week study [136]."

"The present study was performed in order to evaluate the micro- and macrovascular changes that accompany dapagliflozin treatment in patients with type 2 diabetes."

Research Design and Methods

"The study was a prospective, randomised, double-blind, placebo-controlled, crossover phase IIIb trial performed at the Clinical Research Center of Erlangen-Nuremberg, Germany."

"Secondary endpoints included the effects on the micro- and macrovascular parameters of the systemic circulation, including central BP, heart rate, and augmentation pressure, as measured by pulse wave analysis."

"At the randomisation visit, a fasting blood sample was taken in order to measure HbA1c, FPG, lipid levels, and other biochemical safety parameters (e.g. creatinine, liver enzymes)."

"Office BP and heart rate measurements were taken in a seated position after 5 min of rest."

"Using data acquired from a similar study [135], the within standard deviation of RCF was estimated to be 63 AU."

"In order to show a decrease of 25 AU after dapagliflozin as opposed to placebo after 6 weeks, for $\alpha = 0.05$ and $\beta = 0.80$, the required number of patients was calculated to be 52."

Results

"In terms of FPG, the level after dapagliflozin treatment decreased by 18 mg/dl ($p < 0.001$), while that after the placebo did not change from baseline."

"Although both the dapagliflozin and placebo resulted in decreases in PPG, the final values after 6 weeks of treatment were significantly lower for the dapagliflozin (154 vs. 180 mg/dl; $p < 0.001$)."

"Lipid levels remained stable during the study, with the only difference being lower triglycerides after dapagliflozin treatment than after placebo (146 vs. 159 mg/dl; $p = 0.043$)."

"Slight changes in central SBP and DBP values from baseline led to a lower PP after 6 weeks of dapagliflozin treatment compared to 6 weeks of placebo (40.9 vs. 43.6 mmHg; $p = 0.05$)."

Discussion

"The slight increase for placebo and slight decrease for dapagliflozin may indicate an effect of the drug, particularly as FPG and PPG were both significantly lower after the 6 weeks of dapagliflozin treatment."

"Dapagliflozin treatment has previously been shown to reduce BP in patients with type 2 diabetes, likely as a result of its natriuretic and diuretic effects [137]."

"RCF was found to be significantly lower after 6 weeks of treatment with dapagliflozin, while there was little change after placebo treatment."

"In patients with type 2 diabetes, we found that RCF after 6 weeks of treatment with saxagliptin was significantly lower than after 6 weeks of placebo, with this being alongside superior glucose lowering [135]."

"In combination with our work on dapagliflozin, the positive results demonstrate that SGLT2 inhibitors are beneficial for decreasing arterial wall stiffness in patients with type 2 diabetes."

Limitations

"The main limitation to this study is its length; however, in the absence of other anti-diabetic therapies, it would not be ethical to administer a placebo for a longer period of time."

"Further limitations are the small sample size and that findings cannot be extrapolated to type 2 diabetes in general, since patients above 70 years were excluded from the study."

Conclusions

"Six weeks of treatment with the SGLT2 inhibitor, dapagliflozin, resulted in improved diabetic control and reduced ambulatory BP."

"While these findings have been demonstrated previously, we additionally showed that the drug was capable of reducing hyperperfusion of retinal capillaries and arteriole remodelling, factors that contribute to the progression of diabetic retinopathy."

"Dapagliflozin treatment appeared to reduce arterial stiffness, as indicated by lower central PP."

"Although the observed effects were small, they demonstrate the multiple advantageous effects on vascular function and structure by dapagliflozin for patients with type 2 diabetes."

SGLT2 Inhibition with Empagliflozin Attenuates Myocardial Oxidative Stress and Fibrosis in Diabetic Mice Heart [138]

This is a machine-generated summary of:

Li, Chenguang; Zhang, Jie; Xue, Mei; Li, Xiaoyu; Han, Fei; Liu, Xiangyang; Xu, Linxin; Lu, Yunhong; Cheng, Ying; Li, Ting; Yu, Xiaochen; Sun, Bei; Chen, Liming: SGLT2 inhibition with empagliflozin attenuates myocardial oxidative stress and fibrosis in diabetic mice heart [138].

Published in: Cardiovascular Diabetology (2019).

Link to original: https://doi.org/10.1186/s12933-019-0816-2

If you want to cite the papers, please refer to the original.

For technical reasons we could not place the page where the original quote is coming from.

Abstract-Summary "Hyperglycaemia associated with myocardial oxidative stress and fibrosis is the main cause of diabetic cardiomyopathy."

"The aim of this study was to investigate the effect of empagliflozin on myocardium injury and the potential mechanism in type 2 diabetic KK-Ay mice."

"Thirty diabetic KK-Ay mice were administered empagliflozin (10 mg/kg/day) by oral gavage daily for 8 weeks."

"Results showed that empagliflozin improved diabetic myocardial structure and function, decreased myocardial oxidative stress and ameliorated myocardial fibrosis."

"Further study indicated that empagliflozin suppressed oxidative stress and fibrosis through inhibition of the transforming growth factor β/Smad pathway and activation of Nrf2/ARE signaling."

"Glycaemic control with empagliflozin significantly ameliorated myocardial oxidative stress injury and cardiac fibrosis in diabetic mice."

Introduction

"Several reports have shown that an increased level of reactive oxygen species (ROS), induced by hyperglycaemia, leads to impaired contractile function and myocardial fibrosis in the left ventricle of diabetic rats [139, 140]."

"Another study revealed that empagliflozin can ameliorate oxidative stress in aortic vessels and prevent endothelial dysfunction in the aortic rings of streptozotocin-induced type 1 diabetic rats [141]."

"Little is known about whether empagliflozin can reduce the oxidative stress of cardiac tissue and prevent cardiac fibrosis and remodelling in type 2 diabetic patients."

"We assess the efficacy of the SGLT2 inhibitor empagliflozin in reducing oxidative stress and preventing diabetic-induced myocardial fibrosis using the type 2 diabetic KK-Ay mice model."

"We also explore the downstream signalling of myocardial fibrosis activated by oxidative stress in the left ventricle of a type 2 diabetic mice model."

Methods

"The mice with a blood glucose concentration greater than 15 mM (200 mg/dL) for 2 consecutive weeks were used for the following experiments."

"The groups were as follows: (1) control group: healthy C57BL/6J mice with no treatment; (2) DM group: type 2 diabetic KK-Ay mice with no treatment; (3) DM + empagliflozin (DM + EM) group: type 2 diabetic KK-Ay mice treated with empagliflozin (10 mg/kg/day for 10 weeks, oral gavage, 0.5% hydroxyethylcellulose was used as the vehicle)."

"The lipid hydroperoxide level was expressed as nmol/mg protein."

"The sections were then incubated in 3% hydrogen peroxide for blocking endogenous peroxidase activity and incubated with primary antibody (mouse monoclonal antibody to TGF-β1, collagen I and collagen III; Abcam) for 1.5 h, followed by corresponding secondary antibody for 2.5 h at room temperature."

"The total protein concentration was quantified by a BCA Protein Assay Kit (Medchem Express, USA)."

Results

"The body weight gain decreased in the mice of the DM + EM group and was significantly affected by empagliflozin therapy in the DM + EM group."

"Fasting and non-fasting blood glucose levels of mice in the DM + EM group were significantly decreased after 8 weeks of empagliflozin treatment compared with the DM group, but it was still higher than the blood glucose in the control group mice."

"Lipid hydroperoxide concentration and MDA level were significantly higher in DM mice than in control and DM + EM groups ($P < 0.05$), whereas the levels of SOD and GSH-Px were significantly lower in DM mice compared with diabetic mice treated with empagliflozin ($P < 0.05$)."

"We found that the NOX4 was greatly elevated in DM mice compared with the control group, and NOX4 expression in the DM + EM group significantly decreased compared with DM mice ($P < 0.05$)."

Discussion

"We evaluated the influence of the SGLT2 inhibitor empagliflozin on cardiac oxidative stress and remodeling in mice with type 2 DM."

"The key findings of this study were that treatment with empagliflozin significantly ameliorated myocardial fibrosis and oxidative stress in type 2 diabetic mice."

"Accumulating clinical data indicate that empagliflozin reduces body weight and glucose levels in an insulin-independent pattern in type 2 diabetic patients [142–144]."

"We also found that empagliflozin can significantly downregulate the level of NOX4 in the myocardial tissue of diabetic rats, namely, by reducing NADPH oxidase activity."

"We observed that empagliflozin had a negative influence on diabetes-induced oxidative stress in the myocardium of mice."

"In view of the close relationship between Nrf2 and oxidative stress levels in diabetic cardiomyopathy, empagliflozin is a promising drug for reducing oxidative stress in myocardium by targeting Nrf2 signalling."

Conclusions

"The SGLT2 inhibitor empagliflozin ameliorates myocardial fibrosis partly through inhibition of collagen formation and deposition via the classical TGF-β/Smad pathway and decreases oxidative stress via promoting Nrf2 translocation to the nucleus and activating Nrf2/ARE signalling in the type 2 diabetic KK-Ay mice model."

"8 weeks of empagliflozin treatment rescues the LV structure and function in diabetic mice."

"Empagliflozin is a promising agent in the prevention and treatment of diabetic cardiomyopathy."

"More clinical data are needed to verify the safety and efficacy of empagliflozin in treating patients with diabetic cardiomyopathy, and its potential mechanism also needs further exploration."

The Effect of Sodium-Glucose Co-transporter-2 (SGLT-2) Inhibitors on Cardiometabolic Profile; Beyond the Hypoglycaemic Action [145]

This is a machine-generated summary of:

Lioudaki, Eirini; Androulakis, Emmanouil S.; Whyte, Martin; Stylianou, Konstantinos G.; Daphnis, Eugenios K.; Ganotakis, Emmanouil S.: The Effect of Sodium-Glucose Co-transporter-2 (SGLT-2) Inhibitors on Cardiometabolic Profile; Beyond the Hypoglycaemic Action [145].

Published in: Cardiovascular Drugs and Therapy (2017).

Link to original: https://doi.org/10.1007/s10557-017-6724-3

If you want to cite the papers, please refer to the original.

For technical reasons we could not place the page where the original quote is coming from.

Abstract-Summary "Sodium-glucose co-transporter (SGLT)-2 inhibitors are a new drug class in the management of T2DM with a mechanism of action independent of insulin."

"To their hypoglycaemic effect, SGLT-2 inhibitors appear to have haemodynamic and nephroprotective effects."

"Metabolic benefits are also attributed to SGLT-2 inhibitors with a modest but consistent body weight decrease recorded along with improvements in lipid profile and uric acid levels."

"In the kidney, SGLT-2 inhibitors reduce hyperfiltration, a precipitant of diabetic nephropathy."

Introduction

"Sodium-glucose co-transporter (SGLT)-2 inhibitors constitute a newly employed drug class in the management of type 2 diabetes mellitus (T2DM)."

"Most SGLT-2 inhibitors have no significant effect on SGLT-1, but canagliflozin does affect SGLT-1."

"A recent meta-analysis suggested a small benefit of high-dose canagliflozin monotherapy in glucose lowering over other SGLT-2 inhibitors [146]; whether this is related to canagliflozin's dual mechanism of action on both SGLT-1 and SGLT-2 remains unclear."

"Current SGLT-2 inhibitors: canagliflozin, dapagliflozin and empagliflozin, are licensed for the management of diabetes in patients if estimated glomerular filtration rate (eGFR) is greater than 45 mls/min."

"It is therefore unsurprising that SGLT-2 inhibitors have effects on the cardio-renal system independent of that of glucose lowering."

Blood Pressure Effects

"A recent meta-analysis of 13 trials by Shyangdan and others [146] indicated that all SGLT-2 inhibitors given as monotherapy or combined with other antidiabetic agents—usually metformin—led to a reduction in systolic BP (SBP) compared with placebo; reductions from baseline ranged from 2.6 mmHg with empagliflozin (10 mg once daily (OD)) to 6 mmHg with canagliflozin (300 mg OD)."

"A previous meta-analysis had shown that SGLT-2 inhibitors are significantly more effective compared to both placebo and other antihyperglycaemic agents in reducing SBP (mean difference, −3.77 and − 4.45 mmHg, respectively) and diastolic BP (DBP) (mean difference − 1.75 and 2.01, respectively) [147]."

"It might prove useful to assess whether BP-lowering efficacy of SGLT-2 inhibitors varies according to levels of HbA1C. The fact that dapagliflozin showed a more pronounced SBP reduction when added to beta-blockers or calcium channel blockers, compared to thiazides [148], does not come as a surprise, indicating the role of volume contraction in the antihypertensive effect of SGLT-2 inhibitors."

Metabolic Effects

"SGLT-2 inhibition is associated with a series of interrelated metabolic effects, primarily represented by amelioration of adverse lipid profile and body weight reductions."

"SGLT-2 inhibitors reportedly reduce body weight with preferential effect on adipose tissue."

"Several SGLT inhibitors such as canagliflozin, dapagliflozin, luseogliflozin, or tofogliflozin, either as monotherapy or combined with metformin, achieved statistically significant reductions in body weight compared to placebo in RCTs with a consistent dose-related effect and mean difference from placebo ranging from 1.61 kg at lower doses to 2.66 at maximum doses [149–155], frequently followed by a reduction in waist circumference [152, 155–157]."

"Reduction of hepatic fat content can lead to favourable changes in the lipoprotein profile [158], which have been associated with SGLT-2 inhibitors as previously mentioned."

"Among all the above, benefits in body weight and visceral adiposity have been broadly reported with most SGLT-2 inhibitors and merit particular consideration given the high-risk metabolic profile of patients with T2DM."

Renal Effect—'Nephroprotective Effect'

"The same patient group showed an increase in angiotensin II and aldosterone levels as well as reductions in plasma nitric oxide (NO) and effective renal plasma flow with an increase in renal vascular resistance both under euglycaemia and clamped hyperglycaemia [159]."

"Given the prognostic role of hyperfiltration for progression to chronic kidney disease in diabetes [160], this effect of SGLT-2 inhibitors emerges as one of particular importance."

"Cherney and others emphasised in their study that the blunting effect on hyperfiltration was most likely the result of decreased plasma NO and effective renal plasma flow along with an increase in renal vascular resistance as result of increased sodium chloride delivery to the distal tubule [159]."

"The observed increase in reninaldosterone-angiotensin system (RAAS) mediators with empaglifozin in the hyperfiltration group represents the decrease in effective circulating volume via SGLT-2 inhibitors' mild diuretic effect."

Beneficial Effect on Cardiovascular Outcomes

"A subsequent analysis suggested that the composite outcome of heart failure hospitalization and CV death was more frequent in the placebo group compared to the empagliflozin group (8.5 vs 5.7%; HR 0.66, 95% CI 0.55–0.79; $p < 0.001$) with the effect being independent of drug dose or baseline characteristics such as age, race, eGFR and other medications."

"A protective CV effect associated with SGLT-2 inhibition was suggested by significant reductions in the risk for major CV events (RR 0.84, 95% CI 0.75–0.95; p = 0.006); CV death (RR 0.63, 95% CI 0.51–0.77; p < 0.0001) and heart failure (RR 0.65, 95% CI 0.50 to 0.85; p = 0.002)."

Safety Concerns

"This appears to be related to increased glucose excretion especially in the presence of low carbohydrate diet resulting in enhanced ketogenesis [161]."

"Pooled data analysis of empagliflozin showed similar rates to placebo [162]."

"Despite that this class of drugs may induce a degree of volume depletion, their use has not been associated with significantly increased rates of acute kidney injury [8, 163]."

Conclusions

"In the kidney, SGLT-2 inhibitors reduce hyperfiltration, a precipitant of diabetic nephropathy."

"Given reported ameliorating effects on blood pressure, central obesity and adverse lipid profile, one could suggest that patients with the metabolic syndrome (i.e., a constellation of the above) on top of T2DM might get maximal benefit from treatment with SGLT-2 inhibition."

"Prospective studies should examine whether SGLT-2 inhibitors might prevent or retard the development or improve outcomes in kidney disease."

"The results of their combination with RAAS inhibitors may be of particular interest."

Sodium-Glucose Cotransporter-2 (SGLT-2) Inhibitors for Cardiovascular Disease Prevention [164]

This is a machine-generated summary of:

Reid, Jessica; Rana, Khyatiben; Niman, Stephanie; Sheikh-Ali, Mae; Lewis, Todd; Choksi, Rushab R.; Goldfaden, Rebecca F.: Sodium-Glucose Cotransporter-2 (SGLT-2) Inhibitors for Cardiovascular Disease Prevention [164].

Published in: American Journal of Cardiovascular Drugs (2020).

Link to original: https://doi.org/10.1007/s40256-020-00397-y

If you want to cite the papers, please refer to the original.

For technical reasons we could not place the page where the original quote is coming from.

Abstract-Summary "Recent data regarding the use of antidiabetic medications to prevent negative cardiovascular outcomes has revealed a positive association with reduced major adverse cardiovascular events (MACE)."

"One class of medications, sodium-glucose cotransporter-2 (SGLT-2) inhibitors, are at the forefront of the cardiovascular outcomes prevention discussion."

"The clinical data presented in this review indicate the potential cardiovascular benefits of SGLT-2 inhibitors in patients with CVD and its potential value as a treatment option in preventing CVD in various patient populations."

Introduction

"Such considerations have strongly encouraged the American Diabetes Association (ADA) to highlight antidiabetic therapy that not only targets glycated hemoglobin (HbA1c) lowering but also aids in the reduction of blood pressure (BP) and weight, with added benefits for HF and renal disease protection to reduce the risk of CVD complications in patients with T2DM [165]."

"Clinical studies in patients with T2DM and a history of ASCVD taking SGLT-2 inhibitor therapy have shown reduced rates of MACE [165]."

"When studied in patients with T2DM, empagliflozin (Jardiance®) demonstrated a reduction in cardiovascular outcomes, including cardiovascular mortality and HHF, and canagliflozin (Invokana®) displayed a decrease in HHF."

"To date, dapagliflozin (Farxiga®) is the only SGLT-2 inhibitor to show a reduction in cardiovascular death and in worsening of HF (WHF) in patients both with and without T2DM."

Sodium-Glucose Cotransporter-2 (SGLT-2) Inhibitors

"Results from the CREDENCE study released in early 2019 led the FDA to grant another significant indication for canagliflozin: reducing the doubling of serum creatinine and reducing the risk of ESRD, cardiovascular death, and HHF in patients with T2DM and diabetic nephropathy with albuminuria of >300 mg/day [166]."

"The PRESERVED-HF study (target completion date September 2019) is a phase IV study evaluating the effects of dapagliflozin 10 mg once daily versus placebo on the change in NT-proBNP from baseline to 12 weeks in patients with NYHA class II–IV HFpEF with an elevated NT-proBNP presenting with at least one additional risk factor [167]."

"The DELIVER study (target completion date June 2021) is a phase III study evaluating the reduction in the composite of cardiovascular death or HHF/urgent HF visits with dapagliflozin 10 mg once daily versus placebo in 4700 patients with NYHA class II–IV HFpEF who have elevated NT-proBNP levels at baseline [168]."

Discussion

"In the 2018 ADA guidelines, in addition to liraglutide (GLP-1 RA), SGLT-2 inhibitors are recommended as a first-choice add-on treatment in patients with T2DM and established ASCVD who do not achieve adequate glycemic control with metformin monotherapy [169]."

"Clinical studies have consistently demonstrated the significant effects of SGLT-2 inhibitors on the relative risk reduction of HHF and progression of renal disease."

"The cardiovascular benefits of SGLT-2 inhibitors may be due to the glycemic control attained by these agents in patients with diabetes, suggesting that achieving adequate glycemic control may have a greater effect in the reduction of microvascular complications than in macrovascular complications."

"In relation to the possible adverse effects (AEs) of SGLT-2 inhibitors, as a drug class they are well-tolerated in patients with T2DM."

"Patient education on the signs and symptoms associated with DKA for patients taking SGLT-2 inhibitors is crucial because patients are often euglycemic in DKA on these agents."

Conclusions

"The robust data from these large clinical studies of SGLT-2 inhibitors have provided evidence that these agents, unlike other glucose-lowering agents, have a positive benefit in a spectrum of patients with T2DM with and without established CVD, including HF."

"Published data on these agents have also shown significant benefits on cardiovascular outcomes in patients without T2DM."

"Major clinical studies are currently ongoing and will hopefully provide more insight and rigorous data to further support the efficacy of these agents in patients with CVD."

SGLT2 Inhibitors and Mechanisms of Hypertension [170]

This is a machine-generated summary of:

Briasoulis, Alexandros; Al Dhaybi, Omar; Bakris, George L.: SGLT2 Inhibitors and Mechanisms of Hypertension [170].

Published in: Current Cardiology Reports (2018).

Link to original: https://doi.org/10.1007/s11886-018-0943-5

If you want to cite the papers, please refer to the original.
For technical reasons we could not place the page where the original quote is coming from.

Abstract-Summary "We sought to review currently available data on the safety and efficacy of sodium-glucose cotransporter 2 (SGLT2) inhibitors in type 2 diabetes mellitus patients with hypertension."

"Recent randomized clinical trials in high cardiovascular risk patients with type 2 diabetes suggest that the unique effects of SGLT2 inhibitors on blood pressure and body weight may translate into reduced cardiovascular events and slowed kidney disease progression."

"SGLT2 inhibitors are viable second-line glucose-lowering agents for people with type 2 diabetes with high cardiovascular risk."

Introduction

"Hypertension (HTN) and diabetes mellitus (DM) coexist frequently and those with HTN are at substantially higher risk for worsening cardiovascular disease (CVD) and chronic kidney disease (CKD) progression compared with people with type 2 diabetes who are normotensive [171, 172]."

"Among those with type 2 diabetes, approximately 40% have HTN at the time of DM diagnosis [173]."

"The etiology of HTN in DM cannot be explained solely by diabetic kidney disease as in approximately half of these patients as HTN occurs before the onset of moderately increased albuminuria [173]."

"The excess filtered glucose is reabsorbed in the proximal tubule via a sodium-glucose cotransporter (SGLT) and leads to increased sodium reabsorption [174]."

"SGLT2 inhibitors reduce both blood glucose, BP, and weight."

"SGLT2 inhibitors promote the renal excretion of glucose and thereby modestly lower elevated blood glucose levels in diabetic patients [175–178]."

Pharmacology of SGLT2 Inhibitors

"The SGLT transporters are located on the luminal surface of the proximal tubule epithelium and transport glucose into the cells against the concentration gradient by cotransporting glucose with sodium."

"Passive transport of glucose out of the cell is mediated by the basolateral GLUT transporters in the proximal tubule, following the concentration gradient."

"Two of the SGLT transporters are involved in the renal reabsorption of glucose."

"About 90% of the filtered glucose is reabsorbed in the early proximal tubule via the action of SGLT2, a high-capacity, low-affinity transporter selectively expressed in the kidney."

"In the distal segment of the tubule, the low-capacity SGLT1 transports the remaining glucose (about 10% of the total)."

"Of SGLT2 transporter upregulation, glucose excretion in the urine occurs at higher plasma glucose levels in patients with diabetes [179]."

"SGLT2 inhibition decreases glucose reabsorption in the proximal tubule of the kidney and modestly lowers blood glucose levels."

SGLT2 Inhibitors and HTN: Clinical Data

"A more recent meta-analysis of 22,528 patients from 43 randomized control trials demonstrated a significant reduction in SBP (weighted mean difference – 2.46 mmHg (95% CI – 2.86 to −2.06)) and DBP (weighted mean difference of −1.46 mmHg (95% CI – 1.82 to −1.09)) with SGLT2 inhibitors compared to placebo or other agents [180]."

"In a separate study of 20 obese patients with type 2 DM, the diuretic effect of SGLT2 inhibition was noted to wane over time [181], while systolic BP decreased by 5.3 mmHg following 2 weeks of therapy, the reduction mainly correlated with glycosuria ($r = -0.62$, $p = 0.0073$)."

"To further test the effects of SGLT2 inhibitors on 24-h BP profiles, body weight, plasma volume, and GFR, dapagliflozin monotherapy was compared with dapagliflozin (10 mg/day) plus hydrochlorothiazide (25 mg/day) or placebo in a small cohort of type 2 diabetic patients [182]."

SGLT2 Inhibitors and Clinical Outcomes

"The primary composite endpoint of death from cardiovascular causes, nonfatal myocardial infarction, or nonfatal stroke occurred in fewer patients assigned to empagliflozin than to placebo (−1.6% absolute risk reduction), with the results driven by a significant reduction in risk of death from cardiovascular causes (−2.2% absolute risk reduction), without differences between empagliflozin doses."

"In this broad population, 87% of whom did not have a history of CVD, data showed that treatment with SGLT2 inhibitors (canagliflozin in 53%, dapagliflozin in 42%, and empagliflozin in 5% of patients) was associated with a lower rate of hospitalization for heart failure and death from any cause compared with other glucose-lowering agents."

"The primary composite endpoint of death from cardiovascular causes, nonfatal myocardial infarction, or nonfatal stroke occurred in significantly less patients in the canagliflozin group (−4.6% absolute risk reduction)."

Conclusion

"SGLT2 inhibitors are the first class to show reductions in CVD mortality and slowed CKD progression among those with vascular disease that is diabetes."

"They reduce not only glucose but also BP and weight through yet undetermined mechanisms."

"Much of the attributed effects of this class are attributed to glucose loss in the urine; however, the benefits are still seen in people with stage 3 CKD where the osmotic/glucose-lowering effects are negligible [183]."

"More research is needed to help understand why this class is doing more than lowering glucose."

Efficacy and Safety of Dapagliflozin, a Sodium Glucose Cotransporter 2 (SGLT2) Inhibitor, in Diabetes Mellitus [163]

This is a machine-generated summary of:

Fioretto, Paola; Giaccari, Andrea; Sesti, Giorgio: Efficacy and safety of dapagliflozin, a sodium glucose cotransporter 2 (SGLT2) inhibitor, in diabetes mellitus [163].

Published in: Cardiovascular Diabetology (2015).

Link to original: https://doi.org/10.1186/s12933-015-0297-x

If you want to cite the papers, please refer to the original.

For technical reasons we could not place the page where the original quote is coming from.

Abstract-Summary "Although antidiabetic agents have been developed to target one or more of the core defects of type 2 diabetes mellitus (T2DM), many patients do not achieve glycemic goals."

"As the mechanism of action of SGLT2 inhibitors is different from other agents and completely insulin-independent, the use of these drugs might potentially be efficacious alone or in combination with any other antidiabetic drug, including insulin."

"Dapagliflozin is a highly selective and reversible SGLT2 inhibitor approved for use in adult patients with T2DM as monotherapy in patients intolerant of metformin or as adjunctive therapy in patients inadequately controlled on existing antidiabetic medications, including insulin."

"Preliminary data from a phase 2 pharmacokinetic/pharmacodynamic study suggest that dapagliflozin may also improve glycemic control in patients with type 1 diabetes mellitus."

"Clinical trials published to date show that dapagliflozin is safe and effective as monotherapy or as an add-on to insulin or oral antidiabetic agents in patients with T2DM."

Background

"The core defects of T2DM include quantitative and qualitative β-cell dysfunction, peripheral (skeletal muscle) insulin resistance, and elevated glucose production in the liver, as well as increased lipolysis when obesity is present."

"It is becoming accepted that other known mechanisms, including increased glucagon, decreased incretin effect, increased glucose reabsorption in the kidneys and some neurotransmitter dysfunction, are also involved in the pathophysiology of T2DM [184]."

"The currently available antidiabetic agents have been developed to target one or more of the underlying defects or processes involved in T2DM [185]."

"SGLT2 inhibitors currently approved or under investigation include dapagliflozin, canagliflozin, empagliflozin and ipragliflozin; this manuscript will focus on the efficacy and safety of the highly selective and reversible SGLT2 inhibitor dapagliflozin, primarily in patients with T2DM."

Search Strategy

"A literature search was conducted using the PubMed database to identify key papers related to human studies of dapagliflozin in the treatment of patients with diabetes mellitus."

"Additional papers were included from the reference lists of relevant articles sourced from the search."

"The initial search was updated to include articles published up to March 27, 2015."

The Role of the Kidney in Glucose Reabsorption

"Renal glucose reabsorption is achieved through the action of the SGLT family of protein transporters, primarily SGLT1 and SGLT2 [186]."

"In individuals without T2DM, SGLT2 is responsible for the majority (80–90%) of renal glucose reabsorption [186, 187]."

"When the concentration of glucose in plasma exceeds that which can be reabsorbed via the SGLT proteins, the excessive amount of glucose is excreted in the urine [188, 189]."

"Data from animal models of diabetes and from preclinical human models suggest that the hyperglycemic state in T2DM is associated with significantly increased expression of SGLT2 and GLUT2 proteins, together with an increased level of renal glucose reabsorption [188, 190]."

The Role of Glycosuria in Glucotoxicity

"The harmful metabolic effects of chronic hyperglycemia associated with the two core defects of T2DM, insulin resistance and partial β-cell failure, can be described as "glucose toxicity", which contributes in turn to further progression of β-cell dysfunction in a vicious cycle of glucose toxicity-induced pathogenesis [191, 192]."

"Tight glycemic glucose control is, in part, considered essential to reverse or slow the glucotoxic effects of chronic hyperglycemia on the β-cells [193]."

"Glycosuria occurs when the maximal reabsorptive capacity of the glucose transport system in the kidney becomes saturated, above or just below the theoretical plasma glucose threshold of approx 11 mmol/L (198 mg/dL); both the threshold and the transport maximum of glucose are higher in patients with diabetes mellitus [187]."

"Induction of glycosuria without affecting other metabolic parameters has been shown to reduce elevated plasma glucose levels, supporting the hypothesis that glucose toxicity contributes to β-cell dysfunction in patients with T2DM and that reversing glucose toxicity via "therapeutic glycosuria" may improve insulin sensitivity and β-cell function [191, 194, 195]."

Sodium-Glucose Cotransporter 2 Inhibitors

"Inhibition of SGLT2 results in a lowering of the threshold for renal glucose excretion and an increase in urinary glucose excretion, with an associated reduction in plasma glucose levels and the potential to decrease glucose toxicity with chronic administration [188, 196, 197]."

"Weight loss associated with SGLT2 inhibitors is biphasic, with an initial reduction in total body weight which can be attributed to fluid loss and a subsequent gradual continuous reduction resulting from increased urinary glucose excretion with associated loss of calories [195, 197–199]."

"The effects of SGLT2 inhibitors on hyperglycemia, body weight, and blood pressure suggest a favorable effect on cardiovascular risk factors."

"The effects of SGLT2 inhibitors on macrovascular and microvascular outcomes are yet to be determined in human studies; however, adding SGLT2 inhibitors, and specifically dapagliflozin, to the standard of care was recently projected to reduce cardiovascular and microvascular complications associated with T2DM, in a human model study using simulation methodology [200]."

Dapagliflozin in Type 2 Diabetes Mellitus

"Dapagliflozin has been shown to be effective in several large (n > 261), randomized, double-blind, placebo-controlled studies of 12 or 24 weeks' duration in treatment-naïve patients with T2DM [201–203]."

"A recent meta-analysis designed to evaluate whether dapagliflozin is synergistic with other antidiabetic agents without affecting body weight concluded that dapagliflozin in combination with conventional antidiabetic drugs (metformin, glimepiride, pioglitazone, and metformin/sitagliptin) improved glycemic control (the overall effect size was −0.52%) and reduced weight gain in patients with T2DM (the effect size was −2.10 kg) [204]."

"Of interest, dapagliflozin 10 mg treatment significantly improved glycemic control and reduced body weight both in 151 early-stage and in 58 late-stage patients with T2DM, reflecting the usefulness of dapagliflozin as monotherapy in patients in the early stage of T2DM, and as add-on or combination therapy in late-stage patients on high doses of insulin plus oral insulin sensitizers [205]."

Dapagliflozin in Type 1 Diabetes Mellitus

"A pilot study describing 2 weeks of dapagliflozin treatment in 62 patients with T1DM showed dose-related reductions in glycemic variability, 24-h glucose and insulin requirement [206]."

"Patients with T1DM on stable insulin therapy were randomized to dapagliflozin 1, 2.5, 5, or 10 mg or placebo."

"Short-term tolerability was acceptable, and the pharmacokinetic profile was similar to that observed in studies in patients with T2DM, including dose-dependent increases in urinary glucose excretion."

"Changes suggestive of improved glycemic control were observed, which will be further explored in larger trials of longer duration."

Conclusions

“Dapagliflozin is an orally available SGLT2 inhibitor with an insulin independent mechanism of action and a lower risk of hypoglycemia than with conventional anti-diabetic agents such as sulfonylureas and insulin.”

“Clinical trials published to date have shown that dapagliflozin is effective and safe in patients with T2DM, both as monotherapy and in combination with other glucose-lowering agents, and recent data reporting 4-years’ clinical experience support these findings [207].”

“Dapagliflozin is effective in both early and late stages of T2DM, despite differences in disease status and concomitant medications, suggesting that the insulin-independent mechanism of action of dapagliflozin could make it a suitable treatment option throughout the different stages of clinical progression of T2DM.”

“Dapagliflozin is also expected to be effective as an adjunct to insulin for the treatment of T1DM, and may be particularly appropriate in patients with T1DM treated with high doses of insulin or who need weight loss.”

Bibliography

1. Jha KK, Adhikari R, Tasdighi E, Osuji N, Rajan T, Blaha MJ (2022) Transitioning to GLP-1 RAs and SGLT2 inhibitors as the first choice for managing Cardiometabolic risk in type 2 diabetes. Curr Atheroscler Rep 24:925. https://doi.org/10.1007/s11883-022-01066-y
2. McMurray JJ, Gerstein HC, Holman RR, Pfeffer MA (2014) Heart failure: a cardiovascular outcome in diabetes that can no longer be ignored. Lancet Diabetes Endocrinol 2:843–851. https://doi.org/10.1016/S2213-8587(14)70031-2
3. Moss SE, Klein R, Klein BE (1991) Cause-specific mortality in a population-based study of diabetes. Am J Public Health 81(9):1158–1162. https://doi.org/10.2105/ajph.81.9.1158
4. Kranenburg G, van der Graaf Y, van der Leeuw J, Nathoe HM, de Borst GJ, Kappelle LJ et al (2015) The relation between HbA1c and cardiovascular events in patients with type 2 diabetes with and without vascular disease. Diabetes Care 38(10):1930–1936. https://doi.org/10.2337/dc15-0493
5. Sarwar N, Aspelund T, Eiriksdottir G, Gobin R, Seshasai SR, Forouhi NG et al (2010) Markers of dysglycaemia and risk of coronary heart disease in people without diabetes: Reykjavik prospective study and systematic review. PLoS Med 7(5):e1000278. https://doi.org/10.1371/journal.pmed.1000278
6. Lamanna C, Monami M, Marchionni N, Mannucci E (2011) Effect of metformin on cardiovascular events and mortality: a meta-analysis of randomized clinical trials. Diabetes Obes Metab 13(3):221–228. https://doi.org/10.1111/j.1463-1326.2010.01349.x
7. Medicine. USNLo: Investigation of metformin in pre-diabetes on atherosclerotic cardiovascular outcomes. https://clinicaltrials.gov/show/NCT02915198. Accessed 23 Nov 2021
8. Zinman B, Wanner C, Lachin JM, Fitchett D, Bluhmki E, Hantel S et al (2015) Empagliflozin, cardiovascular outcomes, and mortality in type 2 diabetes. N Engl J Med 373(22):2117–2128
9. Lytvyn Y, Bjornstad P, Udell JA, Lovshin JA, Cherney DZI (2017) Sodium glucose cotransporter-2 inhibition in heart failure: potential mechanisms, clinical applications, and summary of clinical trials. Circulation 136(17):1643–1658. https://doi.org/10.1161/circulationaha.117.030012

10. Peters AL, Buschur EO, Buse JB, Cohan P, Diner JC, Hirsch IB (2015) Euglycemic diabetic ketoacidosis: a potential complication of treatment with sodium-glucose cotransporter 2 inhibition. Diabetes Care 38(9):1687–1693
11. Legaspi R, Narciso P (2015) Euglycemic diabetic ketoacidosis due to gastroparesis, a local experience. J Ark Med Soc 112(5):62–63
12. Wiviott SD, Raz I, Bonaca MP, Mosenzon O, Kato ET, Cahn A et al (2019) Dapagliflozin and cardiovascular outcomes in type 2 diabetes. N Engl J Med 380(4):347–357
13. Bhatt DL, Szarek M, Steg PG et al (2021) Sotagliflozin in patients with diabetes and recent worsening heart failure. N Engl J Med 384:117–128
14. Perkovic V, Jardine MJ, Neal B, Bompoint S, Heerspink HJL, Charytan DM et al (2019) Canagliflozin and renal outcomes in type 2 diabetes and nephropathy. N Engl J Med 380(24):2295–2306
15. Cavender MA, Norhammar A, Birkeland KI, Jorgensen ME, Wilding JP, Khunti K et al (2018) SGLT-2 inhibitors and cardiovascular risk: an analysis of CVD-REAL. J Am Coll Cardiol 71(22):2497–2506
16. Kosiborod M, Lam CSP, Kohsaka S, Kim DJ, Karasik A, Shaw J, Tangri N, Goh SY, Thuresson M, Chen H et al (2018) Cardiovascular events associated with SGLT-2 inhibitors versus other glucose-lowering drugs: the CVD-REAL 2 study. J Am Coll Cardiol 71(23):2628–2639
17. Marso SP, Daniels GH, Brown-Frandsen K, Kristensen P, Mann JF, Nauck MA et al (2016) Liraglutide and cardiovascular outcomes in type 2 diabetes. N Engl J Med 375(4):311–322
18. Marso SP, Bain SC, Consoli A, Eliaschewitz FG, Jodar E, Leiter LA et al (2016) Semaglutide and cardiovascular outcomes in patients with type 2 diabetes. N Engl J Med 375(19):1834–1844
19. Giugliano D, Scappaticcio L, Longo M, Caruso P, Maiorino MI, Bellastella G et al (2021) GLP-1 receptor agonists and cardiorenal outcomes in type 2 diabetes: an updated meta-analysis of eight CVOTs. Cardiovasc Diabetol 20(1):189. https://doi.org/10.1186/s12933-021-01366-8
20. FDANewsRelease (2016) FDA approves Jardiance to reduce cardiovascular death in adults with type 2 diabetes. https://www.fda.gov/news-events/press-announcements/fda-approves-jardiance-reduce-cardiovascular-death-adults-type-2-diabetes. Accessed 30 Nov 2021
21. FDANewsRelease (2020) FDA approves new treatment for a type of heart failure. https://www.fda.gov/news-events/press-announcements/fda-approves-new-treatment-type-heart-failure. Accessed 30 Nov 2021
22. FDANewsRelease (2020) FDA approves dulaglutide for adults with T2D, regardless of CVD. https://www.ajmc.com/view/fda-approves-dulaglutide-for-adults-with-t2d-regardless-of-cvd. Accessed 30 Nov 2021
23. Visseren FLJ, Mach F, Smulders YM, Carballo D, Koskinas KC, Bäck M et al (2021) ESC guidelines on cardiovascular disease prevention in clinical practice. Eur J Prev Cardiol 2021:5. https://doi.org/10.1093/eurjpc/zwab154
24. Committee ADAPP (2021) 10. Cardiovascular disease and risk management: standards of medical care in diabetes—2022. Diabetes Care 45(Supplement_1):S144–S174. https://doi.org/10.2337/dc22-S010. This recent guideline (despite the 2021 version) proposed utilizing SGLT2is and GLP1-RAs as the first agent for T2DM treatment in patients with established ASCVD, HF, CKD, and high CV risk
25. Li C, Luo J, Jiang M, Wang K (2022) The efficacy and safety of the combination therapy with GLP-1 receptor agonists and SGLT-2 inhibitors in type 2 diabetes mellitus: a systematic review and meta-analysis. Front Pharmacol 13:838277. https://doi.org/10.3389/fphar.2022.838277
26. ClinicalTrials.gov. A research study to see how semaglutide works compared to placebo in people with type 2 diabetes and chronic kidney disease (FLOW). Identifier: NCT03819153. https://clinicaltrials.gov/ct2/show/NCT03819153. Accessed 16 Oct 2024
27. ClinicalTrials.gov.: renal effects of treatment with empagliflozin alone or in combination with semaglutide in patients with type 2 diabetes and albuminuria (EmpaSema). Identifier: NCT04061200. https://clinicaltrials.gov/ct2/show/NCT04061200. Accessed 16 Oct 2024

28. PCORI.org (2021) PRECIDENTD (PREvention of CardIovascular and DiabEtic kidNey disease in Type 2 Diabetes). https://www.pcori.org/research-results/2021/precidentd-prevention-cardiovascular-and-diabetic-kidney-disease-type-2. Accessed 20 Nov 2021
29. Arbab-Zadeh A, Fuster V (2015) The myth of the "vulnerable plaque": transitioning from a focus on individual lesions to atherosclerotic disease burden for coronary artery disease risk assessment. J Am Coll Cardiol 65(8):846–855. https://doi.org/10.1016/j.jacc.2014.11.041
30. Cardoso R, Dudum R, Ferraro RA, Bittencourt M, Blankstein R, Blaha MJ et al (2020) Cardiac computed tomography for personalized management of patients with type 2 diabetes mellitus. Circ Cardiovasc Imaging 13(9):e011365. https://doi.org/10.1161/circimaging.120.011365
31. Elkeles RS, Godsland IF, Feher MD, Rubens MB, Roughton M, Nugara F et al (2008) Coronary calcium measurement improves prediction of cardiovascular events in asymptomatic patients with type 2 diabetes: the PREDICT study. Eur Heart J 29(18):2244–2251. https://doi.org/10.1093/eurheartj/ehn279
32. Malik S, Zhao Y, Budoff M, Nasir K, Blumenthal RS, Bertoni AG et al (2017) Coronary artery calcium score for long-term risk classification in individuals with type 2 diabetes and metabolic syndrome from the multi-ethnic study of atherosclerosis. JAMA Cardiol 2(12):1332–1340. https://doi.org/10.1001/jamacardio.2017.4191
33. Bittencourt MS, Hulten E, Ghoshhajra B, O'Leary D, Christman MP, Montana P et al (2014) Prognostic value of nonobstructive and obstructive coronary artery disease detected by coronary computed tomography angiography to identify cardiovascular events. Circ Cardiovasc Imaging 7(2):282–291. https://doi.org/10.1161/circimaging.113.001047
34. Cainzos-Achirica M, Patel KV, Quispe R, Joshi PH, Khera A, Ayers C et al (2021) Coronary artery calcium for the allocation of GLP-1RA for primary prevention of atherosclerotic cardiovascular disease. JACC Cardiovasc Imaging 14(7):1470–1472. https://doi.org/10.1016/j.jcmg.2020.12.024
35. Pitt B, Filippatos G, Agarwal R, Anker SD, Bakris GL, Rossing P et al (2021) Cardiovascular events with finerenone in kidney disease and type 2 diabetes. N Engl J Med 385:2252. https://doi.org/10.1056/NEJMoa2110956
36. Bakris GL, Agarwal R, Anker SD, Pitt B, Ruilope LM, Rossing P et al (2020) Effect of finerenone on chronic kidney disease outcomes in type 2 diabetes. N Engl J Med 383(23):2219–2229. https://doi.org/10.1056/NEJMoa2025845
37. Agarwal R (2021) Cardiovascular and kidney outcomes with finerenone in patients with type 2 diabetes and chronic kidney disease: the FIDELITY pooled analysis. Eur Heart J 43:474. https://doi.org/10.1093/eurheartj/ehab777
38. Adminestration USFD (2022) FDA approves novel, dual-targeted treatment for type 2 diabetes. https://www.fda.gov/news-events/press-announcements/fda-approves-novel-dual-targeted-treatment-type-2-diabetes. Accessed 16 Oct 2024
39. Lyu YS, Oh S, Kim JH, Kim SY, Jeong MH (2023) Comparison of SGLT2 inhibitors with DPP-4 inhibitors combined with metformin in patients with acute myocardial infarction and diabetes mellitus. Cardiovasc Diabetol 22(1):185. https://doi.org/10.1186/s12933-023-01914-4
40. International Diabetes Federation (2016) Diabetes and cardiovascular disease report. IDF, Brussels
41. Neal B, Perkovic V, Mahaffey KW, De Zeeuw D, Fulcher G, Erondu N et al (2017) Canagliflozin and cardiovascular and renal events in type 2 diabetes. N Engl J Med 377(7):644–657
42. Cannon CP, Pratley R, Dagogo-Jack S, Mancuso J, Huyck S, Masiukiewicz U et al (2020) Cardiovascular outcomes with ertugliflozin in type 2 diabetes. N Engl J Med 383(15):1425–1435
43. Thygesen K, Alpert JS, Jaffe AS, Simoons ML, Chaitman BR, White HD, Joint ESCAAHAWHFTFfUDoMI, Authors/Task Force, Members C, Thygesen K, Alpert JS et al (2012) Third universal definition of myocardial infarction. J Am Coll Cardiol 60(16):1581–1598

44. Chang T-Y, Lu C-T, Huang H-L, Chou R-H, Chang C-C, Liu C-T, Huang P-H, Lin S-J (2022) Association of Sodium-Glucose cotransporter 2 (SGLT2) inhibitor use with cardiovascular and renal outcomes in type 2 diabetes mellitus patients with stabilized acute myocardial infarction: a propensity score matching study. Front Cardiovasc Med 9:882181
45. Kohsaka S, Lam CSP, Kim DJ, Cavender MA, Norhammar A, Jorgensen ME et al (2020) Risk of cardiovascular events and death associated with initiation of SGLT2 inhibitors compared with DPP-4 inhibitors: an analysis from the CVD-REAL 2 multinational cohort study. Lancet Diabetes Endocrinol 8(7):606–615
46. Persson F, Nyström T, Jørgensen ME, Carstensen B, Gulseth HL, Thuresson M, Fenici P, Nathanson D, Eriksson JW, Norhammar A (2018) Dapagliflozin is associated with lower risk of cardiovascular events and all-cause mortality in people with type 2 diabetes (CVD-REAL Nordic) when compared with dipeptidyl peptidase-4 inhibitor therapy: a multinational observational study. Diabetes Obes Metab 20(2):344–351
47. Zheng SL, Roddick AJ, Aghar-Jaffar R, Shun-Shin MJ, Francis D, Oliver N, Meeran K (2018) Association between use of sodium-glucose cotransporter 2 inhibitors, glucagon-like peptide 1 agonists, and dipeptidyl peptidase 4 inhibitors with all-cause mortality in patients with type 2 diabetes: a systematic review and meta-analysis. JAMA 319(15):1580–1591
48. Habibi J, Aroor AR, Sowers JR, Jia G, Hayden MR, Garro M, Barron B, Mayoux E, Rector RS, Whaley-Connell A, DeMarco VG (2017) Sodium glucose transporter 2 (SGLT2) inhibition with empagliflozin improves cardiac diastolic function in a female rodent model of diabetes. Cardiovasc Diabetol 16:9. https://doi.org/10.1186/s12933-016-0489-z
49. Peterson LR, Herrero P, Schechtman KB, Racette SB, Waggoner AD, Kisrieva-Ware Z, Dence C, Klein S, Marsala J, Meyer T et al (2004) Effect of obesity and insulin resistance on myocardial substrate metabolism and efficiency in young women. Circulation 109(18):2191–2196
50. Peterson LR, Waggoner AD, Schechtman KB, Meyer T, Gropler RJ, Barzilai B, Davila-Roman VG (2004) Alterations in left ventricular structure and function in young healthy obese women: assessment by echocardiography and tissue Doppler imaging. J Am Coll Cardiol 43(8):1399–1404
51. Peterson LR, Soto PF, Herrero P, Mohammed BS, Avidan MS, Schechtman KB, Dence C, Gropler RJ (2008) Impact of gender on the myocardial metabolic response to obesity. JACC Cardiovasc Imaging 1(4):424–433
52. Ren J, Ceylan-Isik AF (2004) Diabetic cardiomyopathy: do women differ from men? Endocrine 25(2):73–83
53. Yue P, Arai T, Terashima M, Sheikh AY, Cao F, Charo D, Hoyt G, Robbins RC, Ashley EA, Wu J et al (2007) Magnetic resonance imaging of progressive cardiomyopathic changes in the db/db mouse. Am J Physiol Heart Circ Physiol 292(5):H2106–H2118
54. Hummel KP, Dickie MM, Coleman DL (1966) Diabetes, a new mutation in the mouse. Science 153(3740):1127–1128
55. Zhang H, Morgan B, Potter BJ, Ma L, Dellsperger KC, Ungvari ZI, Zhang C (2010) Resveratrol improves left ventricular diastolic relaxation in type 2 diabetes by inhibiting oxidative/nitrative stress. Am J Physiol Heart Circ Physiol 299:985–994
56. Durak A, Olgar Y, Degirmenci S, Akkus E, Tuncay E, Turan B (2018) A SGLT2 inhibitor dapagliflozin suppresses prolonged ventricular-repolarization through augmentation of mitochondrial function in insulin-resistant metabolic syndrome rats. Cardiovasc Diabetol 17(1):144. https://doi.org/10.1186/s12933-018-0790-0
57. Aguilar D, Bozkurt B, Ramasubbu K, Deswal A (2009) Relationship of hemoglobin A1C and mortality in heart failure patients with diabetes. J Am Coll Cardiol 54(5):422–428
58. Pocock SJ, Wang D, Pfeffer MA, Yusuf S, McMurray JJ, Swedberg KB, Ostergren J, Michelson EL, Pieper KS, Granger CB (2006) Predictors of mortality and morbidity in patients with chronic heart failure. Eur Heart J 27(1):65–75
59. Khalaf KI, Taegtmeyer H (2012) After avandia: the use of antidiabetic drugs in patients with heart failure. Tex Heart Inst J 39(2):174–178

60. Bilginoglu A, Kandilci HB, Turan B (2013) Intracellular levels of Na(+) and TTX-sensitive Na(+) channel current in diabetic rat ventricular cardiomyocytes. Cardiovasc Toxicol 13(2):138–147
61. Turan B, Desilets M, Acan LN, Hotomaroglu O, Vannier C, Vassort G (1996) Oxidative effects of selenite on rat ventricular contractility and ca movements. Cardiovasc Res 32(2):351–361
62. Olgar Y, Degirmenci S, Durak A, Billur D, Can B, Mutlu GK, Inan EA, Turan B (2018) Aging related functional and structural changes in the heart and aorta: MitoTEMPO improves aged-cardiovascular performance. Exp Gerontol 110:172–181
63. Litvinova L, Atochin DN, Fattakhov N, Vasilenko M, Zatolokin P, Kirienkova E (2015) Nitric oxide and mitochondria in metabolic syndrome. Front Physiol 6:20
64. Mitchell T, Darley-Usmar V (2012) Metabolic syndrome and mitochondrial dysfunction: insights from preclinical studies with a mitochondrially targeted antioxidant. Free Radic Biol Med 52(5):838–840
65. Kusaka H, Koibuchi N, Hasegawa Y, Ogawa H, Kim-Mitsuyama S (2016) Empagliflozin lessened cardiac injury and reduced visceral adipocyte hypertrophy in prediabetic rats with metabolic syndrome. Cardiovasc Diabetol 15:157
66. Lee T-M, Chang N-C, Lin S-Z (2017) Dapagliflozin, a selective SGLT2 inhibitor, attenuated cardiac fibrosis by regulating the macrophage polarization via STAT3 signaling in infarcted rat hearts. Free Radic Biol Med 104:298–310
67. Tanajak P, Sa-Nguanmoo P, Sivasinprasasn S, Thummasorn S, Siri-Angkul N, Chattipakorn SC et al (2018) Cardioprotection of dapagliflozin and vildagliptin in rats with cardiac ischemia-reperfusion injury. J Endocrinol 236:69–84
68. Chen H, Teng D, Xu B, Wang C, Wang H, Jia W, Gong L, Dong H, Zhong L, Yang J (2023) The SGLT2 inhibitor Canagliflozin reduces atherosclerosis by enhancing macrophage autophagy. J Cardiovas Transl Res 16:999. https://doi.org/10.1007/s12265-023-10390-w
69. Cowie MR, Fisher M (2020) SGLT2 inhibitors: mechanisms of cardiovascular benefit beyond glycaemic control. Nat Rev Cardiol 17(12):761–772. https://doi.org/10.1038/s41569-020-0406-8
70. Xu L et al (2017) SGLT2 inhibition by empagliflozin promotes fat utilization and browning and attenuates inflammation and insulin resistance by polarizing M2 macrophages in diet-induced obese mice. EBioMedicine 20:137–149. https://doi.org/10.1016/j.ebiom.2017.05.028
71. Xu L, Ota T (2018) Emerging roles of SGLT2 inhibitors in obesity and insulin resistance: focus on fat browning and macrophage polarization. Adipocytes 7(2):121–128
72. Stawowy P, Meyborg H, Stibenz D et al (2005) Furin-like proprotein convertases are central regulators of the membrane type matrix metalloproteinase-pro-matrix metalloproteinase-2 proteolytic cascade in atherosclerosis. Circulation 111(21):2820–2827
73. He J, Zhang G, Pang Q et al (2017) SIRT6 reduces macrophage foam cell formation by inducing autophagy and cholesterol efflux under ox-LDL condition. FEBS J 284(9):1324–1337
74. Ouimet M, Franklin V, Mak E, Liao X, Tabas I, Marcel YL (2011) Autophagy regulates cholesterol efflux from macrophage foam cells via lysosomal acid lipase. Cell Metab 13(6):655–667
75. Jeong SJ, Lee MN, Oh GT (2017) The role of macrophage lipophagy in reverse cholesterol transport. Endocrinol Metab (Seoul) 32(1):41–46
76. Martinet W, De Meyer I, Verheye S, Schrijvers DM, Timmermans JP, De Meyer GR (2013) Drug-induced macrophage autophagy in atherosclerosis: for better or worse. Basic Res Cardiol 108(1):321
77. Han JH, Oh TJ, Lee G et al (2017) The beneficial effects of empagliflozin, an SGLT2 inhibitor, on atherosclerosis in ApoE(−/−) mice fed a western diet. Diabetologia 60(2):364–376
78. Terasaki M, Hiromura M, Mori Y et al (2015) Amelioration of hyperglycemia with a sodium-glucose cotransporter 2 inhibitor prevents macrophage-driven atherosclerosis through macrophage foam cell formation suppression in type 1 and type 2 diabetic mice. PLoS One 10(11):e0143396

79. Al-Sharea A, Murphy AJ, Huggins LA, Hu Y, Goldberg IJ, Nagareddy PR (2018) SGLT2 inhibition reduces atherosclerosis by enhancing lipoprotein clearance in Ldlr(−/−) type 1 diabetic mice. Atherosclerosis 271:166–176
80. Nasiri-Ansari N, Dimitriadis GK, Agrogiannis G et al (2018) Canagliflozin attenuates the progression of atherosclerosis and inflammation process in APOE knockout mice. Cardiovasc Diabetol 17(1):106
81. Mori K, Tsuchiya K, Nakamura S et al (2019) Ipragliflozin-induced adipose expansion inhibits cuff-induced vascular remodeling in mice. Cardiovasc Diabetol 18(1):83
82. Sawami K, Tanaka A, Node K (2023) Recent understandings about hypertension management in type 2 diabetes: what are the roles of SGLT2 inhibitor, GLP-1 receptor agonist, and finerenone? Hypertens Res 46:1892. https://doi.org/10.1038/s41440-023-01324-9
83. Vaduganathan M, Mensah GA, Turco JV, Fuster V, Roth GA (2022) The global burden of cardiovascular diseases and risk: a compass for future health. J Am Coll Cardiol 80:2361–2371
84. Tatsumi Y, Ohkubo T (2017) Hypertension with diabetes mellitus: significance from an epidemiological perspective for Japanese. Hypertens Res 40:795–806
85. Ahmad E, Lim S, Lamptey R, Webb DR, Davies MJ (2022) Type 2 diabetes. Lancet 400:1803–1820
86. Ferrannini E, Cushman WC (2012) Diabetes and hypertension: the bad companions. Lancet 380:601–610
87. Adler AI (2000) Association of systolic blood pressure with macrovascular and microvascular complications of type 2 diabetes (UKPDS 36): prospective observational study. BMJ 321:412–419
88. UK Prospective Diabetes Study Group (1998) Tight blood pressure control and risk of macrovascular and microvascular complications in type 2 diabetes: UKPDS 38. BMJ 317:703–713
89. Umemura S, Arima H, Arima S, Asayama K, Dohi Y, Hirooka Y et al (2019) The Japanese Society of Hypertension Guidelines for the Management of Hypertension (JSH 2019). Hypertens Res 42:1235–1481
90. Arnett DK, Blumenthal RS, Albert MA, Buroker AB, Goldberger ZD, Hahn EJ et al (2019) 2019 ACC/AHA guideline on the primary prevention of cardiovascular disease: a report of the American College of Cardiology/American Heart Association task force on clinical practice guidelines. J Am Coll Cardiol 74:e177–e232
91. ElSayed NA, Aleppo G, Aroda VR, Bannuru RR, Brown FM, Bruemmer D et al (2023) 10. Cardiovascular disease and risk management: standards of Care in Diabetes-2023. Diabetes Care 46:S158–S190
92. Cosentino F, Grant PJ, Aboyans V et al (2020) 2019 ESC guidelines on diabetes, prediabetes, and cardiovascular diseases developed in collaboration with the EASD. Eur Heart J 41:255–32323
93. Kelsey MD, Nelson AJ, Green JB, Granger CB, Peterson ED, McGuire DK et al (2022) Guidelines for cardiovascular risk reduction in patients with type 2 diabetes: JACC guideline comparison. J Am Coll Cardiol 79:1849–1857
94. Emdin CA, Rahimi K, Neal B, Callender T, Perkovic V, Patel A (2015) Blood pressure lowering in type 2 diabetes: a systematic review and meta-analysis. JAMA 313:603–615
95. Nazarzadeh M, Bidel Z, Canoy D, Copland E, Bennett DA, Dehghan A et al (2022) Blood pressure-lowering treatment for prevention of major cardiovascular diseases in people with and without type 2 diabetes: an individual participant-level data meta-analysis. Lancet Diabetes Endocrinol 10:645–654
96. Davies MJ, Aroda VR, Collins BS, Gabbay RA, Green J, Maruthur NM et al (2022) Management of hyperglycaemia in type 2 diabetes, 2022. A consensus report by the American Diabetes Association (ADA) and the European Association for the Study of Diabetes (EASD). Diabetologia 2022(65):1925–1966
97. Kobayashi K, Toyoda M, Hatori N, Sakai H, Furuki T, Sato K et al (2022) Comparison of the blood pressure management between sodium-glucose cotransporter 2 inhibitors and glucagon-like peptide 1 receptor agonists. Sci Rep 12:16106

98. van Ruiten CC, Smits MM, Kok MD, Serné EH, van Raalte DH, Kramer M et al (2022) Mechanisms underlying the blood pressure lowering effects of dapagliflozin, exenatide, and their combination in people with type 2 diabetes: a secondary analysis of a randomized trial. Cardiovasc Diabetol 21:63
99. Tanaka A, Node K (2019) Evidence-based and tailored medication in type 2 diabetes: a pathway learned from clinical trials. Cardiovasc Diabetol 18:19
100. Gourdy P, Darmon P, Dievart F, Halimi J-M, Guerci B (2023) Combining glucagon-like peptide-1 receptor agonists (GLP-1RAs) and sodium-glucose cotransporter-2 inhibitors (SGLT2is) in patients with type 2 diabetes mellitus (T2DM). Cardiovasc Diabetol 22(1):79. https://doi.org/10.1186/s12933-023-01798-4
101. Sattar N, Lee MMY, Kristensen SL, Branch KRH, Del Prato S, Khurmi NS, Lam CSP, Lopes RD, McMurray JJV, Pratley RE, Rosenstock J, Gerstein HC (2021) Cardiovascular, mortality, and kidney outcomes with GLP-1 receptor agonists in patients with type 2 diabetes: a systematic review and meta-analysis of randomised trials. Lancet Diabetes Endocrinol 9(10):653–662
102. Guo M, Gu J, Teng F, Chen J, Ma X, Chen Q et al (2020) The efficacy and safety of combinations of SGLT2 inhibitors and GLP-1 receptor agonists in the treatment of type 2 diabetes or obese adults: a systematic review and meta-analysis. Endocrine 67(2):294–304
103. Wright AK, Carr MJ, Kontopantelis E, Leelarathna L, Thabit H, Emsley R et al (2022) Primary prevention of cardiovascular and heart failure events with SGLT2 inhibitors, GLP-1 receptor agonists, and their combination in type 2 diabetes. Diabetes Care 45(4):909–918
104. Trombara F, Cosentino N, Bonomi A, Ludergnani M, Poggio P, Gionti L, Baviera M, Colacioppo P, Roncaglioni MC, Leoni O, Bortolan F, Agostoni P, Genovese S, Marenzi G (2023) Impact of chronic GLP-1 RA and SGLT-2I therapy on in-hospital outcome of diabetic patients with acute myocardial infarction. Cardiovasc Diabetol 22:26. https://doi.org/10.1186/s12933-023-01758-y
105. Standl E, Khunti K, Hansen TB, Schnell O (2019) The global epidemics of diabetes in the 21st century: current situation and perspectives. Eur J Prev Cardiol 26(2):7–14
106. Ovbiagele B, Markovic D, Fonarow GC (2011) Recent US patterns and predictors of prevalent diabetes among acute myocardial infarction patients. Cardiol Res Pract 2011:1–8
107. Marenzi G, Cosentino N, Milazzo V et al (2018) Prognostic value of the acute-to-chronic glycemic ratio at admission in acute myocardial infarction: a prospective study. Diabetes Care 41:847–853
108. Marenzi G, Cosentino N, Genovese S et al (2019) Reduced cardio-renal function accounts for most of the in-hospital morbidity and mortality risk among patients with type 2 diabetes undergoing primary percutaneous coronary intervention for st-segment elevation myocardial infarction. Diabetes Care 42:1305–1311
109. Tripolt NJ, Kolesnik E, Pferschy PN et al (2020) Impact of EMpagliflozin on cardiac function and biomarkers of heart failure in patients with acute MYocardial infarction-the EMMY trial. Am Heart J 221:39–47
110. Burgess S, Juergens CP, Yang W et al (2021) Cardiac mortality, diabetes mellitus, and multivessel disease in ST elevation myocardial infarction. Int J Cardiol 323:13–18
111. Milazzo V, Cosentino N, Genovese S et al (2021) Diabetes mellitus and acute myocardial infarction: impact on short and long-term mortality. Adv Exp Med Biol 1307:153–169
112. Kristensen SL, Rorth R, Jhund PS, Docherty KF, Sattar N, Preiss D et al (2019) Cardiovascular, mortality, and kidney outcomes with GLP-1 receptor agonists in patients with type 2 diabetes: a systematic review and meta-analysis of cardiovascular outcome trials. Lancet Diabetes Endocrinol 7(10):776–785
113. Zelniker TA, Wiviott SD, Raz I, Im K, Goodrich EL, Furtado RHM et al (2019) Comparison of the effects of glucagon-like peptide receptor agonists and sodium-glucose cotransporter 2 inhibitors for prevention of major adverse cardiovascular and renal outcomes in type 2 diabetes mellitus. Circulation 139(17):2022–2031

114. Gerstein HC, Colhoun HM, Dagenais GR, Diaz R, Lakshmanan M, Pais P et al (2019a) Dulaglutide and cardiovascular outcomes in type 2 diabetes (REWIND): a double-blind, randomised placebo-controlled trial. Lancet 394(10193):121–130
115. Neuen BL, Ohkuma T, Neal B, Matthews DR, de Zeeuw D, Mahaffey KW et al (2018) Cardiovascular and renal outcomes with canagliflozin according to baseline kidney function. Circulation 138(15):1537–1550
116. Wanner C, Lachin JM, Inzucchi SE, Fitchett D, Mattheus M, George J, Woerle HJ, Broedl UC, von Eynatten M, Zinman B, EMPA-REG OUTCOME Investigators (2018) Empagliflozin and clinical outcomes in patients with type 2 diabetes mellitus, established cardiovascular disease, and chronic kidney disease. Circulation 137(2):119–129. https://doi.org/10.1161/CIRCULATIONAHA.117.028268. Epub 13 Sep 2017
117. Noyan-Ashraf MH, Momen MA et al (2009) GLP-1R agonist liraglutide activates cytoprotective pathways and improves outcomes after experimental myocardial infarction in mice. Diabetes 58:975–983
118. Lønborg J, Vejlstrup N, Kelbæk H et al (2012) Exenatide reduces reperfusion injury in patients with ST-segment elevation myocardial infarction. Eur Heart J 33:1491–1499
119. Andreadou I, Efentakis P, Balafas E et al (2017) Empagliflozin limits myocardial infarction in vivo and cell death in vitro: role of STAT3, mitochondria, and redox aspects. Front Physiol 8:1077
120. Mozawa K, Kubota Y, Hoshika Y et al (2021) Empagliflozin confers reno-protection in acute myocardial infarction and type 2 diabetes mellitus. ESC Hear Fail 8:4161–4173
121. Clinicaltrials.gov. NCT04564742—Dapagliflozin effects on cardiovascular events in patients with an acute heart attack (DAPA-MI). https://clinicaltrials.gov/ct2/show/NCT04564742. Published 2021
122. Mosenzon O, Leibowitz G, Bhatt DL et al (2017) Effect of Saxagliptin on renal outcomes in the SAVOR-TIMI 53 trial. Diabetes Care 40:69–76
123. Rosenstock J, Perkovic V, Johansen OE, Cooper ME, Kahn SE, Marx N, Alexander JH, Pencina M, Toto RD, Wanner C (2019) Effect of linagliptin vs placebo on major cardiovascular events in adults with type 2 diabetes and high cardiovascular and renal risk: the CARMELINA randomized clinical trial. JAMA 321(1):69–79
124. Gore MO, Patel MJ, Kosiborod M et al (2012) National registry of myocardial infarction investigators diabetes mellitus and trends in hospital survival after myocardial infarction, 1994 to 2006. Circ Cardiovasc Qual Outcomes 5:791–797
125. Donahoe SM, Stewart GC, McCabe CH et al (2007) Diabetes and mortality following acute coronary syndromes. JAMA 298:765
126. Kip KE, Faxon DP, Detre KM, Yeh W, Kelsey SF, Currier JW (1996) Coronary angioplasty in diabetic patients. Circulation 94:1818–1825
127. Odegaard AO, Jacobs DR, Sanchez OA, Goff DC, Reiner AP, Gross MD (2016) Oxidative stress, inflammation, endothelial dysfunction and incidence of type 2 diabetes. Cardiovasc Diabetol 15:51
128. Pfeffer MA, Claggett B, Diaz R, Dickstein K, Gerstein HC, Køber LV, Lawson FC, Ping L, Wei X, Lewis EF, Maggioni AP, McMurray J, Probstfield JL, Riddle MC, Solomon SD, Tardif JC, Investigators ELIXA (2015) Lixisenatide in patients with type 2 diabetes and acute coronary syndrome. N Engl J Med 373:2247–2257. https://doi.org/10.1056/NEJMoa1509225
129. Shimizu W, Kubota Y, Hoshika Y et al (2020) Effects of empagliflozin versus placebo on cardiac sympathetic activity in acute myocardial infarction patients with type 2 diabetes mellitus: the EMBODY trial. Cardiovasc Diabetol 19(1):148
130. Trevisan M, Fu EL, Szummer K et al (2021) Glucagon-like peptide-1 receptor agonists and the risk of cardiovascular events in diabetes patients surviving an acute myocardial infarction. Eur Heart J Cardiovasc Pharmacother 7:104–111
131. Longato E, Di Camillo B, Sparacino G, Gubian L, Avogaro A, Fadini GP (2020) Cardiovascular outcomes of type 2 diabetic patients treated with SGLT-2 inhibitors versus GLP-1 receptor agonists in real-life. BMJ Open Diabetes Res Care 8:e001451

132. Baviera M, Foresta A, Colacioppo P et al (2022) Effectiveness and safety of GLP-1 receptor agonists versus SGLT-2 inhibitors in type 2 diabetes: an Italian cohort study. Cardiovasc Diabetol 21:162
133. Patorno E, Pawar A, Bessette LG, Kim DH, Dave C, Glynn RJ et al (2021) Comparative effectiveness and safety of sodium–glucose cotransporter 2 inhibitors versus glucagon-like peptide 1 receptor agonists in older adults. Diabetes Care 44(3):826–835
134. Ott C, Jumar A, Striepe K, Friedrich S, Karg MV, Bramlage P, Schmieder RE (2017) A randomised study of the impact of the SGLT2 inhibitor dapagliflozin on microvascular and macrovascular circulation. Cardiovasc Diabetol 16:26. https://doi.org/10.1186/s12933-017-0510-1
135. Ott C, Raff U, Schmidt S, Kistner I, Friedrich S, Bramlage P, Harazny JM, Schmieder RE (2014) Effects of saxagliptin on early microvascular changes in patients with type 2 diabetes. Cardiovasc Diabetol 13:19
136. Cherney DZ, Perkins BA, Soleymanlou N, Har R, Fagan N, Johansen OE et al (2014) The effect of empagliflozin on arterial stiffness and heart rate variability in subjects with uncomplicated type 1 diabetes mellitus. Cardiovasc Diabetol 13:28
137. Imprialos KP, Sarafidis PA, Karagiannis AI (2015) Sodium-glucose cotransporter-2 inhibitors and blood pressure decrease: a valuable effect of a novel antidiabetic class? J Hypertens 33(11):2185–2197
138. Li C, Zhang J, Xue M, Li X, Han F, Liu X, Xu L, Lu Y, Cheng Y, Li T, Yu X, Sun B, Chen L (2019) SGLT2 inhibition with empagliflozin attenuates myocardial oxidative stress and fibrosis in diabetic mice heart. Cardiovasc Diabetol 18:15. https://doi.org/10.1186/s12933-019-0816-2
139. Wilson AJ, Gill EK, Abudalo RA, Edgar KS, Watson CJ, Grieve DJ (2018) Reactive oxygen species signalling in the diabetic heart: emerging prospect for therapeutic targeting. Heart 104(4):293–299
140. Russo I, Frangogiannis NG (2016) Diabetes-associated cardiac fibrosis: cellular effectors, molecular mechanisms and therapeutic opportunities. J Mol Cell Cardiol 90:84–93
141. Aroor AR, Das NA, Carpenter AJ et al (2018) Glycemic control by the SGLT2 inhibitor empagliflozin decreases aortic stiffness, renal resistivity index and kidney injury. Cardiovasc Diabetol 17(1):108
142. Ferranini E, Solini A (2012) SGLT2 inhibitors in diabetes mellitus: rationale and clinical prospects. Nat Rev Endocrinol 8:495–502
143. Rosas-Guzman J, Rosas-Saucedo J, Romero-Garcia ARJ (2017) SGLT2 inhibitors in diabetes mellitus treatment. Rev Recent Clin Trials 12(1):8–18
144. Hasan FM, Alsahli M, Gerich JE (2014) SGLT2 inhibitors in the treatment of type 2 diabetes. Diabetes Res Clin Pract 104(3):297–322
145. Lioudaki E, Androulakis ES, Whyte M, Stylianou KG, Daphnis EK, Ganotakis ES (2017) The effect of sodium-glucose co-transporter-2 (SGLT-2) inhibitors on Cardiometabolic profile; beyond the Hypoglycaemic action. Cardiovasc Drugs Ther 31:215. https://doi.org/10.1007/s10557-017-6724-3
146. Shyangdan DS, Uthman OA, Waugh N (2016) SGLT-2 receptor inhibitors for treating patients with type 2 diabetes mellitus: a systematic review and network meta-analysis. BMJ Open 6(2):e009417
147. Vasilakou D, Karagiannis T, Athanasiadou E, Mainou M, Liakos A, Bekiari E et al (2013) Sodium-glucose cotransporter 2 inhibitors for type 2 diabetes: a systematic review and meta-analysis. Ann Intern Med 159(4):262–274. https://doi.org/10.7326/0003-4819-159-4-201308200-00007
148. Weber MA, Mansfield TA, Cain VA, Igbal N, Parikh S, Ptaszynska A (2016) Blood pressure and glycaemic effects of dapagliflozin versus placebo in patients with type 2 diabetes on combination antihypertensive therapy: a randomised, double-blind, placebo-controlled, phase 3 study. Lancet Diabetes Endocrinol 4:211–220
149. Bode B, Stenlöf K, Sullivan D, Fung A, Usiskin K (2013) Efficacy and safety of canagliflozin treatment in older subjects with type 2 diabetes mellitus: a randomized trial. Hosp Pract (1995) 41(2):72–84

150. Inagaki N, Harashima S, Maruyama N, Kawaguchi Y, Goda M, Iijima H (2016) Efficacy and safety of canagliflozin in combination with insulin: a double-blind, randomized, placebo-controlled study in Japanese patients with type 2 diabetes mellitus. Cardiovasc Diabetol 15:89
151. Lavalle-González FJ, Januszewicz A, Davidson J, Tong C, Qiu R, Canovatchel W et al (2013) Efficacy and safety of canagliflozin compared with placebo and sitagliptin in patients with type 2 diabetes on background metformin monotherapy: a randomised trial. Diabetologia 56(12):2582–2592
152. Bolinder J, Ljunggren O, Kullberg J, Johansson L, Wilding J, Langkilde AM et al (2012) Effects of dapagliflozin on body weight, total fat mass, and regional adipose tissue distribution in patients with type 2 diabetes mellitus with inadequate glycemic control on metformin. J Clin Endocrinol Metab 97(3):1020–1031
153. Ji L, Ma J, Li H, Mansfield TA, Tjoen CL, Iqbal N et al (2014) Dapagliflozin as monotherapy in drug-naive Asian patients with type 2 diabetes mellitus: a randomized, blinded, prospective phase III study. Clin Ther 36(1):84–100
154. Kaku K, Watada H, Iwamoto Y, Utsunomiya K, Terauchi Y, Tobe K et al (2014) Efficacy and safety of monotherapy with the novel sodium/glucose cotransporter-2 inhibitor tofogliflozin in Japanese patients with type 2 diabetes mellitus: a combined Phase 2 and 3 randomized, placebo-controlled, double-blind, parallel-group comparative study. Cardiovasc Diabetol 13:65
155. Bolinder J, Ljunggren Ö, Johansson L, Wilding J, Langkilde AM, Sjöström CD, Sugg J, Parikh S (2014) Dapagliflozin maintains glycaemic control while reducing weight and body fat mass over 2 years in patients with type 2 diabetes mellitus inadequately controlled on metformin. Diabetes ObesMetab 16(2):159–169. https://doi.org/10.1111/dom.12189. Epub 29 Aug 2013 PMID: 23906445
156. Seino Y, Sasaki T, Fukatsu A, Ubukata M, Sakai S, Samukawa Y (2014) Efficacy and safety of luseogliflozin as monotherapy in Japanese patients with type 2 diabetes mellitus: a randomized, double-blind, placebo-controlled, phase 3 study. Curr Med Res Opin 30(7):1245–1255
157. Kashiwagi A, Kazuta K, Goto K, Yoshida S, Ueyama E, Utsuno A (2015) Ipragliflozin in combination with metformin for the treatment of Japanese patients with type 2 diabetes: ILLUMINATE, a randomized, double-blind, placebo-controlled study. Diabetes Obes Metab 17(3):304–308
158. Fabbrini E, Magkos F (2015) Hepatic steatosis as a marker of metabolic dysfunction. Nutrients 7(6):4995–5019
159. Cherney DZ, Perkins BA, Soleymanlou N, Maione M, Lai V, Lee A et al (2014) Renal hemodynamic effect of sodium-glucose cotransporter 2 inhibition in patients with type 1 diabetes mellitus. Circulation 129(5):587–597
160. Ruggenenti P, Porrini EL, Gaspari F, Motterlini N, Cannata A, Carrara F et al (2012) Glomerular hyperfiltration and renal disease progression in type 2 diabetes. Diabetes Care 35:2061–2068
161. Andrews TJ, Cox RD, Parker C, Kolb J (2016) Euglycemic diabetic ketoacidosis with elevated acetone in a patient taking a sodium-glucose cotransporter-2 (SGLT2) inhibitor. J Emerg Med 52:223
162. Kohler S, Salsali A, Hantel S, Kaspers S, Woerle HJ, Kim G et al (2016) Safety and tolerability of empagliflozin in patients with type 2 diabetes. Clin Ther 38(6):1299–1313
163. Fioretto P, Giaccari A, Sesti G (2015) Efficacy and safety of dapagliflozin, a sodium glucose cotransporter 2 (SGLT2) inhibitor, in diabetes mellitus. Cardiovasc Diabetol 14:142
164. Reid J, Rana K, Niman S, Sheikh-Ali M, Lewis T, Choksi RR, Goldfaden RF (2020) Sodium-glucose Cotransporter-2 (SGLT-2) inhibitors for cardiovascular disease prevention. American journal of cardiovascular. Drugs 20:419. https://doi.org/10.1007/s40256-020-00397-y
165. Furtado RHM, Bonaca MP, Raz I, Zelniker TA, Mosenzon O, Cahn A et al (2019) Dapagliflozin and cardiovascular outcomes in patients with type 2 diabetes mellitus and previous myocardial infarction. Circulation 139(22):2516–2527

166. INVOKANA® (canagliflozin) tablets. 2019. http://www.janssenlabels.com/package-insert/product-monograph/prescribing-information/INVOKANA-pi.pdf. Accessed 20 Dec 2019
167. ClinicalTrialsgov (2017) Dapagliflozin in PRESERVED ejection fraction heart failure (PRESERVED-HF). https://clinicaltrials.gov/ct2/show/NCT03030235. Accessed 20 Dec 2019
168. ClinicalTrials.gob (2018) Dapagliflozin Evaluation to Improve the LIVEs of Patients With PReserved Ejection Fraction Heart Failure. (DELIVER). https://clinicaltrials.gov/ct2/show/NCT03619213. Accessed 20 Dec 2019
169. American Diabetes Association (2018) Standards of medical care in diabetes-2018. https://diabetesed.net/wp-content/uploads/2017/12/2018-ADA-Standards-of-Care.pdf. Accessed 20 Dec 2019
170. Briasoulis A, Al Dhaybi O, Bakris GL (2018) SGLT2 inhibitors and mechanisms of hypertension. Curr Cardiol Rep 20(1):1. https://doi.org/10.1007/s11886-018-0943-5
171. Fuller JH (1985) Epidemiology of hypertension associated with diabetes mellitus. Hypertension 7(6 Pt 2):II3–II7
172. Epstein M, Sowers JR (1992) Diabetes mellitus and hypertension. Hypertension 19(5):403–418. https://doi.org/10.1161/01.HYP.19.5.403
173. Cruickshank K, Riste L, Anderson SG, Wright JS, Dunn G, Gosling RG (2002) Aortic pulse-wave velocity and its relationship to mortality in diabetes and glucose intolerance: an integrated index of vascular function? Circulation 106(16):2085–2090. https://doi.org/10.1161/01.CIR.0000033824.02722.F7
174. Nosadini R, Sambataro M, Thomaseth K, Pacini G, Cipollina MR, Brocco E et al (1993) Role of hyperglycemia and insulin resistance in determining sodium retention in non-insulin-dependent diabetes. Kidney Int 44(1):139–146. https://doi.org/10.1038/ki.1993.224
175. DeFronzo RA, Norton L, Abdul-Ghani M (2016) Renal, metabolic and cardiovascular considerations of SGLT2 inhibition. Nat Rev Nephrol 13:11–26. https://doi.org/10.1038/nrneph.2016.170
176. Bailey CJ (2011) Renal glucose reabsorption inhibitors to treat diabetes. Trends Pharmacol Sci 32(2):63–71. https://doi.org/10.1016/j.tips.2010.11.011
177. Thomson SC, Rieg T, Miracle C, Mansoury H, Whaley J, Vallon V et al (2012) Acute and chronic effects of SGLT2 blockade on glomerular and tubular function in the early diabetic rat. Am J Physiol Regul Integr Comp Physiol 302(1):R75–R83. https://doi.org/10.1152/ajpregu.00357.2011
178. Mancia G, Cannon CP, Tikkanen I, Zeller C, Ley L, Woerle HJ et al (2016) Impact of empagliflozin on blood pressure in patients with type 2 diabetes mellitus and hypertension by background antihypertensive medication. Hypertension 68(6):1355–1364. https://doi.org/10.1161/HYPERTENSIONAHA.116.07703
179. Gerich JE (2010) Role of the kidney in normal glucose homeostasis and in the hyperglycaemia of diabetes mellitus: therapeutic implications. Diabet Med 27:136–142
180. Mazidi M, Rezaie P, Gao H-K, Kengne AP (2017) Effect of sodium–glucose cotransport-2 inhibitors on blood pressure in people with type 2 diabetes mellitus: a systematic review and meta-analysis of 43 randomized control trials with 22 528 patients. J Am Heart Assoc 6:e004007
181. Heise T, Jordan J, Wanner C, Heer M, Macha S, Mattheus M et al (2016) Pharmacodynamic effects of single and multiple doses of empagliflozin in patients with type 2 diabetes. Clin Ther 38(10):2265–2276. https://doi.org/10.1016/j.clinthera.2016.09.001
182. Lambers Heerspink HJ, de Zeeuw D, Wie L, Leslie B, List J (2013) Dapagliflozin a glucose-regulating drug with diuretic properties in subjects with type 2 diabetes. Diabetes Obes Metab 15(9):853–862
183. Yamout H et al (2014) Efficacy and safety of canagliflozin in patients with type 2 diabetes and stage 3 nephropathy. Am J Nephrol 40(1):64–74
184. DeFronzo RA (2009) From the triumvirate to the ominous octet: a new paradigm for the treatment of type 2 diabetes mellitus. Diabetes 58(4):773–795. https://doi.org/10.2337/db09-9028

185. Inzucchi SE, Bergenstal RM, Buse JB, Diamant M, Ferrannini E, Nauck M et al (2012) Management of hyperglycaemia in type 2 diabetes: a patient-centered approach. Position statement of the American Diabetes Association (ADA) and the European Association for the Study of Diabetes (EASD). Diabetologia 55:1577–1596
186. Lu Y, Griffen SC, Boulton DW, Leil TA (2014) Use of systems pharmacology modeling to elucidate the operating characteristics of SGLT1 and SGLT2 in renal glucose reabsorption in humans. Front Pharmacol 5:274
187. DeFronzo RA, Davidson JA, Del Prato S (2012) The role of the kidneys in glucose homeostasis: a new path towards normalizing glycaemia. Diabetes Obes Metab 14:5–14
188. Chao EC, Henry RR (2010) SGLT2 inhibition–a novel strategy for diabetes treatment. Nat Rev Drug Discov 9:551–559
189. Farber SJ, Berger EY, Earle DP (1951) Effect of diabetes and insulin of the maximum capacity of the renal tubules to reabsorb glucose. J Clin Invest 30:125–129
190. Rahmoune H, Thompson PW, Ward JM et al (2005) Glucose transporters in human renal proximal tubular cells isolated from the urine of patients with non-insulin-dependent diabetes. Diabetes 54:3427–3434. https://doi.org/10.2337/diabetes.54.12.3427
191. Giaccari A, Sorice G, Muscogiuri G (2009) Glucose toxicity: the leading actor in the pathogenesis and clinical history of type 2 diabetes—mechanisms and potentials for treatment. Nutr Metab Cardiovasc Dis 19:365–377
192. Rossetti L, Giaccari A, DeFronzo RA (1990) Glucose toxicity. Diabetes Care 13:610–630
193. American Diabetes Association (2015) Standards of medical care in diabetes-2015. Diabetes Care 38(Suppl 1):S3–S93
194. Merovci A, Mari A, Solis C, Xiong J, Daniele G, Chavez A et al (2015) Dapagliflozin lowers plasma glucose concentration and improves beta cell function. J Clin Endocrinol Metab 100:jc20143472
195. Scheen AJ, Paquot N (2014) Metabolic effects of SGLT-2 inhibitors beyond increased glucosuria: a review of the clinical evidence. Diabetes Metab 40:S4–S11
196. Vivian EM (2014) Sodium-glucose co-transporter 2 (SGLT2) inhibitors: a growing class of antidiabetic agents. Drugs Context 3:212264
197. Washburn WN, Poucher SM (2013) Differentiating sodium-glucose co-transporter-2 inhibitors in development for the treatment of type 2 diabetes mellitus. Expert Opin Investig Drugs 22:463–486
198. Scheen AJ (2015) Pharmacodynamics, efficacy and safety of sodium–glucose co-transporter type 2 (SGLT2) inhibitors for the treatment of type 2 diabetes mellitus. Drugs 75(1):33–59. https://doi.org/10.1007/s40265-014-0337-y
199. Hinnen D (2015) Glucuretic effects and renal safety of dapagliflozin in patients with type 2 diabetes. Ther Adv Endocrinol Metab 6:92–102
200. Dziuba J, Alperin P, Racketa J, Iloeje U, Goswami D, Hardy E et al (2014) Modeling effects of SGLT-2 inhibitor dapagliflozin treatment versus standard diabetes therapy on cardiovascular and microvascular outcomes. Diabetes Obes Metab 16:628–635
201. Kaku K, Kiyosue A, Inoue S, Ueda N, Tokudome T, Yang J et al (2014) Efficacy and safety of dapagliflozin monotherapy in Japanese patients with type 2 diabetes inadequately controlled by diet and exercise. Diabetes Obes Metab 16(11):1102–1110
202. Bailey CJ, Iqbal N, T'joen C, List JF. (2012) Dapagliflozin monotherapy in drug-naive patients with diabetes: a randomized-controlled trial of low-dose range. Diabetes Obes Metab 14(10):951–959. https://doi.org/10.1111/j.1463-1326.2012.01659.x
203. Kaku K, Inoue S, Matsuoka O, Kiyosue A, Azuma H, Hayashi N et al (2013) Efficacy and safety of dapagliflozin as a monotherapy for type 2 diabetes mellitus in Japanese patients with inadequate glycaemic control: a phase II multicentre, randomized, double-blind, placebo-controlled trial. Diabetes Obes Metab 15:432–440
204. Sun YN, Zhou Y, Chen X, Che WS, Leung SW (2014) The efficacy of dapagliflozin combined with hypoglycaemic drugs in treating type 2 diabetes mellitus: meta-analysis of randomised controlled trials. BMJ Open 4:e004619

205. Zhang L, Feng Y, List J, Kasichayanula S, Pfister M (2010) Dapagliflozin treatment in patients with different stages of type 2 diabetes mellitus: effects on glycaemic control and body weight. Diabetes Obes Metab 12:510–516
206. Henry RR, Rosenstock J, Edelman S, Mudaliar S, Chalamandaris AG, Kasichayanula S et al (2015) Exploring the potential of the SGLT2 inhibitor dapagliflozin in type 1 diabetes: a randomized, double-blind, placebo-controlled pilot study. Diabetes Care 38:412–419
207. Del Prato S, Nauck M, Duran-Garcia S et al (2015) Long-term glycaemic response and tolerability of dapagliflozin versus a sulphonylurea as add-on therapy to metformin in patients with type 2 diabetes: 4-year data. Diabetes Obes Metab 17:581–590

Chapter 9
A Comprehensive Review of SGLT2 Inhibitor's Effects on Cardiovascular Events, Mortality, and Significant Safety Outcomes in Individuals with Type 2 Diabetes

Mukesh Nandave

Introduction by the Editor

SGLT2 is considered as the main treatment for cardiovascular disorders. Eight Cardiovascular outcomes trials (CVOTS) of SGLT2i were conducted, and the results showed a decrease in mortality, a decrease in cardiovascular events, and a prohibition of heart failure and renal illness. Beyond statistical analysis and observational research, the FDA and EMA were used in this chapter to show the actuality of SGLT2i in those trials. The diuretic activity was also verified by SGLT2i due to its method of action, increasing osmotic diuresis, and its crucial side effects owing to hypovolemia and increased hematocrit. They also provide credence to the idea that beliefs in the morbidity-mortality advantages of SGLT2i are generally exaggerated and based on undemonstrated endpoints. Finally, it is evident that the antidiabetic effect of SGLT2i, which is a byproduct of its renal mechanism of action, plateaued after a few months and sharply reduced over time, casting doubt on its long-term objective of keeping the HbA1c of diabetic patients below 7%. Additionally, this impact is almost nonexistent in people with renal impairment. We believe this chapter will benefit every doctor caring for diabetes patients to balance the perception and reality of SGLT2i prescription effects.

Large-scale cardiovascular outcome studies have shown the effect of SGLT2i pharmacological selectivity on cardiac outcomes in patients with T2D. A more prominent SGLT1 inhibitory property was shown to have no extra influence on most outcomes, but compared to strong pharmacological SGLT2 selectivity, it was substantially related to a decreased risk of stroke. In terms of side effects, non-selective SGLT2 inhibitors seem to have a greater risk of hypotension.

M. Nandave (✉)
Department of Pharmacology and Pharmaceutical Biotechnology, Delhi Pharmaceutical Sciences and Research University (DPSRU), New Delhi, Delhi, India

M. Nandave (ed.), *Sodium-glucose Cotransporter-2 (SGLT2) Inhibitors in Heart Failure*, https://doi.org/10.1007/978-981-97-7568-2_9

Given that people with partially reduced SGLT1 transport activity (corresponding to pharmacological SGLT1 inhibition), but not SGLT2 transport activity, experience significant improvements in their cardiovascular and survival rates when compared to non-affected controls, the notable differences in the degree of pharmacological selectivity of SGLT2i to SGLT2 over SGLT1 may be clinically significant [1]. In terms of the complications of hospitalization for heart failure or cardiac death, a recent meta-analysis of trials specifically focused on heart failure revealed that reduced SGLT2 selectivity was much more favorable. Many preclinical investigations have connected SGLT1 to compulsive processes in the kidney, heart, and brain, which is consistent with our clinical observations. The impact of SGLT2i pharmacological selectivity on clinical outcomes in high-risk T2D patients, however, remains unclear [2].

Based on extensive clinical research, in patients with T2D and increased cardiovascular risk, the pharmacological selectivity of SGLT2i is not significantly correlated with the risk of MACE, cardiac death, fatal and nonfatal MI, survival rate, hospitalization for HF, or the renal composite outcome. It appears that further SGLT1 inhibition added to SGLT2 blockage may not have an impact on these results in the patient groups under investigation. The pharmaceutical SGLT2:SGLT1 selectivity ratio, on the other hand, showed a significant correlation with stroke consequences; a lower SGLT2 selectivity, or a more prominent inhibitory impact on SGLT1, was associated with a lower risk.

Furthermore, this difference held true even for individuals whose baseline eGFR was less than 60 mL/min/1.73 m^2. Consequently, the risk of stroke may be decreased by SGLT2 inhibitors that have a strong SGLT1 inhibitory effect; this effect appears to be less impacted by baseline eGFR.

Only patients with established atherosclerotic cardiovascular disease (ASCVD) benefit from SGLT2 inhibitors concerning atherosclerotic major adverse cardiovascular outcomes, according to prior meta-analyses of large cardiovascular outcome trials. SGLT2i have been demonstrated to dramatically lower the risk of MACE and MI (both fatal and nonfatal) only in type 2 diabetic individuals with established ASCVD, not in those without ASCVD [3].

SGLT2 inhibitors, on the other hand, did not affect the risk of stroke in individuals with or without ASCVD39. Hence, by demonstrating that the selectivity of SGLT2i is a significant predictor of stroke outcomes, our current results may supplement earlier meta-analyses. In T2D individuals who are already at a greater risk, dual SGLT1/2 inhibition may provide a unique pharmaceutical method to reduce unfavourable stroke outcomes.

These outcome trials mostly involved ischemic stroke as the predominate subtype, since SGLT2i in general lower new-onset atrial fibrillation or flutter (AF/AFL), a significant risk factor for ischemic stroke. Only dapagliflozin (DECLARE-TIMI 58 trial) lowered the hazard of AF/AFL at the individual trial level, regardless of the patient's prior history of HF, ASCVD, or AF. Dapagliflozin, however, did not influence the risk of an ischemic stroke. Thus, it seems improbable that therapy with SGLT2i modifies the risk of stroke by lowering the incidence of new-onset AF/AFL.

These include enhanced native glucagon-like peptide-1 levels, which have straight and subsidiary antithrombotic effects, and favourable alteration of the gut microbiome as a result of intestinal inhibition of SGLT1-mediated glucose absorption. Postprandial serum glucose excursions are also blunted. Fascinatingly, tiny animal investigations have connected SGLT1 overexpression after ischemic stroke to neuronal injury, presumably via increased absorption of glucose; its knockdown decreased lesion volume and caused brain injury. The clinical significance and potential impact of pharmacological inhibition of cerebral SGLT1 in stroke prophylaxis remain unknown at this time.

In terms of safety results, people with type 2 diabetes who used both highly selective and non-selective SGLT2 inhibitors had a comparable increase in the incidence of genital infections and diabetic ketoacidosis when compared to placebo. Conversely, there was no significant increase in the incidence of hypoglycemia or lower limb amputation associated with any pharmacological grouping. In contrast to highly selective medicines, non-selective SGLT2 inhibitors were linked to a twice higher risk of hypotension. This may once more be indicative of different mechanisms underlying the actions of selective vs non-selective SGLT2 inhibitors.

In summary, large-scale cardiovascular outcome studies have shown that decreased pharmacological selectivity of SGLT2i with a more significant inhibitory impact on SGLT1 is linked with condensed risk of both fatal and nonfatal stroke in high-risk T2D patients. In these individuals, combined SGLT1/2 inhibition may represent a unique pharmaceutical strategy for stroke prevention. Additional research is necessary to clarify the practical implications of these findings that raise questions.

Machine Generated Summaries

Disclaimer: The summaries in this chapter were generated from Springer Nature publications using extractive AI auto-summarization: An extraction-based summarizer aims to identify the most important sentences of a text using an algorithm and uses those original sentences to create the auto-summary (unlike generative AI). As the constituted sentences are machine selected, they may not fully reflect the body of the work, so we strongly advise that the original content is read and cited. The auto generated summaries were curated by the editor to meet Springer Nature publication standards. To cite this content, please refer to the original papers.

Machine generated keywords: sglti, canvas, mmhg, medical, empareg, empareg outcome, variable, atrial, eligible, patient type, antihypertensive, infection, diabete hypertension, pharmacologic, exclusion.

SGLT2 Inhibitors and Cardiovascular Outcomes: Current Perspectives and Future Potentials [4]

This is a machine-generated summary of:

Jia, Xiaoming; Mehta, Paras B.; Ye, Yumei; Alam, Mahboob; Birnbaum, Yochai; Bajaj, Mandeep: SGLT2 Inhibitors and Cardiovascular Outcomes: Current Perspectives and Future Potentials [4].

Published in: Current Diabetes Reports (2018).

Link to original: https://doi.org/10.1007/s11892-018-1038-9

If you want to cite the papers, please refer to the original.

For technical reasons we could not place the page where the original quote is coming from.

Abstract-Summary "New studies examining SGLT2i action on sodium-hydrogen exchanger proteins in both the heart and the kidney, on myocardial energetics and impact on inflammation and atherosclerosis continue to shed light on the multitude of pleotropic effects of these agents."

"More data is needed to substantiate the safety and efficacy, SGLT2i should be considered as a valuable therapy to help reduce CV risk in patients with diabetes."

"SGLT2i may have utility in preventing progression to diabetes or providing CV protection in patients who do not have diabetes."

Introduction

"Even in trials that did show CV benefit, positive outcomes manifested only after an extended period of time [5, 6]."

"This paradigm shift is poised to continue with the advent of new classes of anti-hyperglycemic medications that have demonstrated CV benefit likely independent of glycemic control."

"While the original purpose of CVOTs for newer agents was to ensure safety and non-inferiority to traditional regimens (e.g., metformin), many of these agents including liraglutide and semaglutide of the GLP1-receptor agonist class and empagliflozin and canagliflozin of the sodium-glucose cotransporter 2 inhibitor (SGLT2i) class have demonstrated superior CV benefit compared to placebo in the background of treating hyperglycemia to goal with standard anti-diabetic medications [7–10••]."

"We focus on the SGLT2i class of medications, starting with the landmark EMPA-REG and CANVAS trials, with discussion of published data regarding CV benefit and potential mechanisms to explain these findings [9••, 10••]."

EMPA-REG, CANVAS, and Beyond

"Outcomes from CANVAS showed significant reduction of primary composite outcome of CV mortality, non-fatal MI, or non-fatal stroke (hazard ratio 0.86; 95% CI 0.75–0.97, $p = 0.02$ for superiority) for canagliflozin compared to placebo."

"Examination of the EASEL population-based cohort study of 25,258 patients showed that as a whole, the SGLT2i group had significant reduction in all-cause mortality (HR 0.57, 95% CI 0.49–0.66, $p < 0.001$) as well as reduction in 3-point major adverse cardiovascular event (MACE) (HR 0.67, 95% CI 0.60–0.75, $p < 0.0001$) and HF hospitalization (HR 0.57, 95% CI 0.45–0.73, $p < 0.0001$), which was consistent with findings of EMPA-REG and CANVAS [11••]."

Proposed Mechanisms

"A study conducted on rodent models demonstrated that empagliflozin inhibited NHE, which led to a decrease in intracellular sodium, reduction in cytoplasmic calcium and increase in mitochondrial calcium within the cardiomyocytes, which improves cardiac mitochondrial function and energetics [12•]."

"In rat heart models, moderate ketosis has been shown to increase cardiac work efficiency and provides an adaptive mechanism to compensate for the dysregulation of fatty acid and glucose metabolism."

"Whereas high levels of ketosis can be detrimental as seen in diabetic ketoacidosis, moderate increases in circulating ketone bodies as seen in patients treated with SGLT2i agents likely exert a cardioprotective effect on the diabetic heart by optimizing myocardial energetics."

"It will be interesting to see in future studies if treatment with SGLT2i can rescue patients with diabetes from myocardial energy deficits as seen previously by magnetic resonance spectroscopy techniques and if so, whether a more efficient energy utilization may lead to improved cardiac function and outcomes [13]."

Clinical Implications

"Given the CV benefits shown in EMPA-REG and CANVAS trials as well as in the EASEL and CVD-REAL cohort studies, we must consider the possibility of SGLT2i as a potential first-line therapy either in conjunction with or instead of metformin in the treatment of T2DM patients with CVD."

"With respect to monotherapy, the argument for SGLT2i and other CV risk reducing anti-hyperglycemic agents over metformin is the presence of more consistent data in CV protection in patients with known CVD."

"Both the mechanism of action of SGLT2i on the cardiovascular system and the consistent benefit shown in CVOT and large community studies among patients with HF suggest that it should be considered over metformin in these patients."

"When lifestyle interventions (which have been proven to be the most effective method for prevention) do not improve glucose metabolism in patients with impaired glucose tolerance, the ADA recommends considering the addition of metformin in certain populations who benefitted most during the Diabetes Prevention Program [14–16]."

Conclusion

"SGLT2i is a class of anti-hyperglycemic agents that has been shown to also confer significant cardiovascular protection in patients with T2DM."

"With a multitude of pleotropic effects as outlined in this review, SGLT2i provides a valuable therapy for clinicians that bridge two major needs in the treatment of T2DM, glycemic control and reduction of CVD risk."

"Taken as a whole, the results of recent CVOTs support the use of agents from the SGLT2i as second-line therapy after metformin, though an argument can be made that SGLT2i should already be considered as a first-line agent in patients with heart failure."

"More long-term evidence on efficacy and safety and better understanding of these newer medications are likely needed to validate their inclusion as first-line interventions in the guidelines and in clinical practice."

SGLT2 Inhibition and Cardiovascular Events: Why Did EMPA-REG Outcomes Surprise and What Were the Likely Mechanisms? [17]

This is a machine-generated summary of:

Sattar, Naveed; McLaren, James; Kristensen, Søren L.; Preiss, David; McMurray, John J.: SGLT2 Inhibition and cardiovascular events: why did EMPA-REG Outcomes surprise and what were the likely mechanisms? [17].

Published in: Diabetologia (2016).

Link to original: https://doi.org/10.1007/s00125-016-3956-x

For technical reasons we could not place the page where the original quote is coming from.

Abstract-Summary "While the modest reduction in the primary composite outcome of myocardial infarction, stroke or cardiovascular death in the EMPA-REG Outcomes trial was welcome, the 30–40% reductions in heart failure hospitalisation (HFH) and cardiovascular and all-cause deaths in patients treated with empagliflozin were highly impressive and unexpected."

"We discuss briefly why cardiovascular endpoint trials for new diabetes agents are required and describe the results of the first four such trials to have reported, as a precursor to understanding why the EMPA-REG Outcomes results came as a surprise."

"We discuss potential mechanisms that could explain the EMPA-REG Outcomes results, concentrating on non-atherothrombotic effects."

"We suggest that the main driver of benefit may derive from the specific effects of sodium-glucose linked transporter-2 (SGLT2) inhibition on renal sodium and glucose handling, leading to both diuresis and improvements in diabetes-related maladaptive renal arteriolar responses."

Introduction: Cardiovascular Endpoint Trials for New Diabetes Agents

"Recent epidemiological studies indicate that diabetes approximately doubles cardiovascular risk [18]."

"Cardiovascular and mortality risks have declined over recent decades, due to reductions in atherogenic lipids, blood pressure and smoking rates, and better glycaemia management."

"The results of recent trials comparing intensive glucose control with standard control led to some concern that aggressive lowering of glucose levels in some individuals may increase short-term mortality, as seen in the Action to Control Cardiovascular Risk in Diabetes (ACCORD) study [19], even though meta-analyses of such trials did confirm a modest reduction in coronary events."

"Initial concerns (now largely refuted [20]) about the cardiovascular safety of rosiglitazone led the US Food and Drug Administration to mandate that all new glucose-lowering agents must be tested for cardiovascular safety in post-marketing endpoint trials."

What Did the Trials with DPP-4 Inhibitors and GLP-1 Receptor Agonists Show?

"The results of the first two DPP-4 inhibitor trials (Saxagliptin Assessment of Vascular Outcomes Recorded in Patients with Diabetes Mellitus [SAVOR]–Thrombolysis in Myocardial Infarction [TIMI] 53 [21] and Examination of Cardiovascular Outcomes with Alogliptin versus Standard of Care [EXAMINE]

[22], testing saxagliptin and alogliptin, respectively, as add-on therapies) were presented at the European Society of Cardiology annual meeting in September 2014."

"The trials reported modest HbA_{1c} differences between treatment arms and demonstrated non-inferiority for cardiovascular events (SAVOR–TIMI 53, HR 1.00 [95% CI 0.89, 1.12]; EXAMINE, HR 0.96 [upper boundary of one-sided repeated CI 1.16])."

"The results showed neutrality with respect to cardiovascular outcomes (HR 0.98 [95% CI 0.88, 1.09]) and there was no evidence for an increase in HFH."

"The trial demonstrated non-inferiority for cardiovascular events (HR 1.02 [95% CI 0.89, 1.17]) with no suggestion of benefit."

The Value of Cardiovascular Endpoint Trials for New Glucose-Lowering Agents

"Although assessing safety is critically important, trials of agents with modest effects on HbA_{1c} which are conducted in specific high-risk populations (e.g. those with recent acute coronary syndrome, arguably limiting the ability to impact upon major cardiovascular events within the first year) over relatively short durations seem unlikely to have the capacity to show benefit, even if the agent in question is superior to standard practice."

"It is important to stress that the results of Liraglutide Effect and Action in Diabetes: Evaluation of Cardiovascular Outcome Results (LEADER; testing liraglutide; ClinicalTrial.gov registration no. NCT01179048 [23]) and Exenatide Study of Cardiovascular Event Lowering Trial (EXSCEL; testing once-weekly exenatide; ClinicalTrial.gov registration no. CT01144338).

SGLT2 Inhibitor Class: EMPA-REG Outcomes

"The aforementioned neutral results of trials might explain why, when EMPA-REG Outcomes data were reported at the EASD annual meeting in Stockholm in 2015, the audience were highly surprised with the reductions in cardiovascular mortality, all-cause mortality and HFH for empagliflozin vs placebo."

"EMPA-REG Outcomes tested empagliflozin at two doses (10 and 25 mg daily) vs placebo in patients with existing cardiovascular disease over about 3 years."

"The primary outcome of this trial was the 'MACE' (major adverse cardiac events) composite of death from cardiovascular causes, non-fatal myocardial infarction or non-fatal stroke, recommended in the US Food and Drug Administration's guidance on evaluating new glucose-lowering agents and used in most of the other trials discussed earlier."

"While the primary outcome was reduced by empagliflozin (HR 0.86 [95 CI 0.74, 0.99]), myocardial infarction was not significantly reduced (HR 0.87 [95% CI 0.70, 1.09]), although it was directionally concordant, and stroke was non-significantly increased (HR 1.18 [95% CI 0.89, 1.56]) despite the fall in blood pressure [9]."

What Potential Mechanisms Could Explain the Benefits?

"It can arise as a result of almost any abnormality of the structure, mechanical function or electrical activity of the heart and is the common, end-stage, manifestation of many cardiovascular diseases including myocardial infarction."

"Once heart failure ensues, reduced systolic (contraction) and/or diastolic (relaxation) function may lead to sodium and fluid retention, due to renal haemodynamic changes and as a result of activation of the renin—angiotensin—aldosterone system, sympathetic nervous system (SNS) and other neurohumoral systems."

"Heart failure is characterised by a trajectory of deteriorating cardiac output and declining renal function leading to fluid retention, peripheral oedema and pulmonary congestion, which if severe may lead to hospitalisation and treatment with intravenous diuretic."

"10% of EMPA-REG Outcomes participants were clinically recorded as having heart failure, and it is likely that a further proportion of this high cardiovascular risk population had subclinical cardiac dysfunction."

Relevance of Blood Pressure and Renal Effects

"Whether the blood pressure-lowering effects of empagliflozin alone can explain the observed benefit is worthy of consideration since reducing blood pressure (even by small amounts) can influence heart failure risks, although not necessarily as rapidly as seen in EMPA-REG Outcomes."

"Empagliflozin also induces a considerable diuresis, with early loss of urinary glucose in particular and subsequently of sodium as reflected by a sizeable increase in the haematocrit (~4%) compared with placebo, and certainly adequate dosage of diuretics can rapidly reduce heart failure risks, or risks for HFH [24]."

"In the Antihypertensive and Lipid-Lowering Treatment to Prevent Heart Attack Trial (ALLHAT), in which just over one-third of patients had type 2 diabetes, use of the thiazide diuretic chlorthalidone was associated with a 28% (95% CI 20, 34) lower risk of heart failure compared with amlodipine despite only a 0.8 mmHg difference in achieved systolic blood pressure [25]."

Other Important Lessons from EMPA-REG Outcomes

"Heart failure remains an under-recognised complication of diabetes and one which carries a poor prognosis [26]."

"In a recent observational analysis of patients with diabetes, heart failure was found to be the second-most common type of first cardiovascular disease presentation (after peripheral vascular disease) [27]."

"It is therefore increasingly apparent that therapeutic approaches that also reduce the development and progression of heart failure (i.e. beyond atherothrombotic targeting) are crucial in patients with diabetes."

Unanswered Questions

"Why stroke risk in EMPA-REG Outcomes did not decline on empagliflozin, when the risk of stroke is normally very sensitive to reductions in blood pressure, is not clear."

"Meta-analysis of trials suggests that stroke risks can be significantly lowered even when baseline systolic blood pressure is <140 mmHg [28] and so further investigations are clearly required."

"That the haemoconcentration effect of SGLT2 inhibition may have balanced out the blood pressure-lowering effect is plausible, and results from other major ongoing trials will yield valuable data."

Will Other SGLT2 Inhibitors Give the Same Results as EMPA-REG Outcomes?

"If we assume that the explanations for the benefit of empagliflozin revolve around its effects principally on diuresis (driven by promoting both glucose and sodium loss) and via blood pressure reductions, then other SGLT2 inhibitors should yield directionally similar outcomes."

"That noted, available SGLT2 inhibitors have differential specificities for SGLT2 and SGLT1 [29], the relevance of which is not clear for the moment."

"We will not have to wait too long before know the results of the ongoing trials for canagliflozin (Canagliflozin Cardiovascular Safety Assessment [CANVAS] due to be completed in 2017; ClinicalTrial.gov registration no. NCT01032629) [30] and dapagliflozin (Dapagliflozin Effect on CardiovascuLAR Events [DECLARE]-TIMI 58, due to be completed in 2019; ClinicalTrial.gov registration no. NCT01730534)" [31].

Summary

"The effects of empagliflozin on important secondary endpoints in EMPA-REG Outcomes, namely HFH, cardiovascular and all-cause death, were unexpected."

"The rapid emergence of these benefits points strongly towards non-atherothrombotic mechanisms, perhaps principally haemodynamic effects."

"Further mechanistic studies will be needed to identify these mechanisms and further clinical trials of SGLT2 inhibitors in patients with and without heart failure, with and without cardiovascular disease and, potentially, with and without diabetes, will likely ensue."

SGLT2 Inhibitors and Atrial Fibrillation in Type 2 Diabetes: A Systematic Review with Meta-Analysis of 16 Randomized Controlled Trials [31]

This is a machine-generated summary of:

Li, Wen-jie; Chen, Xing-qing; Xu, Ling-ling; Li, Yuan-qing; Luo, Bi-hui: SGLT2 inhibitors and atrial fibrillation in type 2 diabetes: a systematic review with meta-analysis of 16 randomized controlled trials [31].

Published in: Cardiovascular Diabetology (2020).

Link to original: https://doi.org/10.1186/s12933-020-01105-5

If you want to cite the papers, please refer to the original.

For technical reasons we could not place the page where the original quote is coming from.

Abstract-Summary "Type 2 diabetes is closely related to an increased risk of atrial fibrillation (AF) and atrial flutter (AFL)."

"We searched electronic databases (PubMed, Embase and ClinicalTrials.gov) from their inception to January 2020 for trials evaluating the AF outcomes of SGLT2 inhibitors in patients with type 2 diabetes."

"Incorporated data demonstrated that compared to placebo, SGLT2 inhibitors significantly reduced AF/AFL (RR: 0.76; 95% CI 0.65–0.90; $p=0.001$) and all-cause mortality (RR: 0.91; 95% CI 0.83–0.99; $p=0.03$)."

"AF/AFL reductions were not modified by age, body weight, glycated haemoglobin (HbA1c), or systolic blood pressure (SBP) at baseline (all p-interactions >0.3)."

"SGLT2 inhibitors also significantly reduced heart failure events (RR: 0.73; 95% CI 0.64–0.84; $p<0.00001$), HbA1c (WMD: −0.62%; 95% CI −0.89 to −0.34; $p<0.00001$), body weight (WMD: −2.12 kg; 95% CI −2.91 to −1.34; $p<0.00001$),

SBP (WMD: −3.34 mmHg; 95% CI −4.12 to −2.56; $p<0.00001$), and diastolic blood pressure (DBP) (WMD: − 1.11 mmHg; 95% CI − 1.62 to − 0.60; $p<0.0001$)."

"SGLT2 inhibitors may confer a specific AF/AFL-reduction benefit in the susceptible type 2 diabetes population, regardless of age, body weight, HbA1c, and systolic blood pressure at baseline."

"Such an AF/AFL-reduction benefit may be partly attributed to pharmacological effects on reductions in HbA1c, body weight, blood pressure, and the occurrence of heart failure."

Introduction

"HF and AF/AFL are closely aligned and share risk factors such as diabetes, obesity and hypertension [32, 33]."

"We hypothesize that at the same time, pharmacologic therapies for HF could contribute to the reduced AF/AFL risk."

"Such findings also imply crucial roles of SGLT2 inhibitors in AF/AFL improvement."

"No RCTs to date, other than a post hoc analysis of the DECLARE-TIMI 58 trial [34] address the relationship between SGLT2 inhibitors and the risk of AF/AFL in the population."

"The overarching purpose of the present meta-analysis was to pool data from all placebo-controlled RCTs that evaluated AF/AFL outcomes of SGLT2 inhibitors, from which we gained more reliable assessments of the efficacy and safety of specific results overall and in relevant subgroups."

Methods

"Data sources and search strategy, data acquisition, inclusion and exclusion criteria, outcome measurements, quality assessment and statistical methods in the present report were performed in accord with the Preferred Reporting Items for Systematic Reviews and Meta-analysis (PRISRM) guidelines [35]."

"We included studies if: they were RCTs published in English, enrolled patients aged 18 years or older who had type 2 diabetes mellitus, were performed in out- or inpatient-settings, compared SGLT2 inhibitors with placebo, and reported outcomes of interest."

"Using a standardized form, 2 independent reviewers (WJL and XQC) manually extracted information from the included studies as follows: (1) study design, patient characteristics, follow-up durations; (2) comparisons, interventions, background intervention, outcomes at different time points or with different agent types; and (3) related items for outcomes of interest."

"Two reviewers (WJL and XQC) independently assessed the risk of bias of the included studies at the study, intervention and outcome levels."

Results

"Pooling 16 studies assessing the incidence of AF/AFL (SGLT2 inhibitors, 20,914 patients; placebo, 17,421 patients) showed that SGLT2 inhibitors significantly decreased the incidence of reported AF/AFL events compared with placebo (RR: 0.76; 95% CI 0.65–0.90; $p = 0.001$; high SOE)."

"Ten studies [36–44] including 35,186 patients evaluated heart failure (SGLT2 inhibitors, 18,701 patients, 356 events; placebo, 16,485 patients, 459 events)."

"The aggregated data showed a significantly lower rate of heart failure in patients treated with SGLT2 inhibitors than in those treated with placebo (RR: 0.73; 95% CI 0.64–0.84; $p < 0.00001$; high SOE)."

"Apart from 1 trial [42], fifteen studies including 21,174 patients evaluated the urinary tract infection rate (SGLT2 inhibitors, 12,332 patients, 657 events; placebo, 8842 patients, 395 events)."

"Meta-regression was used to investigate the heterogeneity source of included studies that evaluated HbA1c change from baseline for high dosage SGLT2 inhibitors."

Discussion

"The present meta-analysis outlined that SGLT2 inhibitors had great benefit in reducing the risk of AF/AFL."

"The present incorporated data demonstrated favourable effects on reducing HbA1c, blood pressure and body weight in patients randomized to SGLT2 inhibitors, which might be of importance in attenuating AF/AFL progression."

"This finding implied that the AF/AFL-reduction effects of SGLT2 inhibitors may be partly independent of HF improvement."

"The data presented herein indicated that SGLT2 inhibitors should be considered in populations with type 2 diabetes for AF/AFL prevention, given that they safely reduced HbA1c, body weight, and blood pressure and widely reduced the risk of HF across the spectrum of these patients."

"Although this meta-analysis provides the first evidence for a favourable effect of SGLT2 inhibitors on reducing AF/AFL risk, several limitations in our work should be emphasized."

Efficacy and Safety Evaluation of SGLT2i on Blood Pressure Control in Patients with Type 2 Diabetes and Hypertension: A New Meta-Analysis [45]

This is a machine-generated summary of:

Zhang, Qin; Zhou, Siyuan; Liu, Lijun: Efficacy and safety evaluation of SGLT2i on blood pressure control in patients with type 2 diabetes and hypertension: a new meta-analysis [45].

Published in: Diabetology & Metabolic Syndrome (2023).

Link to original: https://doi.org/10.1186/s13098-023-01092-z

If you want to cite the papers, please refer to the original.

For technical reasons we could not place the page where the original quote is coming from.

Abstract-Summary "The clinical efficacy and safety of SGLT2i in treating patients with type 2 diabetes mellitus and hypertension lack immense data support."

"To systematically evaluate the clinical efficacy and safety of SGLT2i in patients with type 2 diabetes mellitus and hypertension by collecting the previously published randomized controlled trials on SGLT2i to provide data support for SGLT2i as an adjuvant in the first-line antihypertensive regimen in patients with type 2 diabetes mellitus and hypertension."

"Randomized controlled trials comparing SGLT2i with a placebo in treating type 2 diabetes with hypertension were screened strictly according to inclusion and exclusion criteria."

"SGLT2i is effective in reducing blood pressure compared with placebo in patients with type 2 diabetes and hypertension, 24HSBP (−5.06 mmHg, 95% CI [−7.10, −3.01], $t=-6.19$, $P<0.05$), 24HDBP (−2.39 mmHg, 95% CI [−4.11, −0.67], $t=-4.15$, $P=0.004$), Office SBP (−4.53 mmHg, 95% CI [−5.66, −3.40], $t=-9.50$, $P<0.05$), Office DBP (−2.12 mmHg, 95% CI [−3.42, −0.82], $t=-4.88$, $P=0.001$)."

"For patients with type 2 diabetes mellitus and hypertension with a low risk of genital infection, SGLT2i should be considered as an adjuvant drug for a first-line antihypertensive regimen."

Introduction

"Hypertension and diabetes mellitus are independent risk factors for cardiovascular disease [46]."

"The risk of cardiovascular complications in patients with type 2 diabetes and hypertension is 2 to 4 times higher than in patients with common diabetes mellitus or hypertension, and the risk of all-cause mortality and cardiovascular events is 1.7 times and 1.5 times higher, respectively, than in patients with normal blood pressure [47]."

"The high incidence of hypertension and cardiovascular risk in type 2 diabetes mellitus urges us to find a safe and effective antihypertensive drug."

"There is still a lack of big data to support how to guide the use of such drugs in patients with type 2 diabetes mellitus and hypertension, as well as the discussion on the safety and effectiveness of SGLT2i as an add-on to first-line antihypertensive drugs in patients with diabetes mellitus and hypertension."

Methods

"Further full-text assessments are obtained for relevant citations that appear in the literature. (1) Comparative analysis of the efficacy of SGLT2i (any dose) and control group (placebo or no SGLT2i) in patients with type 2 diabetes mellitus and hypertension, efficacy measures including blood pressure (24HSBP/DBP or average office SBP/DBP). (2) The study type is a randomized controlled intervention study. (3) The shortest follow-up time was 4 weeks. (4) The research data are accurate and complete, and the research subjects are at least 18 years old and above, regardless of region, country, nationality, and language. (1) Non-randomized controlled trials. (2) Conference documents and other data are incomplete. (3) The same experimental data were published repeatedly. (4) The sample size is less than 60 cases. (5) The loss to follow-up rate during follow-up is more than 20%."

Result

"The results showed that SGLT2i could reduce office SBP by 4.53 mmHg compared with placebo, 95% CI [−5.66, −3.40], $t = -9.50$, $P < 0.05$, and the difference was statistically significant."

"The results showed that SGLT2i reduced office DBP by 2.12 mmHg compared with placebo, 95% CI [−3.42, −0.82], $t = -4.88$, $P = 0.001$, and the difference was statistically significant."

"The results showed that SGLT2i could reduce HbA1c by 0.57% compared with placebo, with 95% CI [−0.60, −0.54], $z = 37.02$, $p < 0.1$, and the difference was statistically significant."

"A total of 8 pieces of literature were included in the study, and the heterogeneity test showed $I^2 = 5.5\%$, $P = 0.39$, indicating no heterogeneity, RR = 1.22, 95% CI [0.916, 1.621], $z = 1.36$ $p = 0.174$."

Discussion

"WHO recommends that antihypertensive drugs be started when systolic blood pressure is 130–139 mmHg in patients diagnosed with hypertension, concomitant cardiovascular disease, or high cardiovascular risk (such as diabetes mellitus or chronic kidney disease).In the initial treatment, any two of angiotensin-converting enzyme inhibitors (ACEIs)/angiotensin-receptor blockers (ARBs), diuretics (thiazide or thiazide-like) and long-acting dihydropyridine calcium channel blockers (CCBs) can be selected for combination therapy."

"Limitations of this study: (1) the included studies were few, and it was not possible to study the effect of SGLT2i on blood pressure control based on baseline blood pressure and the impact of cardiovascular risk factors. (2) The number of studies included was minimal, and the screening criteria for the literature were too wide, failing to analyze subgroups by geography, disease duration, gender, age, concomitant underlying condition, ethnicity, blood pressure, and underlying antihypertensive drug status. (3) The results of this study are somewhat biased due to the tiny study base, diverse location, ethnicity, and sample size. (4) The majority of research times ranged from 4 to 12 weeks, and SGLT2i's long-term antihypertensive effectiveness is uncertain. (5) To further address these issues, additional clinical studies with sizable sample sizes, multicenter, prolonged study periods, and thorough study methods must be added."

The Role of SGLT-2 Inhibitors as Part of Optimal Medical Therapy in Improving Cardiovascular Outcomes in Patients with Diabetes and Coronary Artery Disease [48]

This is a machine-generated summary of:

Mosleh, Wassim; Sharma, Abhinav; Sidhu, Mandeep S.; Page, Brian; Sharma, Umesh C.; Farkouh, Michael E.: The Role of SGLT-2 Inhibitors as Part of Optimal Medical Therapy in Improving Cardiovascular Outcomes in Patients with Diabetes and Coronary Artery Disease [48].

Published in: Cardiovascular Drugs and Therapy (2017).

Link to original: https://doi.org/10.1007/s10557-017-6729-y

If you want to cite the papers, please refer to the original.

For technical reasons we could not place the page where the original quote is coming from.

Abstract-Summary "The optimal treatment approach to patients with coronary artery disease (CAD), including those with type 2 diabetes mellitus (T2DM), has been extensively evaluated."

"Several trials of stable ischemic heart disease including patients with T2DM have demonstrated that medical management is comparable to revascularization in terms of mortality and rates of major adverse cardiovascular events (MACE)."

"It is vital to target T2DM patients to prevent or delay MACE events through advanced OMT, ultimately delaying if not avoiding the need for revascularization."

"There has been significant evolution in the development of pharmacologic management of T2DM patients."

"SGLT2-inhibitors have great potential in reducing MACE in patients with T2DM and CAD."

"If results similar to the EMPA-REG OUTCOMES trial are replicated in other trials, the use of these pharmacologic agents as a part of OMT may narrow the gap between revascularization and OMT alone in patients with T2DM and multi-vessel disease."

Introduction

"Coronary artery disease (CAD) is a major clinical consequence of T2DM and is the leading cause of death in diabetic patients."

"Several trials of stable ischemic heart disease (SIHD) including patients with T2DM have demonstrated that medical management is comparable to revascularization in terms of mortality and rates of major adverse cardiovascular events (MACE) [49, 50]."

"Since the Clinical Outcomes Utilizing Revascularization and Aggressive Drug Evaluation (COURAGE) trial, which evaluated outcomes in patients with and without DM randomly assigned to optimal medical therapy (OMT) alone or OMT plus PCI [50], guideline recommendations place OMT as an equivalent to PCI for SIHD."

"The Bypass Angioplasty Revascularization Investigation 2 Diabetes (BARI-2D) [49] and Fractional Flow Reserve versus Angiography for Multivessel Evaluation 2 (FAME-2) [51] trials also addressed the role of revascularization versus an initial conservative approach of OMT in SIHD patients with and without DM, showing no incremental benefit in long-term major cardiovascular event rates with the revascularization arm."

"Diabetic patients have higher rates of cardiovascular death than non-diabetics regardless of treatment strategy (OMT, PCI, and coronary artery bypass grafting (CABG)) [52]."

Mechanism of Action of SGLT2 Inhibitors

"SGLT2-inhibitors work by inhibiting SGLT2 in the proximal convoluted tubule."

"SGLT2-inhibitors have several potential effects."

"SGLT2-inhibitors are also associated with significant reductions in systolic and diastolic blood pressure (BP) independent of glycemic or body weight reduction, and the reductions in BP are greater in patients with high baseline systolic BP [53]."

"The mechanism of BP reduction in SGLT2-inhibitors happens primarily through osmotic diuresis and reduction in plasma volume [54]."

"Some SGLT2-inhbitors such as canagliflozin increase high-density lipoprotein cholesterol (HDL-C) and reduce triglyceride levels [55, 56]."

"The unique mechanism of SGLT2 inhibitors along with their pleiotropic effects on weight, BP, and HDL-C makes them attractive options for add-on therapy in patients with cardiovascular risk factors not well controlled on other medications, especially those with higher baseline weight and BP."

Review of SGLT2 Inhibitors in Cardiovascular Outcome Trials

"There is still a need to further elucidate the potential physiologic mechanisms of SGLT2 inhibitors on HF, including the impact on effective circulating volume, myocardial perfusion, and coronary flow reserve."

"The EMPA-REG OUTCOME trial [9] studied the effects of empagliflozin, an SGLT2-inhibtor, compared to standard of care, on cardiovascular morbidity and mortality in patients with T2DM at high cardiovascular risk."

"There are a number of ongoing clinical trials that will study the effect of other SGLT2-inhibitors on cardiovascular events including CV death, MI, hospitalization for HF, hospitalization for unstable angina pectoris, or hospitalization for any revascularization."

"These include the Multicenter Trial to evaluate the Effect of Dapagliflozin on the Incidence of Cardiovascular Events (DECLARE –TIMI 58), the CANagliflozin cardioVascular Assessment Study (CANVAS trial), and the Safety and Effectiveness of SGLT-2 Inhibitors in Patients With Heart Failure and Diabetes (REFORM) trial."

"These trials could prove the effectiveness of SGLT-2 inhibitors in reducing mortality in patients with HF."

SGLT2-Inhibitors Close the Gap Between Optimal Medical Therapy Versus Revascularization

"Similar baseline findings were also seen in a pooled analysis [57] which evaluated the proportion of patients achieving guideline-based, protocol-driven treatment targets for systolic blood pressure, low-density lipoprotein cholesterol, smoking cessation, and HbA1c in the COURAGE, BARI2D, and FREEDOM trials."

"Patients with up to two uncontrolled risk factors had double the risk of death (hazard ratio 2.0 [1.3 to 3.3], p = 0.0031) and 1.7 times the risk of the composite outcome of death, myocardial infarction, and stroke (hazard ratio: 1.7 [1.2 to 2.5], p = 0.0043) in comparison with patients with all risk factors controlled (smoking, HbA1c <7%, hypertriglyceridemia, non-HDL-C < 130 mg/dL, systolic blood pressure < 130 mmHg, and diastolic blood pressure < 80 mmHg) [58, 59]."

"In the SYNTAX post hoc study [60], a randomized comparison of PCI vs CABG in 1800 patients with and without diabetes, revealed that OMT was underutilized in patients undergoing revascularization."

"These findings highlight that the role OMT plays in reducing the risk of subsequent cardiac events, even among those patients treated with revascularization."

SGLT2 Inhibitors as Potential Insulin Sparing Agents

"It has been shown that patients treated with insulin have worse outcomes than non-insulin-treated diabetics."

"A secondary analysis of the FREEDOM trial investigated the long-term CV outcome of PCI versus CABG in insulin-treated and non-insulin-treated diabetic patients [61]."

"Other studies have demonstrated no difference in cardiovascular outcomes between insulin-treated patients versus non-insulin-treated patients with diabetes [49, 62]."

"Regardless of whether worse clinical outcomes in insulin-treated diabetic patients are due to a direct adverse effect of insulin or rather a more aggressive disease state, a novel hypoglycemic agent such as SGLT2-inhibitors that significantly reduces the need for insulin and its possible adverse cardiovascular effects may improve clinical outcomes."

SGLT2-Inhibitors' Impact on Heart Failure as an Outcome in Clinical Trials

"Since one of the main principles in the management of these patients has been revascularization directed at flow-limiting coronary stenosis will more effectively treat myocardial ischemia and thereby preserve ventricular systolic function, studying HF as an outcome in DM patients managed with OMT alone vs OMT plus revascularization is an important outcome to evaluate."

"HF hospitalizations have only recently been prespecified in clinical trials of medical therapy among patients with DM; however, this is predominantly in the form of an adverse event, and not as a component of a composite or primary outcome [63]."

"Evaluating hospitalization due to HF as a component of the primary outcome in trials of revascularization in patients with DM is warranted."

Role of Left Ventricular Ejection Fraction as an Outcome in Clinical Trials

"An objective in the management of patients with DM and CAD should be to prevent a decline in left ventricular ejection fraction (LVEF)."

"Revascularization among patients with DM and CAD has been shown to potentially prevent a decline in LVEF."

"Preventing a decline in LVEF remains an important yet understudied objective among patients with DM."

"Given the prognostic importance of LVEF, a decline in LVEF should be considered as an endpoint in clinical trials of patients with DM and CAD."

Conclusion

"SGLT2-inhibitors may have tremendous potential in reducing adverse CV outcomes and improving HF outcomes in patients with T2DM and CAD."

"Empagliflozin should be considered as a part of OMT among patients with T2DM and pre-existing cardiovascular disease."

"If results similar to the EMPA-REG OUTCOMES trial are seen with other SGLT-2 inhibitor trials, the use of these pharmacologic agents as a part of OMT may narrow the gap between revascularization and OMT alone in patients with T2DM and MVD."

"Future studies on the role of SLGT-2 inhibitors with regard to HF outcomes are needed to elucidate the mechanisms and clinical effects in this vulnerable population."

External Applicability of SGLT2 Inhibitor Cardiovascular Outcome Trials to Patients with Type 2 Diabetes and Cardiovascular Disease [64]

This is a machine-generated summary of:

Smidt, Lisanne C. A.; Visseren, Frank L. J.; de Ranitz-Greven, Wendela L.; Nathoe, Hendrik M.; Kappelle, L. Jaap; de Borst, Gert J.; de Valk, Harold W.; Westerink, Jan: External applicability of SGLT2 inhibitor cardiovascular outcome trials to patients with type 2 diabetes and cardiovascular disease [64].

Published in: Cardiovascular Diabetology (2021).

Link to original: https://doi.org/10.1186/s12933-021-01373-9

If you want to cite the papers, please refer to the original.

For technical reasons we could not place the page where the original quote is coming from.

Abstract-Summary "Recent treatment guidelines support the use of sodium-glucose cotransporter 2 inhibitors (SGLT2i) in patients with type 2 diabetes and cardiovascular disease based on the results of cardiovascular outcome trials (CVOTs)."

"Applicability of these trials to everyday patients with type 2 diabetes and cardiovascular disease is however unknown."

"Trial in- and exclusion criteria from EMPA-REG OUTCOME, CANVAS, DECLARE-TIMI 58 and VERTIS-CV were applied to 1389 type 2 diabetes patients with cardiovascular disease in the Utrecht Cardiovascular Cohort-Secondary Manifestations of ARTerial disease (UCC-SMART)."

"After applying trial in- and exclusion criteria, 48% of UCC-SMART patients with type 2 diabetes and cardiovascular disease would have been eligible for DECLARE-TIMI 58, 35% for CANVAS, 29% for EMPA-REG OUTCOME and 21% for VERTIS-CV."

"For all trials the observed risk for cardiovascular events and all-cause mortality was similar in eligible and ineligible patients after adjustment for age and gender."

"A large proportion of patients with type 2 diabetes and cardiovascular disease in daily clinical practice would have been eligible for participation in the SGLT2i CVOTs."

Introduction

"Four cardiovascular outcome trials (CVOTs) have been conducted to assess the safety and efficacy of sodium-glucose cotransporter 2 inhibitors (SGLT2i) on cardiovascular end-points in high risk type 2 diabetes patients (EMPA-REG OUTCOME, DECLARE-TIMI 58, CANVAS and VERTIS-CV) [9, 65–67]."

"Meta-analysis of the first three of these trials has shown a reduced risk for cardiovascular events and mortality, especially in type 2 diabetes patients with cardiovascular disease at baseline [68]."

"In order to quantify the applicability of SGLT2i CVOTs to real world patients, several studies have been conducted in which trial in- and exclusion have been applied to populations of type 2 diabetes patient both with and without cardiovascular disease [69–76]."

"The objective of this paper is to assess the external applicability of guideline-informing SGLT2i CVOTs in a real-world cohort consisting of patients with type 2 diabetes and concomitant cardiovascular disease."

Methods

"These in- and exclusion criteria where applied to all type 2 diabetes patients with cardiovascular disease in the UCC-SMART, to assess the eligibility of UCC-SMART patients for each trial."

"Due to extensive availability of baseline data of patients in the UCC-SMART, a wide variety of inclusion and exclusion criteria including HbA1c, age, cardiovascular history, blood pressure, eGFR, BMI but also alcohol abuse or triglyceride level could be used in the current analysis."

"The number of patients in the UCC-SMART eligible or ineligible for participation in each trial was calculated."

"Cumulative incidence of MACE and all-cause mortality and individual MACE components for patients that were eligible and ineligible for each trial were plotted for the first 15 years of follow-up in UCC-SMART."

"The crude hazard ratio for 15 year risk on MACE, all-cause mortality and individual MACE components for trial eligible vs ineligible patients, as well as a hazard ratio adjusted for age and sex was calculated using a Cox proportional hazard model."

Results

"In the UCC-SMART 823 patients (59%) had a HbA_{1c} below 53 mmol/mol (7%), which was the lower inclusion limit for EMPA-REG OUTCOME, VERTIS-CV and CANVAS and 512 patients (37%) had a HbA_{1c} below 48 mmol/mol (6.5%), which was the lower inclusion limit for DECLARE-TIMI 58."

"For each CVOT the mean HbA_{1c} was higher amongst eligible patients compared to ineligible patients [HbA_{1c} difference: 12.1 mmol/mol (95% CI 11.0, 13.2) or 1.1% (95% CI 1.0, 1.2) for EMPA-REG OUTCOME; 16.2 mmol/mol (95% CI 15.1, 17.3) or 1.5% (95% CI 1.4, 1.6) for CANVAS; 12.1 mmol/mol (95% CI 10.9, 13.3) or 1.1% (95% CI 1.0, 1.2) for DECLARE-TIMI 58; and 11.9 mmol/mol (95% CI 10.6, 13.1) or 1.1% (95% CI 1.0, 1.2) for VERTIS-CV)."

Discussion

"The current study distinguishes itself from earlier applicability studies by assessing the risk on MACE and all-cause mortality in patients with type 2 diabetes and concomitant cardiovascular disease eligible and ineligible for SGLT2i CVOT participation based long-term cohort follow-up data."

"The current analysis does not raise major concerns regarding applicability of SGLT2i CVOT results to a larger population of type 2 diabetes patients with cardiovascular disease, as the only differences in outcome data between eligible and ineligible patients—a lower risk on MACE and all-cause mortality for patients eligible for DECLARE-TIMI 58—did not remain significant after adjustment for age and sex."

"Future studies on real-world of applicability SGLT2i CVOTS should consist of larger (international) cohorts of type 2 diabetes patients, that also have follow-up data available to calculate the risk on adverse (cardiovascular) outcome for trial eligible and ineligible patients."

Conclusions

"A large proportion of patients with type 2 diabetes and cardiovascular disease in daily clinical practice would have been eligible for participation in the SGLT2-inhibitor CVOTs."

"Main reason for trial ineligibility is the level of HbA_{1c}."

"Trial eligible and ineligible patients have the same risk for MACE and all-cause mortality."

"Based on the current analysis, trial selection criteria are unlikely to confine the applicability of SGLT2i CVOT results to a larger population of type 2 diabetes patients with established cardiovascular disease."

Bibliography

1. Pitt B, Bhatt DL, Metra M (2022) Does SGLT1 inhibition add to the benefits of SGLT2 inhibition in the prevention and treatment of heart failure? Eur Heart J 43(45):4754–4757
2. Cardoso R, Graffunder FP, Ternes CM, Fernandes A, Rocha AV, Fernandes G, Bhatt DL (2021) SGLT2 inhibitors decrease cardiovascular death and heart failure hospitalizations in patients with heart failure: a systematic review and meta-analysis. EClinicalMedicine 36:100933
3. Sayour AA, Oláh A, Ruppert M, Barta BA, Merkely B, Radovits T (2024) Effect of pharmacological selectivity of SGLT2 inhibitors on cardiovascular outcomes in patients with type 2 diabetes: a meta-analysis. Sci Rep 14(1):2188
4. Jia X, Mehta PB, Ye Y, Alam M, Birnbaum Y, Bajaj M (2018) SGLT2 inhibitors and cardiovascular outcomes: current perspectives and future potentials. Curr Diab Rep 18:63. https://doi.org/10.1007/s11892-018-1038-9

5. UK Prospective Diabetes Study (UKPDS) Group (1998) Intensive blood-glucose control with sulphonylureas or insulin compared with conventional treatment and risk of complications in patients with type 2 diabetes (UKPDS 33). Lancet 352(9131):837–853
6. Holman RR, Paul SK, Bethel MA, Matthews DR, Neil HA (2008) 10-year follow-up of intensive glucose control in type 2 diabetes. N Engl J Med 359(15):1577–1589
7. Marso SP, Daniels GH, Brown-Frandsen K, Kristensen P, Mann JF, Nauck MA et al (2016) Liraglutide and cardiovascular outcomes in type 2 diabetes. N Engl J Med 375(4):311–322
8. Marso SP, Holst AG, Semaglutide VT (2017) Cardiovascular outcomes in patients with type 2 diabetes. N Engl J Med 376(9):891–892
9. Zinman B, Wanner C, Lachin JM, Fitchett D, Bluhmki E, Hantel S et al (2015) Empagliflozin, cardiovascular outcomes, and mortality in type 2 diabetes. N Engl J Med 373(22):2117–2128
10. Neal B, Perkovic V, Mahaffey KW, De Zeeuw D, Fulcher G, Erondu N et al (2017) Canagliflozin and cardiovascular and renal events in type 2 diabetes. N Engl J Med 377(7):644–657
11. Udell JA, Yuan Z, Rush T, Sicignano NM, Galitz M, Rosenthal N (2018) Cardiovascular outcomes and risks after initiation of a sodium glucose cotransporter 2 inhibitor: results from the easel population-based cohort study (evidence for cardiovascular outcomes with sodium glucose cotransporter 2 inhibitors in the real world). Circulation 137(14):1450–1459
12. Baartscheer A, Schumacher CA, Wüst RCI, Fiolet JWT, Stienen GJM, Coronel R et al (2017) Empagliflozin decreases myocardial cytoplasmic Na(+) through inhibition of the cardiac Na(+)/H(+) exchanger in rats and rabbits. Diabetologia 60:568–573
13. Levelt E, Rodgers CT, Clarke WT, Mahmod M, Ariga R, Francis JM et al (2016) Cardiac energetics, oxygenation, and perfusion during increased workload in patients with type 2 diabetes mellitus. Eur Heart J 37(46):3461–3469
14. Gillies CL, Abrams KR, Lambert PC, Cooper NJ, Sutton AJ, Hsu RT et al (2007) Pharmacological and lifestyle interventions to prevent or delay type 2 diabetes in people with impaired glucose tolerance: systematic review and meta-analysis. BMJ 334(7588):299
15. Knowler WC, Barrett-Connor E, Fowler SE, Hamman RF, Lachin JM, Walker EA et al (2002) Reduction in the incidence of type 2 diabetes with lifestyle intervention or metformin. N Engl J Med 346(6):393–403
16. American Diabetes Association (2016) Standards of medical care in diabetes-2016: summary of revisions. Diabetes Care 39(Suppl 1):S4–S5
17. Sattar N, McLaren J, Kristensen SL, Preiss D, McMurray JJ (2016) SGLT2 inhibition and cardiovascular events: why did EMPA-REG outcomes surprise and what were the likely mechanisms? Diabetologia 59:1333–1339. https://doi.org/10.1007/s00125-016-3956-x
18. Sarwar N, Gao P, Kondapally Seshasai SR et al (2010) Diabetes mellitus, fasting blood glucose concentration, and risk of vascular disease: a collaborative meta-analysis of 102 prospective studies. Lancet 375:2215–2222. https://doi.org/10.1016/S0140-6736(10)60484-9
19. Gerstein HC, Miller ME, Byington RP, Goff DCJ, Bigger JT, Buse JB et al (2008) Effects of intensive glucose lowering in type 2 diabetes. N Engl J Med 358(24):2545–2559
20. Home PD, Pocock SJ, Beck-Nielsen H et al (2007) Rosiglitazone evaluated for cardiovascular outcomes—an interim analysis. N Engl J Med 357:28–38
21. Scirica BM, Bhatt DL, Braunwald E, Steg PG, Davidson J, Hirshberg B, Ohman P, Frederich R, Wiviott SD, Hoffman EB, Cavender MA, Udell JA, Desai NR, Mosenzon O, McGuire D, Ray KK, Leiter LA, Raz I, SAVOR-TIMI 53 Steering Committee and Investigators (2013) Saxagliptin and cardiovascular outcomes in patients with type 2 diabetes mellitus. N Engl J Med 369:1317–1326. https://doi.org/10.1056/NEJMoa1307684
22. White WB, Cannon CP, Heller SR, Nissen SE, Bergenstal RM, Bakris GL, Perez AT, Fleck PR, Mehta CR, Kupfer S, Wilson C, Cushman WC, Zannad F, EXAMINE Investigators (2013) Alogliptin after acute coronary syndrome in patients with type 2 diabetes. N Engl J Med 369:1327–1335. https://doi.org/10.1056/NEJMoa1305889
23. Marso SP, Poulter NR, Nissen SE et al (2013) Design of the liraglutide effect and action in diabetes: evaluation of cardiovascular outcome results (LEADER) trial. Am Heart J 166:823–830

24. Abraham WT, Adamson PB, Bourge RC et al (2011) Wireless pulmonary artery haemodynamic monitoring in chronic heart failure: a randomised controlled trial. Lancet 377:658–666
25. The ALLHAT Officers and Coordinators for the ALLHAT Collaborative Research Group (2002) Major outcomes in high-risk hypertensive patients randomized to angiotensin-converting enzyme inhibitor or calcium channel blocker vs diuretic. The Antihypertensive and Lipid-Lowering Treatment to Prevent Heart Attack Trial (ALLHAT). JAMA 88:2981–2997
26. McMurray JJ, Gerstein HC, Holman RR, Pfeffer MA (2014) Heart failure: a cardiovascular outcome in diabetes that can no longer be ignored. Lancet Diabetes Endocrinol 2:843–851. https://doi.org/10.1016/S2213-8587(14)70031-2
27. Shah AD, Langenberg C, Rapsomaniki E et al (2014) Type 2 diabetes and incidence of cardiovascular diseases: a cohort study in 1·9 million people. Lancet Diabetes Endocrinol 3:105–113
28. Emdin CA, Rahimi K, Neal B, Callender T, Perkovic V, Patel A (2015) Blood pressure lowering in type 2 diabetes: a systematic review and meta-analysis. JAMA 313:603–615
29. Washburn WN, Poucher SM (2013) Differentiating sodium-glucose co-transporter-2 inhibitors in development for the treatment of type 2 diabetes mellitus. Expert Opin Investig Drugs 22:463–486
30. Neal B, Perkovic V, de Zeeuw D, Mahaffey KW, Fulcher G, Stein P et al (2013) Rationale, design, and baseline characteristics of the Canagliflozin Cardiovascular Assessment Study (CANVAS)-a randomized placebo-controlled trial. Am Heart J 166(2):217–223
31. Li W-j, Chen X-q, Xu L-l, Li Y-q, Luo B-h (2020) SGLT2 inhibitors and atrial fibrillation in type 2 diabetes: a systematic review with meta-analysis of 16 randomized controlled trials. Cardiovasc Diabetol 19:130. https://doi.org/10.1186/s12933-020-01105-5
32. Kotecha D, Piccini JP (2015) Atrial fibrillation in heart failure: what should we do? Eur Heart J 36(46):3250–3257
33. Trulock KM, Narayan SM, Piccini JP (2014) Rhythm control in heart failure patients with atrial fibrillation: contemporary challenges including the role of ablation. J Am Coll Cardiol 64(7):710–721
34. Zelniker TA, Bonaca MP, Furtado RHM, Mosenzon O, Kuder JF, Murphy SA, Bhatt DL, Leiter LA, McGuire DK, Wilding JPH et al (2020) Effect of dapagliflozin on atrial fibrillation in patients with type 2 diabetes mellitus: insights from the DECLARE-TIMI 58 trial. Circulation 141(15):1227–1234
35. Liberati A, Altman DG, Tetzlaff J, Mulrow C, Gotzsche PC, Ioannidis JP, Clarke M, Devereaux PJ, Kleijnen J, Moher D (2009) The PRISMA statement for reporting systematic reviews and meta-analyses of studies that evaluate healthcare interventions: explanation and elaboration. BMJ 339:b2700
36. Perkovic V, Jardine MJ, Neal B, Bompoint S, Heerspink HJL, Charytan DM, Edwards R, Agarwal R, Bakris G, Bull S et al (2019) Canagliflozin and renal outcomes in type 2 diabetes and nephropathy. N Engl J Med 380(24):2295–2306
37. A study of the effects of canagliflozin (JNJ-28431754) on Renal endpoints in adult participants with type 2 diabetes mellitus (CANVAS-R). https://www.clinicaltrials.gov/ct2/show/NCT01989754?cond=NCT01989754&draw=2&rank=1
38. CANVAS—CANagliflozin cardiovascular assessment study. ClinicalTrials.gov. https://www.clinicaltrials.gov/ct2/show/NCT01032629
39. A Phase III Study of BMS-512148 (dapagliflozin) in patients with type 2 diabetes who are not well controlled with diet and exercise. ClinicalTrials.gov. https://www.clinicaltrials.gov/ct2/show/NCT00528372
40. Leiter LA, Cefalu WT, de Bruin TW, Gause-Nilsson I, Sugg J, Parikh SJ (2014) Dapagliflozin added to usual care in individuals with type 2 diabetes mellitus with preexisting cardiovascular disease: a 24-week, multicenter, randomized, double-blind, placebo-controlled study with a 28-week extension. J Am Geriatr Soc 62(7):1252–1262
41. Yale JF, Bakris G, Cariou B, Nieto J, David-Neto E, Yue D, Wajs E, Figueroa K, Jiang J, Law G et al (2014) Efficacy and safety of canagliflozin over 52 weeks in patients with type 2 diabetes mellitus and chronic kidney disease. Diabetes Obes Metab 16(10):1016–1027

42. Multicenter trial to evaluate the effect of dapagliflozin on the incidence of cardiovascular events (DECLARE-TIMI58). https://www.clinicaltrials.gov/ct2/show/NCT01730534?cond=NCT01730534&draw=2&rank=1
43. Bode B, Stenlof K, Harris S, Sullivan D, Fung A, Usiskin K, Meininger G (2015) Long-term efficacy and safety of canagliflozin over 104 weeks in patients aged 55–80 years with type 2 diabetes. Diabetes Obes Metab 17(3):294–303
44. Barnett AH, Mithal A, Manassie J, Jones R, Rattunde H, Woerle HJ, Broedl UC (2014) Investigators E-RRt: efficacy and safety of empagliflozin added to existing antidiabetes treatment in patients with type 2 diabetes and chronic kidney disease: a randomised, double-blind, placebo-controlled trial. Lancet Diabetes Endocrinol 2(5):369–384
45. Zhang Q, Zhou S, Liu L (2023) Efficacy and safety evaluation of SGLT2i on blood pressure control in patients with type 2 diabetes and hypertension: a new meta-analysis. Diabetol Metab Syndr 15:118. https://doi.org/10.1186/s13098-023-01092-z
46. Viigimaa M, Sachinidis A, Toumpourleka M, Koutsampasopoulos K, Alliksoo S, Titma T (2020) Macrovascular complications of type 2 diabetes mellitus. Curr Vasc Pharmacol 18(2):110–116
47. Chen G, McAlister FA, Walker RL, Hemmelgarn BR, Campbell NR (2011) Cardiovascular outcomes in Framingham participants with diabetes: the importance of blood pressure. Hypertension 57(5):891–897
48. Mosleh W, Sharma A, Sidhu MS, Page B, Sharma UC, Farkouh ME (2017) The role of SGLT-2 inhibitors as part of optimal medical therapy in improving cardiovascular outcomes in patients with diabetes and coronary artery disease. Cardiovasc Drugs Ther 31:311–318. https://doi.org/10.1007/s10557-017-6729-y
49. Frye RL, August P, Brooks MM, Hardison RM, Kelsey SF, MacGregor JM et al (2009) A randomized trial of therapies for type 2 diabetes and coronary artery disease. N Engl J Med 360(24):2503–2515
50. Boden WE, O'Rourke RA, Teo KK, Hartigan PM, Maron DJ, Kostuk WJ et al (2007) Optimal medical therapy with or without PCI for stable coronary disease. N Engl J Med 356(15):1503–1516
51. De Bruyne B, Pijls NH, Kalesan B, Barbato E, Tonino PA, Piroth Z et al (2012) Fractional flow reserve-guided PCI versus medical therapy in stable coronary disease. N Engl J Med 367(11):991–1001
52. Lima EG, Hueb W, Garcia RM, Pereira AC, Soares PR, Favarato D et al (2013) Impact of diabetes on 10-year outcomes of patients with multivessel coronary artery disease in the medicine, angioplasty, or surgery study II (MASS II) trial. Am Heart J 166(2):250–257
53. Vasilakou D, Karagiannis T, Athanasiadou E, Mainou M, Liakos A, Bekiari E et al (2013) Sodium-glucose cotransporter 2 inhibitors for type 2 diabetes: a systematic review and meta-analysis. Ann Intern Med 159(4):262–274. https://doi.org/10.7326/0003-4819-159-4-201308200-00007
54. Lambers Heerspink HJ, de Zeeuw D, Wie L, Leslie B, List J (2013) Dapagliflozin a glucose-regulating drug with diuretic properties in subjects with type 2 diabetes. Diabetes Obes Metab 15(9):853–862
55. Musso G, Gambino R, Cassader M, Pagano G (2012) A novel approach to control hyperglycemia in type 2 diabetes: sodium glucose co-transport (SGLT) inhibitors: systematic review and meta-analysis of randomized trials. Ann Med 44(4):375–393. https://doi.org/10.3109/07853890.2011.560181
56. Sha S, Devineni D, Ghosh A, Polidori D, Hompesch M, Arnolds S et al (2014) Pharmacodynamic effects of canagliflozin, a sodium glucose co-transporter 2 inhibitor, from a randomized study in patients with type 2 diabetes. PLoS One 9(8):e105638
57. Farkouh ME, Boden WE, Bittner V, Muratov V, Hartigan P, Ogdie M et al (2013) Risk factor control for coronary artery disease secondary prevention in large randomized trials. J Am Coll Cardiol 61(15):1607–1615

58. Bittner V, Bertolet M, Barraza Felix R, Farkouh ME, Goldberg S, Ramanathan KB et al (2015) Comprehensive cardiovascular risk factor control improves survival: the BARI 2D trial. J Am Coll Cardiol 66(7):765–773
59. Maron DJ, Boden WE (2015) Why optimal medical therapy should be a universal standard of care. J Am Coll Cardiol 66(7):774–776
60. Iqbal J, Zhang YJ, Holmes DR, Morice MC, Mack MJ, Kappetein AP et al (2015) Optimal medical therapy improves clinical outcomes in patients undergoing revascularization with percutaneous coronary intervention or coronary artery bypass grafting: insights from the synergy between percutaneous coronary intervention with TAXUS and cardiac surgery (SYNTAX) trial at the 5-year follow-up. Circulation 131(14):1269–1277
61. Dangas GD, Farkouh ME, Sleeper LA, Yang M, Schoos MM, Macaya C et al (2014) Long-term outcome of PCI versus CABG in insulin and non-insulin-treated diabetic patients: results from the FREEDOM trial. J Am Coll Cardiol 64(12):1189–1197
62. Investigators OT, Gerstein HC, Bosch J, Dagenais GR, Diaz R, Jung H et al (2012) Basal insulin and cardiovascular and other outcomes in dysglycemia. N Engl J Med 367(4):319–328
63. Sharma A, Bhatt DL, Calvo G, Brown NJ, Zannad F, Mentz RJ (2016) Heart failure event definitions in drug trials in patients with type 2 diabetes. Lancet Diabetes Endocrinol 4(4):294–296
64. Smidt LCA, Visseren FLJ, de Ranitz-Greven WL, Nathoe HM, Kappelle LJ, de Borst GJ, de Valk HW, Westerink J (2021) External applicability of SGLT2 inhibitor cardiovascular outcome trials to patients with type 2 diabetes and cardiovascular disease. Cardiovasc Diabetol 20:181. https://doi.org/10.1186/s12933-021-01373-9
65. Neal B, Perkovic V, Matthews DR, Mahaffey KW, Fulcher G, Meininger G et al (2017) Rationale, design and baseline characteristics of the CANagliflozin cardioVascular Assessment Study-Renal (CANVAS-R): a randomized, placebo-controlled trial. Diabetes Obes Metab 19(3):387–393
66. Wiviott SD, Raz I, Bonaca MP, Mosenzon O, Kato ET, Cahn A et al (2019) Dapagliflozin and cardiovascular outcomes in type 2 diabetes. N Engl J Med 380(4):347–357
67. Cannon CP, Pratley R, Dagogo-Jack S, Mancuso J, Huyck S, Masiukiewicz U et al (2020) Cardiovascular outcomes with ertugliflozin in type 2 diabetes. N Engl J Med 383(15):1425–1435
68. Zelniker TA, Wiviott SD, Raz I, Im K, Goodrich EL, Bonaca MP et al (2019) SGLT2 inhibitors for primary and secondary prevention of cardiovascular and renal outcomes in type 2 diabetes: a systematic review and meta-analysis of cardiovascular outcome trials. Lancet 393(10166):31–39. https://doi.org/10.1016/S0140-6736(18)32590-X. Erratum in: Lancet (2019) 393(10166):30
69. Wittbrodt ET, Eudicone JM, Bell KF, Enhoffer DM, Latham K, Green JB (2018) Eligibility varies among the 4 sodium-glucose cotransporter-2 inhibitor cardiovascular outcomes trials: implications for the general type 2 diabetes US population. Am J Manag Care 24(8 Suppl):S138–S145
70. Wittbrodt E, Chamberlain D, Arnold SV, Tang F, Kosiborod M (2019) Eligibility of patients with type 2 diabetes for sodium-glucose co-transporter-2 inhibitor cardiovascular outcomes trials: an assessment using the diabetes collaborative registry. Diabetes Obes Metab 21(8):1985–1989
71. Pintat S, Fenici P, Hammar N, Ji L, Khunti K, Medina J et al (2019) Eligibility of patients with type 2 diabetes for sodium-glucose cotransporter 2 inhibitor cardiovascular outcomes trials: a global perspective from the DISCOVER study. BMJ Open Diabetes Res Care 7(1):e000627
72. Birkeland KI, Bodegard J, Norhammar A, Kuiper JG, Georgiado E, Beekman-Hendriks WL et al (2019) How representative of a general type 2 diabetes population are patients included in cardiovascular outcome trials with SGLT2 inhibitors? A large European observational study. Diabetes Obes Metab 21(4):968–974
73. Nicolucci A, Candido R, Cucinotta D, Graziano G, Rocca A, Rossi MC et al (2019) Generalizability of cardiovascular safety trials on SGLT2 inhibitors to the real world: implications for clinical practice. Adv Ther 36(10):2895–2909

74. Canivell S, Mata-Cases M, Vlacho B, Gratacòs M, Real J, Mauricio D et al (2019) How many patients with type 2 diabetes meet the inclusion criteria of the cardiovascular outcome trials with SGLT2 inhibitors? Estimations from a population database in a mediterranean area. J Diabetes Res 2019:2018374–2018379
75. Hinton W, Feher M, Munro N, Joy M, de Lusignan S (2020) Sodium-glucose co-transporter-2 inhibitor cardiovascular outcome trials and generalizability to English primary care. Diabet Med 37(9):1499–1508
76. Shao S-C, Lin Y-H, Chang K-C, Chan Y-Y, Hung M-J, Kao Yang Y-H et al (2019) Sodium glucose co-transporter 2 inhibitors and cardiovascular event protections: how applicable are clinical trials and observational studies to real-world patients? BMJ Open Diabetes Res Care 7:e000742. https://doi.org/10.1136/bmjdrc-2019-000742
77. Committee ADAPP (2021) 10. Cardiovascular disease and risk management: standards of medical care in diabetes—2022. Diabetes Care 45(Supplement_1):S144–SS74. https://doi.org/10.2337/dc22-S010. This recent guideline (despite the 2021 version) proposed utilizing SGLT2is and GLP1-RAs as the first agent for T2DM treatment in patients with established ASCVD, HF, CKD, and high CV risk

Correction to: Sodium-Glucose Cotransporter-2 (SGLT2) Inhibitors in Heart Failure

Mukesh Nandave

Correction to: M. Nandave (ed.), *Sodium-Glucose Cotransporter-2 (SGLT2) Inhibitors in Heart Failure*, https://doi.org/10.1007/978-981-97-7568-2

The original version of this book was inadvertently published with errors. The titles of Chapters 3–9 have been updated after publication.

In the book, the titles of the chapters have been corrected as follows:

Chapter 3: SGLT2 Inhibitors for Primary and Secondary Protection from Cardiovascular and Renal Diseases in Type 2 Diabetes

Chapter 4: SGLT2 Inhibitors: Emerging Opportunities for the Treatment of Myocardial Infarction

Chapter 5: Potential Role of SGLT2 Inhibitors in the Treatment and Prevention of Diabetic Cardiomyopathy

Chapter 6: Role of Therapeutic Potential, Contemporary Management, Unmet needs of SGLT2 Inhibitors in Congestive Heart Failure

Chapter 7: A Comprehensive Review of Preclinical and Clinical Information on the Cardiovascular Advantages of SGLT2 Inhibitors

Chapter 8: Exploring the Current Selective Drugs of SGLT2 Inhibitors for the Treatment of Cardiovascular Disease in Type 2 Diabetes

Chapter 9: A Comprehensive Review of SGLT2 Inhibitor's Effects on Cardiovascular Events, Mortality, and Significant Safety Outcomes in Individuals with Type 2 Diabetes

---

The updated version of the book can be found at
https://doi.org/10.1007/978-981-97-7568-2

M. Nandave (ed.), *Sodium-glucose Cotransporter-2 (SGLT2) Inhibitors in Heart Failure*, https://doi.org/10.1007/978-981-97-7568-2_10

The manufacturer's authorised representative in the EU is Springer Nature Customer Service Centre GmbH, Europaplatz 3, 69115 Heidelberg, Germany. If you have any concerns regarding our products, please contact ProductSafety@springernature.com

Printed and bound by CPI Group (UK) Ltd, Croydon, CR0 4YY

30/09/2026

02225298-0019